Public health nutrition in developing countries

Part - I

Edited by
Sheila Chander Vir

WOODHEAD PUBLISHING INDIA PVT LTD
New Delhi • Cambridge • Oxford • Philadelphia

Published by Woodhead Publishing India Pvt. Ltd.
Woodhead Publishing India Pvt. Ltd., G-2, Vardaan House, 7/28, Ansari Road
Daryaganj, New Delhi – 110002, India
www.woodheadpublishingindia.com

Woodhead Publishing Limited, 80 High Street, Sawston, Cambridge,
CB22 3HJ UK

Woodhead Publishing USA 1518 Walnut Street, Suite1100, Philadelphia

www.woodheadpublishing.com

First published 2011, Woodhead Publishing India Pvt. Ltd.

Woodhead Publishing India Pvt. Ltd. ISBN: 978-93-80308-06-7

Woodhead Publishing Ltd. ISBN: 978-0-85709-004-1

Typeset by Sunshine Graphics, New Delhi
Printed and bound by Replika Press Pvt. Ltd.

Dedicated to my mother
Shanta Metre and father, Padma Bhushan W. B. Metre,
in fond memory of their love, blessings, inspiration and
encouragement.

Contents

Part - II

Preface

Public health nutrition has increasingly gained attention as an important subject in the field of development. It is recognized as a specialized discipline of nutrition that deals with expanding and integrating the understanding of nutrition issues across various levels – individual, family, community, national and global – geared towards solving nutrition problems of individuals and communities.

Malnutrition is known to contribute to approximately one-third of child deaths. High levels of malnutrition in developing countries are a major area of concern inhibiting achievement of the Millennium Development Goals (MDGs). Alleviation of malnutrition in developing countries poses to be a major challenge and needs urgent attention.

In the developing world, a total of 129 million children under the age of five years are underweight; 27 percent of these are in Asia and 21 percent in Africa. Stunting affects 195 million children under the age of five years in the developing world, and more than 90 percent of stunted children live in Asia and Africa. Many of these children have a poor start in life, with 13 million infants being born with intrauterine growth restriction annually, resulting in low birth weight. Deficiencies of micro-nutrients, such as iodine, iron, vitamin A, folic acid and zinc, caused mainly due to inadequate dietary intake and frequent infections, affect the population in developing world.

There is immense hope in reducing malnutrition in a positive international development environment. The multiple causes of malnutrition are well known, new technologies are available and vast knowledge has been generated on effective interventions from programmes that have successfully accelerated reduction of malnutrition in countries such as Thailand, and more recently, Vietnam and Brazil. Experiences from successful programmes emphasize that political commitment and support, leadership and strategic capacity development, provision of basic and essential services, combined with community ownership for improving nutrition indicators are key ingredients for accelerated reduction of malnutrition. The enormous challenge for the developing world is the scaling up of malnutrition reduction programmes

Foreword

Public health nutrition has increasingly gained attention as an important subject in the field of development. It is recognized as a specialized discipline of nutrition that deals with expanding and integrating the understanding of nutrition issues across various levels – individual, family, community, national and global – geared towards solving nutrition problems of individuals and communities.

Malnutrition is known to contribute to approximately one-third of child deaths. High levels of malnutrition in developing countries is a major area of concern inhibiting achievement of the Millennium Development Goals (MDGs). Alleviation of malnutrition in developing countries poses to be a major challenge and needs urgent attention.

In the developing world, a total of 129 million children under the age of five years are underweight; 27 percent of these are in Asia and 21 percent in Africa. Stunting affects 195 million children under the age of five years in the developing world; and more than 90 percent of stunted children live in Asia and Africa. Many of these children have a poor start in life with 13 million infants being born with intrauterine growth restriction annually, resulting in low birth weight. Deficiencies of micro-nutrients, such as iodine, iron, vitamin A, folic acid and zinc, caused mainly due to inadequate dietary intake and frequent infections, affect the population in developing world.

There is immense hope in reducing malnutrition in a positive international development environment. The multiple causes of malnutrition are well known, new technologies are available and vast knowledge has been generated on effective interventions from programmes that have successfully accelerated reduction of malnutrition in countries such as Thailand, and more recently, Vietnam and Brazil. Experiences from successful programmes emphasize that political commitment and support, leadership and strategic capacity development, provision of basic and essential services, combined with community ownership for improving nutrition indicators are key ingredients for accelerated reduction of malnutrition. The enormous challenge for the developing world is the scaling up of malnutrition reduction programmes in order to achieve multiple MDGs. Adaptations of known effective interventions in the national and local context would save time and reduce the risk of implementing strategies that are unlikely to yield results. Understanding existing gaps and the key elements of successful programming are critical for formulating, implementing and evaluating effective programmes.

This book on Public Health Nutrition is timely and collates information on the current situation of malnutrition in the developing world. It not only presents recent technical developments in nutrition science but also highlights the application of proven sound recommendations for programme implementation. The book will be helpful to health and nutrition professionals, as well as, policy makers, programme designers and project implementers, in dealing with various nutrition issues effectively. The editor, taking into consideration the defined scope and focus of the book, has brought together authors who not only have in-depth technical knowledge of the subject but also have first-hand experience in planning and implementation of public health nutrition programmes. The book is reader friendly and the lessons learned from programmes are emphasized in box formats where appropriate. It also focuses on broader health and social issues that need to be addressed for achieving the goal of reducing malnutrition. Interestingly, the book also covers other issues of public health nutrition that relate to a wide variety of situations such as neonatal care, safe drinking water, diarrhoea and HIV. In addition, one section of the book concentrates on programming, with chapters on programme planning and implementation, communication, monitoring and evaluation, linking evidence-based research to programming. These chapters will enable practitioners to apply nutrition science to appropriate programme designing and its implementation.

The editor, Dr Sheila C. Vir, has over 25 years of experience working with UNICEF and has contributed significantly in the field of public health nutrition. The passion in the subject is evident from the effort put in by her for undertaking this monumental task of bringing together over thirty selected experts to contribute to this book. She should be congratulated for this exceptional publication in public health nutrition.

The book will be a very useful reference not only for nutritionists and public health specialist but also for pediatricians, development professionals, programmers and international agencies. It should be of interest to politicians, policy makers, bureaucrats, economists and agriculture scientists. Non-government organizations and civil society organizations will also find this book interesting, informative and thought provoking. It is hoped that this book will help adaptation of proven successful interventions from across the developing world and accelerate and scale up their implementation towards reducing malnutrition.

It is indeed my great pleasure and honour to write the foreword for this book.

10th October 2010

Prof Emeritus Kraisid Tontisirin MD, Ph D
Chairman of the Policy Board,
The Thailand Research Fund, Bangkok
Formerly Director Nutrition and Consumer Protection Division,
Food and Agriculture Organisation of the United Nations (FAO), Rome

Preface

Public Health Nutrition in Developing Countries focuses on application of public health and nutrition sciences for formulating strategies and actions for preventing and solving the serious problem of malnutrition in developing countries. Presented are experiences, evidences and developments in addressing public health nutrition problems over the last three to four decades. The lessons learnt from past experiences are highlighted to facilitate understanding of the basis of policy formulation, development of strategies, design and implementation of programmes within a result-based framework. Along with these, a description of universally recommended process and impact indicators is presented for measuring progress and outcomes of a wide range of public health nutrition interventions. In this context, the metabolism of a few selected nutrients are described to explain the rationale for the selection of a specific set of indicators in relation to specific nutrition intervention programmes.

This book presents an update on public health nutrition problems of developing countries along with a description of approaches used and efficacy of trials undertaken for addressing them. It highlights the experiences emerging from up-scaling intervention trials to programme models and elaborates on the principles of public health nutrition programme planning and implementation. The book covers emerging global experiences for a wide spectrum of public health nutrition issues, ranging from those addressing women and child undernutrition and micronutrient deficiencies, nutrition care in HIV and management of nutrition in emergency situations. It therefore aims to provide not only an update on current knowledge but also to generate interest in upcoming challenges and scenarios for future programmes. Presentation of case studies from developing countries is incorporated to draw the attention of policy makers and programmers, and academics to actual experiences, processes, value additions, lessons learned and to potential challenges that remain to be addressed. The book intends to elaborate on the 'how' of addressing public health nutrition programming, to inform strategic planning, design and implementation of effective plans that would accelerate the reduction of malnutrition. Specific reference is made to policy formulation processes

Preface

Public Health Nutrition in Developing Countries focuses on application of public health and nutrition sciences for formulating strategies and actions for preventing and solving the serious problem of malnutrition in developing countries. Presented are experiences, evidences and developments in addressing public health nutrition problems, over the last three to four decades. The lessons learnt from past experiences are highlighted to facilitate understanding of the basis of policy formulation, development of strategies, designing and implementation of programmes within a result-based framework. Along with these, a description of universally recommended processes and impact indicators is presented for measuring progress and outcomes of a wide range of public health nutrition interventions. In this context, the metabolism of a few selected nutrients are described to explain the rationale for the selection of a specific set of indicators in relation to specific nutrition intervention programmes.

This book presents an update on public health nutrition problems of developing countries along with a description of approaches used and efficacy of trials undertaken for addressing them. It highlights the experiences emerging from up-scaling intervention trials to programme models and elaborates on the principles of public health nutrition programme planning and implementation. The book covers emerging global experiences for a wide spectrum of public health nutrition issues, ranging from those addressing women and child undernutrition and micronutrient deficiencies, nutrition care in HIV, and management of nutrition in emergency situations. It therefore aims to provide not only an update on current knowledge but also to generate interest in upcoming challenges and scenarios for future programmes. Presentation of case studies from developing countries is incorporated to draw the attention of policy makers and programmers, and academics to actual experiences, processes, value additions, lessons learned and to potential challenges that remain to be addressed. The book intends to elaborate on the 'how' of addressing public health nutrition programming, to inform strategic planning, design and implementation of effective plans that would accelerate the reduction of malnutrition. Specific reference is made to policy formulation processes and programme experiences in India since the country has historically taken a global lead in launching various public health nutrition programmes.

The book highlights the emerging double-burden of undernutrition and overnutrition in developing countries. The association of malnutrition with the increasing challenge of communicable and non-communicable diseases has also been described. Additionally, the problem of nutrition of the aged population faced by many countries undergoing demographic transition is also dealt with. Separate sections are devoted to nutritional epidemiology, undernutrition in children and women and major micronutrient deficiency programmes such as iron, vitamin A, iodine and zinc. However, there is some intended overlap in micronutrient sections since different perspectives of similar subjects are addressed.

It is envisaged that this book, produced in two volumes, will provide public health experts, nutrition programmers, medical and nutrition graduates, nurses, programme managers with NGOs, or food industry and policy makers with information on technical and programmatic aspects of public health nutrition and thereby enhances skills in formulating and implementing appropriate solutions and actions.

I am indebted to innumerable women living in the developing world who greatly inspired me to address issues of public health nutrition with a new perspective. Women play a central role in influencing the nutrition status not only of children but of the entire family. This is well reflected in the profound statement of Swami Vivekananda, "there is no chance for the welfare of the world unless the condition of women is improved. It is not possible for the bird to fly on one wing". For improving nutrition situation in developing countries, we need to move beyond accessibility to food. Simultaneously, the social, educational and economic empowerment of women needs to be addressed. A multi-dimensional approach is essential for overcoming malnutrition.

As editor, I would like to acknowledge the contributors who are eminent scholars and leading programme specialists for their excellent contributions to this book. Their deep knowledge and vast experience has added immense value to the content of the book. I am particularly grateful to the authors for the colossal effort they have put in preparing the manuscripts. Furthermore, I would like to express my appreciation for the support provided by my team at the Public Health Nutrition and Development Centre (PHNDC), New Delhi. The invaluable assistance of Ms. Ritu Jain, Research Nutritionist, PHNDC, in reviewing literature and analyzing data, as well as, her continuous support in networking with the authors is appreciated. The support of Ms. Rachita Gupta, Research Nutritionist, PHNDC, in the final stage of this book is valued. I sincerely appreciate the contribution of Ms. Falguni Gokhale (Director, Design Directions) for the design of the cover page of this book.

I am deeply indebted to my mentor, late Professor A.H.G. Love, for his guidance during my doctoral work at the Institute of Clinical Sciences, Queen's University of Belfast, and for generating my interest in the subject of public health nutrition. The production of this book would not have been possible without the untiring love, care and support of my husband Dr. Chander Vir whose constant and unrelenting motivation helped me work towards my mission to promote public health nutrition issues in developing countries. My special thanks to my brother-in-law, Dr. Ishwar Dass, IAS, who constantly inspired and encouraged me to complete this book. The support, enthusiasm, patience and understanding of my daughters Parul and Anubha and my son-in-law Amit Garg is appreciated and acknowledged. I also sincerely appreciate and acknowledge the support, understanding and continuous encouragement from my extended family.

My special acknowledgement to the United Nations Children's Fund (UNICEF) with whom I have been associated for almost three decades, first as Project officer and now as a consultant. This association has provided me with the opportunity to learn in an ever evolving development environment.

This book could not have been produced without the cooperation of the publishers, Woodhead Publishing India Ltd. My sincere thanks to the publishing house team members—Mr. Ravindra Saxena and Mr. Sumit Aggarwal.

Sheila C. Vir MSc Ph D
Director,
Public Health Nutrition and Development Centre,
New Delhi, India
January 2011

List of Contributors

Prof Bhattacharya Madhulika
Professor
Community Health Administration
National Institute of Health and Family Welfare(NIHFW)
New Delhi, India

Dr Bulusu Saraswati
Nutrition specialist,
UNICEF Field Office
Hyderabad, India

Dr Casanova Ines G.
Department of Nutrition and Health Sciences
Rollins School of Public Health
Emory University
Atlanta, USA

Dr Chaddha Ravinder
Associate Professor
Department of Food and Nutrition
Lady Irwin College
University of Delhi
New Delhi, India

Dr Chaudhary Deepika Nayar
Deputy Regional Director, Asia
The Micronutrient Initiative
New Delhi, India

Prof Das Tara Gopal
Director
Tara Consultancy Services
Bengaluru, India

Dr Dhingra Pratibha
Senior Research Scientist
Center for Micronutrient Research
New Delhi, India

Prof Dwivedi Shraddha
Professor and Head
Department of Preventive and Social Medicine
MLN Medical College
Allahabad, India

Ms Garg Aashima
Nutrition Specialist
UNICEF Field Office
Jaipur, India

Dr Gera Tarun
Consultant
Department of Pediatrics
Fortis Hospital
New Delhi, India

Prof Godbole Madan M
Professor and Head
Department of Endocrinology
Sanjay Gandhi Post Graduate Institute of Medical Sciences
Lucknow, India

Gulati Deepti
Senior Programme Associate,
Global Alliance for Improved Nutrition (GAIN)
New Delhi, India

Ms Jain Ritu
Research Nutritionist
Public Health Nutrition and Development Centre
New Delhi, India

Prof Kanani Shubhada
Professor
Department of Foods and Nutrition
Faculty of Home Science Maharaja
Sayajirao University of Baroda
Gujarat, India

Prof Kapur Deeksha
Professor
Department of Nutritional Sciences
School of Continuing Education
Indira Gandhi National Open University
New Delhi, India

Ms. Kathuria Ashi K.
Senior Nutrition Specialist
The World Bank
New Delhi, India

Dr Khanna Kumud
Director
Institute of Home Economics
University of Delhi
New Delhi, India

Dr Kotecha Prakash V
Country Representative
A2Z
USAID Micronutrient Project
Academy for Education Development
New Delhi, India

Dr Krishnaswamy Kamala
Former Director
National Institute of Nutrition
Hyderabad, India

Prof Kurpad Anura
Dean and Professor
Department of Nutrition
St. John's Research Institute
Bengaluru, India

Dr Lakshaman Anand
Coordinator, Planning and Knowledge Management
The Micronutrient Initiative (Asia office)
New Delhi, India

Dr Laxmaiah Avula
Deputy Director (Epidemiology)
Division of Community Studies
National Institute of Nutrition
Hyderabad, India

Dr Mathews Minnie
Former Senior Program Advisor
United Nations World Food Programme
New Delhi, India

Dr Menon Purnima
Senior Research Fellow
Division of Poverty, Health and Nutrition
International Food Policy Research Institute
New Delhi, India

Mr Mukherjee Ashish
Executive Director
Centre for Development Finance
Institute of Financial Management and Research
Chennai, India

Dr Nair K. Madhavan
Scientist and Head
Micronutrient Research Group
Department of Biophysics National Institute of Nutrition
Hyderabad, India

Prof Nandan Deoki
Director
National Institute of Health and Family Welfare (NIHFW)
New Delhi, India

Dr Nigam Arun K
Executive President
Institute of Applied Statistics & Development Studies
Lucknow, India

Dr Paintal Kajali
Nutrition Specialist
UNICEF
New Delhi, India

Prof Pandav Chandrakant
Head and Professor
Centre for Community Medicine
AIIMS
New Delhi, India

Dr Puri Seema
Associate Professor
Department of Food and Nutrition
Institute of Home Economics
University of Delhi
New Delhi, India

Dr Vijayaraghavan Kamasamudram
Former Head
Department of the Division of Community studies
National Institute of Nutrition
Hyderabad, India

Dr Raj Kamal
Emergency Nutrition Specialist
Child Nutrition & Development Section
UNICEF,
New Delhi, India

Dr Ramachandran Prema
Director
Nutrition Foundation of India
New Delhi, India

Dr Ramakrishnan Usha
Associate Professor
Hubert Department of Global Health
Rollins School of Public Health
Emory University
Atlanta, USA

Prof Ramji S
Professor
Department of Pediatrics
Maulana Azad Medical College
New Delhi, India

Prof Sachdev Harshpal S.
Senior Consultant
Pediatrics and Clinical Epidemiology
Sitaram Bhartia Institute of Research and Science
New Delhi, India

Dr Sankar Rajan
Regional Manager and Special Adviser in South Asia
Global Alliance for Improved Nutrition (GAIN)
New Delhi, India

Dr Sazwal Sunil
Associate Professor
Department of International Health
Program on Global Disease Epidemiology and Control
Johns Hopkins Bloomberg School of Public Health
USA

Prof Selvam Jerard M.
Professor and Head
Department of Epidemiology
The Tamil Nadu DrMGR Medical University
Chennai, India

Prof Seshadri Subadra
Senior Nutrition Consultant
Former Professor and Head at Department of Food and Nutrition
Faculty of Home Science Maharaja Sayajirao University of Baroda
Gujarat, India

Dr Seth Veenu
Associate Professor,
Department of Food and Nutrition
Lady Irwin College
University of Delhi
New Delhi, India

Dr Shah Dheeraj
Associate Professor
Department of Pediatrics,
University College of Medical Sciences
New Delhi, India

Dr Singh Padam
Head
Research & Evaluation
EPOS Health India
New Delhi, India

Dr Pandey Richa S.
Nutrition Specialist
UNICEF Field Office
Lucknow, India

Dr Swaminathan Sumathi
Research Supervisor
Department of Epidemiology and Statistics
St. John's Research Institute
Bengaluru, India

Dr Mannar M.G. Venkatesh
President
The Micronutrient Initiative
Ottawa, Canada

Dr Vir Sheila C.
Former Programme Officer ,UNICEF (India)
Director
Public Health Nutrition and Development Centre
New Delhi, India

Dr Wesley Annie S.
Senior Program Specialist
The Micronutrient Initiative
Ottawa, Canada

Dr Yunuss Shariqua
Programme Officer – Health and Nutrition
United Nations World Food Programme
New Delhi, India

Prof Zodpey Sanjay P.
Director, Public Health Education
Public Health Foundation of India and
Director, Indian Institute of Public Health, Delhi
New Delhi, India

* The content of the text presents views of the author and not necessarily reflect outlook of the organization.

1 Principles of epidemiology and epidemiologic methods

Sanjay P. Zodpey

Sanjay P. Zodpey, MBBS, MD, PhD, is a Public Health Specialist and Epidemiologist. Currently, he is Director, Public Health Education, Public Health Foundation of India (PHFI), New Delhi and Director at Indian Institute of Public Health, Delhi. Earlier, he was Vice Dean at the Government Medical College, Nagpur, Maharashtra, India. His areas of interest include clinical epidemiology, evidence-based health care, health policy, health systems research, program evaluation and public health governance. Dr Zodpey has been involved in several major international and national research initiatives that have contributed significantly to the field of public health.

1.1 Introduction

The scientific progress in health care research, application and policy formulation begins with a study among the population. The understanding of health events and outcomes in larger groups facilitates researchers in obtaining the 'true' and 'complete' picture of the situation. Several methods of scientific enquiry have been devised for the study among populations. Based upon the nature of enquiry, the study methods are broadly categorized as qualitative and quantitative. Qualitative methods equip researchers to gather an in-depth understanding of human behaviour and the reasons that govern human behaviour. Quantitative studies involve an ardent numerical foundation and seek to provide 'hard' and measurable evidence. Nutrition lends itself to several exploratory and explanatory tools. These tools aim to capture the health status of the population and measure its determinants.

1.2 What is epidemiology?

The term 'epidemiology' is coined from the Greek, implying 'study among the population'. Indeed, the science of epidemiology is essentially based on the study of phenomena that affect the population at large. A widely quoted definition is offered by Last in 'The Dictionary of Epidemiology' where the term is defined as "The study of the distribution and determinants of health-related states or events in specified populations, and the application of this study to control of health problems". The definition succeeds in capturing the essence of epidemiology as based among the people at large. It aims to study not just disease or disease processes, but it is directed towards the entire gamut of health related states across the spectrum. It also addresses events that may influence the presence in such a state or which may force a departure from it. Lastly, it completes the picture by emphasizing upon the very purpose of epidemiology of working towards the control of health problems. The history of advancement in the science of epidemiologic methods has been hand-in-hand with public health. Epidemiology is a rapidly expanding and essential quantitative tool in the wide science of public health.

1.3 Development in epidemiologic methods

Contrary to popular belief, the epidemiologic method of scientific enquiry is not a recent addition in the repertoire of the expert. In 1747, James Lind conducted his famous study with 12 participants

Box 1.1 Aims of epidemiology [5]

First, to identify the *etiology* or *cause* of a disease and the relevant risk factors, i.e. factors that increase a person's risk for a disease.
Second, to determine the extent of disease found in the community.
Third, to study the natural history and prognosis of disease.
Fourth, to evaluate both existing and newly developed preventive and therapeutic measures and modes.
Fifth, to provide the foundation for developing public policy relating to environmental problems, genetic issues, and other considerations regarding disease prevention and health promotion.

Uses of epidemiology

- Identifying health related event
- Identifying the risk factor and its linkages
- Establishing the causal relationship between risk factors and health related events
- Completing the natural history and clinical picture of disease
- Designing an intervention for addressing the problem
- Evaluating the effectiveness of intervention

aboard a naval ship. He tried to address scurvy, a significant public health problem among the sailors at that time. The understanding of the basic principles of epidemiology has undergone a significant refinement since this experiment by James Lind. Rapid strides have been made, especially in the last 50 years. The advent of computers and the ability to handle complex mathematical processes has fuelled the recent advancements. It is now practically impossible to imagine this progress in public health practices without any assistance from epidemiological methods.

The science of epidemiology is a reflection of the inquisitiveness of human nature. It seeks out answers to the elementary questions that are posed to researchers and policy-makers. In this attempt, epidemiology has been influenced by several other scientific domains. The rapid expansion of this field and the need for specialized methods has promoted several new offshoots. The trial conducted by James Lind was a foray into alleviating a nutritional problem by using scientific techniques. Similarly, the means to study chronic diseases and account for multifactorial causation and long latency assisted the development of multivariate methods in epidemiology. Likewise, several fields like infectious diseases, geriatrics, cancer, nutrition, occupational and environmental medicine are developing and contributing to the development of tools and measures. The influence of these disciplines on epidemiology is immense and a welcome addition. Before embarking upon a discussion on the basic principles of the subject, the readers may bear in mind that although epidemiology is a large contributor towards the advancement of public health, it is not the only contributor. The creation of a complete picture for a public health problem mandates an understanding of the social and behavioural sciences as well. These may be studied by their unique methods, not necessarily just epidemiology.

1.4 Epidemiological reasoning

Epidemiological thinking follows a set pattern. Epidemiological reasoning attempts to rule out alternate explanations for the association between the cause and the effect. Let us understand this reasoning with an example from nutrition. For example, we may want to study the relationship between dietary fat consumption and obesity. The systematic collection and analysis of epidemiological data involves the determination of whether the probability of development of obesity in the presence of high dietary fat consumption is merely a chance or random event. The two conditions could be absolutely unconnected and by a stroke of luck may have been present in the study sample. There could be other alternate explanations. A systematic error that has crept into the study (bias) may be responsible for the conclusion. This systematic error could be due to a faulty ascertainment of dietary fat intake in all the study subjects. Alternatively, the association between high dietary fat consumption and obesity may be due to the effects of additional factors (confounding) like physical inactivity. If the issues of chance, bias and confounding can be satisfactorily addressed in the study, the investigators seek to make a judgment on causality that is, attributing a cause–effect relationship between high dietary fat consumption and obesity. Such a judgment would be made after considering several ancillary factors like the strength of the association, consistency of findings from all other studies and biologic plausibility. These factors are considered in tandem before arriving at a judgment of causality between the exposure and the outcome. The stronger the association between the cause and the effect, the higher is the likelihood of a causal relation between the exposure and the outcome. The presence of a biologic explanation for the purported causal effect (biologic plausibility) may aid in the process of attributing causality. Also, there must be a temporal sequence between the cause and the effect. The causal factor must precede the effect before attributing a causal relationship between the factors. The judgment of causality also considers the specificity of the association between the cause and the effect. The inference of causality is further strengthened by examining the coherence and analogy of the association between the cause and the effect. Similarly, if a particular finding is evidenced in several studies, in different locations and by different researchers, there is a stronger possibility of the existence of a causal relationship.

1.5 Classifying epidemiologic study methods

The simplest classification of epidemiologic studies is into observational and experimental studies (Table 1.1). Observational studies are those studies where the investigator observes and reports on the events without attempting to alter or control the events. On the other hand, in the experimental studies, the researcher controls the intervention within the study participants. The investigator offers the specific intervention under study and proceeds to study the change in the outcome. These studies or methods often compliment one another.

Table 1.1 Study designs in epidemiology

I. Observational designs	(a) Case reports and case series
	(b) Ecologic studies
	(c) Cross-sectional studies
	(d) Cohort studies
	(e) Case-control studies
II. Experimental studies	Controlled trials and uncontrolled trials

The study methods that are close approximations to the ideal experimental conditions are considered relatively higher in the chain of evidence. For example, a double-blinded randomized controlled trial

(RCT) substantiating the beneficial effects of oral zinc supplementation in the treatment of acute diarrhea is considered superior to a simple longitudinal study on the problem. This hierarchy of study designs which rates experimental studies over observational studies may have some relevance, but it is necessary to understand that the choice of study designs must not be influenced by the hierarchy of evidence alone. The actual choice of a certain epidemiologic design is influenced by the current state of knowledge about the disease and the nature of the research question. There may be instances where a well-conducted case-control study may provide sufficient evidence and may not warrant the conduction of a RCT. Research usually proceeds from simpler designs that serve to identify and describe the problem to complex designs that address causality. The choice of a study design is also influenced by the frequency of the disease in the community, the ability to quantify the variables linked to the disease and the operational feasibility.

1.5.1 Observational designs

Case reports and case series

Though conventionally not classical epidemiologic in their origins, these represent the earliest evidence that is accumulated within clinics and hospitals. Case reports are narratives of unique or rare occurrences during routine practice. Their uniqueness may represent a chance occurrence or may be an unrecognized dimension of a disease. For example, a case report may detail a case of vitamin B_{12} deficiency associated with severe depression. This severe depression may be actually linked to the B_{12} deficiency or may be a chance occurrence. A case-series lists similar experiences in several patients. Both forms may serve as initial pointers towards identifying newer effects of a disease or even the emergence of a totally unrelated new disease. A case-series of clustering of *pneumocystis carinii* pneumonia (a rare cause of pneumonia) was published from Los Angeles, United States in 1981. Subsequent research led to the identification of a new virus which was called as the HIV virus. The case report and case series may thus be viewed as the earliest descriptors of a disease. They serve to provide the foundation and rationale for the conduction of further epidemiologic studies.

Ecological study

Ecological studies are population-level studies that assist primarily in hypothesis generation. Ecological studies, unlike other study forms, are not conducted at the individual level. These are conducted at the population level. For example, an ecological study may be conducted to explore the relationship between food prices and the occurrence of vitamin deficiency in the pediatric age group. This comparison may be drawn between various states in the country and it may be evident that with a rise in price of food grains, there is a corresponding elevation in the vitamin deficiency rate. Such a study may therefore yield ground to base a new hypothesis which may be examined by a study design. Because this study is conducted at the population level, it is not possible to draw interpretations at the individual level. This is because it is not possible to state with certainty that the particular child who is suffering from vitamin deficiency is so affected because of food prices or some other cause. This ecological fallacy is the chief drawback in this study design.

Cross-sectional studies

Cross-sectional studies seek to collect information about a health event and its putative risk factors or outcomes at an individual level and at a specific point of time. In this respect, these studies closely resemble a photograph as they capture all the essential information in a single brief contact with the participant. Cross-sectional studies are distinguished from longitudinal studies by providing only a single opportunity for collecting the information on the disease and the outcome. They do not have a built-in directionality like the prospective study designs and retrospective study designs to be discussed later in this chapter. They differ from ecological studies in studying the health event within individual participants, in contrast to ecological studies which attempt to study the relationships at group level. Cross-sectional studies may have a descriptive as well as an analytical component associated with it. The descriptive component attempts to explore the 'what', 'when' and 'where' of a disease. The cross-sectional studies are well-developed to answer this descriptive dilemma. The cross-sectional studies may also be analytical in seeking to provide information about the presence and strength of association between the disease and the study variable, thus permitting the testing of a hypothesis. Analytical cross-sectional studies describe as to 'why' the disease in occurring.

The study is conducted within a population that is well-enumerated and described. Though it is not an absolute necessity, the conduction within a known group greatly facilitates in drawing inferences about the possible relationship between a variable and the health status. At the time of the data collection, instant estimate (summary) of the presence or absence of the disease is linked with the presence or absence of the variable that

Box 1.2

Descriptive study – A study designed only to describe the distribution of an event (exposure or outcome), to describe the frequency of specific events or diseases in a particular population without seeking to explain the distribution by looking for association. The descriptive component attempts to explore the 'what', 'when' and 'where' of a disease.

Analytical study – A study designed to examine associations, often with the aim of identifying possible causes for an outcome. Analytical cross-sectional studies describe as to 'why' the disease is occurring.

seeks to describe the disease. This summary at a point of time is collected for every individual to yield the pattern of the disease in the entire community. By providing this summary measure (prevalence), the cross-sectional study gives a representative picture of the disease status in the entire community.

Box 1.3

Prevalence is concerned with quantifying the number of existing cases in a population at a designated time. The prevalence of disease in a population is defined as the total number of cases of the disease in the population at a given time.

When this estimate is derived for an exact time period, like on a specific date, the measure is more accurately referred to as a point-prevalence measure. The analogous term for a longer time interval like a season or a week may be referred to as period-prevalence.

Incidence is the frequency of occurrence of the new cases in a defined population, arising during a given time period. Incidence, in contrast to prevalence, is a measure of new cases that occur in a population.

The rate that is thus calculated is referred to as cumulative incidence rate (Number of incident cases/ total population at risk at beginning of follow-up period). Cumulative incidence assumes that there is a uniform and complete follow-up of the entire population at risk, from the beginning of the observation period to the end of the observation period. Incidence density, a similar measure, overcomes this contextual difficulty by substituting the exact amount of time for which each individual is followed-up in the study.

Box 1.4 Basic steps in conduction of a cross-sectional study

- Defining the target population and baseline characteristics of the area and population.
- Conducting literature review to understand current state of knowledge upon subject.
- Formalizing the study objectives and methodology.
- Sampling the study population and identifying the study participants.
- Developing the study tools and standard operating procedures for data collection.
- Analysing data and interpreting results.

The preliminary step before the conduction of any population-based epidemiologic study, including cross-sectional studies, is to obtain the basic characteristics of the area (defining the population) where the study is planned. This preliminary step is vital because it provides a proper perspective to the study by justifying its need. It also assists in the process of planning the data-collection mechanisms that can be employed within the setting. Finally, at the stage of drawing interpretations, it assists the researcher in providing the appropriate context for formulation of the recommendations. The second step is also common to all studies. It involves the conduction of a thorough literature review. Literature reviews involve searching the print and electronic media for information and research conducted upon the subject. A thorough literature review facilitates the subsequent steps in the study conduction and also clarifies to the researcher the current state of knowledge upon the subject. The search should not be limited to indexed journals or to the print media alone. Adequate references may also be searched using online databases.

After the researcher is well-acquainted with the study problem and the current status of knowledge on the subject, the researcher may embark upon formalizing the objectives for the study. The study objectives are a set of well-defined and usually quantifiable measures. The study design and methods are planned in accordance with these objectives. Subsequent to the finalization of the objectives, the study methods are formalized. These involve the selection of a study tool and the necessary training of the data collection team. The choice of standard operating procedures for data collection would contribute towards the internal validity of the findings. Internal validity is the approximate truth about inferences drawn from a study. It refers to the confidence we place in the findings of a study. Internally valid studies would generate results/findings which would be applicable to the participating population. External validity, on the other hand, deals with the generalizibility of the study results, in populations that are distinct from the study population. In other words, if the findings of a study demonstrate an increase in the growth velocity of malnourished children with the feeding of energy – protein dense diet, external validity answers the question about whether malnourished children in other locations, countries and conditions will respond similarly with an improvement in the growth velocity as predicted by the study.

The analysis of a cross-sectional study proceeds along two general lines. These are guided as to whether the cross-sectional study is planned to be a descriptive cross-sectional study or an analytical cross-sectional study. A descriptive cross-sectional study will seek to provide a preliminary analysis by the calculation of means, medians or ratios as appropriate. The most commonly used measure is a prevalence measure that is derived and can be stratified for age, sex and other demographic variables.

An analytical cross-sectional study, in addition to the prevalence measure, will seek to identify the absence or presence of association between the putative exposure factor and the outcome measure. If an association is present, it then seeks to quantify the strength of the association. This may be in the form of odds ratio or rate ratio. For example, in a study addressing association between increased cholesterol and Coronary Heart Disease (CHD), we can calculate prevalence of CHD disease in those exposed to high-cholesterol diet and compare it with prevalence with those not consuming high-cholesterol diet to estimate the odds of suffering from CHD given high-cholesterol intake. Also, we can do stratified analysis for various level of cholesterol (high, medium, low) for presence or absence of CHD to estimate the strength of association.

The cross-sectional study (Table 1.2) has several points of interest. The chief advantage of this form of study is that it is a one-time exercise. As a result, it has a high degree of operational advantages for the research team. It is also a valuable exercise in generating a preliminary hypothesis. But it suffers from a disadvantage in being unable to attribute the exposure to the effect. For example, a cross-sectional study may identify that there is an association between a mal-absorption syndrome and vitamin D deficiency. The study is however unable to determine whether the vitamin D deficiency is caused by the mal-absorption per se. It may also be that the vitamin D deficiency may have caused enzymatic changes and then may have contributed to mal-absorption. Thus, the one-time visit of the investigator for a cross-sectional study may be an operational advantage, but fails to establish the sequence of events.

Cohort study

Cohort studies are a frequently encountered research design in public health nutrition literature. The basic constituent of a cohort study is a follow-up of a group of people who constitute the 'cohort'. A cohort is a group of people with some common characteristic. If this common characteristic is chosen to be year of birth, we may have a cohort of all the children born in 2008. If this characteristic selected is the area of residence, we could constitute a cohort of all the residents of a particular locality or township. Consider a research question where the investigator plans to determine whether the rates of vitamin D deficiency are similar or different in those consuming calcium supplements. The first step in a cohort study would be to define the cohort. This could be done to include all the residents of a fixed geographical area, say village X. The subsequent step would be to classify the members of the cohort (village X) into two groups on the basis of the particular exposure factor (calcium supplementation; taken or not taken) into exposed and the un-exposed groups. We can classify all the people taking calcium supplements as the 'exposed' group

Table 1.2 Effect measures in cross-sectional studies and definitions of common terms[3]

	Disease (+)	Disease (–)	Total
Exposure (+)	A	b	a+b
Exposure (–)	C	d	c+d
Total	a+c	b+d	a+b+c+d

Measure	Formula
Means and standard deviations	
Medians, percentiles and other quantiles	
Proportions and ratios	
Odds Ratio	ad/bc
Prevalence ratio	{a/(a+b)}/{c/(c+d)}
Rate Ratio (exposure)	{a/(a+c)}/{b/(b+d)}
Rate Differences (prevalence difference)	{a/(a+b)} - {c/(c+d)}
Rate Differences (exposure difference)	{a/(a+c)} - {b/(b+d)}
Excess risk among exposed	{a/(a+b)} - {c/(c+d)}
Population Excess Risk	{(a+c)/n} - {c/(c+d)}
Attributable fraction (exposed)	{a/(a+b) - c/(c+d)}/ {a(a+b)} × 100
Population attributable fraction	{(a+c)/n - c/(c+d)}/ {(a+c)/n} × 100
Prevented fraction (exposed)	[{c/(c+d) - a/(a+b)}/{c/(c+d)}] × 100
Prevented fraction (population)	[{c/(c+d) - (a+c)/n}/{c/(c+d)}] × 100

Definitions of common terms

Mean is the sum of the values for observations/number of observation. It is well-suited for mathematical manipulation.

Median is the point where the number of observations above equals the number below. It is not easily influence by extreme values.

Mode is most frequently occurring value. It has simplicity of meaning.

Range is from lowest to highest value in distribution. It include all values.

Standard deviation is the absolute value of the average difference of individual values from the mean. It is also well-suited for mathematical manipulation.

Percentile, deciles, and quartiles are proportions of all observations falling between specified values. They describe the "unusualness" of a value without assumptions about the shape of a distribution.

Rate measures the occurrence of an event (disease) per unit of person-time.

Proportion measures the percentage/fraction of people who develop new event (disease) during a specified period of time.

Ratio measures the odds of having an event in question (disease) relative to not having the event.

Risk Ratio: Compares the incidence of risk of an outcome in two groups/ populations. It measures how much more likely members of one group develops outcome of interest than members of the other group. It estimates the magnitude if the effect of the exposure on the outcome.

Rate Ratio: Compares the incidence rate of an outcome in two groups, one exposed to factor under study and other not exposed. It is only measure that takes into account the person-time risk in each exposure group.

Relative risk. For rare outcomes there are few people entering and leaving different exposure groups, the risk ratio and rate ratio are numerically similar. Both ratios in these circumstances are called as relative risk. However, it is better to specify which measure of effect we are using.

Odds ratio is defined as the ratio of the odds of development of disease in exposed persons to the odds of development of disease in non-exposed persons.

Prevalence ratio is used to compare the burden if disease in different group. It is neither an estimate of the magnitude of effect of exposure nor a measure of strength of association between an exposure and outcome.

An alternative way to compare the occurrence of an outcome in a group that has been exposed to a particular factor with the occurrence in group that has not been exposed is to use a difference measure. *Absolute difference* is calculated by subtracting the occurrence in the unexposed group from the occurrence in the exposed group.

Risk difference compares the incidence risk of an outcome in two populations.

Rate difference compares the incidence rate of an outcome in two populations.

When there is a causal relationship between an exposure and an outcome, the difference measure is sometimes called as the *attributable risk* or *attributable rate*.

The *attributable risk* is defined as the amount or proportion of disease incidence (or disease risk) that can be attributed to a specific exposure.

The attributable risk *in the total population* also called the *population attributable risk* – or the *PAR* "population attributable risk" or "population attributable fraction" as the reduction in incidence that would be achieved if the population had been entirely unexposed, compared with its current (actual) exposure pattern.

and the ones who do not as the 'unexposed' group. Both these groups would then be followed for about 6 months and the rates of occurrence of vitamin D deficiency in both these groups would be compared. The design thus seeks to establish a relationship between a risk factor (calcium supplementation) and the subsequent development of a disease (vitamin D deficiency).

Cohort studies can be conducted in clinical or community settings. In clinical settings, these studies may be employed to study the mechanisms of disease causation or the treatment effects. In community settings, these studies are usually employed to study the population health impact of exposures. This study form may also be used to study occupational and environmental exposures responsible for disease causation. The cohort studies are referred to as longitudinal studies, implying that the studies involve a prospective follow-up from purported cause to the effect. Cohort studies are best suited for studying common diseases or where a sufficient number of cases will accumulate at the end of the follow-up period. As discussed in the vitamin D example in the earlier section, this design draws its conclusions after a lengthy period of time. The loss of patients to follow-up (due to death, migration etc.) thus presents serious challenges to this study design. All cohort studies incorporate a detailed follow-up plan to meet with such contingencies. These studies can also be undertaken to study multiple common outcomes in the general populations. Special cohorts may also be constituted to study rare exposures, for example, cohorts constructed after the Bhopal gas tragedy (rare exposure) attempt to document the effects of exposure to methyl iso-cynate.

Box 1.5 Basic steps in conducting cohort studies

- Defining the study question
- Defining and identifying appropriate cohort
- Selecting the study population, selection and enrolment of participants
- Defining and measuring the exposure
- Developing the study tools and Standard Operating Procedures for data collection
- Follow-up of participants
- Ascertaining outcome
- Analysing data and interpreting results

Cohort studies are classified according to the follow-up schedules for the study participants. If the follow-up is done entirely in the future, the study is referred to as a prospective cohort study. If a part of the study is conducted in the past and part in the future, it is referred to as an ambispective cohort study. A cohort study wherein the follow-up was conducted entirely in the past is referred to as a retrospective cohort study. Although prospective cohort studies are the classical form of the study, they may involve excessively long-waiting periods. This is because once the cohort is established and the cohort members are segregated as exposed and non-exposed, we have to essentially wait for the development of the outcome in both these groups. This duration varies between situations and may be relatively short in the development of food allergies, but may be as long as 5 years as in the case of vitamin B_{12} deficiency. The latter situation will warrant a follow-up of at least about an equal duration in all the study participants.

After the identification of an appropriate cohort, the success of the study depends upon the nature of the cohort. Cohorts may be classified as 'open' cohorts or 'closed' cohorts. A cohort is labeled as 'open' or 'dynamic' when it permits new entrants into the follow-up group provided they fulfill specific criteria. For example, an open cohort of school children would permit new entrants/admissions into the school to be a part of the subsequent follow-up. The school drop-outs would be likewise omitted from the analysis. A 'closed' cohort of the same school children, in contrast to open or dynamic cohorts would not permit any changes to the original participant list of the study. Both forms of cohorts have specific advantages and disadvantages and are used in very different situations. The choice of the group to be selected for a cohort study is chiefly influenced by the ease and the practicality of the follow-up procedure. This is because for the accrual of sufficient outcomes/cases at the end of the follow-up period, it is essential to ensure a high follow-up rate among the study participants. Successful cohort studies like the Framingham heart study enrolled population from a relatively stable community near Boston which agreed to the study. The Nurses' health study has studied the relationship between diet, physical activity, weight gain and the risk of chronic diseases. The success of this cohort lay in the ready accessibility of this group to the investigators and the provision of a high follow-up rate. The cohort may thus be chosen from the general population or from a specific population group.

After the selection and enrollment of the study participants, the next step in a cohort study is to determine the exposure status of the participants. It may be noted that the cohort study bases its analysis on the determination of the outcomes in two groups: exposed and the unexposed. The determination of the exposure status at the commencement of the study is useful for the segregation of the participants into the two groups. It is mandatory to have a good operational definition of the exposure for the purpose of the study. The investigators must formulate a detailed, accurate, objective and unambiguous definition for the exposure. The criteria for the establishment of the exposure status should also be uniform across all the study subjects. For example, if the nutritional status of a group of under-5 children is to be studied, the investigators must clearly state the classification being used to assign children as under-nourished. It must also state the cut-off between normal and under-nourishment. The measurement of weight must be done according to uniform criteria, for example on the same brand of weighing scale. The methods to determine the exposure status should be similar for all the participants of the study. The exposed group should ideally be similar to the unexposed group in all factors except the exposure under study.

After classifying the study participants into the two groups, the investigators proceed with the collection of the base-line information about the study participants. For example, in order to study the relationship between diet in antenatal women (exposure) and birth-weight (outcome), a cohort of women attending antenatal clinic in a district hospital may be formulated. In addition to the exposure we aim to study, there are several additional factors that may influence the causation of low birth weight among the newborns. These could vary from cultural habits in the household, socio-economic status, cooking practices and so on. All these factors could also independently influence the occurrence of the outcome. Data-collection methods employed must therefore also collect information about these factors. This information may be collected formally as a part of the study or it may be collected from pre-existing records. For example, the information about the health status of the individual mother in a cohort may be collected from the previous antenatal health records. Hospitalization records may be collected from the hospitals within the geographic limits of the cohort. However, this information must be accurate and more importantly, should be easily linked to the specific mother/child in the survey. The commonly used methods for procuring information involve the conduction of personal interviews, questionnaires dispatched by post and telephonic interviews. These methods have varying rates of response with the highest response rates achieved on personal interview. Medical examinations may be necessary to obtain information of which the subject cannot be expected to be aware. For example, no participant can be assumed to be aware about the serum level of vitamin D. A study on such substrates may necessitate the collection of biological specimens. Direct examinations can also be used to validate information obtained from interviews. However, use of all such techniques contributes towards increasing the cost of the study. Investigator time may also need to be devoted towards the training and the standardization of the biological measurements as well as the quality-check processes.

The follow-up schedule for the study participants must be chalked out well in advance. Follow-up must be identical for all members in both the groups of the cohort. A differential plan of follow-up may inadvertently introduce a bias in the study. It is usually recommended to ensure the highest possible follow-up rates in both the groups. This may be facilitated by designing a comprehensive follow-up plan that may utilize several strategies. Chief among them include periodic re-examination of the subjects, postal or telephonic reviews and indirect surveillance of hospital records and death certificates. The duration of follow-up usually depends on the natural history of disease and length of latent period.

Cohort studies basically provide estimates of incidence. Incidence, in contrast to prevalence, is a measure of new cases that occur in a population. The burden of disease in a community is composed of 'old' (already existent) and 'new' (newly developed, during the course of the study) cases. A cohort study aims to determine whether there are differential incidence rates between the exposed and the unexposed groups. The rates thus calculated are referred as cumulative incidence rate and incidence density (Refer to Box 1.3). Incidence density measures the exposure in terms of person-time or person-years to keep the contribution of each individual commensurate with their follow-up period. For example, an individual followed for 10 years without outcome event contribute 10 person-years, where as an individual followed for 1 year contributes one person-year to the denominator (Number of incident cases/ total person year follow-up).

Cohort studies permit study progression in the same direction as would occur in nature. This study design allows a complete description of the individuals' experiences subsequent to exposure, including the natural history of disease. As a result, they can convincingly state the temporal sequence and help add this information to the causal chain. Cohorts once set up and adequately followed-up, are a wealth of information. They may investigate the causation of multiple outcomes. For example, a cohort of obese men may yield information not just on the incidence of myocardial infarction in obese men, but may also yield information on the incidence of colonic carcinoma. A cohort study is ideally suited for an investigation into rare exposures. A specially constructed cohort of individuals subjected to a rare exposure may help unravel the health effects of the exposure on the population at large. In general, cohort studies are usually for a long duration, mandating the set-up of a detailed follow-up plan for the study participants. The loss to follow up can be a significant deterrent to the drawing of valid conclusions and must be specifically observed as a part of the study. Thus the chief limitations of this study design are operational and administrative. In addition, ethical considerations also assume great significance in cohort studies.

Table 1.3 Effect measures in cohort studies [4]

	Disease +	Disease –	Total
Exposure +	a	b	m1
Exposure -	c	d	m0
Total	n1	n0	t

Cumulative incidence rate/ incidence density

Incidence ratio $IR_E = (I_E / I_0)$

Where I_0 = incidence rate in standard non-exposed group; I_E = incidence rate in exposed group

Relative risk (risk ratio) $RR_E = (R_E / R_0)$

Cumulative incidence relative risk (a/n1) / (b/n0)

	Disease +	Disease –	Total
Cases	a	b	m1
Person time	n1	n0	t

Incidence density relative risk (a/n1) / (b/n0)

Incidence difference $ID_E = I_E - I_0$

$ID_E = I_0(IR_E - 1)$

Attributable risk (risk difference) $RD_E = R_E - R_0$

$RD_E = R_0(RR_E - 1)$

Etiological fraction $AF = (I_T - I_0)/ I_T$

I_T = incidence rate in total population; I_0 = incidence rate in group without exposure

Case-control study

A case-control study is an efficient analytical study design. The study population in a case-control study consists of groups who either have (cases) or do not have a particular health problem or outcome (controls). Case-control studies, in contrast to cohort studies, proceed from the effect to the cause. In other words, the disease has already occurred when this study is conducted. This is a highly efficient study design for examining rare diseases and diseases with long incubation periods. This is unlike a classical cohort study which would have to either recruit a magnanimous number of participants (for yielding sufficient outcomes) or would have to undertake extremely long follow-ups for the long latent periods. This is deemed unnecessary by the proponents of a case-control design which overcomes these shortcomings and successfully identifies the differences in the presumed causal factors between the cases and controls.

A case-control study can be conducted over a variety of settings. They are commonly employed in clinical as well as community research. Additionally, this design is often used to study occupational and environmental diseases. The choice of the case-control study design, like all other study designs, is strongly guided by the factors common for other designs. These include the current state of knowledge on the study problem, the availability of an institutional framework and the resources to conduct the study. They may be employed in clinical settings to outline the mechanism of disease causation or in community settings to identify the population health impact of exposure.

Box 1.6 Basic steps in conduction of case-control study

- Defining the study question
- Developing criteria for identification and selection of the cases
- Selecting appropriate controls and matching for efficiency
- Measuring exposure
- Analysing data
- Interpreting the results, and assessing the potential sources of error

The case-control study proceeds with the investigator attempting to determine the presence or absence of the putative risk-factor(s) in either group and then comparing them. The intention of this comparison is to determine whether the exposure is responsible for the given disease. The case-control study commences with the identification of the cases and the controls for the purpose of the study. A 'case' is defined as a specific outcome. It may be the presence of the disease or condition of interest, a complication etc. This case selection must be done using the standard definitions for diseases and must follow uniform criteria as outlined under cohort studies. A set of operational definitions must be set-up. Diagnostic methods employed for the purpose of the study must also be defined and included in the study protocol. It is usually recommended that case-control studies should recruit newly diagnosed cases or incident cases as a 'case' for these studies. The reason for such a recommendation stems from the knowledge that prevalent cases, in contrast to the incident cases, are a product of factors that cause a disease and also factors that govern the duration of illness. For example, consider the relationship between cases of colorectal cancer and sex. The occurrence of cases of colorectal cancer is higher among males than among females. But the survival is better in females than in males. Consequently, at any given point in time, if the prevalence of colorectal cancer is assessed in a community, it would yield a higher proportion of the disease in the females. This can result in a systematic error in the study. It can be however minimized by considering incident cases rather than prevalent cases. So the inclusion of incident cases as 'case' in a case-control study is backed by sound reasoning. Additionally, the incident cases being relatively recent, the cases can be expected to easily recall the influencing factors in a questionnaire. The cases may be registered from hospital admission or registry records, physician records, pathology records, clinic notes/ case-file or from clinics with a good follow-up or recording system.

The selection of controls is a critical issue in case-control studies and it depends on the setting in which the study is being conducted. The controls must be free of the disease. Specific inclusion and exclusion criteria are framed to identify controls. The criteria used to select controls should be comparable in all ways with the criteria used to select cases, except disease status. In hospital-based studies, the controls are usually selected from the hospital attendees. Controls may also be selected from the same neighbourhood as the cases or from the relatives of the cases. Such controls will possibly have similar environmental exposures as the cases and may be suited for the study of certain exposure–effect relationships. Alternately, controls may also be selected from the general population; random digit dialing on the telephone can help in identifying potential study participants. Comparison of cases with specific controls contributes towards the study efficiency. In studies with small sample sizes, selection of more than one control per case helps to improve the statistical power of the study. This increase in statistical power is observed up to a 1:4 ratio between cases and controls. Beyond this number, there is hardly any gain in statistical power per new control.

Case-control studies may employ matching between cases and control as another unique feature. Matching is performed for certain characteristics or variables of interest. For example, cases and controls may be matched for age and sex, socio-economic variables, literacy and so on. It is usually employed only for the known risk-factors for the outcome. Matching must be performed for only those variables which improve the statistical efficiency of the study. An overzealous attempt at matching for all possible variables must be avoided. This is important because an overmatched study may under-estimate the true odds associated with the outcome. Also, once matching has been accomplished, it is not possible to separate the effect of the matched variables. The subsequent step in the study is exposure assessment. It is done using a variety of methods. This can be accomplished through interviews or by utilizing medical or occupational records/histories. Biological markers may also be used whenever feasible. The study proceeds by a calculation of the odds ratio. This statistic, also referred to as a cross-product ratio, is an estimate of the relative risk obtained in cohort studies. The interpretation of this measure is relatively simple. For example, if the odds ratio for sepsis in low birth weight babies is 3, it means that the low birth weight babies are 3 times more likely to suffer from sepsis than normal weight babies.

The study quality may be compromised by the presence of unique biases. Case-control studies are conducted after the disease or event of interest has occurred. As a result, the in-depth interview and examination for the exposure having occurred may be followed up with differing vigor in cases and controls. For example, the history of immunization with vitamin A may be queried and checked with great detail in a known case of malnutrition than in a normal weight child. Such biases can be controlled by blinding the data collecting team of the specific objective of the study. Alternatively, the study instrument may be so prepared and the questions may be so objectively included that there is no variability in the questioning style among the cases and the controls. This measure will ensure a uniform method of data collection regarding exposure status in both the groups. Biases can be minimized by the careful planning, design and appropriate analysis in the study. These biases are classified as selection bias, misclassification (information) bias and confounding bias.

Box 1.7 Biases that may occur in case-control design [5]

Selection bias refers to error due to systematic differences in characteristic between who take part in study and those who do not, such that the people selected to participate in a study are not representative of the reference population or the comparison groups are not comparable.

Mis-classification bias refers to error in the measurement of exposure or outcome that results in systematic difference in the accuracy of information collected between comparison groups.

Confounding bias is about alternative explanations for an association between an exposure and an outcome. It is the situation where an association between an exposure and an outcome is entirely or partially due to another exposure (called confounder). In order to be a confounder, the variable must be associated with exposure of interest, must be a risk factor for outcome of interest, and must not be on casual pathway between exposure and outcome.

Minimizing such biases is an important challenge in the conduction of case-control studies. However, in-spite of these limitations, the case-control study offers significant methodological advantages to the researcher. Newer hybrid designs, like nested case-control studies combine the advantages of cohort and case-control studies for investigating into exposure–outcome associations (Table 1.4).

1.5.2 Experimental studies – controlled and uncontrolled trials

Experimental studies are characterized by the prerogative of the investigator in assigning the participants to a particular intervention. This distinguishing feature characterizes experimental studies from the other types of epidemiologic studies. The investigator allocates the participants

Table 1.4 Effect measures in case-control studies

	Disease (+)	Disease (–)	Total
Exposure (+)	a	b	a+b
Exposure (–)	c	d	c+d
Total	a+c	b+d	a+b+c+d
Exposure rates			(a/a+b) and (c/c+d)
Odds ratio			[a / c] / [b / d] = ad / bc
Attributable risk proportion			(OR-1)/OR
Population attributable risk proportion			1-[b(c+d) /d(a+b)]

into groups and also determines which study participants receive the intervention. These studies progress forward in time, in a sense; they are longitudinal or prospective like the cohort studies. In the causal chain, experimental studies are said to provide the strongest evidence of disease causation. Although rated high on the causal chain, their inherently complex nature makes them a difficult proposition for researchers. Experimental studies may be carried out in several settings. They are often carried out in hospital settings as clinical trials to evaluate therapeutic regimes. Equally common are community-based study designs which may or may not employ control subjects. In communities they may be used to examine population-level interventions.

Box 1.8 Following basic steps are critical for experimental studies

- Formulating the hypothesis / Defining the study question
- Developing the study protocol
- Selecting the study population
- Randomization and allocation of the intervention
- Follow-up of participants
- Measuring outcome
- Analysing data and Interpreting results

The first step in the conduction of an experimental study is the formulation of a hypothesis. The hypothesis is the very basic premise on which the study is based. Experimental studies are an operational, financial and ethical challenge. Consequently, they are conducted in situations where there is an uncertainty which can be addressed by the conduction of this study. An experimental design is then constructed to study the hypothesis. The methodology and the steps to be followed in the study are enumerated and described in the study protocol. This protocol is implemented subject to ethical clearance by the institutional review board or ethics committee. Using specific inclusion and exclusion criteria, the investigators seek to recruit participants for this study. These criteria ensure the participation of individuals who would be capable of withstanding the intervention as well as the subsequent assessment of the outcome. The participants who meet the eligibility criteria must then consent to their participation in the experimental study. Consider an experimental design constructed to study the effect of a dietary intervention on anemia in pregnant women. The inclusion criteria for such a study would include the mothers registering in antenatal clinics over the study area. After determination of their hemoglobin status, the women with hemoglobin levels below 11 g% would be classified as anemic and therefore eligible to participate in the interventional study. Women with normal hemoglobin levels would be excluded from such a study. The informed consent procedure must be strictly monitored and non-consent for participation must not adversely affect the treatment of the individual. The informed consent must not be blanket consent for participation into the study but must clearly mention the interventions to which the participant will be subjected. The consenting participants may then be allocated into the study arms using random or non-random allocation depending on the design of the study.

Randomization is a method to allocate individual subjects who have been accepted for a study into one of the groups (arms) of a study. The process of randomization is akin to tossing a coin for allocating the participants into groups. It may be pre-decided that all participants who toss a heads may be allocated to one group and all the participants who toss tails may be allocated to the other group. Alternatively, randomization may also be carried out using random-number tables. The usage of such tables is easy and ensures random distribution of the participants into the groups. Many studies employ computer-generated random allocation sequences which may be used for classifying the study participants into groups. Essentially, all these procedures ensure that every individual has an equal chance of being a participant in either of the two groups: the study or the control group.

Consequent to randomization, the basic explanatory factors get divided evenly among the two groups. This similarity between the two groups is what makes randomization so crucial in experimental studies. Out of a total of 100 children, after randomization it may be expected that there will be near equal number of boys and girls in either group. Similarly, there would be a near equal number of underweight children in both these groups. Such a balance between the two groups extends not only between the known etiological factors or causal factors, but also between the unknown causes or contributors of a disease. For example, it may be known that the nutritional status of a child is influenced by the total daily caloric intake of the child. Randomization of participating children will achieve a near equivalence in the caloric status between the two groups. It also ensures that if there is any other confounder that is present, it too will get equally distributed between the experimental and the control groups. This division of measured/non-measured, visible/invisible, known/unknown variables will be approximately equal between the two arms in the presence of a big sample.

The procedure of randomization helps to minimize selection bias in the study. It does so by ensuring allocation of the study participants into the groups using a pre-defined method. Thus, a conscious or sub-conscious bias on part of the investigator can be minimized. In the evaluation of two dietary supplementation plans for mal-nourished children, randomization assures that the investigator does not show a conscious or sub-conscious preference for any dietary plan by allotting the healthier children to that group. Additionally randomization meets the assumption of statistical tests used to compare the two groups. The group to which a particular participant is allocated may alternatively be concealed from the study investigator whenever possible. Once registered the patient remains irrevocably in the study. Such a process in which the group assignment of the next patient remains undisclosed (or concealed) from the recruiting physician is termed, 'concealed randomization' or 'allocation concealment'.

There are several issues that must be considered when undertaking randomization. This procedure yields the intended results only when the randomizing method is strictly followed and is adhered for each and every participant. There must be no break in the sequence or the technique for any participant. The randomization is employed only when the subject is a part of the study and must not be employed prior to the participation of the study subject.

Another procedure frequently encountered in experimental studies is blinding. Blinding is done so that the prejudices or enthusiasms of the subjects don't result in behaviour that promotes or inhibits the recognition of disease outcomes. It can be performed in three ways: single blind (The trial is so planned that the participant is not aware whether he/she belongs to the study group or control group); double blind (The trial is so planned that neither the doctor/investigator nor the participant is aware of the group allocation and the treatment received); or triple blind (The participant, the investigator and the person analyzing the data are all blind as far as group allocation is concerned). Triple blinding is considered as ideal but can be infrequently employed. It is necessary to understand that 'concealed randomization' is not 'blinding'. Concealed randomization is to take place before initiation of treatment whereas blinding involves steps at and after initiation of treatment.

It must be attempted to reduce or minimize a contamination in a clinical trial. This occurs when the control group receives part or all of the intervention. When the comparison is between two active treatments, contamination occurs when patients in one arm receive the treatment of the other arm. Such contamination tends to blur the difference between the treatments. A genuine effect may be completely obscured or may be underestimated.

Controlled trials may proceed in several ways. In the parallel design, they begin with the participants of the trial being classified into the two groups (group A receiving intervention, i.e. experimental group and group B not receiving intervention, i.e. control group) according to randomization sequence. Subsequently, the two groups are followed up for the occurrence of the outcome which is compared between the groups. Outcome ascertainment is carried out in the follow up period. This outcome is defined according to the study objectives and is preferably done using objective and specific criteria. Alternatively in cross-over studies, the two groups would proceed as mentioned earlier and after ascertaining outcomes, the groups are exchanged. That is, the exposed group now participates as the control group and the original control group as the experimental group. This cross-over is permissible after a wash-out period that guarantees that the original intervention group is now free of the effects of the intervention.

However, not all experimental studies are randomized or employ controls. Non-randomized trials are also frequently encountered in scientific literature. Due to several logistic and operational issues, it may not always be possible to randomize participants into groups. For example, when evaluating impact of national initiatives like implementation of Integrated Child Development Services (ICDS) on nutritional status at district level since all districts, it is not possible to employ a control district group. This is not possible because the intervention is administered across the country in all districts where only some blocks may not be covered. In such circumstances, epidemiologists conduct a type of experimental study referred to as a before–after study. This means that a study is conducted where in data on the nutritional status of the children is compared before and after the intervention is applied within the community. After allowing sufficient time for the intervention to cause an effect, we evaluate the population for any change in the nutritional status of the children. Any change in the nutritional status between these two time intervals is carefully examined for the possible causes. Another variety of non-randomized studies are studies of natural phenomena and their descriptions. For example the famous experiment by John Snow to identify the etiology of cholera was a natural experiment. This form of study makes use of the naturally occurring phenomena and making a careful record of the observation to arrive upon justified conclusions. Follow-up is also an integral part of any experimental study. It implies examination of the experimental and control group subjects at defined intervals of time, in a standard manner, with equal intensity, under the same given circumstances. The outcome of the study may include positive as well as negative events. These must preferably be objective and determined for all participants in the study. Investigators pay special attention towards ensuring a high degree of compliance among the study participants in order to facilitate assessment of the outcome.

Experimental studies when conducted in this fashion provide an estimate of the *efficacy* of an intervention. They attempt to determine whether the intervention works under ideal, highly controlled and optimal conditions. Ideally, the determination of efficacy is based on the results of an RCT. But eventually, all interventions are employed in the larger population or community. The extent to which a specific intervention when deployed in the field does what it is intended to do for a defined population is distinct from validity and is referred to as the *effectiveness* of an intervention (Box 1.9).

1.5.3 Hybrid study designs

There has been recent attention towards the development of study designs that employ the advantages of more than one study design. Such designs are either combinations of study designs or modifications in the study methods. Such observational hybrid designs include nested case-control studies, follow-up prevalence study, selective prevalence study, case-crossover studies and so on. In nested case-control studies for example, a cohort is constructed and duly followed up for the occurrence of the outcome. Those participants of the cohort who experience the outcome are designated as cases while the participants who do not experience the outcome constitute the controls. Such studies are being increasingly conducted in the nutritional field.

Box 1.9

Efficacy is the effect of the intervention under trial conditions, the maximum benefit under ideal conditions.

Effectiveness is the effect of the intervention under operational conditions, such as would be the effect of intervention into routine practice.

For example, the effect of nutritional supplementation for HIV-infected individuals may have positive impact (weight gain) in trial conditions, but when translated in clinical practice, we would expect it to be less effective because the population is less carefully selected; adherence would be low, resulting in reduced benefits.

Table 1.5 Effect measures in experimental studies

Risk difference (absolute risk reduction) where R_t is the risk/probability of outcome in the treatment group and R_c is the risk/probability of outcome in the control group	=	$R_t - R_c$
Risk ratio (Relative risk)	=	R_t / R_c
Relative risk reduction percent) or 1 – RR (in	=	100 – RR (in decimals)
Number needed to treat	=	1/ Risk difference

References

1. STOLLY PD, LILIENFELD DE (1994). *Foundations of Epidemiology*. Oxford University Press.
2. MCEWEN, BEAGLEHOLE, TANAKA, DETELS, (eds). Oxford Textbook of Public Health. Oxford University Press, 2002.
3. ABRAHAMSON JH. *Survey Methods in Community Medicine*. Churchill Livingstone, 1999.
4. HENNEKENS CH, BURING JE. *Epidemiology in Medicine*. Williams and Wilkins, 1987.
5. GORDIS L. *Epidemiology*. Elsevier Saunders, 2004.
6. ASCHENGRAU A, GEORGE R. SEAGE III. *Essentials of epidemiology in Public Health*. Jones and Bartlett Publishers, 2003.
7. BONITA R, BEAGLEHOLE R, and KJELLSTRÖM T. *Basic Epidemiology*. World Health Organization, 2007.

2

Nutrition epidemiology for developing countries

Usha Ramakrishnan and *Ines G. Casanova*

Usha Ramakrishnan, MSc, PhD, is Associate Professor at the Hubert Department of Global Health, and Director of the Doctoral Program in Nutrition and Health Sciences (NHS) at Emory University. Dr. Ramakrishnan is internationally known for her expertise in maternal and child nutrition and for her research is focused on the functional consequences of micronutrient malnutrition during pregnancy and early childhood in developing countries.

Ines G. Casanova, MS (Nutrition), worked at the Department of Community Nutrition at the Mexican National Institute of Public Health (INSP) for 3 years. She is currently a doctoral student in the NHS Program at Emory University.

2.1 Introduction

Epidemiology is defined as "the study of the distribution and determinants of health-related states or events in specified populations, and the application of this study to control health problems" [1]. Meanwhile, nutrition is "the process by which substances in food are transformed into body tissues and provide energy for the full range of physical and mental activities that make up human life". Nutritional sciences primarily involve the study of biological processes, but also integrate fields like anthropology and psychology that play an important role in the determining patterns of dietary intake and health in large groups or people, i.e. populations [2]. The application of epidemiological principles to human nutrition has resulted in the unique field of "Nutritional Epidemiology" which provides the necessary tools to generate scientifically valid information that advances our understanding of the role of nutrition in human health and/or disease [3]. Nutritional epidemiology is defined as "all the studies between diet and health in human populations" [4].

The purpose of this chapter is to provide a general understanding of "Nutritional Epidemiology" by describing the main concepts and features that define this discipline, and to focus on the application of the science of nutritional epidemiology to the nutritional and health problems that the less developed countries face. The first section is a review of different types of epidemiologic studies and their application to the methods used to assess nutritional status at a population level. This is followed by a discussion of the issues related to measurement error and the assessment of validity and precision at a population level. Finally, the last two sections focus on the role of nutrition epidemiology in a) addressing the determinants and dynamics of nutrition in developing countries and b) in public health nutrition towards the goal of improving the health and well-being of populations.

2.2 Epidemiological studies

Epidemiology as a science has five major objectives: (i) to identify risk factors for disease; (ii) to determine the extent of disease in a community; (iii) to study the natural history and prognosis of disease; (iv) to evaluate preventive and therapeutic methods of health care delivery; and (v) to provide the foundation for developing public policy. The two key constructs in epidemiological research are "exposure" and "outcome". Exposure is typically defined as the variable believed to be associated with the presence or absence of the disease. In the case of nutritional epidemiology the main exposure of interest is dietary intake (including nutritional supplements), while the outcome is its effect on human health [1, 5]. The relation between dietary intake and child health is illustrated well in the UNICEF conceptual framework; inadequate food intake is directly related to disease, and both are direct causes of children malnutrition, disability and death (Figure 2.1). Nutritional epidemiology allows us to examine the nature of these associations [6]. For example, dietary fat intake or frequency of consumption of animal foods could serve as exposures of interest whereas the outcome is the disease itself (or the absence of it); such as presence/absence of stunting and/or anemia. The dynamics between exposure and outcome are central to epidemiologic studies which can be conducted using different kinds of study design. The most common classification of studies based on their design is either "observational" or "experimental". A description of the different types of study design under the above two categories is provided in the following section with examples of their application to nutritional epidemiology.

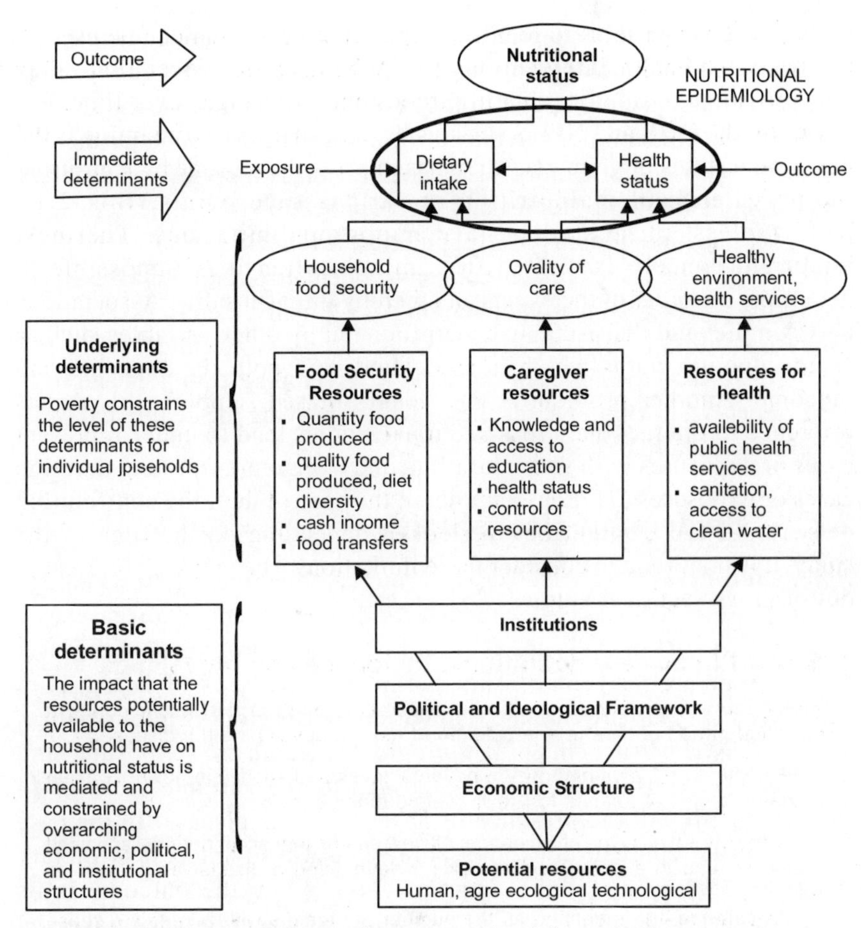

2.1 UNICEF Malnutrition Framework – an example of dietary intake as an exposure.

2.2.1 Observational studies

Cross-sectional studies

This study design is mainly used to estimate prevalence. Typically both exposure and disease are assessed at the same point (or period) of time in all subjects or a representative sample [7]. Examples of cross-sectional studies in nutritional epidemiology are the national health and nutrition surveys that many countries periodically implement to describe the nutritional and health status at a specific point of time. These include the Demographic Health Surveys (DHS) in many developing countries including the National Health and Family Survey (NFHS) in India, that obtain anthropometric and hemoglobin measurements in women of reproductive age and young children, the National Nutrition Surveys in Mexico, and the Nutrition and Health Examination Surveys (NHANES) in the United States of America. These surveys are very useful to identify population needs and can be used as the basis for health interventions [5]. When repeated over time, they also provide a basis of estimating trends and/or changes over time. For example, the DHS and NFHS surveys have been useful to examine if the nutritional status of young children has improved over time by measuring the prevalence of malnutrition at various time points (Box 2.1). Nevertheless, these studies have important limitations. The most important concern is related to "timing"; often it is impossible to determine the order of the events and thereby infer causality. Associations between diet and disease may be confounded by other variables such as socioeconomic status which is associated with both the exposure and outcome. Another problem is the "length-biased sample", this makes reference to the fact that cross-sectional studies tend to under-represent cases or exposures with short duration, and over-represent long duration cases or exposures [7]. For example, in the case of diet, the contribution of seasonal foods might be overlooked depending on the time of the study. It is important to consider these limitations when making inferences out of cross-sectional studies.

Box 2.1 Important definitions: incidence and prevalence

Incidence – It is defined as all new cases of a disease that occur during a specified period of time in a population at risk for developing the disease.

- Example: In a 6-month period 66 patients developed anemia in "town X". Then the incidence of anemia for "town X" in 6 months is 66.

Mortality – It is a type of incidence. All new deaths that occur during a specified period of time in a population at risk for developing a disease is defined as mortality.

Prevalence – It is defined as the number of persons with a certain disease present in a population at a specific time divided by the number of persons in the population at that time.

- Example: A survey conducted on 26th of February in "town X" determined that 3000 persons had anemia at that time. The city has 30000 habitants; then the prevalence of anemia in "town X" is 0.10 or 10%.

Ecologic studies

This design differs from all other epidemiologic studies in the unit of observation. Ecologic studies focus on groups of people instead of on individuals. The most common use of this type of studies is to compare between countries; sometimes they have been used to compare other defined groups like schools, workplaces, organizations, cities, etc. Both exposure and outcome are measured at a population level. Food consumption or availability is an example of the data that is often used. The data are typically from cross-sectional and obtained from national nutrition surveys or food production statistics. The information is expressed per capita, where the amount of total food available is divided by the number of people and does not necessarily reflect individual intake [1, 5, 7]. Food balance sheets that describe all food and nutrient availability at the national level [8] are often used; for example, the grams of fat consumed per capita in China, India and Japan can be related to the prevalence of obesity in each of these countries.

Cohort studies

In a cohort study the researcher classifies the participants in two groups based on exposure status and then follows both groups to compare the incidence of disease. A positive association between exposure and disease is represented by a greater incidence in the exposed group compared to the unexposed [1]. The main strength of this design is the ability to make inferences about etiology [3]. It is possible to determine timing and directionality because exposure is assessed before the onset of the disease. These studies are useful to determine the relation between diet and disease [5]. The main limitation however is that they may be time consuming and expensive especially when you are examining conditions that may take a long time to develop such as cancers and/or are rare in which case you need a very large sample size. A well known example of cohort studies in the field of nutrition is the Nurses Health Study in the United States. Other examples of cohort studies include the INCAP longitudinal study from Guatemala [9, 10], the Pelotas Birth Cohort in Brazil that followed children born in 1982 in the city of Pelotas up to adulthood [11], and the Japan Collaborative Cohort Study for Evaluation of Cancer (JACC) [12]. Many of these studies have followed up their subjects for several decades either from early childhood to adulthood, young adulthood to later adulthood which have allowed them to examine the role of early nutrition in the etiology of chronic disease and other health outcomes.

Case-control studies

In case-control studies, the investigators first identify a group of individuals with a specific disease/condition (cases), following which they randomly select a group of individuals with similar characteristics but are disease free (controls). This is followed by the assessment of one or more exposures of interest which are then compared in both groups. For example, dietary exposures are established using surveys or medical records. Diet can be assessed at four different levels: individual, household, institutions and national. These studies, particularly in the case of dietary intakes, often suffer from recall problems and/or low quality data because of the retrospective design. Another concern in case control studies is the appropriate selection of the control group. These potential sources of bias, referred to as systematic error often result in incorrect conclusions about the nature of the associations being examined. It is therefore important to consider these limitations and interpret the results of these studies cautiously. However, these studies are logistically more feasible than prospective studies (i.e. cohort studies) and can provide relevant information to assess the diet-disease interactions [1, 3, 5, 7, 13].

2.2.2 Experimental studies

An experiment is understood as a trial where the investigator(s) manipulates the exposure of interest. Experimental studies are typically preferred in a scientific setting but often difficult and expensive to carry out. Nevertheless, studying human beings involves many factors that the researcher is unable to control; this is true particularly for nutritional epidemiology [5]. Experimental epidemiology is also limited ethically to studies in which exposures are expected to cause no harm. The other important ethical consideration is the appropriate use of a placebo and need to ensure that all participants are assured "the standard of care" in the specific setting where the study is being conducted. For example, iron supplementation is routine during pregnancy in many developing countries and denying this could be regarded as "unethical" [7].

Randomized controlled trials (RCTs) – Randomized controlled trials are considered the gold standard in assessing the effect of an intervention. In these trials, subjects are randomly assigned either to an exposed (treatment) or unexposed (control or placebo) group. Clinical trials in nutrition typically include a baseline and a follow up measurement of nutrition or health related exposures and outcomes. The greatest advantage of these studies is their effectiveness in assessing causality.

Box 2.2 Reporting clinical trials – the Consolidated Standards of Reporting Trials (CONSORT) Statement

CONSORT was designed by a group of clinical trial researchers, statisticians, epidemiologists, and biomedical editors and has been supported by a growing number of medical and health care journals. CONSORT encourages transparency with reporting of the methods and results, so that reports of RCTs can be better interpreted. The use of CONSORT also reduces inadequate reporting. Most importantly, evidence suggests that the use of CONSORT could positively influence the way in which RCTs are conducted, by setting standards that should be considered during the design stage. [14–16]. The CONSORT checklist comprises 22 items that include information on reporting the design, analysis and interpretation of the trial. This includes specific details on the objectives, nature of the intervention, randomization and blinding, data collection and analysis. The flow diagram provides information on how to report the changes in sampling and the study population (Figure 2.2).

Randomization is the assignment by chance to the treatment or to the control group. This tool helps reduce the chances of selection bias, and also helps to control for confounding factors that otherwise could be overlooked by the researcher [1]. Details on the ideal ways to randomize and allocate treatments are described in The CONSORT (Consolidating Standards of Reporting Trials) statement that was developed and published in the mid 1990s with the aim of improving the quality of the reports of clinical trials [14–16] (Box 2.2).

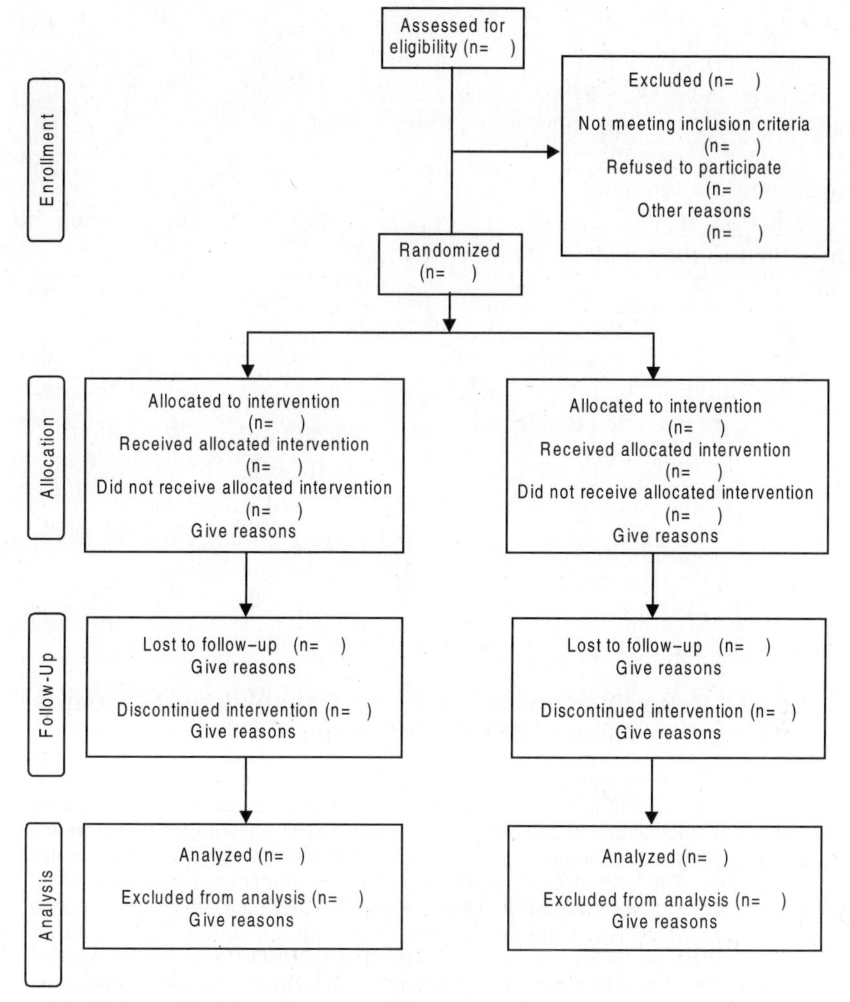

2.2 CONSORT Statement 2001 flow diagram.

Another advantage of RCTs is the usage of a placebo (indistinguishable from the treatment), which allows blinding to the treatment. In a single blinded study the subjects are unable to distinguish if they are taking the treatment or the placebo; while in a double blinded study, neither the subjects or the researchers know the assignation to the groups. Blinding eliminates the possibility of bias induced by modification of the behavior of subjects or researchers related to the grouping [5, 13]. The chances for differential bias in the measurement of outcomes are reduced which increases the validity of the findings. It may however be difficult to conduct placebo-controlled RCTs when food based interventions are being evaluated. Although the participants cannot be blinded to the treatment, the inclusion of a control group and blinding of the personnel who collect and analyze the data are recommended to minimize bias. The inclusion of a control group allows one to compare changes over time in a group that did not receive the treatment and determine if the treatment group fared better. For example, if the prevalence of anemia did not decline in women who received multiple-micronutrient supplements but increased in the control group over the same time period, it would be easier to interpret that the treatment group still benefited as the supplements prevented the increase in anemia that would have otherwise occurred. Another major advantage of including control groups is to minimize the effect of confounding variables that may be associated with the outcome of interest. Another element of clinical trials is the utilization of "intention to treat' principle in the analysis of outcomes. This concept is related to adherence to the treatment and is used in efficacy trials; "Intention to treat" means that groups are analyzed as initially assigned, independent of adherence [1]. For example, in a study of comparing the effects of consuming multiple micronutrients to iron only supplement in women of reproductive age, if 600 women were originally randomized to treatment but only 550 actually received the treatment and 400 consumed at least 80% of the intended dose, intention to treat analysis will compare the outcome of interest for e.g. prevalence of anemia in all 600 women who were originally randomized to either the treatment or control groups irrespective of how many doses they consumed. Comparing the benefits of the intervention only among those who consumed at least 80% of the intended dose would be treated as a sub-analysis.

Community interventions

Community intervention trials are an important tool in nutrition epidemiology. They are similar to clinical trials, except that the interventions are targeted to groups of individuals, for e.g. villages or organizations such as schools etc (as opposed to individuals). An exposure is introduced to a whole community or group of people, and a similar community is used as a control. When more than two communities or large groups of people are intervened, the assignment to the groups should be by randomization. Examples of community interventions are environmental changes like water fluoridation, increasing fruit and vegetable availability by building a market, etc. Dietary interventions may be more convenient at a family, household or community level [7].

2.3 Nutritional epidemiology – measurement

Careful consideration of the methods selected to assess nutritional status in terms of their suitability (see Box 2.3) as well as accuracy and precision are important for nutrition epidemiologic studies. This is especially critical in the case of the exposure and outcome variables. Today, nutritional assessment in many low income countries emphasizes new simple, noninvasive approaches. These methods are used to assess nutritional deficiencies or excesses, as well as to monitor or evaluate the effect of interventions aimed to improving nutrition and health outcomes [17]. Inadequate measurement however can lead to inappropriate conclusions, and waste valuable resources [3]. Nutritional assessment is defined as "the interpretation of information from dietary, laboratory, anthropometric and clinical studies", where this information is used to determine the nutritional status of individuals or populations [18]. These procedures were typically use to describe the nutritional status of populations since the 1960s but more recently have been used to examine the relationship between diet (or nutritional supplements) and disease.

Box 2.3 Nutritional assessment in developing countries

At a population level, nutritional assessment systems are classified in surveys, surveillance systems, screening and interventions.

- Nutrition surveys are cross sectional studies, mainly used to identify groups at risk of nutritional deficiencies.
- Nutritional surveillance is a continuous monitoring of the nutritional status of selected groups (usually high-risk groups).
- Nutritional screening is the identification of malnourished individuals or groups that require an intervention.
- Nutrition interventions are evaluated by nutritional assessment methods [3].

2.3.1 Methods to assess nutritional status

The selection of appropriate nutritional assessment methods is one of the most important elements in nutrition epidemiology. These methods have been traditionally used to characterize deficiency stages; and lately, to establish associations between health maintenance and risk factors for chronic diseases. The most common methods, as stated above, of nutrition assessment include

(a) Dietary assessment in which information about food intakes is obtained and often used to calculate intake of nutrients

(b) Biochemical measures of blood or other body tissues that provide indications of nutritional status and diet composition.
(c) Anthropometric assessment that includes measures of body dimensions that reflect long-term effects of diet including growth and body composition.
(d) Clinical assessment that includes clinical signs of severe deficiency.

A description of nutritional assessment methods and its applications to nutritional epidemiology is presented in the following sections [18].

Dietary methods

As mentioned before, the main exposure in nutritional epidemiology is diet. However, diet is not a single exposure but a complex set of exposures that vary over time and in different places. Measurement of dietary intakes is complicated and requires well trained personnel and validated methods. Estimation of continuous levels of exposure to specific dietary variables, like food patterns, is complicated by the daily variation of food intake. Also, the inter-correlation of dietary variables complicates the study of effects associated to independent factors. Individuals are usually unaware of the composition of the foods they consume; hence nutrient composition is usually determined indirectly [5, 7, 13].

In general, in nutritional epidemiology, diet has been studied in terms of nutrient intakes; diet however can also be described in terms of foods, food groups or dietary patterns. Several dietary methods are available; the choice should be guided by the objectives of the study and the characteristics of the study group [5, 7, 13]. The main tools used to assess dietary intakes are short-term recall methods and food frequency questionnaires.

- *Short time recalls and diet records* – The most widely used dietary assessment method is the 24 hours recall. It is the basis of several national nutrition surveys and many cohort studies. This method consists of an interview by a nutritionist or trained personnel. The interviewer, generally with the help of food models or standard quantities, collects information on the participant intake in the last 24 hours. The interview lasts approximately 20 minutes and has the advantage that minimum effort is required on the part of the participant [7]. The validity of 24 hours recalls have been assessed by observation in a controlled environment, and application of the questionnaire next day. The results yield that subjects both reported foods that they had not consumed and forgot foods that they had actually eaten [19]. The main limitation of the 24 hours recall method is that food consumption is high variability from day to day. An alternative to address this problem are food diaries. Dietary records or food diaries are detailed meal by meal registers of types and quantities of food consumed during an specific time, generally 3–7 days. Subjects weight each portion before eating, or alternatively household measures can be used. These methods however are time-consuming and typically require literacy compared to 24 hour recalls. The application of short time and diet recall methods to epidemiologic studies is also inappropriate for case control studies, because the exposure of interest might have occurred earlier or later, and the recall might not register it. Multiple 24 hours recalls can be useful for cohort studies; however the costs may be a limitation, particularly in developing countries. These methods can be used for validation or calibration of other methods of dietary assessment more practical for nutritional epidemiology in developing countries [17,18].

- *Food frequency questionnaires* – The food frequency questionnaire (FFQ) approach was developed as a means to measure long term dietary intake. A FFQ has two main components: a list of foods and beverages and a time scheme for the subject to indicate how often he/she consumes each food. A comprehensive assessment of the diet is desirable whenever possible. This is because it is generally impossible to anticipate all the information regarding diet that will be important at the end of data collection. A limited list of foods may leave out items that in retrospect result important. Additionally, sometimes total diet composition is necessary to prevent confounding by other dietary factors (i.e. total energy). Food frequency questionnaires are classified as quantitative and semi-quantitative. The difference between the two is that quantitative questionnaires provide additional information on serving sizes; whereas semi-quantitative questionnaires only assess the type of food and frequency of intake. Evidence suggests that including serving sizes does not represent a significant improvement in assessing diet. Food frequency questionnaires are widely used in nutritional epidemiology. They have great advantages for assessing diet at a population level: they are easy from subjects to complete, often self-administered, and processing is relatively inexpensive [7, 20, 21].

Biochemical methods

Gibson [18] classifies biochemical tests as (a) static and (b) functional tests. Static biochemical tests measure a nutrient or a metabolite in fluids or tissues and are useful in identifying intermediate stages of nutrition deficiencies when the body stores become depleted. These methods can also be used to assess excess of nutrients (i.e. cholesterol) or reactions to the intake of a specific nutrient (allergic reactions). Static biochemical tests are useful at a population level and have been used in national nutrition surveys. Functional tests assess specific nutrient dependent functions, for example activity of a nutrient dependent enzyme such as Flavin Adenine Dehyrdogenase (FAD) that requires riboflavin [5, 18]. These tests however are not suitable for large-scale nutrition surveys especially in resource poor environments.

Anthropometric methods

Anthropometric methods involve measurement of physical dimensions of the body and gross composition of the body [18]. These methods are used to assess moderate to severe malnutrition; nevertheless it is impossible to identify specific nutrition deficiencies. The main advantage of anthropometric methods is that they can detect chronic malnutrition. Body composition reflects very accurately nutritional history. Another advantage is that these methods can be performed relatively quickly and inexpensively. Examples of these measures are height, weight, body circumferences, etc. The measurement then are interpreted using indexes like the Body Mass Index (BMI), height to weight circumference or height for age, amongst others [5, 18].

Clinical methods

The aim of these methods is to detect signs (manifestations that can be observed) and symptoms (reported by the patients). The assessment is done by physical examination or medical history. Clinical manifestations appear at advanced stages of nutritional deficiencies and often are not very specific. These signs however have become less common with improvements in nutritional status and often require screening large samples. It is recommended to use these methods in combination with laboratory, clinical and/or anthropometric methods [5].

2.3.2 Indices and indicators

Construction of indices is often necessary for the interpretation and the grouping of the four methods previously described. Indices are continuous variables, formed by the combination of two or more measurements, which can be related to characteristics like age, sex or race. Indices are often evaluated at a population level by comparison with predetermined cutoff points. When used to assess the nutrition status at a population level indices become indicators. Nutritional indicators are widely used in public health or for decision making at a population level. For example, iodine deficiency at the population level is defined as a total goiter rate over 5% in school age children. The proportion of the population with nutrient intakes below the Estimated Average Requirement can also be an indicator of dietary inadequacy. For nutritional epidemiology the selection of indicators is a key issue in the design of studies and evaluations [18, 22, 23]. Inappropriate conclusions may be made if the correct indicator is not selected. For example, body mass index (BMI) which is widely used as an indicator of body composition and overweight (BMI>25) may not be appropriate in pregnant women and/or special populations like athletes. Similarly, certain biochemical indicators of micronutrient status such as serum ferritin and retinol may not work well in populations where infections are common.

2.3.3 Study design

Study design is a critical in nutritional epidemiology and is influenced by a variety of factors. The first element to consider is the purpose or the reason to conduct the research which will determine the type of design (cross-sectional, cohort, case-controls, experimental, etc) and choice of measurements, indices and indicators. The next and equally important consideration is the availability of resources that include time, money and expertise available [3]. Typically, logistic and economic limitations make it impossible to include the entire population in the study. Consequently, as part of the study design, it is important to develop a sampling protocol to select a group of individuals. This sample of individuals ideally should be an accurate representation of the source population and of an adequate size to respond to the objectives of the study. The information obtained in the study will depend on the way these individuals are selected. Hence, it is important to carefully develop a sampling system. The first element to consider in developing a sampling protocol is the availability of a sample frame, or a list of all the individual parts of the population (persons, schools, hospitals, etc). If this information is not available, it is necessary to select the sample using non-probabilistic methods; on the other hand if the sample frame is available it is possible to use probability based sampling protocols. These procedures are usually conducted by people trained in sampling techniques. Several statistical packages (for e.g. EPI-INFO, SAS, STATA) and specialized software packages (e.g. PASS) are available to calculate sample sizes. The World Health

Organization (WHO) also has a useful resource for calculating a sample size on their website (Box 2.4). Finally, an adequate study design provides the researcher elements of validity, precision and accuracy which are important to minimize bias. A brief description of these constructs is presented in the following sections.

Box 2.4 A tool to calculate sample size

The STEP-wise approach to surveillance is a program of the WHO to collect standardized information in different countries. This program provides two useful tools to calculate sample size and to determine a sampling frame: the "Sample Size Calculator" and the "Sampling Spreadsheet" which are available online. (http://www.who.int/chp/steps/resources/sampling/en/).

The *sample size calculator* describes the application of the formula that requires information on the level of confidence (for e.g. 95 % confidence), the margin of error (< 0.05) and expected baseline level of the indicators which is assumed to be 0.5 if no information is available. This is followed by adjusting for other factors such as the design effect in case a complex sample design is used, age-sex strata and expected response rate.

The *sampling spreadsheet* provides additional information that is useful for using the following different approaches to obtaining the sample.

- Probability proportional to size sampling
- Simple random sampling
- Weighing your data

Validity is defined as the capacity of reflecting the true situation of the population that is being studied. For a study to have high validity it must measure the exposure, for example diet, at a relevant time, in a relevant population or sample using methods that reflects adequately the exposure and outcome. Validity also assumes that there is no error in the way the information is collected, analyzed and interpreted. Validity can be classified as internal or external. Internal validity refers to the quality of the measurements and procedures inside the study. External validity is the generalizability of the study. In order to have external validity is necessary to first have internal validity. However, a study that is internally valid may have limited external validity which means that the results cannot be applied to the general population [1, 3, 13, 18].

Validity is also used to describe the methods used to assess the exposure or the disease. A valid test is able to distinguish accurately between who has the disease and who does not, or who is exposed and who is not. When validating a test there are two elements to consider: sensitivity and specificity. Sensitivity is defined as the ability of a test to identify correctly those who have the disease (or exposure); while specificity refers to the ability to identify correctly those who do not have the disease (or exposure) (see Box 2.5).

Box 2.5 Test validation – sensitivity, specificity, positive and negative predictive value

		Gold Standard	
		+	-
New Test	+	True Positives	False Positives
	?	False Negatives	True Negatives

Sensitivity= True Positives / (True Positives+ False Negatives)
Specificity= True Negatives / (True Negatives+ False Positives)
Positive Predictive Value= True Positives /(True Positives+ False Positives)
Negative Predictive Value= True Negatives /(True Negatives+ False Negatives)

Usually it is necessary to trade sensitivity for specificity; this trade is related to the cut-off points. A low cut-off point classifies more persons as diseased when they are actually not diseased (low specificity), but captures all individuals with the disease (high sensitivity). When the cut-off point is raised the test will start missing persons that have the disease (low sensitivity), but most of the negative results will actually be disease free (high specificity). For example, increasing the cut-off value for blood glucose from 75 to 130 mg/dl increases the specificity of this test in diagnosing diabetes but decreases the sensitivity as shown in Box 2.6.

Box 2.6 A trade-off – sensitivity and specificity

The following figure illustrates the changes in sensitivity and specificity depending on the cut-off point. In this example the diagnostic test is blood glucose and the outcome diabetes.

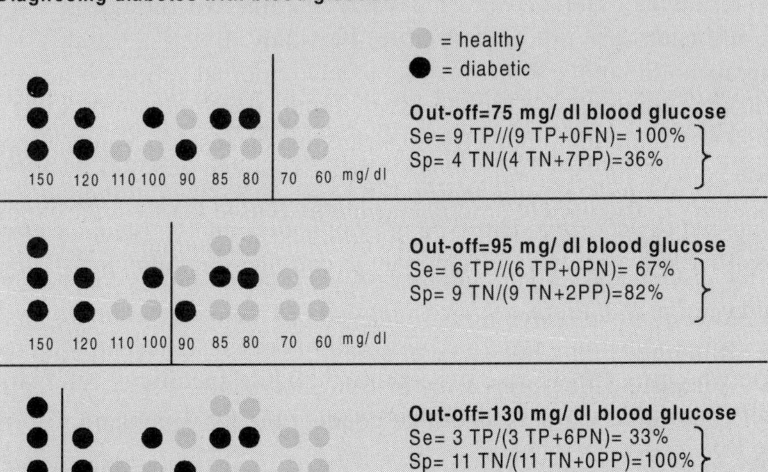

A test can also be evaluated by considering its predictive value; this is described as the proportion of individuals classified by the test as diseased that actually have the disease (positive predictive value), or the proportion of individuals classified by the test as not having the disease that are truly disease free (negative predictive value). These two values depend also on the prevalence of the disease: when prevalence is high it is more probable to correctly identify subjects as diseased [1, 3, 13, 18].

Precision is defined as the degree to which repeated measures of the same variable yield the same value. This is also known as reproducibility or reliability. For a study to achieve internal validity it is necessary to consider the assessment of precision during the study design. Typically, replicate observations are recommended. A way to determine the reproducibility of the measures is by using the coefficient of variation (CV = standard deviation*100%/mean). Precision is a function of two elements: the random measurement error and the actual change in the measurement induced by time. Both factors should be considered by the study design. Some strategies have been proposed to increase the precision of measurements related to nutrition:

- Compiling an operations manual with clear guidelines for taking each measurement.
- Training all the examiners to use the standardized techniques consistently. The measurements should be consistent between different examiners.
- Selecting and standardizing all the instruments used by data collection.
- Testing, refining and validating questionnaires.
- Reducing the effect of random errors by repeating all the measurements (when possible) [24, 25].

Accuracy is used to describe the extent to which the measurement is close to the true value. An accurate measurement needs to be precise, but a precise measurement is not necessarily accurate; it might be that the procedure always yields the same result (precise) but the result might not be the correct (inaccurate). This type of error is defined as systematic error or bias. To achieve accuracy is important to consider the following strategies:

- Making unobtrusive measurements,
- Blinding,
- Adequate calibration of the instruments, and
- Training of the personnel that conduct the measurements.

Because an accurate result requires precision the recommendations described earlier also apply to this section.

Sources of measurement error – Error in nutritional epidemiology is classified as "random" or "systematic". Random error is the one that generates a deviation from the correct result only by chance and can result from (a) individual biological variation, (b) an inadequate sampling procedure or (c) a non systematic measurement error. Random error is very common in diet assessment; the high individual variations during time may lead to inaccurate conclusions, by showing associations with outcomes that are only product of chance. Random error can be minimized by increasing precision and accuracy; nevertheless, it can never be completely eliminated [1, 3, 13, 18].

As mentioned before, bias is defined as a systematic error. The most common biases are selection and information bias. Selection bias happens when the subjects included in the study are systematically different than those that were not included; this makes it impossible to generalize the results to the entire population. An example is when people that have an inadequate dietary intake consistently refuse to participate in the study; in that case, the results can only be applied to the sector of the population that has adequate dietary intakes. Information or misclassification bias can be introduced on a variety of ways: not calibrated instruments, inaccurate tests, observer bias, untrained personnel, etc. An example is a 24 hours recall that consistently underestimates fat intake [18].

Confounding is a type of bias that masks the true relationship between an exposure and an outcome. A confounder is a variable that is distributed differently in the exposed and unexposed groups, and that affects the outcome being assessed. For example, in a study looking at the relationship between alcohol consumption and colon cancer, the association might be confounded by smoking: smoking increases the risk of colon cancer and people than drink are more likely to smoke. In this case alcohol consumption might appear to cause colon cancer, but the actual factor increasing the risk among the exposed is smoking. For a variable to be a confounder it must be related to the outcome, related to the disease but not be an intermediate in the causation pathway. For example, HDL cholesterol is not a confounder in the relationship between physical activity and cardiovascular diseases: physical activity prevents cardiovascular diseases by increasing HDL cholesterol. Typical confounders are age, gender and race/ethnicity. It is important to consider all possible confounders since the design stage to be able to account for them during the analysis and interpretation of the results. A statistical term that also influences the relationships between exposure and outcome is the interaction or effect modification. Interaction happens when the outcome in the presence of two or more risk factors differs from the outcome expected from the individual effects. There are many methods to control for confounding or address effect modification during the analysis; nevertheless none of these methods can be used if confounding and interaction are not considered in the stage of design of the study [1, 3, 13, 18].

2.3.4 Interpretation of findings

The presentation of findings from epidemiological studies varies widely; it typically includes measures of variability and statistical significance of the associations. For example, inclusion of 95% confidence intervals for estimates is highly recommended rather than just 'p' values. The measures of variability can be calculated for either measures of central tendency such as group means, or for measures of association such as an odds ratio or relative risk as shown in Box 2.7.

Box 2.7 Important definitions: measures of association

Risk- it is defined as the incidence of disease in a population and is primarily used in cohort studies, where it is possible to estimate the incidence in the total population. For example if 10 patients experience a heart-attack in a cohort of 100 patients, the risk is 10/100=0.1.

Relative risk (RR) – this measure of association is defined as the risk in the exposed divided by the risk in the unexposed. For example if the incidence of heart attacks in the exposed group was 20/50=0.4 and the incidence in the unexposed group was 10/50 = 0.2 resulting in a RR = 0.4/0.2 = 2. The exposed have twice the risk of the unexposed of suffering a heart attack.

Odds – it is the probability of an event happening divided by the probability of the event not happening. For example, the probability of having a heart attack of 50-year-old man is 0.1. Then the odds of having a heart attack are 0.1/(1 - 0.9)=0.11.

Odds ratio (OR) – this measure of association is primarily used in case control studies, where the risk cannot be determined. It is obtained by dividing the odds of being exposed of the cases by the odds of being exposed of the controls. For example, the odds of being a high fat consumer (or being exposed) for persons that suffered a heart attack (cases) is 0.33; while the odds of being a high fat consumer in persons that did not suffer a heart attack is 0.11, then the OR=0.33/0.11= 3. When the sample is big, the OR approximates the relative risk.

Since there is considerable variability in how studies are conducted both in terms of the study design and study population, tools such as meta-analyses that combine the results of several studies have become popular. They are particularly useful to guide policy and reduce problems associated with inadequate power due to limited sample size and contradictory findings. Typically meta-analyses have been done primarily using data from well designed RCTs. Estimates from each study are included and weighted to generate weighted mean difference or risk ratio. The Cochrane Group is known for conducting this kind of analysis and provides stringent criteria for the inclusion of well designed intervention trials in the calculation of the weighted estimates. Several methodological issues including the role of publication bias need to be considered while interpreting results from systematic review and meta-analysis [26]. There are several examples of meta-analyses in public health nutrition that have important policy implications. Of note is the meta-analysis that evaluated several large community-based trials of vitamin A supplementation on child mortality and found a protective effect [27]. In contrast, a recent meta-analysis evaluated the impact of micronutrient interventions on child growth and found that only multiple micronutrient interventions were beneficial but the effect size was small indicating the need for other strategies [28].

2.4 Importance of nutrition epidemiology in developing countries

Nutritional epidemiology in developing countries faces greater and more demanding challenges. The health status of developing countries has historically been characterized by predominant infectious diseases. In this context, undernutrition and micronutrient deficiencies are the main focus of nutritional epidemiology, since they aggravate the severity and duration of infectious diseases. Malnutrition also slows economic growth and perpetuates poverty; recent work has shown the direct and indirect effects on productivity that are mediated via poor physical status and/or poor cognitive function as well as increased health care costs [29]. More recently, however, chronic diseases that were considered characteristic of industrialized countries [30] have dramatically increased in the less developed countries (LDC). Cardiovascular disease (CVD) is the leading cause of death worldwide and LDC account for ~80% of all these deaths [31]. The traditional approach to understanding nutrition related problems is therefore no longer adequate in the developing world that is facing the dual burden of undernutrition and overnutrition. "Transitional societies" who were previously low-income societies now face significant improvements in income that affect disease and dietary patterns [32–34]. Epidemiologic transition is defined as the shift in morbidity and mortality causes, from mainly communicable infectious diseases to non communicable chronic diseases. This transition is intimately related to the nutrition transition, defined as the rapid changes in dietary patterns, characterized by an increase in fat intake and a decrease in the consumption of traditional foods; that changes modify the epidemiology of overweight and undernutrition. In low income countries these changes are occurring in an accelerated and polarized way. Communities with both under and overweight individuals are common in many developing countries like India, Brazil, China and the Russian Federation. This phenomenon may be explained by dramatic changes in dietary patterns and physical activity. Rapid shifts in income, educational levels, urbanization, globalization, and major sources of energy are some of the explanations for the rapid changes in dietary patterns. Technological resources, less activity at work and at school, insecurity and unplanned urbanization decrease physical activity, contributing also to nutritional and epidemiologic transitions [35, 36]. Another important factor in the rapid onset of obesity and nutrition related chronic diseases are demographic changes. An increase in life expectancy and a decrease in birth rates have changed the age distribution of transitional societies. The proportion of the population over 60 years of age is growing in these countries. This sector of the population is at a higher risk to suffer chronic diseases and impose a higher burden to the health system [30].

Nutritional epidemiology thus plays a key role in addressing the challenges faced by developing countries. Three main challenges have been identified: addressing the pending burden of undernutrition and micronutrient deficiencies; prevention of diet related chronic diseases with a life-course perspective; and achieving nutrition for optimal health and well-being across the lifespan or healthy aging. Nutrition status of the population is determined by complex interactions of socioeconomic and environmental factors, along with genetic determinants. It is impossible to address the current challenges without knowledge and understanding of nutrition and epidemiologic determinants. Nutritional epidemiology provides scientific tools to better understand these determinants and implement cost-effective approaches; evidence based interventions and policies that will be more effective in improving nutritional status of the population [29] which calls for the timely and appropriate application of nutritional epidemiology in developing countries that are undergoing nutritional and epidemiologic transitions.

2.5 Nutrition epidemiology and public health nutrition

Nutritional epidemiology is the basis for public health nutrition. Studies conducted at a population level relating diet and nutrition with health outcomes provide scientific information to develop interventions and policies which in turn can improve the nutritional and health status of the population. In light of the nutritional and epidemiologic panorama and the limited resources available to address these situations, nutritional epidemiology is an important tool in designing, evaluating and renewing interventions and policies. The information obtained by this discipline can be use to improve the design and implementation of programs. For developing countries the application of nutritional epidemiology in the form of public health nutrition is especially relevant considering all the challenges that were previously described. For these countries it is important to find cost effective interventions; that is, interventions that provide greater benefits than the economic, human and material resources invested in their implementation. The high cost benefit of several nutrition interventions (like promoting breastfeeding) has been estimated using well designed epidemiological studies [29].

Currently, programs that can prevent or reduce malnutrition are not being effectively implemented or scaled up in most regions of the world; particularly in developing countries where service delivery mechanism is inadequate and utilization of identified solution is low. The development and implementation of health and nutrition programs depends on policy makers, program planners and implementers, markets and civil society, along with the behaviours of households and individuals. Research focused on delivery, utilization and evaluation of nutrition programs and services helps to build evidence base information to guide decisions and select the best options for delivering interventions [13, 29, 37].

The crucial element in the development of effective interventions is the translation from scientific research, discussion and assessment, to government, industry and civil society. It has been proposed that the main challenges for public health nutrition are to agree on a suitable evidence based approach, develop a conceptual framework (Box 2.8) for decision making, and act professionally. Decisions in public health nutrition should be rational and evidence based. Nevertheless, this raises the concern of the quality and quantity of the information available for decision-makers. The scientific arena is filled with contradictions, and judgments are usually cautious with lack of adequate convincing information to policy makers. Also, it is hard to define the amount of information needed to undertake an action. A way around these limitations is designing research that can be applied to develop nutrition interventions [38–40].

Box 2.8 Definition of conceptual framework

A conceptual or logical framework is used in research to define a problem, outline an approach to an idea, or to define a course of action. All the components of the research, the approach to the problem or hypothesis and the potential course should be represented in the conceptual framework. It can be used as a planning and guiding tool throughout all the research process: before research, during research and after research. A well designed framework is important for nutritional epidemiology to analyze the results from epidemiological trials; and for public health nutrition in the translation of these results into programs and interventions.

The WHO in its "Progress newsletter", 2005 states that "in using a conceptual framework it is advisable to see it not as a prescriptive model but rather as a framework for stimulating thinking about the potential options and opportunities for enhancing the chances for research utilization". It also proposes six guiding principles to develop a framework with practical applications:

1. The different models presented in the literature share common underlying concepts and elements. It is possible to take that elements and use their essence for practical application.
2. Models created for research utilization are often complex and thus hard to use for research application. A practical model simplifies the pathways to facilitate implementation.
3. It is possible to identify common factors that facilitate or impede research utilization.
4. It is useful to classify the different factors and elements influencing research in three phases: pre-research, during research and after research. Although, it is important to consider that in the practicum they represent a continuous.
5. A conceptual framework can be utilized to assess research utilization along different application of research results for example "initiation of further research; advocacy or a new program, policy or practice".
6. A conceptual framework should be able to capture broader contextual factors that can influence research and research implementation and "should refrain from imposing a false sense of order on what is often a chaotic and seemingly non-rational process" [41].

An example of a well designed conceptual framework in nutrition is the UNICEF malnutrition framework presented on Figure 2.1.

There are many examples of the application of nutritional epidemiology to public health. The most well known is the development of nutritional guidelines. The constant improvement and reassessment of nutritional guidelines is based in epidemiologic studies that assess the relationship between diet and health. An extensive discussion on the influence of nutritional epidemiology on the development of dietary guidelines in the United States was published by Byers in 1999 [4]. Examples of the applications of nutritional epidemiology to public health also exist in developing countries. A compilation of science based nutrition and physical activity interventions can be found in the report of the Pan-American Health Organization (PAHO), "Nutrition and an Active Life: from Knowledge to Action" [41]. Some of the conclusions of this compendium are the following:

- There is sufficient evidence on the impact of malnutrition on the health of individuals and populations to confirm the need for effective, low-cost programs to reduce its prevalence.
- The successful experiences described on the book are flexible enough to adapt to a wide variety of circumstances. These models hold great potential for successful adoption in other parts of the world.
- To achieve the expected results, technical expertise and support of diverse disciplines are required.
- All the experiences required the collaboration of a broad segment of interests in the design and implementation of the interventions.
- One of the essential elements to success is the full empowerment of all the institutions involved and the civil society in terms of project objectives and their active participation.

- To demonstrate their achievements, programs should conduct impact evaluations [42].

In conclusion, a good understanding and appropriate application of the principles of nutritional epidemiology is crucial for developing countries to improve the health status and well-being of their populations. This chapter provides an overview of the main elements and uses of nutritional epidemiology in developing countries and shows how it can be used in many aspects of nutritional sciences: from improvements in nutritional assessment to the application of research to public health nutrition that are urgently needed.

References

1. GORDIS L (2008). *Epidemiology*, 4th edition, Saunders (ed), Philadelphia.
2. *Encyclopaedia Britannica*.
3. MARGETTS BM and NELSON M (1997). *Design Concepts in Nutritional Epidemiology*, 2nd edition, Oxford: Oxford University Press.
4. BYERS T (1999). The role of epidemiology in developing nutritional recommendations: past, present, and future. *Am J Clin Nutr* **69**, no. 6, pp. 1304S–1308S.
5. ZIEGLER EE and LJ FILER (1996). *Present Knowledge in Nutrition*, 7th edition, Washington: ILSI Press.
6. VENEMAN AM (2007). UNICEF report on state of the world children 2007: the double advantage of gender equality. *Assist Inferm Ric* **26**, no. 1, pp. 46–50.
7. ROTHMAN KJ, GREENLAND S, and LASH TL (2008). *Modern Epidemiology*, 3rd edition, Philadelphia: Lippincot Williams and Wilkins.
8. FAO, *Food Balance Sheets*. 2009.
9. RAMAKRISHNAN U, BARNHART H, SCHROEDER DG, STEIN AD, MARTORELL R (1999). EARLY CHILDHOOD NUTRITION, education and fertility milestones in GUATEMALA. *J NUTR* **129**, no. 12, pp. 2196–2202.
10. STEIN AD, MELGAR P, HODDINOTT J, MARTORELL R (2008). Cohort Profile: the Institute of Nutrition of Central America and Panama (INCAP) Nutrition Trial Cohort Study. *Int J Epidemiol* **37**, no. 4, pp. 716–720.
11. BARROS FC, VICTORA CG and VAUGHAN JP (1990). The Pelotas (Brazil) birth cohort study 1982-1987: strategies for following up 6,000 children in a developing country. *Paediatr Perinat Epidemiol* **4**, no. 2, pp. 205–220.
12. TAMAKOSHI A, YOSHIMURA T, INABA Y, ITO Y, WATANABE Y, FUKUDA K, ISO H; JACC Study Group (2005). Profile of the JACC study. *J Epidemiol* **15**, no. 1, pp. S4–8.
13. LANGSETH L (1996). *Nutritional Epidemiology: Possibilities and Limitations*, Belgium: ILSI Europe.
14. HOPEWEL S, CLARKE M, MOHER D, WAGER E, MIDDLETON P, ALTMAN DG, SCHULZ KF, The CG (2008). [CONSORT for reporting randomized controlled trials in journal and conference abstracts: explanation and elaboration]. *Zhong Xi Yi Jie He Xue Bao* **6**, no. 3, pp. 221–232.
15. KNOBLOCH K, GOHRITZ A and VOGT PM (2008). CONSORT and QUOROM statements revisited: standards of reporting of randomized controlled trials in general surgery. *Ann Surg* **248**, no. 6, pp. 1106–1107; discussion 1107–1108.

16. MOHER D, SCHULZ KF and ALTMAN DG (2001). The CONSORT statement: revised recommendations for improving the quality of reports of parallel group randomized trials. *BMC Med Res Methodol* **1**, p. 2.
17. SOLOMONS NW and VALDES-RAMOS R (2002). Dietary assessment tools for developing countries for use in multi-centric, collaborative protocols. *Public Health Nutr* **5**, no. 6A, p. 955–968.
18. GIBSON R (2005). *Principles of Nutritional Assessment*, 2nd edition, Oxford: Oxford University Press.
19. KARVETTI RL and KNUTS LR (1992). Validity of the estimated food diary: comparison of 2-day recorded and observed food and nutrient intakes. *J Am Diet Assoc* **92**, no. 5, pp. 580–584.
20. WILLETT WC and HU FB (2007). The food frequency questionnaire. *Cancer Epidemiol Biomarkers Prev* **16**, no. 1, pp. 182–183.
21. DELCOURT C, CUBEAU J, BALKAU B, PAPOZ L (1994). Limitations of the correlation coefficient in the validation of diet assessment methods. CODIAB-INSERM-ZENECA Pharma Study Group. *Epidemiology* **5**, no. 5, pp. 518–524.
22. HABICHT JP (2000). Comparing the quality of indicators of nutritional status by receiver operating characteristic analysis or by standardized differences. *Am J Clin Nutr* **71**, no. 3, pp. 672–673.
23. HABICHT JP and STOLTZFUS RJ (1997). What do indicators indicate? *Am J Clin Nutr* **66**, no. 1, pp. 190–191.
24. CUMMINGS GS and CROWELL RD (1998). Source of error in clinical assessment of innominate rotation. A special communication. *Phys Ther* 68, no. 1, p. 77–78.
25. CUMMINGS KM, KIRSCHT JP, BECKER MH and LEVIN NW (1984). Construct validity comparisons of three methods for measuring patient compliance. *Health Serv Res* **19**, no. 1, pp. 103–116.
26. STERNE JAC and EGGER M (2005). Regression methods to detect publication and other bias in meta-analysis. In: ROTHSTEIN HR, SUTTON AJ, BORENSTEIN M (eds.) *Publication Bias in Meta-Analysis: Prevention, Assessment and Adjustment.* New York: John Wiley & Sons, pp. 99–110.
27. FAWZI WW, CHALMERS TC, HERRERA MG, MOSTELLER F (1993). vitamin a supplementation and child mortality. A meta-analysis. *JAMA* **269**, no. 7, pp. 898–903.
28. RAMAKRISHNAN U, NGUYEN P and MARTORELL R (2009). Effects of micronutrients on growth of children under 5 years of age: meta-analyses of single and multiple micronutrient interventions. *Am J Clin Nutr* **89**, pp. 191–203.
29. *Repositioning nutrition as central to development. A strategy for large-scale action* (2006). The World Bank.
30. UAUY R and KAIN J (2002). The epidemiological transition: need to incorporate obesity prevention into nutrition programmes. *Public Health Nutr* **5**, no. 1A, pp. 223–229.
31. REDDY KS and YUSUF S (1998). Emerging epidemic of cardiovascular disease in developing countries. *Circulation* **97**, pp. 596–601.
32. POPKIN BM and DU S (2003). Dynamics of the nutrition transition toward the animal foods sector in China and its implications: a worried perspective. *J Nutr* **133**, Suppl. 2, pp. 3898S–3906S.
33. POPKIN BM and GORDON-LARSEN P (2004). The nutrition transition: worldwide obesity dynamics and their determinants. *Int J Obes Relat Metab Disord* **28**, Suppl 3, pp. S2–S9.

34. POPKIN BM, LU B and ZHAI F (2002). Understanding the nutrition transition: measuring rapid dietary changes in transitional countries. *Public Health Nutr* **5**, no. 6A, pp. 947–953.
35. POPKIN BM (2003). Dynamics of the nutrition transition and its implications for the developing world. *Forum Nutr* **56**, pp. 262–264.
36. POPKIN BM (2004). The nutrition transition: an overview of world patterns of change. *Nutr Rev* **62**, no. 7 Pt 2, pp. S140–S143.
37. LABARTHE MC (2008). [1/10. Nutrition, a public health priority]. *Soins* **722**, pp. 59–60.
38. Unknown. Nutrition and health transition in the developing world: the time to act. *Public Health Nutr* **5,** no. 1A, pp. 279–280.
39. MADANAT HN, TROUTMAN KP and AL-MADI B (2008). The nutrition transition in Jordan: the political, economic and food consumption contexts. *Promot Educ* **15**, no. 1, pp. 6–10.
40. VERHEIJDEN MW and KOK FJ (2005). Public health impact of community-based nutrition and lifestyle interventions. *Eur J Clin Nutr* **59**, Suppl 1, pp. S66–S75; discussion S76.
41. WHO (2005). The challenge of putting research to use. Progress in Reproductive Health Research, p. 70.
42. FREIRE W (2005). *Nutrition and Active Life: From Knowledge to Action,* Paho (ed), Washington DC.

3 Undernutrition in children

Sheila C. Vir

Sheila C Vir, MSc, PhD, is a senior nutrition consultant and Director of Public Health Nutrition and Development Centre, New Delhi. Following MSc (Food and Nutrition) from University of Delhi, Dr Vir was awarded PhD by the Queen's University of Belfast, United Kingdom. Dr. Vir, a past secretary of the Nutrition Society of India, is a recipient of the fellowship of the Department of Health and Social Services, UK, and Commonwealth Van den Bergh Nutrition Award. Dr Vir worked briefly with the Aga Khan Foundation (India) and later with UNICEF. As a Nutrition Programme Officer with UNICEF for twenty years, Dr. Vir provided strategic and technical leadership for policy formulation and implementation of nutrition programmes in India.

3.1 Undernutrition, child survival and millennium development goals

The term 'undernutrition' comprises both protein energy malnutrition (PEM) and micronutrient malnutrition (MNM). "Undernutrition includes being underweight for one's age, too short for one's age (stunting), dangerously thin for one's height (wasting) and deficient in vitamins and minerals (micronutrient deficiencies)" [1]. Malnutrition is commonly used as an alternative to undernutrition but technically it is a broad term which also refers to overnutrition [1].

Undernutrition, as presented in Fig. 3.1, contributes to more than one-third of child deaths and more than 10% of the global disease burden [1, 2, 3]. This implies that one in three children who die from pneumonia, diarrhea and other illness would survive if these children were not undernourished. Children with severe acute malnutrition are at the highest risk of dying – over nine times more likely to die than children who are not undernourished [3]. On the other hand, moderate and mildly undernourished children are at lower risk of dying but are large in numbers in developing countries [1]. Undernourished children who survive may suffer irreversible damage to their development.

Undernutrition, an important determinant of maternal and child health, has significant adverse effect on survival and growth as well as cognitive and physical development [3]. Overcoming undernutrition is critical with

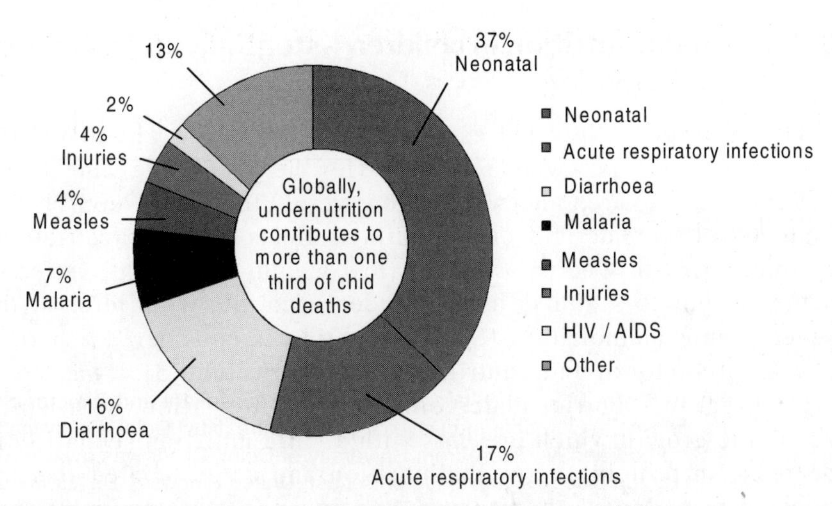

3.1 Undernutrition and mortality in children under-5 years old [1].

reference to not only the first Millennium Development Goal (MDG) to eradicate extreme poverty and hunger [4] – the specific target of the first Millennium Development Goal is to reduce the prevalence of underweight by 50 per cent among children younger than 5 years between 1990 and 2015 – but influences the achievement of the other MDG goals pertaining to child survival, maternal health, education, gender equity (Table 3.1) [5]. Undernutrition slows down national progress. "One underweight or one undernourished child is an individual tragedy. But multiplied by tens and millions, undernutrition becomes a global threat to societies, to economies and to generations to come" [6].

Table 3.1 Millennium Development Goals (MDG) and Nutrition Effect [5]

	MDG Goal	Nutrition Effect (if Goal not achieved)
Goal 1	Eradicate extreme poverty and hunger	decreased human capital, adverse impact on cognitive and physical development
Goal 2	Achieve universal primary education	reduced school attendance, retention and performance
Goal 3	Promote gender equality and empower women	reduced access to food, health and care resources – female biases
Goal 4	Reduce child mortality	increased burden of disease and death
Goal 5	Improves maternal health	compromised maternal health – maternal stunting and iron and iodine deficiencies
Goal 6	Combat HIV/AIDS, malaria and other diseases	increased risk of HIV transmission, compromise antiretroviral therapy, and hasten the onset of full blown AIDS and premature deaths

This chapter focuses on undernutrition with special reference to stunting, underweight and wasting. Details on micronutrient deficiencies in children are covered in other chapters of this book.

3.2 Undernutrition in children – stunting, underweight and wasting

UNICEF Report 2009 [1] estimates that there are globally 195 million under 5 years who are stunted (low height for age) and about 129 million who are underweight (low weight for age). Weight is an indicator of acute deficiencies. Stunting reflects a chronic restriction of linear growth whereas wasting (low weight for height) reflects acute weight loss and is used for identification of children with severe acute malnutrition (SAM). Stunting is considered a better overall predictor of undernutrition than underweight [3]. It has been argued that in countries undergoing nutrition transition, with rapid economic growth which presents with a child nutrition scenario of decrease in protein energy malnutrition and an associated rise in obesity prevalence, monitoring stunting and wasting in young children is more appropriate than monitoring underweight, a composite measure of both stunting and wasting [7]. Stunting is considered an appropriate measure since in a developing country situation, the environment is often not conducive for children who are stunted early in life to gain optimum height. On the other hand, underweight can be overcome with appropriate nutrition and health improvements. An underweight child at the age of 4–5 years may present with normal weight for age despite slow growth and development that may have occurred due to deficiencies during pregnancy or infancy [1]. A child who is underweight can also be stunted or wasted or both. It has been observed that severe wasting is not accompanied by stunting in 80–100% of younger children and 40–50% of older children [2]. Moreover, countries with similar stunting rates can have vast difference in prevalence rates of severe wasting [8].

3.3 Undernutrition and age trend

Earlier analysis of growth faltering in children, using the National Centre for Health Statistics (NCHS) reference with primary focus only on assessment of weight for age, had indicated that faltering starts at about three months of life in developing country settings [9–12]. Pattern of growth faltering with age was studied in 2001 by Shrimpton et al [13] by analyzing data of 39 national surveys. It was observed that at birth the average weight for age, length for age and weight for length were quite close to NCHS reference (Figure 3.2). However, these three growth indices presented a different growth pattern in the first three months of life. As indicated in Fig. 3.2, mean weight for age (underweight) was noted to start faltering at about three months of age and there was continuous and rapid decline until about 12 months. The

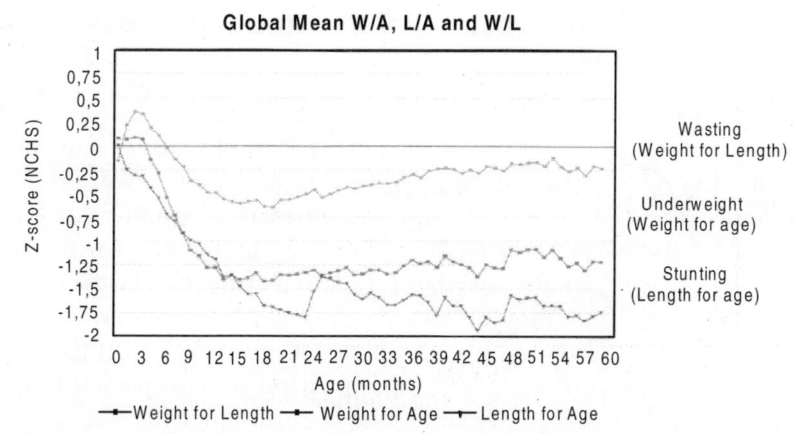

3.2 Mean anthropometric z scores by age for all 39 studies (children 0–59 months), relative to the NCHS reference [13].

decline was observed to continue but was slower until about 18–19 months of age. On the other hand, the process of stunting began at birth and continued during the first 3 years of life. After the first three months, fall in stunting and underweight was noted to be very similar upto 12 months. Stunting continued to decrease upto 40 months of age. Stunting that occurred in the first 3 years was reported to be irreversible. On the other hand, weight for length (wasting) decrease was concentrated in the period 3–15 months followed by rapid improvement.

The age-wise prevalence of undernutrition in developing countries at the national or regional level, using NCHS reference, has traditionally been reported for six monthly or 12 monthly intervals and not month-wise. In India, the analysis of national data of child undernutrition revealed that undernutrition (weight for age) prevalence in children was highest in the age group 12–24 months as compared to 6–12 months or > 24–36 months, >36–48 months or >48–60 months. Based on this interpretation, a shift in the national programme focus to children under 2 years instead of those under 5 years has been recommended.

In 2001, an analysis of month-wise data (Figure 3.3) of underweight children between 3 and 24 months was reported from Uttar Pradesh, India [14]. The analysis, using NCHS standards, z scores classification (median, –2 SD, –3 SD), revealed that the highest proportion of underweight children were in the age group of 8–11 months [14]. This problematic age of late infancy was observed to coincide with a significant increase in nutritional requirement of infants during this period which are often not met due to poor complementary feeding practices, limited capacity for mastication and stomach volume as well as increased activity, exposure to environment and susceptibility to diarrhea. It was emphasized that actions for preventing undernutrition in children should concentrate efforts primarily on under ones [15].

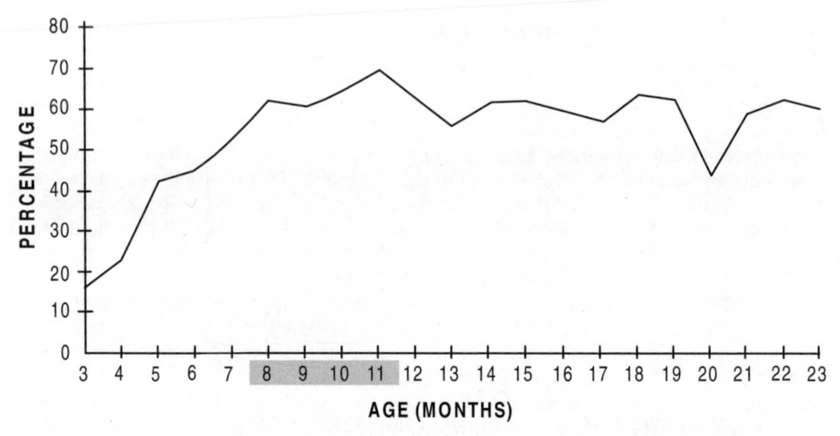

3.3 Month-wise undernutrition prevalence in children 3–23 months [14].

Using the revised WHO Child Growth Standards, it is now evident that undernutrition in the first six months of life itself is a serious problem [16]. It was emphasized in 2008 that such a growth trend in the first half of pregnancy was not apparent earlier with the limitation of using the National Centre for Health Statistics (NCHS) reference which incorrectly made it appear that growth was protected during the first months of life [16]. This is possibly due to the fact that NCHS reference used measured length at birth and 3 months, while a curve fitting method was used for intermediate ages [17, 18]. The WHO standard (Box 3.1), on the other hand, provides a better description of physiological, growth since the standard is based on empirical data at birth, weeks 2, 4 and 6 and monthly thereafter in the first year [17, 18].

Using the WHO standards, it is now observed (Figure 3.5) that stunting prevalence increases progressively and reaches a plateau at around 24 months of age while the prevalence of severe wasting is higher at younger age and then declines and reaches a plateau at 24 months [8]. The worldwide growth faltering pattern study, based on analysis of data of 54 countries using WHO standards show "that growth faltering in early childhood is even more pronounced than suggested by previous analysis based on the National centre for Health Statistics reference" [17].

Analysis of India's third National Health and Family Survey (NFHS3) data on month-wise prevalence of undernutrition in Indian children below 5 years, using WHO standards, for the period 2005–2006 presents a similar trend as noted in the global analysis [21] – Fig. 3.4. The NFHS 3 data was also analysed to study the month-wise trend of severely wasted, severely stunted and severely underweight children [22]. The findings are presented in Figs. 3.4 and 3.5. As indicated in Fig. 3.4, the proportion of children with stunting and underweight continued to increase and was highest by 24 months of age while the trend in

Box 3.1 WHO growth standards

National Centre for Health Statistics (NCHS) reference, also known as NCHS/WHO International Growth Reference, was recommended three decades ago by WHO [19]. The NCHS reference was based on data on longitudinal study of children of European ancestry from a single community in the United States which was collected between 1929 and 1975 [20]. These children were measured every three months. Majority of these infants were fed artificial milk. The limitation of NCHS was that the measurement was not adequate to describe the rapid and changing rate of growth in early infancy. Additionally, there were shortcomings inherent in the statistical methods available and used.

In 1990, following an in-depth analysis of growth data from breastfed infants, a review group recommended that a new growth standard be constructed. The emphasis was on standard rather than a reference to be constructed. A reference is simply applied for comparison whereas a standard serves for both comparison as well as a basis for assessing the adequacy of growth. The standard could therefore be used as a tool for value judgement. Between July 1997 and December 2003, a WHO Multicentric Growth Reference Study (MGRS) was thus conducted [20]. The study involved exclusive breastfed children in six sites of different regions of the world – Brazil, Ghana, India, Norway, Oman and the USA. In Ghana, India and Oman, children from effluent economic groups whose growth was not environmentally constrained were selected. Term low birth weight (<2500 grams) were not excluded. The MGRS comprised information from a longitudinal follow-up from birth to 24 months with a cross-sectoral component of children 18–71 months. The study showed that children everywhere grow in similar pattern when their nutrition, health and care needs are met.

In 2006, new World Health Organisation standards (WHO standard) were introduced on the basis of the MGRS. The new WHO growth standard identifies breastfed child as the normative model for growth and development standards, depicts normal early childhood growth under optimal environmental conditions, and can be used to assess children regardless of ethnicity, socioeconomic status and type of feeding. The WHO standard describes how children should grow when not only free of disease but also when reared following healthy practices such as breastfeeding and non-smoking environment.

Differences of WHO standard compared to previously recommended NCHS/WHO international reference are particularly important in infancy. According to WHO Multicentric Growth Reference Study Group [20], the following differences are considered noteworthy – stunting will be greater throughout childhood, substantial increase in underweight rates during 0–6 months and a decrease thereafter, wasting rates will be substantially higher during infancy (i.e. up to 70 cm length).

severe wasting showed a decreasing trend in the first 12 months. Severe undernutrition prevalence, as measured by all the three indicators, is about 10 percent in the first six months of life [22]. Severe wasting shows a decreasing trend upto 16 months of age while in the first 22–24 months, severe stunting and severe underweight show an increasing trend. The analysis clearly reveals that undernutrition sets in the first two months of life itself. The findings reveal that undernutrition during the first six months of life is a much greater problem and needs attention.

It is evident from these analysis using WHO standards that low birth rate (LBW) (Box 3.2) and its association with neonatal deaths (Fig. 3.6) and undernutrition in the first six months of life cannot be ignored. For preventing growth failure in children, prenatal and early life interventions are critical.

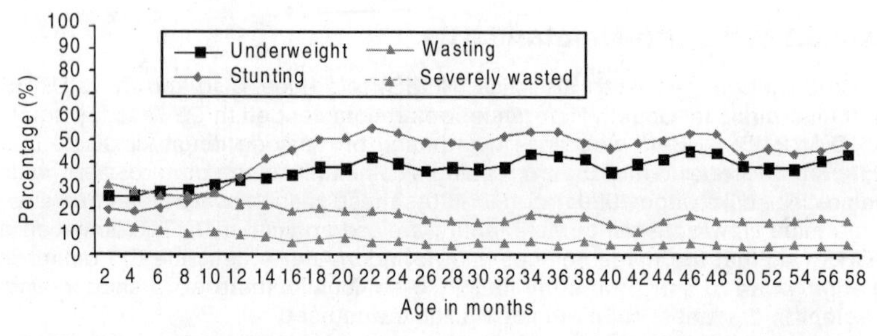

3.4 Prevalence of underweight by age in children below 5 years [21, 22].

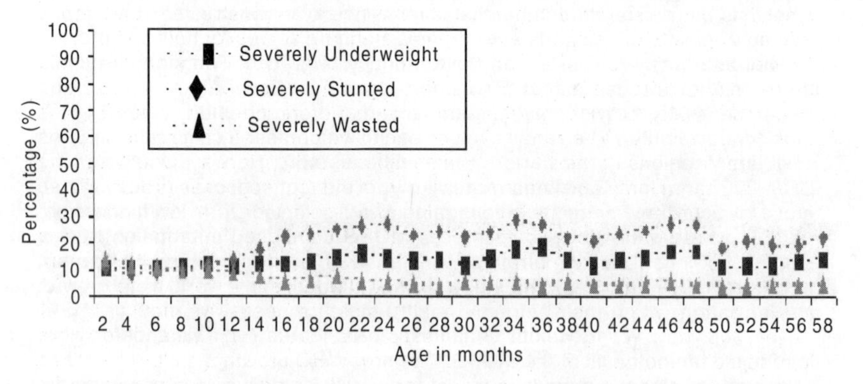

3.5 Month-wise prevalence of severe undernutrition in children in India [22].

A total of 19 million newborns per year are born LBW. India accounts for 7.8 millions LBW babies born per year in developing world (Figure 3.7). India and Pakistan together contribute to almost half of the world's LBW each year. India contributes to 39% while Pakistan contributes to 9%. The estimations on LBW incidence rate reported have limitations since almost 60% of newborns in developing countries are not weighed at birth [1].

3.4 Stunting, underweight and wasting – an overview of the global situation

UNICEF report 2009 on undernutrition [1] indicates that of the 195 million stunted children under 5 years of age in developing world, 90% live in Asia and Africa. Eighty percent of the world's stunted children live in 24 countries. Five countries together (four of these 5 countries being from Asia) contribute to almost 50% of the global under 5 years stunted children – India (31.2%), China (6.5%), Nigeria (5.2%), Pakistan (5.1%) and Indonesia (3.9%) – Table 3.3.

Box 3.2 Low birth weight (LBW)

Low birth weight has been defined by the World Health Organisation [23] as weight at birth, irrespective of gestation age, of less than 2500 g (upto and including 2499 g). Birth weight is governed by two major processes: duration of gestation and intrauterine growth rate. LBW is either the result of preterm birth (before 37 weeks of gestation) or due to restricted foetal (intrauterine) growth or intrauterine growth restriction (IUGR). In developed countries, IUGR (birth weight <2500 g and gestation age ≥37weeks) is far less prevalent. Most LBW babies in developed world are premature rather than growth retarded. In contrast in developing countries, IUGR accounts for the majority of LBW [24]. Small for gestational age (SGA) is often used as a proxy for IUGR. WHO defines SGA as birth weight below the tenth percentile for gestational age based on sex-specific reference. Some SGA infants may be constitutionally small and not truly growth restricted.

The determinants of IUGR are low energy intake, poor weight gain during pregnancy, low pre-pregnancy BMI, short stature, malaria, cigarette smoking, pregnancy induced hypertension, ethnic origin and other genetic factors.

LBW contributes to a range of poor health outcomes. Infants born at term weighing 1500–1999 grams are 8.1 times more likely to die and those weighing 2000–2099 who are 2.8 times more likely to die from all causes during the neonatal period than are those weighing 2499 g at birth [3]. LBW, which is related to maternal malnutrition, is a causal factor in 60–80% neonatal deaths (Figure 3.6) [25]. LBW who survive have a higher chance of facing compromised health care and entering a vicious cycle of ill health and undernutrition.

The level of LBW in developing countries is 16.5% – almost the double in the developed regions with 7% LBW [26]. There is significant variation in LBW incidence across six main geographical regions [26]. LBW rate is estimated to be 18% in Asia, 14 % in Africa and 6.4% in Europe (Table 3.2).

Direct causes of neonatal deaths, 200*

Low birth weight, which is related to maternal malnutrition, is a causal factor in 60-80 per cent of neonatal deaths.

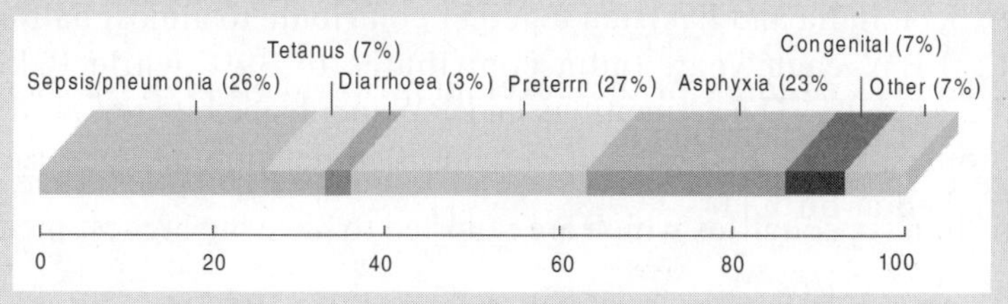

* Percentages may not total 100% because of rounding.

3.6 Direct causes of neonatal deaths [25].

The proportion of children who are moderately underweight or moderately stunted is higher in LBW babies. Figure 3.9 presents an association of LBW with nutritional status of children below 2 years.

In nine countries, every second child is reported to be stunted with prevalence rates higher than 50% – Afghanistan (59%), Yemen (58%), Guatemala and Timor-Leste (54%), Burundi, Madagascar, Malawi (53%) and Ethiopia and Rwanda (51%). India has a lower stunting prevalence rate of 48.1% but has the largest number of stunted children – 61 million Indian children are estimated to be stunted and contribute to almost a third

Table 3.2 Global and regional estimate of LBW [26]

	% Low birth weight infants	Number of low birth weight infants (1000s)
World	15.5	20, 629
More developed	7.0	916
Less developed	16.5	19, 713
Least developed countries	18.6	4, 968
Africa	14.3	4, 320
Asia	18.3	14, 195
Europe	6.4	460
Latin America and Caribbean	10.0	1, 171
North America	7.7	343
Oceania	10.5	27

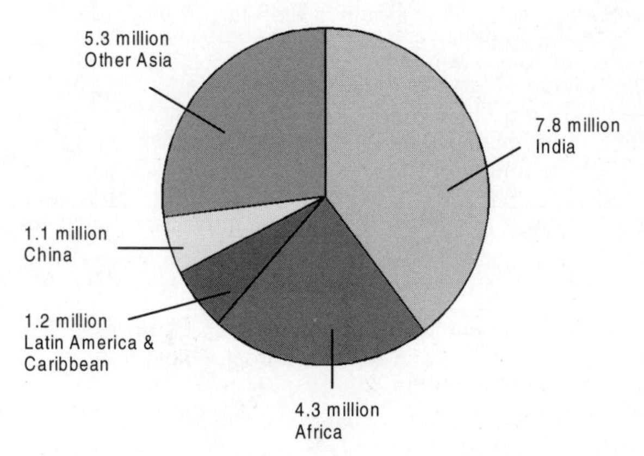

3.7 Low birth weight infants (millions) in developing countries [26].

of the stunted children in the developing world (Box 3.3 presents an overview of undernutrition in India).

Figure 3.8 presents the percentage of infants weighing less than 2,500 g at birth in six countries which are reported to have the highest incidence rate of LBW [1].

In developing countries, on the whole, stunting prevalence rate in under-5 children is estimated to be 34 percent. The stunting prevalence rate is 40 percent in Africa and 36 percent in Asia (Figure 3.10).

In developing world, underweight prevalence rate in children under 5 years is 21 percent. Unlike stunting, the underweight rate is higher in Asia than in Africa (Figure 3.10). Underweight prevalence rates of over 30% are reported from 17 countries which includes three countries from Asia – India, Nepal and Bangladesh [1]. The four following countries have underweight prevalence rates higher than 40% – Timor-Leste (49%), India and Yemen (43%) and Bangladesh (41%). In the global context, India contributes to 42 percent of the total estimated 129 million underweight children in developing

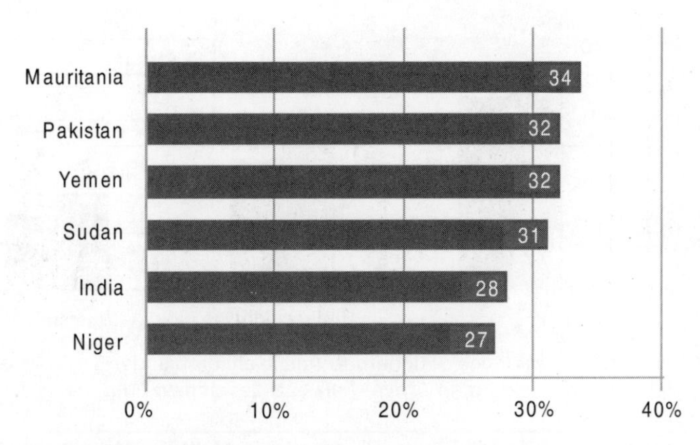

3.8 Percentage of infants weighing less than 2,500 g at birth in countries with highest rates [1].

Note: Estimates are based on data collected in 2003 and later with the exception of the Sudan (1999) and Yeman (1997).

Table 3.3 Details of five countries that together contribute to half of world's stunted under-5-year children [1]

Country	Rank	Stunting prevalence (%)	% of developing world total (195.1 million)	Number of children who are stunted (Thousands, 2008)
India	1	48	31.2	60, 788
China	2	15	6.5	12, 685
Nigeria	3	41	5.2	10, 158
Pakistan	4	42	5.1	9, 868
Indonesia	5	37	3.9	7, 688
Total			51.9	101187

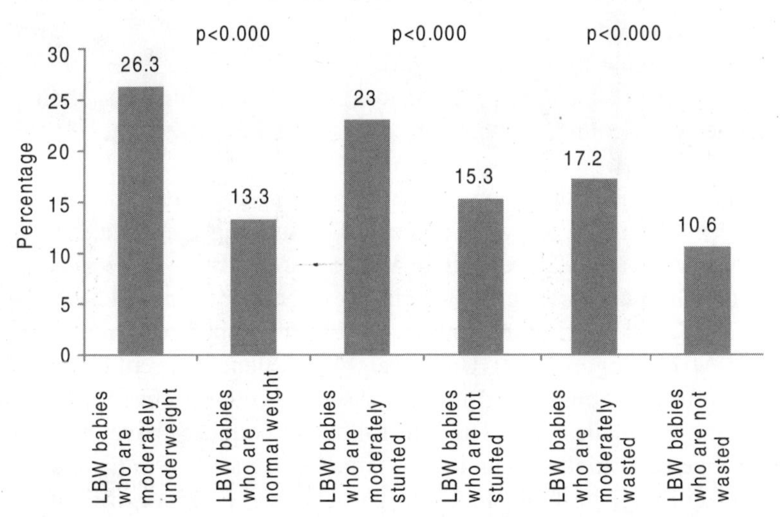

3.9 Association of Low Birth Weight (LBW) and nutritional status of children < 2 years [22].

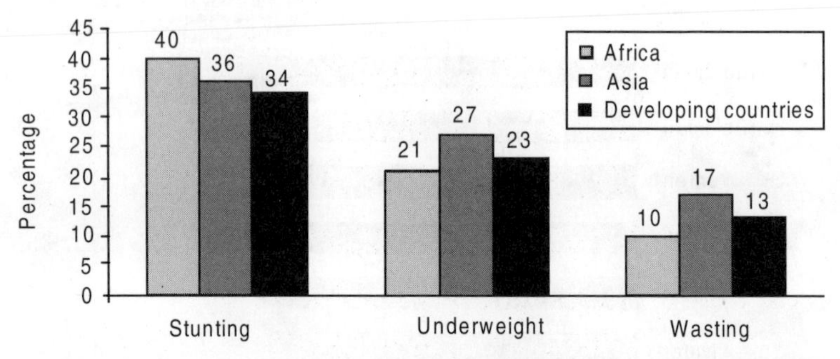

3.10 Percentage prevalence of undernutrition in children under-5 years, based on WHO Growth Standard, in Africa, Asia and developing countries [1].

world under fives while Pakistan, Bangladesh and Nigeria each contribute to 5 percent (combined 15 percent) and the remaining 43 percent underweight children are from other developing countries.

As presented in Figure 3.10, 13% of children under 5 years in developing world are wasted while the wasting prevalence rate is 17 percent in Asia and 10 percent in Africa [1]. Ten countries account for 60% of under 5 year children who suffer from wasting and eight of these countries have moderate wasting prevalence rates higher than 10 percent_while 2–7 percent children in these countries are severely wasted (Figure 3.11). These estimated 26 million severely wasted children from developing world are nine times at higher risk of dying compared to normal children [1].

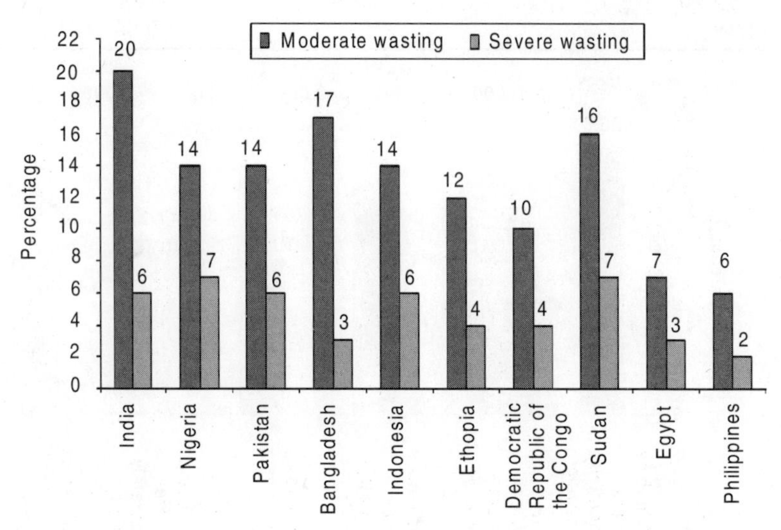

3.11 Ten countries which contribute to sixty percent of the global under 5 years of wasted children [1].

The greatest reduction in underweight prevalence in children under 5 years, between the period 1990 and 2008, has been reported in five countries – Bangladesh, Mauritania, Viet Nam, Indonesia and Malaysia. During this period, three countries (Bangladesh, Mauritania and Viet Nam) are reported to have not only the highest decline in underweight in under-5-year children but also over 20 percentage points decline in stunting prevalence rates (Figure 3.12). Unlike Bangladesh and Mauritania, the percentage prevalence rate of stunting in children in Vietnam continues to be higher than underweight prevalence rate. Box 3.5 at the end of the chapter presents the factors contributing to higher rate of decline in underweight or stunting noted in selected countries in the last two decades.

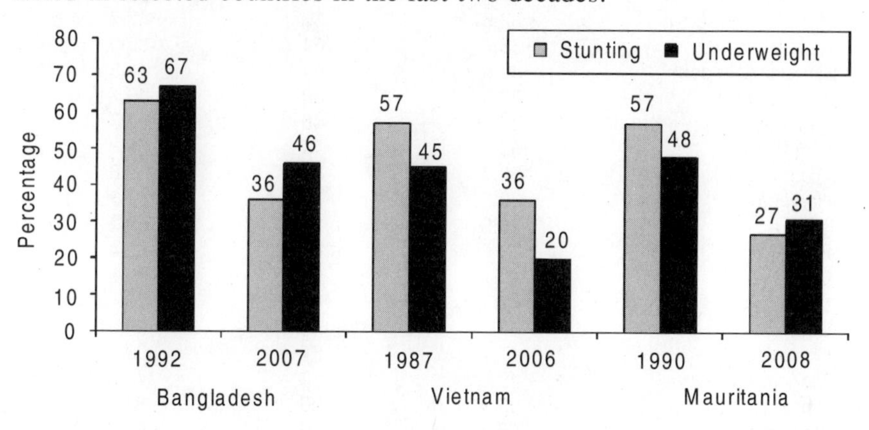

3.12 Stunting and underweight (percentage of children) under 5 years – declining trends in stunting and underweight [1].

3.5 Determinants of undernutrition

The cause of undernutrition is not limited to inadequate access to food. UNICEF conceptual framework of malnutrition in children and women (Figure 3.14) presents a number of varied factors which influence the maternal and child nutrition status [29]. Undernutrition is a result of multiple, complex, interactive causes which influences food, care and health of an individual and the nutritional status. Immediate causes of undernutrition in children are lack of proper infant and young child feeding resulting in low intake of nutrients and loss of nutrients due to frequent infections such as diarrhea, acute respiratory infections, measles, sepsis, etc.

Nutrition status of children resulting from immediate causes is aggravated by underlying factors operating at households and community levels such as household food insecurity, inadequate care of women and children combined with unhealthy environment with lack of ready access to safe drinking water and environmental sanitation. The underlying

Table 3.4 Undernutrition in India [21, 28]

States	Underweight (%)	IMR	U5MR
Sikkim	19.7	33	40.1
Mizoram	19.9	37	52.9
Manipur	22.1	14	41.9
Kerala	22.9	12	16.3
Punjab	24.9	41	52.0
Goa	25.0	10	20.3
Nagaland	25.2	26	64.7
Jammu & Kashmir	25.6	49	51.2
Delhi	26.1	35	46.7
Tamil Nadu	29.8	31	35.5
Andhra Pradesh	32.5	52	63.2
Arunachal Pradesh	32.5	32	87.7
Assam	36.4	64	85.0
Himachal Pradesh	36.5	44	41.5
Maharashtra	37.0	33	46.7
Karnataka	37.6	45	54.7
Uttaranchal	38.0	44	56.8
West Bengal	38.7	35	59.6
Haryana	39.6	54	52.3
Tripura	39.6	34	59.2
Rajasthan	39.9	63	85.4
Orissa	40.7	69	90.6
Uttar Pradesh	42.4	67	96.4
Gujarat	44.6	50	60.9
Chhattisgarh	47.1	57	90.3
Meghalaya	48.8	58	70.5
Bihar	55.9	56	84.8
Jharkhand	56.5	46	93.0
Madhya Pradesh	60.0	70	94.2
India	42.5	53	74.3

causes of undernutrition in children are linked to basic causes such as poverty and lack of education which are influenced by larger political, economic, social and cultural environment.

Poor access to safe source of water increases transmission of water borne diseases and contributes in setting up a cycle of infection and undernutrition (Figure 3.15). Eighty-eight percent cases of diarrhea world-wide are attributed to unsafe water, inadequate sanitation and poor hygiene [30]. The practice of hand washing after defecation is critical. In northern states of India, with over 50 percent undernutrition, less than 30 percent mothers washed hands after defecation [15, 31]. In such situations, diarrhea and other infections in children are common and result in increased loss of nutrients from the body as well as lower the immune defences. Moreover, children who are sick often have low appetite which aggravates poor intake of food. A vicious cycle of undernutrition and infection is set up (Figure 3.15).

Box 3.3 Undernutrition in children in India

In India, in 2005–2006, 40 percent children below 3 years of age and 42.5 percent children below 5 years of age are reported to be underweight [21]. The percentage of stunted children under 3 years is 44.9 percent while 48 percent children under 5 years are stunted. The proportion of underweight children below 3 years has decreased from 42.7 percent in 1998–1999 [27] to 42 percent in 2005–2006. On the other hand stunting in the same period has decreased by a larger margin from 51 percent to 44.9 percent in under 3 years children (Figure 3.13). Severe wasting has increased from 6.7 percent to 7.9 percent in this decade indicating possibly a better survival of wasted children under the ongoing health programmes.

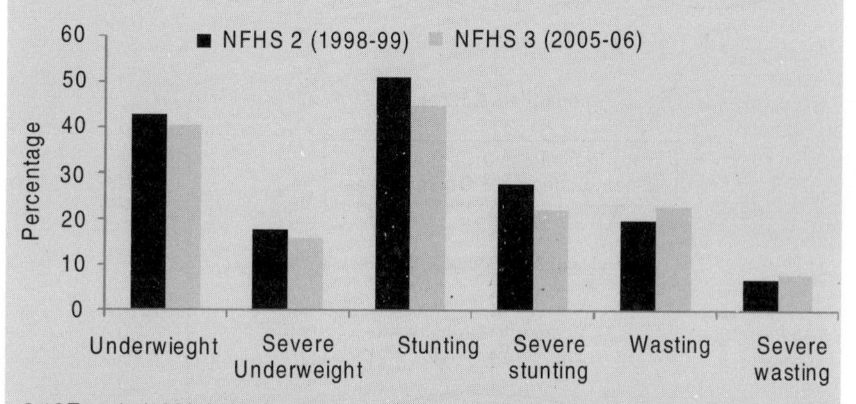

3.13 Trends (1998-2006) in nutritional status in children < 3 years [21, 27].

Child undernutrition is a problem throughout India, but the situation is considerably better in some states than in others. Table 3.4 shows that underweight percentage is higher than 40 percent in eight states – Madhya Pradesh, Bihar, Gujarat, Chhattisgarh, Jharkhand, Orissa, Uttar Pradesh and Meghalaya. These eight states have a high under-5 mortality rate (U5MR) ranging from 60.9 to 94.2 and infant mortality rate (IMR) between 46 and 70 (Table 3.4). The proportion of children under 3 years with stunting rate of over 50% are from five states – Gujarat, Chhattisgarh, Meghalaya, Bihar, Uttar Pradesh while underweight of over 50% is reported from three states – Madhya Pradesh, Bihar and Jharkhand. Children in states of Mizoram, Sikkim, Manipur and Kerala have comparatively better nutritional status.

Besides unsafe drinking water and poor sanitation, the other important underlying causes of undernutrition are inadequate availability of food through the year, poor maternal health and nutrition as well as inadequate and timely access to health services. Agriculture productivity, food policy and food prices influence food availability. It is well established that environmental factors and not genetic endowment are the principal determinants in disparities in child growth [32].

Poor stature, low pre-pregnancy weight or low body mass index combined with conception at young age below 18 years, poor care during pregnancy with inadequate weight gain, poor spacing between pregnancies, high level

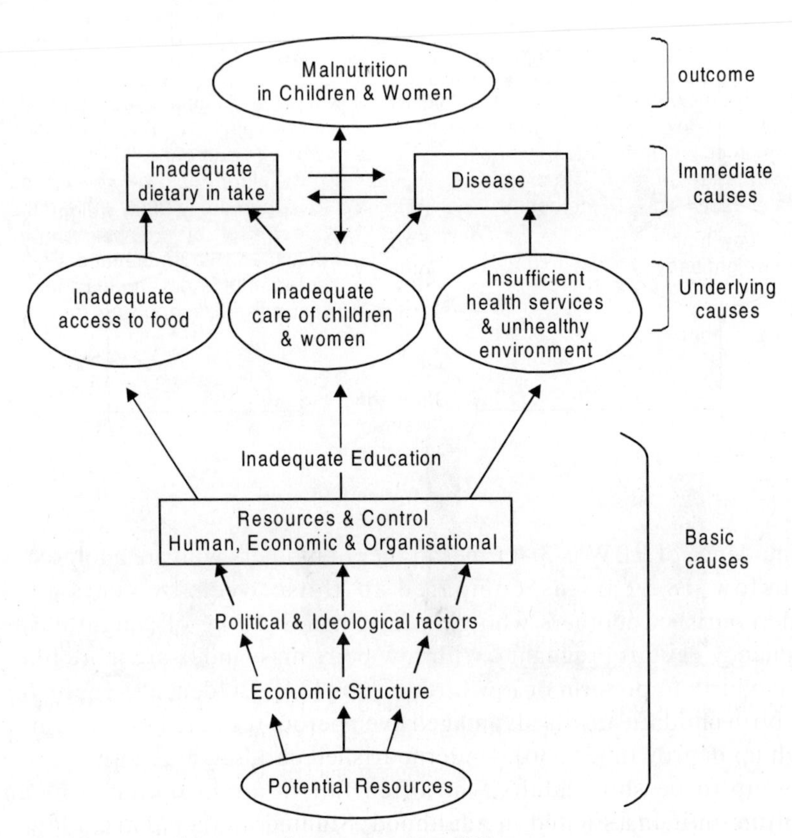

3.14 Conceptual framework of malnutrition [29].

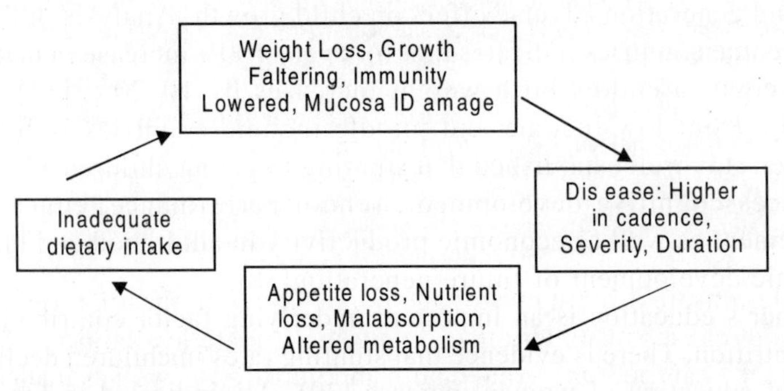

3.15 Undernutrition and infection cycle [29].

of energy expenditure by women in undertaking physical stressful chores such as carrying water, cooking fuel etc contributes to undernutrition and sets up an inter-generational cycle of low birth weight, growth failure and undernutrition – a cycle of undernutrition to be repeated over generations (Figure 3.16).

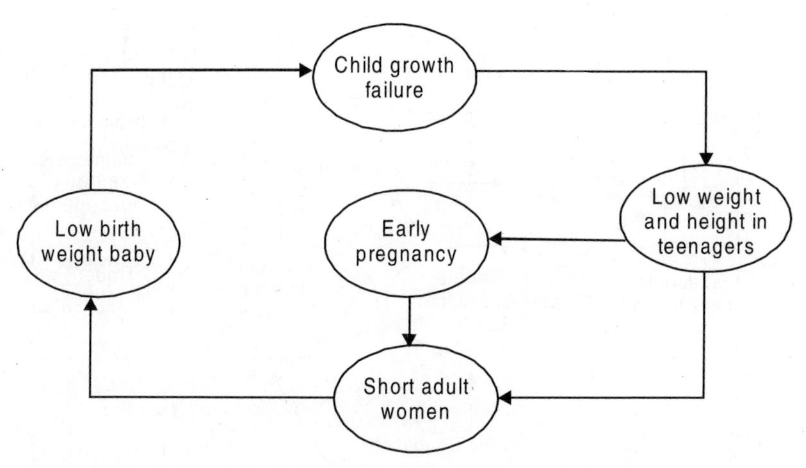

3.16 Intergenerational cycle of undernutrition [29].

Incidence of LBW is 3–4 times higher in mothers who are adolescents or below 18 years as compared to those over 18 years [33]. Undernourished mothers who gain less than 8–10 kg of weight during pregnancy or start pregnancy with low body mass index are more likely to give birth to preterm or low birth babies [34]. Evidence suggests that low birth children are disadvantaged even before they are born and rarely catch up in growth [35, 36]. Undernourished children are more likely to grow up to be short adults who often fail to attain optimum height resulting in being stunted in adulthood. Stunted mothers have a higher chance of giving birth to small babies or low birth weight babies resulting in second generation adverse effect on child growth. Analysis of data of high-income countries indicates that for every 100 g increase in maternal birth weight, a child's birth weight increases by 10–20 g [37]. Such evidence from low-income and middle-income countries is limited. However, it is well established that stunting in young children adversely influences cognitive development, school performance, educational achievement as well as economic productivity in adulthood and hinders economic development of future generation[38].

Mother's education is an important underlying factor contributing to undernutrition. There is evidence that stunting rates in children decline as levels of education of women increase [39]. As indicated in Fig. 3.17 higher level of education which can be considered a proxy indicator of the decision making power with women, is associated with a reduction in percentage of adolescence marriage, low BMI and underweight prevalence in children [21]. Empowered women, who have control over their incomes, are more likely than men to invest in food, nutrition, health and education of children and self care. The social context in which women reside

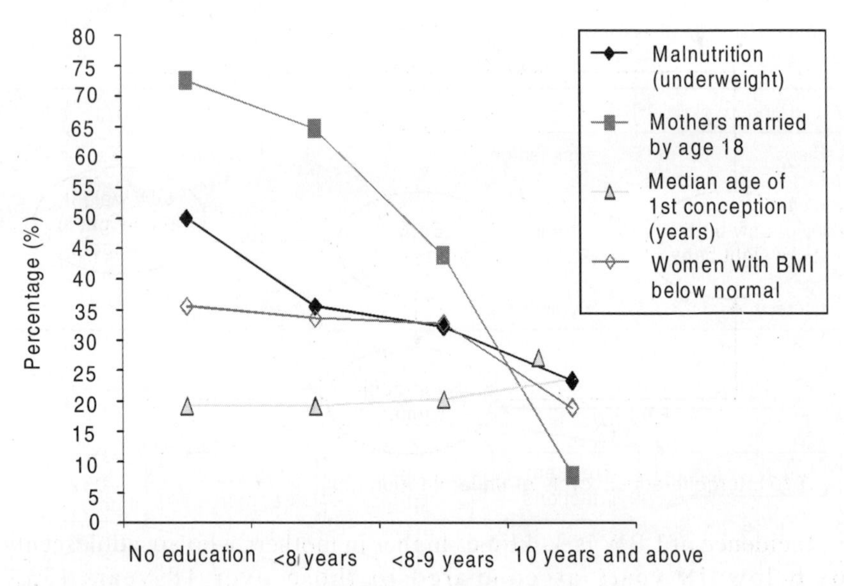

3.17 Women's education and trend in BMI and underweight in children – Rajasthan, India [21].

influence their power to take decisions regarding health and other care-seeking behaviours. An analysis of India data reveals that the risk of underweight in children has a significant association with domestic violence experienced by women [22]. The low status of women in many developing countries is considered to be one of the primary reasons for undernutrition across the life cycle.

A regression analysis of risk factors of undernutrition in children indicates that the primary risk factors associated with underweight in developing regions, such as India, in order of magnitude of risk, are body mass index (BMI) of mothers, occurrence of childhood diseases, child's age 12–35 months and illiteracy of mothers (Table 3.5). As presented in Table 3.5, poor hygiene practices are observed to be important contributory factors of stunting in children. Occurrence of child diseases contributes to highest risk to wasting in children [14, 40].

Poverty is a basic cause of undernutrition in children. Poverty and low income contributes to undernutrition by adversely influencing food and nutrition security, housing and living environment with increased risk of infections. Poor population have a lower access to health and family planning services and are often involved in hard physical labour which also contributes to poor nutrition. The vicious cycle of poverty and undernutrition (Figure 3.18) adversely influence the nutritional status of children and economic development of future generation [41].

Table 3.5 Risk factors for underweight, stunting and wasting in children – an analysis of situation in Uttar Pradesh, India [40]

Underweight		Stunting		Wasting	
Risk factor	Factor loading	Risk factor	Factor loading	Risk factor	Factor loading
BMI	1.63	BMI	1.30	Disease	1.64
Disease	1.58	Literacy	1.27	BMI	1.29
Child's age	1.41	Child's age	1.26	Child's age	1.19
Literacy	1.28	Hygiene	1.19	Literacy	1.17

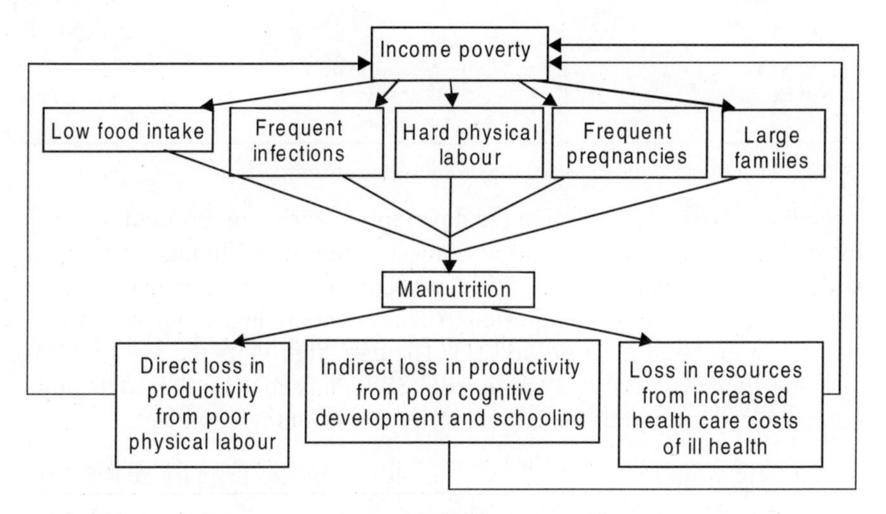

3.18 Vicious cycle of poverty and malnutrition [41].

However, poverty resulting in poor purchasing power of the family and poor access to food by family is not the sole cause of undernutrition in children. Data from nine states of India (Table 3.6) indicates that 59.2–93.1 percentage of adult women in these states consume over 70% recommended dietary allowances (RDA) of energy and protein as compared to only 19.4–52.3% of children 1–3 years of age in those families consuming over 70% RDA [42]. The data highlights the fact that young children below 3 years of age who need much less food as compared to adults are often deprived of food in the crucial stage of growth not necessarily due to lack of access of food by family but very often due to inadequate knowledge regarding appropriate feeding and care practices to be followed for young children, i.e. exclusive breastfeeding in the first six months followed by complementing breastfeed with right quantity of food of right composition with adequate energy density as well as right consistency and right frequency of feeding.

Table 3.6 Undernutrition and percentage of adults and children with protein–calorie adequacy [42]

States	Prevalence of undernutrition (%) in children	Distribution (%) protein calorie adequacy – sedentary adult women[(a)]	Distribution (%) protein calorie adequacy – 1–3 year children
Andhra Pradesh	36.5	87.7	52.3
Gujarat	47.4	69.8	24.2
Karnataka	41.1	80.2	25.5
Kerala	28.8	78.6	19.4
Madhya Pradesh	60.3	77.6	33.7
Maharashtra	39.7	59.2	30.8
Orissa	44.0	93.1	24.9
Tamil Nadu	33.2	80.6	23.2
West Bengal	43.5	84.8	37.1
Pooled	41.6	80.0	30.1

[(a)] 70% requirement defined as energy protein adequacy

Undernourished children in the developing world are reported not only in the low wealth quintile but also the top quintile – though the gap is wide. As presented in Table 3.7, 56.6 percent children in India in the lowest socio-economic group are reported to be undernourished compared to 19.7 percent in the wealthiest group [21]. The data highlights the fact that it is not only food insecurity or hunger per se which is contributing to the high percentage of undernourished children in developing countries.

Table 3.7 Prevalence of underweight by location, wealth quintile, gender and caste

	Underweight Prevalence 2005–06	Severe underweight Prevalence 2005–06
Total	42.5	15.8
Urban	32.7	10.8
Rural	45.6	17.5
Female	43.1	16.4
Male	41.9	15.3
Scheduled caste	47.9	18.5
Scheduled tribe	54.5	24.9
Other castes	33.7	11.1
Quintile 1 (Poorest)	56.6	24.9
Quintile 2	49.2	19.4
Quintile 3	41.4	14.1
Quintile 4	33.6	9.5
Quintile 5 (Wealthiest)	19.7	4.9

3.6 Maternal and child undernutrition – evidence for actions

"Too early, too close, too many and too late pregnancies adversely affect nutrition and health status of mother child dyad" [42]. Poor nutritional status of mother, including chronic energy deficiency and micronutrient deficiencies, before and during pregnancy is critical to successful outcome of pregnancy. Birth weight is influenced by the nutrition and health status of mother. Mother's weight and height at conception influences birth weight to a great extent. A number of studies have demonstrated a good correlation between birth weight and maternal weight as well as poor pre-pregnancy weight gain. Maternal body size is strongly associated with size of newborn children [24]. Risk of intrauterine growth restriction (IUGR) is associated with short stature of mother and poor maternal nutrition stores [3, 43]. Data from India reports an association between mother's weight and birth weight as well as an association of birth weight with economic situation – the latter in turn is observed to be associated with lower height and weight of mothers (Tables 3.8 and 3.9).

Table 3.8 Effect of maternal body weight on birth weight [44]

Mother weight (kgs)	No.	Mean birth weight (gm)
<45	128	2639.6
45-54	251	2779.1
>=55	96	3009.41
Total	475	2788.0

Table 3.9 Birth weight and socio-economic status [45]

	Poor income	Middle Income	High income
Age (years)	24.1	24.3	27.8
Parity	2.41	1.96	1.61
Height (cm)	151.5	154.2	156.3
Weight (kg)	45.7	49.9	56.2
Hb (g/dl)	10.9	11.1	12.4
Birth weight (kg)	2.70	2.90	3.13

In a developing country, such as India, maternal situation such as adolescence marriage (a proxy for adolescence conception), height, level of education, access and use of health services (such as consumption of full dose of iron–folic acid supplement, antenatal care and institutional delivery) have been observed to have a significant association with underweight prevalence rates in children below 2 years of age (Table 3.10).

LBW children in a developing country, as stated earlier, are often full term newborns with intrauterine growth retardation. The survival chance of these children is much better than pre-term newborns. However, these surviving children are at higher risk of poor nutritional and health. Full term LBW children have been reported to have a low trajectory for growth in infancy and childhood (Figure 3.19) – resulting in increasing the chances of prevalence of undernutrition in young children [46]. Figure 3.9

Table 3.10 Maternal factors significantly associated[(a)] with underweight in children in Uttar Pradesh, India [22]

Maternal situation	% of underweight children	Level of significance[(a)]
■ Age of marriage <18	43.1	0.000
>18	35.1	
■ Height of mother <145 cm	50.0	0.000
> 145 cm	38.5	
■ No education	46.2	0.000
10 years and above education	23.8	
■ Emotional violence	47.5	0.035
No emotional violence	41.5	
■ Consumption of IFA tablets for <90 days	39.8	0.000
Consumption of IFA tablets for >90 days	22.0	
■ <3 ANC check-ups	44.6	0.000
>3 ANC check-ups	28.8	
■ No institutional delivery	43.3	0.000
Institutional delivery	29.1	

[(a)]Level of significance < 0.05 indicates significant association

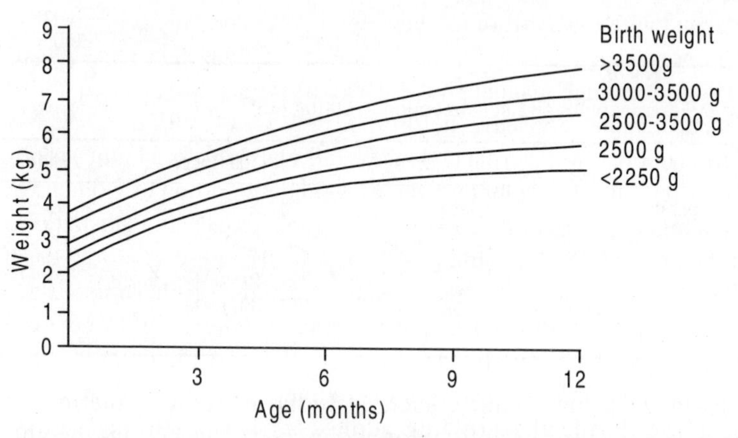

3.19 Growth in relation to birth weight [46].

(presented earlier in Box 3.2) highlights the association of LBW with nutritional status of young children. Birkin et al [47] in a study of association between birth weight and growth concluded that infants with lower birth weights are likely to remain shorter and lighter throughout childhood, especially those who are intrauterine growth retarded rather than premature. Conversely, those infants with higher birth weights are likely to remain taller and heavier and have a higher risk of obesity. The study indicates birth weight is a strong predictor of weight and height in early childhood, not only for low birth weight children but also for those of normal and high birth weight.

Undernutrition in children begins with the mother [2]. Mother's own foetal growth and her diet from birth to pregnancy affect birth weight. Studies from India and other developing countries indicate that reduction in dietary intake below habitual levels or increase in work load above habitual levels as well as adolescent pregnancy is associated with worsening in maternal nutrition status and low birth weight. Deterioration in maternal nutritional status has been reported with reduction in normal habitual diet during drought or pre-harvest season, increase in work with induction of new manual labour and adolescent pregnancy [41]. An analysis of 36, 555 birth records from North India revealed seasonal variations in birth weights. The incidence of LBW was reported to be minimal in post winter births. It was observed that these mothers in the third trimester not only had a better appetite in the winter season but also consumed much higher quantities of fresh vegetables and fruits which were easily accessible in the winter season [48].

Women's nutrition and health status through out the life cycle from childhood through adolescence and into adulthood is critical in determining maternal and neonatal health outcomes. Intrauterine growth restriction is associated with low BMI of mothers, mothers conceiving prior to 18 years of age, poor food availability during pregnancy, suboptimal energy intake along with continued high manual physical activity, high parity, inadequate rest and absence of maternity leave before delivery [3, 49, 50, 51, 52]. Maternal undernutrition, low maternal body mass index (BMI <18.5 kg/m^2) is prevalent in many regions of developing countries. The proportion of women with low BMI is higher in South Asia – 14.3% in Nepal, 20.4% in Pakistan, 28.5% in Bangladesh and 35.6% in India (13, 21, 53, 54).

The social practice of early marriage and high rates of teenage pregnancy is a major factor contributing to poor height and low BMI. Amongst girls living in disadvantaged situations, the velocity of growth during adolescence is slower and is extended for a longer period. Early conception during the growing adolescent period in these girls often results in arresting growth of adolescent mothers [36]. Undernourished girls in developing countries who become pregnant in the growing adolescent phase are at much higher risk of LBW. Children born to teenage mothers are 40% more likely to die in their first year than those born to women in their twenties [36]. The proportion of such women who begin child bearing below 18 years is high in developing countries – 16 % in India [21], 20% in Nepal [53] and 37% in Bangladesh [54]. Several studies indicate adult height is positively associated with birth weight and length. Many countries in south-central Asia have more than 10% women with short stature [16]. The percentage of women with short stature, height below 145 cm is 11.4% in India and 14.2% in Nepal and

15.7% in Bangladesh [16, 53, 54]. Short stature of mother and poor maternal nutrition stores are associated with increased risk of intrauterine growth restriction. An increase in adult height of 0.7–1.0 cm is associated with 1 cm increase in birth length [38].

Improving nutritional status of mother before and during pregnancy is critical for reducing undernutrition in children [24, 55, 56]. A study from Gambia demonstrated that prenatal dietary supplementation reduced retardation in intrauterine growth when effectively targeted at risk mothers. Gambia study was a 5-year controlled trial of all pregnant women in 28 villages who were provided with daily supplement of high energy groundnut biscuits (4.3 MJ/day) for about 20 weeks before delivery. Food supplement to mothers increased weight gain in pregnancy. The birth weight increased significantly during the nutrition deprived season of June to October – weight gain increased by 201 grams in the hungry season, 94 grams in the harvest season and by 136 g for the whole year. Birth length and gestation were not affected [57]. In India, a variation in mean birth weight of babies born during different time periods has been reported. Highest mean birth weight was observed in March (post-winter) and lowest in August (post-summer and dry season) and an association with availability of fresh fruits rich in minerals and vitamins was indicated [48]. In 13 trials (4665 women), modest increase in maternal weight gain and mean birth weight was observed with balance energy–protein supplement. A substantial reduction in risk of small for gestational age (SGA) birth was also observed. High protein or balance protein supplement alone was not beneficial [58].

Kusin et al [59] in a controlled randomised trial in Madura, East Java studied the impact of high energy (1950 kJ/465 kcal) and low-energy supplement (218 kJ/52 kcal) to pregnant women in the last trimester of pregnancy. The effect of this intervention on the children's growth was assessed longitudinally for the first 5 years of life in the mothers who had consumed the supplement for at least 90 days. Infants entered the study at birth and their growth was measured at 4-week intervals until 12 months old; thereafter they were measured every 3 months. The birth weight in such cases is increased by nearly 100 g [59]. It was observed that up to the age of 24 months, children of mothers receiving high energy supplement were significantly heavier than the other group with low-energy supplement. The high-energy group children were also taller throughout the first 5 years. There was a 20% reduction in stunting at 5 years of age. Weight-for-height was similar in both groups, but stunting (height-for-age) was less prevalent in high energy supplement group. The study concluded that in a community characterized by chronic energy deficiency among women of reproductive age, energy supplementation of women for the last 90 days of pregnancy, was effective in the promotion of postnatal growth and reduction in undernutrition in preschool children. A study in Guatemala also demonstrated that children born to women who had received high protein-moderate energy supplement were taller than those receiving non-protein–low-energy supplement [60].

Besides inadequate consumption of energy and protein, deficiency of micronutrient is common in women in developing countries. Globally almost half of pregnant women, about 56.4 million are estimated to be anemic [61]. Iron deficiency is often the primary cause of anemia. Anemia accounts for 20% maternal mortality and contributes to lowering birth weight. Low birth weight can be attributed to anemia per se or combined effect of poor nutritional status of mother or poor access to antenatal services. It has been reported that the incidence of LBW doubles when haemoglobin level is <8 g/dl (Figure 3.20) [62].

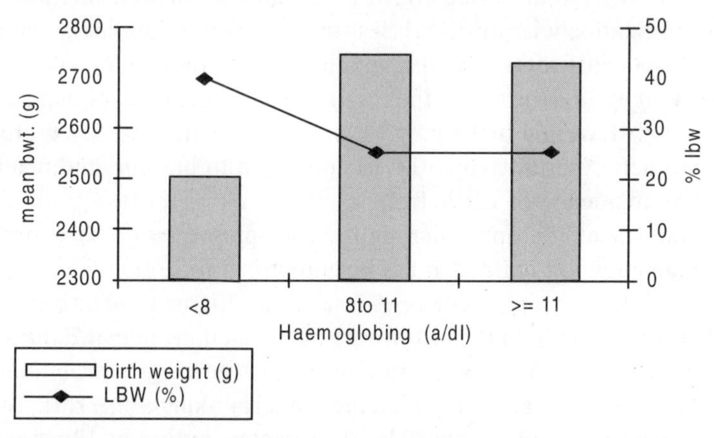

3.20 Effect of maternal Hb on birth weight [62].

Intervention measures are important prior to onset of pregnancy for building iron stores and preventing severe anemia. Building iron stores right from adolescence age itself has been recommended [63]. Iron supplementation study from Vietnam has demonstrated that weekly iron–folic acid prior to and during pregnancy is associated with better iron stores in the first and second trimester of pregnancy and with reduced prevalence of low birth weight compared with pregnant women who receive daily iron-folic acid supplementation during pregnancy [64]. Iron supplementation has been demonstrated to improve birth weight, even in non-anemic women [65]. Deworming in the second trimester of pregnancy in Nepal has been reported to lowering the rate of severe anemia during the third trimester and improving birth weight [66].

Besides iron, pregnant women are often deficient in several other micronutrients such as iodine, zinc, calcium, vitamin A. These deficiencies are often "not visible" but can result in health problems in mothers and intra-uterine growth restriction [2, 67, 68]. Addressing micronutrient deficiencies during pregnancy in mother increases birth weight [67]. Fall et al [69] in a meta-analysis on impact of multiple micronutrient supplementation during pregnancy in low income countries on birth size and length of gestation observed a mean increase in birth weight of 22 g with a range in birth weight increase across studies from 4.9 to 75.5 g. The study concluded that "the effect on birth weight is greater in women with higher BMI and is very small in energy deficient mothers". This increase was in comparison to what was achieved by iron-folic acid supplement. Shrimpton et al [67] observed that the increase in birth weight achieved by the multiple micronutrient supplements is of similar order of magnitude as that reported to be achieved with food supplementation during pregnancy. A hospital-based trial in pregnant women enrolled at 24–32 weeks of gestation with low BMI (less than 18.5) and anemia (haemoglobin level of 7–9 g/dl) showed that a supplement containing 29 vitamins and minerals taken in addition to the regular iron–folic acid supplementation increased birth weight by 98 g, increased birth length by 0.80 cm, reduced early neo-natal mortality by 50% as compared to placebo and resulted in decline in incidence of LBW from 43.1% to 16.2% [70].

The impact of multiple micronutrient supplementation on growth and development later in childhood has been reported from follow up studies in Nepal, Bangladesh and Vietnam [71, 72, 73]. Vietnam effectiveness trial reported not only reduction in LBW rate but on stunting rate at 2 years of age [72]. The Nepal study [73] reported no impact on height but influence on weight, head and mid-arm circumference while the Bangladesh study reported positive impact on motor skills [71]. A systematic review of 12 efficacy and 6 effectiveness trials covering 12 countries from three continents (Asia, Latin America and Sub-Saharan Africa) concludes "multiple micronutrient supplement during pregnancy in developing countries contribute significantly to a body of evidence which shows that supplementing women in pregnancy can improve outcomes beyond anemia, including deficiencies of other minerals and vitamins and birth weights" [74].

Based on the review of the meta-analysis results of comparing multiple micronutrients with daily iron folic acid supplementation during pregnancy, it has been proposed to replace iron folic acid supplements with multiple micronutrient supplement in the package of nutrition and health interventions during antenatal care [67]. Box 3.4 presents details of micronutrient supplements used in the various trials that were covered under the meta-analysis. The findings stress the need to improve nutritional

Box 3.4 Micronutrient supplements used in efficacy and effectiveness trials

In 1999 UNICEF, the World Health Organization (WHO) and the United Nations University (UNU) jointly proposed a standard composition of multi-micronutrient supplement for pregnant women comprising 15 vitamins and minerals. The supplement was proposed to be used in efficacy and effectiveness trials to assess its impact on pregnancy and birth outcome. This supplement is referred to as United Nations International Multiple Micronutrient Preparation (UNIMMAP). Nine trials in eight countries (Bangladesh; Burkino Faso; China; Guinea-Bissau; Indonesia (Lombok and Indramayu); Nepal (Janakpur); Niger; Pakistan) used UNIMMAP as antenatal supplements. The other three trials conducted in Mexico, Nepal (Sarlahi) and Zimbabwe used other multiple micronutrient supplement formulation as presented below (Table 3.11) [75].

Table 3.11 Micronutrient composition of supplements used in 12 trials

Micronutrient	UNIMMAP"	Mexico	Sarlahi, Nepal	Zimbabwe
Iron (mg)	30	62.4	60	0"
Zinc (mg)	15	12.9	30	15
Copper (mg)	2.0	—	2.0	1.2
Selenium (ug)	65	—	—	65
Magnesium (mg)	—	252	10	—
Iodine(ug)	iso	—	—	—
Vitamin A (ug RE)	800	2,150 (1U)	1,000	3,000
p-Carotene (mg)	—	—	—	3.5
Vitamin B. (mg)	1.4	0.93	1.6	1.5
Vitamin B, (mg)	1.4	1.S7	1.8	1.6
Folic acid (ug)	400	215	400	0
Niacin (mg)	18	15.5	20	17
Vitamin B_6 (mg)	1.9	1.94	2.2	2.2
Vitamin B,2 (ug)	2.6	2.04	2.6	4.0
Vitamin C (mg)	70	66.5	100	80
Vitamin D (ug)	5	7.7	10	10
Vitamin E (mg)	10	5.7 (IU)	10	10
Vitamin K (ug)	—	—	6S	—

* RE, retinol equivalent; UNIMMAP, United Nations International Multiple Micronutrient Preparation

status before as well as during pregnancy. Besides supplementing with multiple micronutrients in situations with a high number of undernourished women, supplementary feeding is considered an important intervention.

3.7 Addressing undernutrition in children – a life cycle approach

World-wide growth faltering analysis using WHO standards stress the significance of prenatal and early life interventions to prevent the growth failure that mainly happens during the first 2 years of life [17]. The need to concentrate on the "critical window from conception to 24 months of age" for targeting interventions is recommended [2, 5]. Successful implementation of intervention measures during pregnancy and lactation, together with appropriate infant and young child feeding as well as care of infants, young children and adolescent girls is essential for reduction in the level of stunting in young children. It has been proposed that intensive timely actions concentrate on population group "at risk" of undernutrition such as pregnant mothers and children below 12 months [14]. Reaching this "risk" group is feasible through the primary health care system. Contacts during antenatal care (ANC) services and routine immunisation provide opportunity for promoting and monitoring appropriate feeding practices and adoption of health and hygiene practices (Table 3.12). ANC services need to systematically include interventions such active promotion of minimum weight gain of 10–12 kg through adoption of practices such as intake of additional diet (additional food equal to one pre-pregnancy major meal) during pregnancy, ensuring minimum 2 hours day rest and regular consumption of iron or multiple micronutrient supplements. It has been emphasized that any delay beyond infancy, may be too late for effective prevention of undernutrition in children [14].

As presented in Table 3.13, the Lancet series on maternal and child undernutrition has identified the following evidence-based direct interventions with demonstrated effectiveness [77]. These interventions are included in the recent strategies at the global level [78].

Interventions to improve nutritional status (Figure 3.21) need to stress on a package of selected actions, through the life cycle, to be effectively implemented in the entire region or a country [1]. Registering and reaching newly married women is critical for introducing intervention measures for preventing adolescent pregnancy as well as for improving health and nutritional status prior to onset of pregnancy. All these efforts for reduction of undernutrition need to be complemented with access to safe drinking water since evidence shows that hygiene interventions can reduce stunting at 36 months by 2–4% [78].

In addition to the above referred package of intervention, basic causes at societal level such as improved women's status are critical [22, 79]. It is well established that women who have control over income are more likely than men to invest in their children's education, health and nutrition [80, 81, 82, 83]. Conditional Cash Transfer (CCT) programme of Mexico is an example of an effort to reduce poverty and food insecurity along with an emphasis for poor women to invest in betterment of the children [84]. Efforts for accelerated and sustainable reduction in undernutrition in children requires long-term investments for improving women's education, empowering women and implementing measures for reducing poverty and ensuring food and nutrition security [22, 80].

Table 3.12 Linking promotion of appropriate infant and young child feeding with immunization contact points [76]

Pregnant women Immunization contacts	Counselling and monitoring
Tetanus toxoid 1st dose Tetanus toxoid 2nd dose	Antenatal care Promote and monitor • Increase in energy dense food • Regular intake of iron folic acid (or multiple micronutrient) • Minimum 2 hours day rest • Weight gain 10–12 kg Preparing for breastfeeding • Initiate breastfeeding within 1 h of birth • Significance of colostrum feeding • Promote exclusive breastfeeding (EBF) for 6 months • No water in first 6 months Institutional delivery • Preparing for institutional delivery

Infants Immunization Contacts	Age	Counselling and monitoring
BCG OPV (O dose)	At birth or along with DPT 1 At birth or within 28 days of birth	Newborn and infant care Promote and monitor • Ensure newborn care intervention package being followed • Record birth weight • Initiate BF within 1 hour of birth – ensure appropriate position / breast attachment • Ensure colostrum feeding Advice • EBF continued for 6 months • No introduction of water with EBF • Hygiene and hand washing • Introduce family spacing measures
OPV 1, DPT 1 OPV 2, DPT 2	6 weeks (1.5 months) 10 weeks (2.5 months)	Promote and monitor • EBF continued (no water) • Check growth – height / weight of child Advice • Continue EBF during illness / diarrhoea • Advice hygiene / hand washing
OPV 3, DPT 3	14 weeks (14.5 months)	Promote and monitor • EBF to be continued up to 6 months Advice • Continue EBF during illness • Sensitize on introduction of appropriate complementary feeding (CF) and continued Breastfeeding (BF) at 6 months • Hygiene / hand-washing practices • Diarrhoea prevention and management
Measles + 1st dose of vitamin A	9 months	Promote and monitor • Complementary feeding (Amount, type, frequency) • Continued BF Advice • Continue BF up to 2 years or beyond • Record child's height / weight

Table 3.13 Direct interventions with demonstrated effectiveness on maternal and child undernutrition [77]

Evidence	Maternal and birth outcomes	Newborn babies	Infants and young children
Evidence sufficient for implementation in all developing countries	Iron–folate supplementation Maternal supplements of multiple micronutrients Maternal iodine through iodization of salt Maternal calcium supplementation Interventions to reduce tobacco consumption or indoor air pollution	Promotion of breastfeeding (individual and group counselling)	Promotion of breastfeeding (individual and group counselling) Behaviour change communication for improved complementary feeding for infants Zinc supplementation Zinc in management of diarrhoea Vitamin A fortification or supplementation Universal salt iodization Hand washing or hygiene interventions Treatment of severe acute malnutrition
Evidence for implementation in specific situational context	Maternal supplements of balanced energy and protein Maternal iodine supplements Maternal deworming in pregnancy Intermittent preventive treatment for malaria Insecticide treated bednets	Neonatal vitamin A supplementation Delayed cord clamping	Conditional cash transfer programmes (with nutritional education) Deworming Iron fortification and supplementation programmes Insecticide treated bednets

Addressing undernutrition is complex and involves a diversity of approaches for achieving success (Box 3.5). A strong government action at various levels, leadership at the highest level, mobilization and information sharing with vulnerable groups, appropriate monitoring and evaluation system with timely corrective actions and significant allocation of resources and public spending is critical for addressing undernutrition in children.

Adolescence / Pre-Pregnancy

- Delay age of marriage / first pregnancy >18 years
- Promote healthy weight
- Weekly iron folic acid supplementation
- Consumption of iron / multiple micro nutrient fortified food
- Education, family life education and empowerment of women

Pregnancy

- Energy dense food/ targeted energy food supplement (undernourished and deprived women) and adequate protein
- Iron folic acid / micro nutrient supplement
- Daily intake of iodized salt
- Deworming (if required)
- Treatment of night blindness in pregnancy
- Malaria prophylaxis and intermittent therapy
- Reduce work load and energy expenditure
- Hand washing and hygiene
- Reduce smoke laden home environment / tobacco
- Adequate day rest

Birth

- Initiate breast feeding withing 1 hour (including colostrum feeding)

Infants <6 months

Interventions for infants

- Exclusive breast feeding (no water)
- Appropriate feeding of HIV exposed infants

Interventions for the mother

- Energy dense food
- Increase quality proteins
- IFA supplements / multi-micronutrient supplementation
- Daily use of iodised salt
- Use of fortified food such as iron fortified flour
- Space pregnancies (>2 years) family planning services

Children 6-23 months

Interventions for young children

- Complementary feeding
- Continued breast-feeding
- Iron folic acid supplement
- Vitamin A supplementation
- Daily intake of iodized salt
- Zinc treatment and feeding during diarrhea
- Deworming
- Hand washing with soap
- Use of safe drinking water
- Full immunization

Interventions for the mother

- Energy dense fortified foods and
- Hand washing with soap. Food hygiene

3.21 Prevention of undernutrition – a life cycle approach (Adapted from [1]).

Box 3.5 Reduction of undernutrition – success factors – interventions – country case studies

The success factors for reduction of child undernutrition are primarily adequate and defined comprehensive policies which are not limited to provision of food supplements alone. Effective implementation of policies through well defined service delivery systems and effective management as well as availability of sufficient resources are critical. Analysis of factors contributing to accelerated progress in nutrition situation of children in Thailand, China, Brazil and Vietnam is presented below [80].

In Thailand, child malnutrition reduced from 50% in 1982 to 25% in 1986. The 2nd National and Health Policy (1982–86) focused on targeted nutrition interventions to eliminate severe malnutrition and effective implementation of behaviour change and communication to prevent mild to moderate malnutrition. The focus of the intervention was on social mobilization – one community volunteer for 20 households – through community-based primary health care delivery system. One of the major factors contributing to the success was high political priority, a large investment of 20% of total government expenditure and integrating nutrition within the National Economic and Social Development Plan.

In China, malnutrition reduced from 25% to 8% between 1990 and 2002. The success is attributed to successful poverty alleviation strategy as well as rapid economic growth along with implementation of nutrition, health and family planning programmes at large scale. Additionally, focusing on important interventions such as sanitation and mother's education. This combined with central leadership, local government ownership and effective monitoring and feed back mechanism were the primary success factors.

In Brazil, 60% reduction in malnutrition was reported between 1975 and 1989. Following sharpest economic growth and poverty alleviation, substantial national resource was invested in food distribution and nutrition programmes as well as water, sanitation and health .Social sector input for education increased significantly. Since 2004, nutrition policy efforts have been intensified with high resource investment.

In Viet Nam, the prevalence of underweight has decreased from 51.5% in 1985 to 24.6% in 2006 – a reduction of 1.3% per year. The prevalence of stunting decreased at the rate of 1.5% per year during this period – from 59.7% in 1985 to 27.9% in 2006 [85]. In the early phase, risk factors were analysed and special attention was accorded to maternal health and nutritional status and child health and family planning services. Family planning programme resulted in creating opportunities to families for better investment in child nutrition and health care. Additionally, poverty alleviation programmes combined with high investment in PEM control programme since 1999 contributed in reducing undernutrition. Reducing child malnutrition was a goal in the 10th Party Conference's document with a revised strategy for Child Malnutrition Control Programme for the period 2006–2010. Stunting Reduction Plan of 2008–2013 gives special focus to pre-pregnant and pregnant women and reducing LBW to under 6%.

References

1. UNICEF (2009). Tracking progress on child and maternal nutrition: a survival and development priority, November 2009.
2. BLACK R. (2008). Nutrition interventions that can accelerate the reduction of maternal and child undernutrition. *SCN News* vol. 36, pp. 17–20.
3. BLACK RE, ALLEN LH, BHUTTA ZA, CAULFIELD LE, DEONIS M, EZZATI M, COLIN M, RIVERA J; maternal and child undernutrition study group (2008). Maternal and child undernutrition 1, maternal and child undernutrition: global and regional experiences and health consequences vol. 371, pp. 243–260.

4. United Nations (2002). Millennium Development Goals www.un.org/millenniumgoals.
5. GRAGNOLATI M, SHEKAR M, GUPTA MS, BREDAN KC and LEE Y (2005). India's undernourished children: A call for reform and actions, HNP discussion paper.
6. VENAMANN AM (2008). 35th SCN session opening speech by the SCN chair. *SCN News* vol. 36, pp. 4–6.
7. UAUY R and KAIN J (2002). The epidemiological transition: need to incorporate obesity prevention into nutrition programme. *Public health Nutrition* vol. 5, pp. 23–29.
8. WHO (2008). WHO Global Database on child growth and malnutrition. www.who.int/nutgrowthdb
9. WHO (1995). Expert committee on nutrition, physical: uses and interpretations of anthropometry. Geneva, Switzerland, World Health Organisation 1995, WHO Technical report series, report No 854.
10. WATERLOW JC and THOMSON AM (1979). Observations on the adequacy of breastfeeding. *Lancet* vol. 2, pp. 238–242.
11. ROGERO JS, EMMETT PM, GOLDING J (1979). The growth and nutritional status of the breastfed infants. *Early Human Dev* vol. 49, pp. S157–S174.
12. BEATON GH (1989). Small but healthy: Are we asking the right question. *Eur J Clin Nutr* vol. 43, pp. 863–875.
13. SHRIMPTON JR, VICTORIA CG, DEONIS M, LIMA RC, BLOSSNER M, TROPH DOEC and GLUGSTON G (2001). Worldwide timings of growth faltering: implications for nutrition interventions. *Pediatrics* vol. 107, pp. 1–7.
14. VIR SC (2001). Nutritional status of children in Uttar Pradesh, NFI Bulletin, January 2001.
15. VIR SC, JAIN A and SINGH R (2006). Mission Poshan – Project to redesigning state programme for addressing malnutrition in under three years in Uttar Pradesh. Report of the Nutrition Foundation of India on "Late infancy and early childhood (6–24 months). Nutrition Foundation of India, New Delhi.
16. VICTORA CG, DE ONIS M, HALLAL PC, BLOSSSNER M, TROPH D and SHRIMPTON R (2010). Worldwide Timing of growth Faltering: Revisiting Implications for interventions Pediatrics vol. 125, pp. 473–480.
17. DE ONIS M, ONYANGO AW, BORGHI E, GARZA C, YANG H (2006). WHO multicentre Growth Reference Study Group, Comparison of the World health Organisation (WHO) child growth standards and the National Centre for Health Statistics/ WHO international growth reference implications for child health programmes. *Public Health Nutrition* vol. 7, pp. 942–947.
18. WATERLOW JC, BUZINA R, KELLER W, LANE JM, NICHAMAN MZ, TANNER JM (1977). The presentation and use of height and weight data for comparing the nutritional status of groups of children under the age of 10 years. *Bull World Health Organ* vol. 55, pp. 489–498.
19. WHO Multicentric Growth Reference Study group (2006). WHO Child growth standards based on length/heights weight and age. *Acta Paediatrica Supple* vol. 450, pp. 76–85.
20. DE ONIS M (2008). Child undernutrition based on the new WHO growth standards and rates of reduction to 2015. *SCN News* vol. 36, pp. 12–16.
21. International Institute for Population Sciences (IIPS) and ORC Macro (2007). National Family Health Survey (NFHS) III, 2005–06, India, Mumbai: IIPS.
22. VIR SC, JAIN R, ADHIKARI T, PANDEY A and YADAV RJ (2010). Undernutrition in young children under 2 years in Uttar Pradesh state, India – an analysis of determinants and proposed actions. Under publication.

23. WHOSIS (2008). WHO Statistical Information System. Low birth weight newborns (percentage), 2008. http://www.who.int/whosis/indicators/compendium/2008/2bwn/en/
24. KRAEMER MS (1987). Determinants of low birth weight: methodological assessment and meta analysis. *Bull World Health Organisation* vol. 65, pp. 663–737.
25. UNICEF (2009). State of the world's children – maternal and new born health. UNICEF, December 2008.
26. WHO and UNICEF (2004). Low birthweight – country, regional and global estimates, UNICEF, New York (2004).
27. International Institute for Population Sciences (IIPS) and ORC Macro, 1999. National Family Health Survey (NFHS) II, 1998–99, India, Mumbai: IIPS.
28. Government of India (GoI). SRS Bulletin (October 2009). Office of Registrar General of India, Ministry of Home Affairs, GoI.
29. UNICEF (1998). The state of world's children report, UNICEF, New York.
30. PRES-USTON A, BOS R, GORE F, BARTRAM H (2008). Safe water, better health, costs, benefits, sustaining of interventions to protect and promote health. WHO, Geneva, 2008.
31. Evaluation report of community based maternal child health nutrition (MCHN) project, Uttar Pradesh, Government of Uttar Pradesh, Operation research Group and UNICEF (2006).
32. WHO (2008). Child growth and development webpage www.who.int/nutrition/topics/childgrowth.
33. UNICEF (2000). Technical consultation on low birth weight. Jointly organised by USAID, World Bank and UNICEF.
34. UNICEF (2004). Mapping India's Children, UNICEF in Action.
35. GILLESPIE S (2002). UNICEF staff working papers, Nutrition series, number 97-improving adolescent and maternal nutrition – An overview of benefits and outputs.
36. VIR S (1990). Adolescent growth in girls – the Indian perspective – editorial. *Indian Pediatrics* vol. 17, p. 1249.
37. RAMAKRISHNAN U, MARTORELL R, SCHOEDER DG, FLORES R (1999). Role of intergenerational effects on linear growth. *J Nutr* vol. 129, pp. 544S–549S.
38. VICTORA CG, ADAIR L, FALL C, HALLAL PC, MARTORELL R, RICHTER L, SACHDEV HPS; the maternal and child undernutrition study group. Maternal and child undernutrition 2. Maternal and child undernutrition, consequences for adult health and human capital. *Lancet* 371.
39. DE ONIS M (2003). Socio economic inequalities and child growth. *Int J Epidemiology* vol. 32, pp. 503–505.
40. Department of women and child development, Government of Uttar Pradesh (GoUP), India, Institute of Applied Statistics and Development (IASDS) and UNICEF (Lucknow). Profile of women and children in Uttar Pradesh, GoUP, 1999.
41. RAMACHANDRAN P (2007). Nutrition transition in India. Nutrition Foundation of India, New Delhi, 2007.
42. National Nutrition monitoring Bureau (2006). Diet and nutritional status of population and prevalence of hypertension amongst adults in rural areas, NIN, ICMR.
43. LEARY S, FALL C, OSMOND C LOVEL H, CAMPBELL D, ERIKSSON J, FORRESTER T, GODFREY K, HILL J, JIE M, LAW C, NEWBY R, ROBINSON S, YAJNIK C (2006). Geographical variation in relationships between parental body size and offspring phenotype at birth. *Acta Obstet Gynaecol* vol. 85, pp. 1066–1079.

44. RAMACHANDRAN P (1989). Nutrition in pregnancy in women and nutrition in India. C. GOPALAN, SUMINDER KAUR (eds). Special publication No. 5. Nutrition Foundation of India, New Delhi.
45. National Nutrition Monitoring Bureau (NNMB) 1979–2006. NNMB Reports. National institute of Nutrition, Hyderabad.
46. GHOSH S, BHARGAVA SK, MADHAVAN S, TASKAR AD, BHARGAVA V and NIZZAM SK. Intrauterine growth of north-Indian babies (1971). *Pediatrics* vol. 47, no. 5, pp. 826–830.
47. BIRKIN NJ, YIP R, FLESHOOD L and TRANSBRIDGE FL (1988). Birthweight and childhood growth. *Pediatrics* vol. 82, no. 6, pp. 824–834.
48. TAMBER B (2006). Seasonality and maternal factors affecting pregnancy an outcome – A study. PhD Thesis, Delhi University.
49. TAFAN N, NAETE RL, GOBEZIE A (1980). Effects of maternal undernutrition and heavy physical workload during pregnancy on birthweight. *Brit J Obstet Gynae* vol. 87, pp. 222–226.
50. RAO S, KANADE A, MARGETTE BM, YAJNIK CS, LUBREE H, REGE S, DESAI B, JACKSON A, FALL CHD (2003). Maternal activity in relation to birth size in rural India. The Pune Maternal Nutrition Study. *Eur J Clin Nutr* vol. 57, pp. 531–542.
51. NOEYE RI and PETERS EC (1982). Working during pregnancy. Effects on foetus. *Pediatrics* vol. 69, pp. 724–727.
52. DINH PH, VUONG TH, HOJER B and PERSSON LA (1996). Maternal factors influencing the occurrence of low birth weight in northern Vietnam. *Ann Trop Pediatr* vol. 16, no. 4, 327–33.
53. Ministry of Health and Population (MDHP), Nepal, New era, macro International Nepal Demographic and Health Survey, 2006, Kathmandu, Ministry of Health and Population, New ERA, and Calverton, Md, USA: Macro International, 2007.
54. National Institute of Population Research and training (NIPORT). Mitra and associates and Macro International, Bangladesh Demographic and Health Survey 2007, Dhaka, National Institute of Population Research and Training, Mitra and associates and Calverton, Md, Macro International 2009.
55. KRAMER M and VICTORIA C (2001). Low birth weight and prenatal mortality: In Semba RD and Bloem M (eds). *Nutrition and Health in Developing Countries.* Humana Press: Totowa.
56. KRAMER MS (2005). Maternal nutrition and adverse pregnancy outcome: lessons from epidemiology. Nestle Nutrition Workshop Series – Paediatric Programme, vol. 55, pp. 1–15. Honstra G, Uauy R and Yang X (eds). In: The Impact of Maternal Nutrition on offspring. Karger: Switzerland.
57. CEESAY SM, PRENTICE AM, COLE TJ, FOORD F, POSKITT EME, WEAVER LT, WHITEHEAD RG (1997). Effects on birth weight and perinatal mortality of maternal dietary supplement in rural Gambia: 5 year randomised trial. *BMJ* vol. 315, pp. 786–790.
58. KRAEMER MS and KAKUMA R (2009). Energy and protein intake in pregnancy (Review). The Cochrane Collaboration published by John Wiley and Sons Ltd, 2009.
59. KUSIN JA, KARDJATI S, HOUTKOOPER JM, RENQVIST UH (1992). Energy supplementation during pregnancy and postnatal growth. *Lancet* vol. 340, pp. 623–626.
60. STEIN AD, BARNHART HX, HICKEY M, RAMAKRISHNAN U, SCHROEDER DG, MARTORELL R (2003). Prospective study of protein energy supplementation early in life and of growth in the subsequent generation in Guatemala. *Am J Clin Nutr* vol. 78, pp. 162–167.
61. MCLEAN E, EGLI I, BENOIST DE, WOJDYLA D (2007). Worldwide prevalence of anemia in preschool aged children, pregnant women and non-pregnant women of

reproductive age. In: Nutritional anaemia. Kraemer K and Zimmerman BMB (eds). Sight and Life Press, 2007.
62. Nutrition Foundation of India. Twenty Five Years Report 1980–2005, New Delhi 2005.
63. WHO (2009). Weekly iron folic acid supplementation in women of reproductive age: its role in promoting optimum maternal and child health. http://www.who.int/
64. BEREGER J, THANH T, CAVALLI-SFORZA T, SMITASIRI S, KHAN NC, MILANI S, HOA PT, QUANG NT, VITERI F (2005). Community mobilisation and social marketing to promote weekly iron–folic acid supplementation in women of reproductive age in Vietnam: impact on anemia and iron stores. *Nutr Rev* vol. 6, pp. S95–S108.
65. RASMUSSEN KM, STOLZFUS RJ (2003). New evidence that iron supplementation during pregnancy improves birth weight: new scientific questions. *AJCN* vol. 78, pp. 673–674.
66. CHRISTIAN P, KHATRY SK, WEST K (2004). Antenatal anti-helminthic treatment, birthweight, infant survival in rural Nepal. *Lancet* vol. 364, pp. 981–983.
67. SHRIMPTON R, HUFFMAN SL, ZEHNER ER, DARNTON-HILL I, DALMIYA N (2009). Multiple micronutrient supplementation during pregnancy in developing country settings. Policy and programme implications of the results of meta-analysis. *FNB* vol. 30, pp. S556–S573.
68. RAMAKRISHNAN U, UUFFMAN SL (2008). Multiple micronutrient malnutrition: What can be done? In: Semba R and Bloem M (eds). *Nutrition and health in Developing Countries*, 2nd edition. Totowa: Humana press.
69. FALL CHD, FISHER DJ, OSMOND C, MARGETTS BM; Maternal micronutrient supplementation study group (MMSSG) (2009). Multiple micronutrient supplementation during pregnancy in low income countries: A meta-analysis of effects on effects on birth size and length of gestation. *FNB* vol. 30, pp. S533–S546.
70. GUPTA P, RAY M, DUA T, RADHAKRISHNAN G, KUMAR R, SACHDEV HPS (2007). Multi-micronutrient supplementation for undernourished pregnant women and birth size of their offspring: A double blind randomised placebo control trail. *Arch Pediatr Adolesec Med* vol. 161, pp. 58–64.
71. TOFAIL F, PERSSON LA, ELARIFEEN S, HAMADONI JD, MEHRIN F, RIDOUT D, EKSTROM EC, HUDNA SN, GRANTHAM-MCGREGOR SM (2008). Effects of prenatal food and micronutrient supplementation in infant development: a randomised trail from the maternal and infant nutrition intervention, Matlab (MINIMat) study. *AJCN* vol. 87, pp. 704–711.
72. HUY ND, HOP LT, SHRIMPTON R, HOA CV, ARTS M (2009). An effectiveness trial of multiple micronutrient supplementation during pregnancy in Vietnam: impact on birth weight and on stunting in children at around 2 years of age. *FNB* vol. 30, pp. S506–S516.
73. VAIDYA A, SAVILLE N, SHRESHTHA BP, COSTELLA AM, MANANDHAR DS, OSRIN D (2008). Effects of antenatal multiple micronutrient supplementation on children's weight and size at 2 years of age in Nepal: follow up of a double blind randomised control trial. *Lancet* vol. 371, pp. 492–499.
74. DALMIYA N, DARNTON-HILL I, SCHULTINK W AND SHRIMPTON R (2009). Multiple micronutrient supplementation during pregnancy: a decade of collaboration in action. *FNB* vol. 30, pp. S477–S479.
75. MARGETTS BM, FALL CHD, RONSMANS C, ALLEN LH, FISHER DJ; the Maternal Micronutrient Supplementation Study Group (MMSSG) (2009). Multiple micronutrient supplementation during pregnancy in low-income countries:

review of methods and characteristics of studies included in the meta-analyses. *Food and Nutrition Bulletin* vol. 30, no. 4, pp. S517–S526.
76. VIR S (1990). Women's nutrition – convergence of programmes, a critical issue. *Indian Journal of Maternal and Child Health* vol. 1, no. 3, p. 74.
77. ZULFI QAR A BHUTTA, TAHMEED AHMED, ROBERT E BLACK, SIMON COUSENS, KATHRYN DEWEY, ELSA GIUGLIANI, BATOOL A HAIDER, BETTY KIRKWOOD, SAUL S MORRIS, H P S SACHDEV, MEERA SHEKAR, for the Maternal and Child Undernutrition Study Group.
78. DFID (2010). The neglected crisis of undernutrition: DFID's strategy.
79. DE ONIS (2003). WHO Global database on child growth and malnutrition, methodology and applications. *Int J Epidemiology* vol. 32, pp. 518–526.
80. RUEL MT (2008). Addressing the underlying determinants of undernutrition: examples of successful integration of nutrition in poverty reduction and agriculture strategies. *SCN News* vol. 36, pp. 21–29.
81. HODDINOT J and HADDAD L (1994). Woman's income and boy girl anthropometric status in the Coto d'voire. *World Development* vol. 22, no. 4, pp. 543–553.
82. KATZ E (1994). The impact of non-traditional export agriculture on income and food availability in Guatemala: an intrahousehold perspective. *FNB* vol. 15, no. 4.
83. QUISUMBING A (2003). Household decisions, gender and development. A synthesis of recent research. IFPRI: Washington DC / Johns Hopkins University Press: Baltimore, MD.
84. LEV S (2006). Progress against poverty. Sustaining Mexico's PROGRESSA – opportunities program. Booking Institution Press: Washington DC.
85. KHAN NC, HOP LH, TUYEN LD, KHOI HH, SON TH, DUONG PH (2008). A national action plan to stunting reduction in Vietnam. *SCN News* vol. 36, pp. 31–37.

4

Dual nutrition burden in women: causes, consequences, and control measures

Prema Ramachandran

Prema Ramachandran, MD in Obstetrics and Gynaecology, is currently the Director of Nutrition Foundation of India. She was an advisor with the Planning Commission (Health, Nutrition and Family Welfare) for nine years and gave the lead to prepare the drafts for the Ninth and Tenth Plan chapters on these sectors. Prior to joining the Planning Commission. Dr Ramachandran was with the Indian Council of Medical Research (ICMR) for 25 years, carrying out clinical and operational research studies on health and nutrition services.

4.1 Introduction

Women especially pregnant and lactating women, form one of the most vulnerable segments of the population from nutritional point of view. Numerous studies in India and elsewhere have shown that in chronically undernourished women, subsisting on unchanged low dietary intake, pregnancy and lactation have an adverse effect on maternal nutritional status. Maternal undernutrition is associated with low birth weight and all its attendant adverse consequences. Epidemiological studies from India during seventies and eighties documented the magnitude and adverse consequences of chronic energy deficiency (CED) on the mother–child dyad and paved way for intervention programmes to address undernutrition during pregnancy and lactation. "Too early, too close, too many and too late" pregnancies adversely affect nutrition and health status of the mother–child dyad. Timely contraceptive care has become an indirect effective intervention to prevent deterioration in maternal and child nutrition. Yet another important indirect cause of undernutrition continues to be infections. Undernutrition increases the susceptibility to infections – infections aggravate undernutrition. While undernutrition continues to be a major problem as in the earlier decades, the current decade has witnessed the progressive rise in overnutrition in women during reproductive age especially among the affluent segments of population both in urban and rural areas and associated increase in the prevalence of non-communicable diseases. A review of the available data on the quantum of under and overnutrition in women, the factors responsible for the emerging problem of dual burden of malnutrition, health hazards associated with it, prevention, early detection and effective management of dual nutrition burden in women is presented.

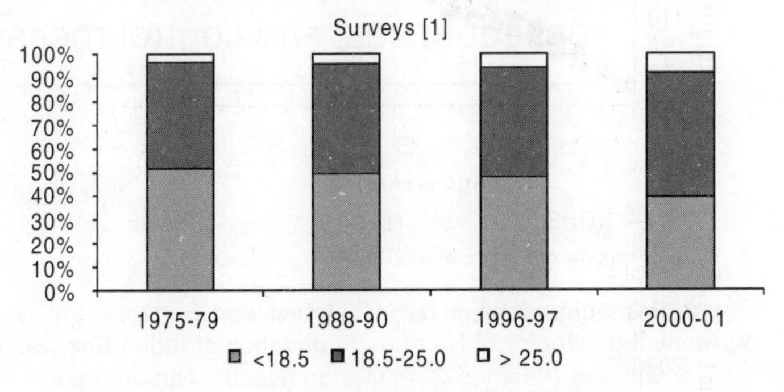

4.1 Time trends in nutritional status of women [1].

4.2 Emergence of dual nutrition burden in India

Data from the National Nutrition Monitoring Bureau (NNMB) on nutritional status of rural women as assessed by BMI over the last three decades is shown in Fig. 4.1. It is obvious that over this period there has been a reduction in undernutrition and increase in the prevalence of overnutrition.

Data NNMB rural surveys on time trends in weight, height and triceps fat fold thickness in all age groups in females is shown in Figs. 4.2, 4.3, and 4.4, respectively. In rural population there is an increase of about three cms in adult height while the increase in body weight over the period is much greater. This increase in body weight is mainly due to fat deposition as apparent from the progressive increase in the fat fold thickness over this period. The increase in fat fold thickness begins in childhood.

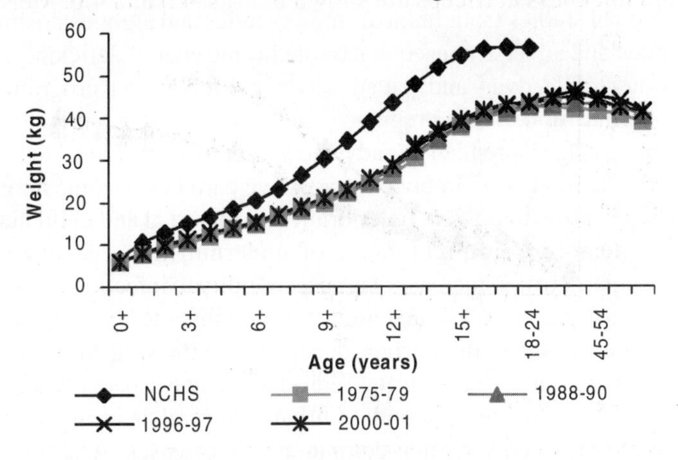

4.2 Time Trends in mean weights in rural women [1].

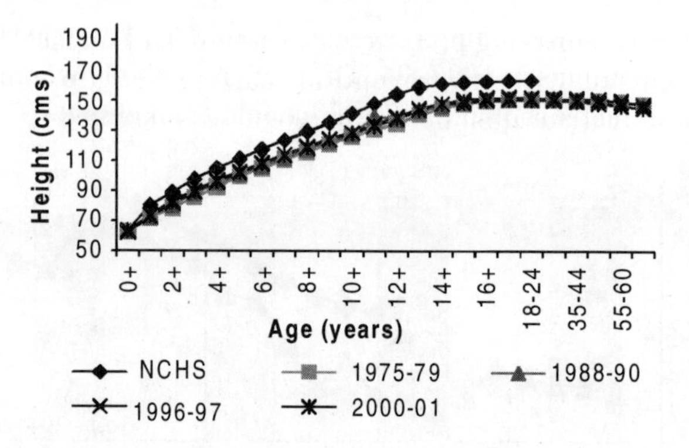

4.3 Time Trends in mean heights in rural women [1].

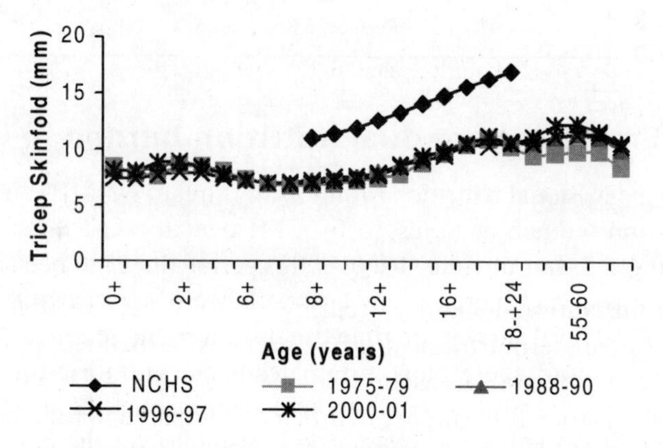

4.4 Time Trends in mean tricep fatfold in rural women [1].

Data from NNMB surveys in urban slums on time trends in weight and fat fold thickness at triceps are shown in Figs. 4.5 and 4.6. Mean body

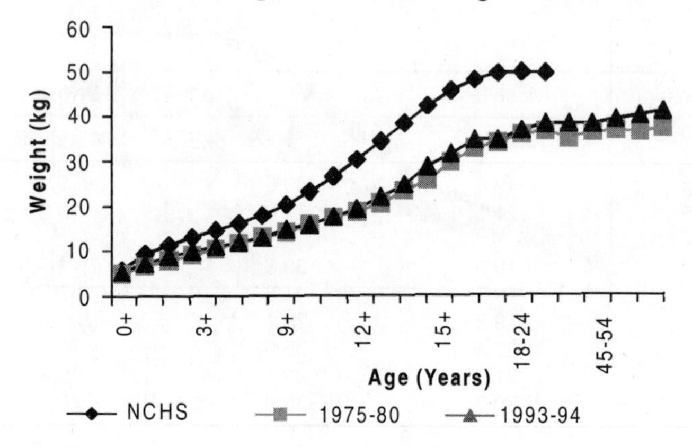

4.5 Time Trends in mean weights in Urban women [1].

weight, mid upper arm circumference and fat fold thickness at triceps were higher in all age groups in 1993–94. The increase in body weight is mainly due to increase fat as shown by rising fat fold thickness.

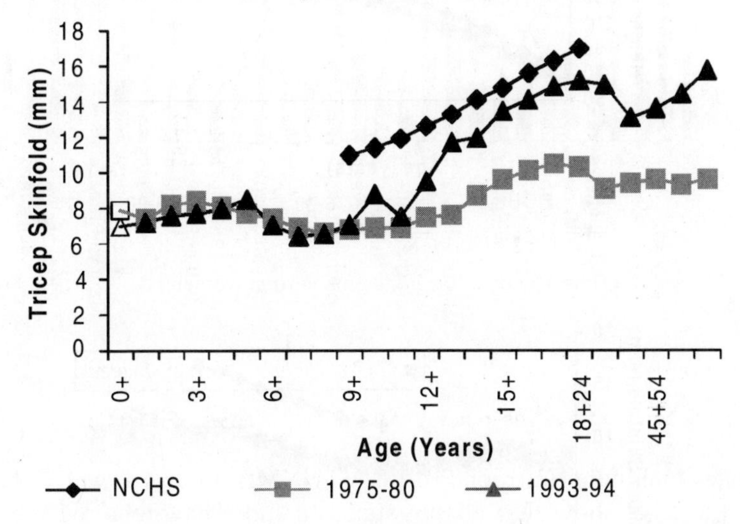

4.6 Time Trends in mean triceps fatfold thickness in Urban women [1].

Data from National Family Health Survey-2 [2] indicates that the prevalence of undernutrition in urban areas is half of the prevalence of undernutrition in rural areas in 1998–1999 (Table 4.1). Prevalence of overnutrition is four-folds higher in urban as compared to rural areas. There is a progressive decline in the prevalence of undernutrition and progressive increase in the prevalence of overnutrition in adult women with increase in age. Data from NFHS-3 show that prevalence of both under and overnutrition in women is higher than men [3].

Table 4.1 Prevalence of undernutrition and overnutrition among women [5, 5–45]

Characteristic	Mean BMI	BMI < 18.5	BMI □ 25
	1998–99	1998–99	1998–99
Rural	19.6	40.6	5.9
Urban	21.1	22.6	23.5
Age			
15–19	19.3	38.8	1.7
20–24	19.3	41.8	3.6
25–29	19.8	39.1	7.3
30–34	20.4	35.0	11.7
35–49	21.1	31.1	16.8
All	20.3	35.8	10.6

Interstate differences in dual nutrition burden

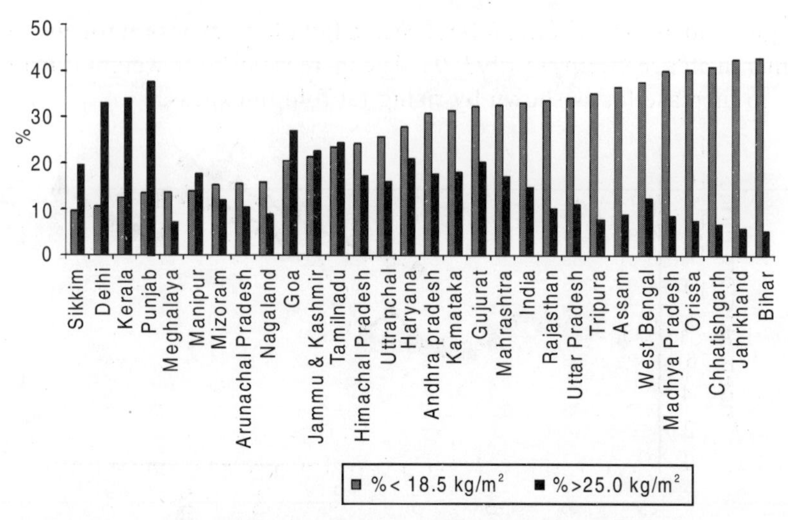

4.7 Interstate differences in nutritional status of women NFHS-3 [6].

Data from India Nutrition Profile and NNMB surveys as well as NFHS data [2, 3, 4] show that all the states in India have entered the dual nutrition burden era but there are substantial interstate differences in prevalence of under and overnutrition (Figure 4.7). Populous states like Uttar Pradesh, Bihar, Madhya Pradesh, Rajasthan and Orissa have high undernutrition and low overnutrition rates. States like Delhi, Punjab has low undernutrition and high overnutrition rates. However, states like Goa, Tamil Nadu and Himachal Pradesh have relatively high undernutrition and overnutrition rates.

4.3 Nutritional status of pregnant and lactating women

4.3.1 Dietary intake in pregnant and lactating women

Data between 1975 and 2006 from NNMB and Indian Nutrition Profile (INP) surveys [5] (using 24-hour dietary recall method) show that between 1975 and 1995 there has been some increase in dietary intake. By the mid-nineties average intake of cereals almost met the RDA. However, data of early 2000 indicates a reduction in cereal intake inspite of the fact that cereals are available, accessible and affordable. There has been a progressive reduction in the pulse intake, which might be related to the rise in the cost of pulses. Intake of vegetables and fruits continue to be low (Table 4.2). Dietary intake of pregnant and lactating women is not different from that of the non-pregnant and non-lactating women (NPNL).

Table 4.2 Time trends in dietary intake (g/day) in pregnant and lactating women [1]

Groups	Year	Cereals and millets	Pulses and legumes	Milk and milk products	GLV's	Roots and tubers	Other vegetables	Fruits	Fats and oil	Sugar and jaggery
Non-pregnant and non-lactating women	1975–79	386	31	56	11	51	47	11	9	16
	1996–97	434	29	72	16	53	49	24	13	21
	2000–01	389	26	67	18	69	50	20	12	16
	2005–06	365	27	80	18	63	52	26	13	14
Pregnant women	1975–79	359	34	75	12	58	44	11	12	19
	1996–97	463	29	70	17	34	42	26	12	15
	2000–01	408	28	77	15	69	44	21	12	17
	2005–06	362	27	87	16	55	49	25	14	14
Lactating women	1975–79	436	30	58	15	48	45	13	10	16
	1996–97	518	34	67	11	43	42	34	13	19
	2000–01	442	28	65	18	69	54	24	13	13
	2005–06	406	30	80	17	63	56	24	14	13

Nutrient intake in pregnant and lactating women over the last three decades is presented in Table 4.3. Between 1975 and 1996 there was an increase in the total energy, protein and fat intake. However, over the last decade there has been a reduction in the energy intake. This might be due to the increasingly sedentary lifestyle in majority of the population and consequent reduction in energy requirement. In each of the four periods of time there is no difference in nutrient intake of pregnant and lactating women and non-pregnant, non-lactating (NPNL). All these data clearly indicate that in India women do not consume more food during pregnancy and lactation.

Table 4.3 Time trends in nutrient intake in non-pregnant non-lactating (NPNL) and pregnant and lactating women (NNMB) [1]

Groups	Years	Protein (g)	Total fat (g)	Energy (kcal)	Calcium (mg)	Iron (mg)	Vitamin A (µg)	Thiamin (mg)	Riboflavin (mg)	Niacin (mg)	Vitamin C (mg)
NPNL women	1975–79	45.4	17.1	1698	330	21.0	118.0	1.00	0.70	11.0	24
	1996–97	49.9	24.5	1983	382	22.0	148.0	0.90	0.80	12.0	32
	2000–01	48.2	27.6	1878	445	14.1	219.8	1.20	0.60	14.9	45
	2005–06	46.5	21.8	1738	443	13.8	254.0	1.10	0.60	14.2	47
Pregnant Women	1975–79	40.8	18.8	1597	390	20.0	160.0	1.00	0.60	10.0	21
	1996–97	47.2	21.5	1994	339	23.0	142.0	0.90	0.80	11.0	28
	2000–01	49.7	25.9	1933	463	14.0	227.0	1.20	0.70	15.1	45
	2005–06	46.8	22.5	1726	456	14.0	261.0	1.10	0.60	13.7	42
Lactating Women	1975–79	47.6	18.3	1797	358	23.0	133.0	1.10	0.70	12.0	23
	1996–97	56.5	24.6	2243	373	23.0	162.0	1.10	0.90	14.0	29
	2000–01	50.3	25.9	2028	408	14.6	212.0	1.30	0.60	16.3	48
	2005–06	49.6	22.1	1878	447	14.7	249.0	1.20	0.60	15.5	46

Studies carried out at National Institute of Nutrition, Hyderabad, in late seventies [6] showed that there was a socio-economic gradient in dietary intake in majority of women. In all the three groups, dietary intake was not higher in pregnant women as compared to non-pregnant women from the same income group. The low income group women weighed 10 kg less than high income group of women and the birth weight of the offspring was only 2.7 kg (Table 4.4). Women from the upper income group consumed 2000 to 2500 kcal per day during pregnancy. In middle and high income groups, pregnant women do not perform hard physical labour during pregnancy and there was reduction in physical activity during pregnancy. The pre-pregnancy weight in this population group ranged between 45-55 kg and pregnancy weight gain was 11 kg. The mean birth weight of infants was 3.1 kg (Table 4.4).These data suggest that among habitually well-nourished women who eat to appetite, there is no increase in dietary intake during pregnancy; unchanged dietary intake did not have any adverse effect either on their own nutritional status or on the course and outcome of pregnancy.

Table 4.4 Effect of socio-economic status on maternal nutrition [63]

	No. (N)	Age (years)	Parity	Height (cm)	Weight (kg)	Hb (g/dl)	Birth weight (kg)
Low income	1468	24.1	2.41	151.5	45.7	10.9	2.7
Middle income	108	24.3	1.61	156.3	49.9	11.1	2.9
High income	63	27.8	1.61	156.3	56.2	12.4	3.13

Studies carried out by National Institute of Nutrition (NIN) during the seventies and early eighties [6] confirmed that among urban and rural low-income group population in Hyderabad, there was no increase in dietary intake during pregnancy and lactation. Dietary intake ranged from 1200 to 1800 kcal per day. Pregnant women continued to look after the household and

Table 4.5 Changes in anthropometric indices during pregnancy [6]

	Weight (kg)	Arm circumference (cm)	FFT (Fat fold thickness) (mm)
NPNL	42.3	22.5	10.5
1st trimester	41.5	22.2	9.6
2nd trimester	44.6	22.1	9.7
3rd trimester	46	21.7	9.2

other activities and remained moderately active throughout pregnancy. These women weighed an average 43 kg prior to pregnancy and gained 6 kg during pregnancy. There was however a reduction in fat fold thickness (FFT) during pregnancy suggesting that the fat was getting mobilised to meet the gap in energy requirement (Table 4.5). There was no obvious deterioration in the maternal nutritional status during pregnancy or following repeated pregnancies provided the inter birth interval is longer than 24 months.

4.3.2 Factor associated with deterioration of maternal nutritional status

Studies from India and other developing countries have shown that reduction in dietary intake below habitual levels or increased workload above the habitual levels were associated with deterioration in maternal nutritional status and reduction in birth weight. Some readily identifiable situations associated with deterioration in maternal nutritional status and reduction in birth weight are

- reduction in habitual dietary intake (during drought and the pre-harvest season),
- increase in work (e.g., newly inducted manual laborers),
- combination of both the above (food for work programmes) during drought,
- adolescent pregnancy,
- pregnancy in lactating women,
- short inter-pregnancy interval and
- infections during pregnancy.

Effect of work status

There is a progressive increase in women's participation in labor force partly due to economic reasons. The economic returns are sometimes essential for improving the dietary intake of the family but the dual burden of work at home and at the work place has resulted in some deterioration in maternal nutrition status as indicated by body weight (Figure 4.8).

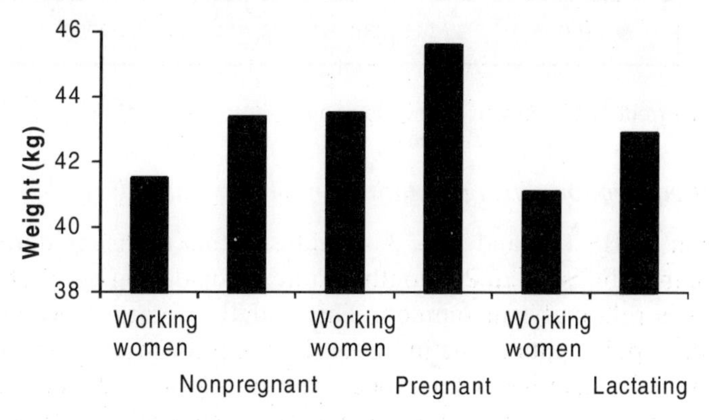

4.8 Nutritional Status of Rural Women (Low Income) [6].

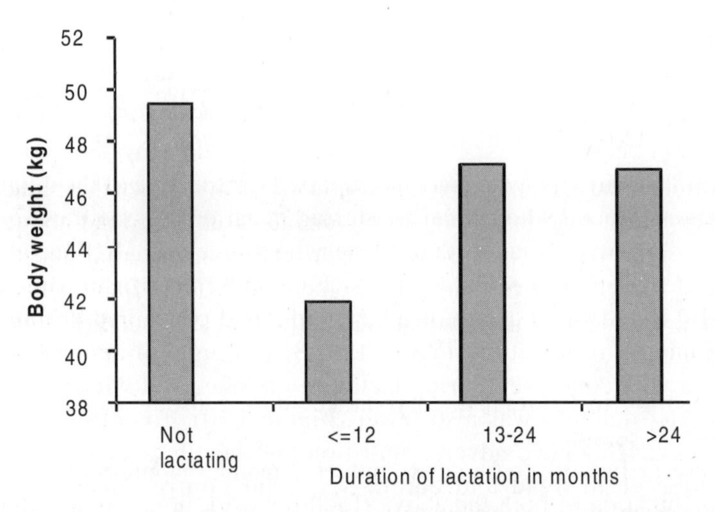

4.9 Weight of pregnant women who concieved during lactation [6].

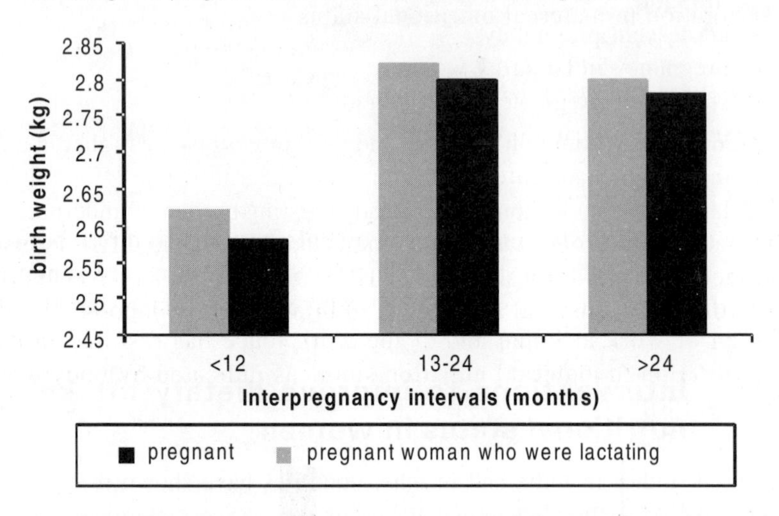

4.10 Effect of conception during lactation on birth weight of infants.

Effect of conception during lactation on mother-child dyad

Data from NFHS 1, 2 and 3 [2, 3, 4] indicate that the mean duration of lactation in India is about 24 months. Conception during the first year of lactation is relatively uncommon. This usually occurs in women who introduce supplements to the infant early, i.e. prior to six months. Most conceptions in lactating women occur during the second and third year of lactation. Studies on dietary intake of women who had conceived during lactation have shown that their dietary intake is essentially similar to the dietary intake of non-pregnant women from similar income groups.

The average calorie intake is no more than 1200–1800 kcal/day, and is inadequate with respect to all the nutrients. The dual stress of pregnancy and lactation widens the already existing gap between dietary intakes and nutrient requirements. Investigations undertaken by the National Institute of Nutrition, Hyderabad, has reported irrespective of the duration of lactation, women who conceived during lactation weighed less in all the trimesters of pregnancy than those who conceived after lactation. The difference in body weight was more marked in the third trimester, especially in the small group of women who had conceived during the first six months of lactation (Figure 4.9). Birth weight of neonates born to women who conceived during lactation or conceived within first 12 months after delivery was also lower (Figure 4.10). Too close and too many pregnancies have adverse nutrition and health consequences on the mother–child dyad and emphasizes that contraceptive care at appropriate time is an indirect but effective intervention to prevent deterioration in maternal nutritional status.

Infections and undernutrition

Morbidity due to common bacterial and viral infections are higher in under nourished women and infections aggravate undernutrition. HIV infection is a relatively new addition to the already existing burden of undernutrition associated with chronic wasting infections like TB. Maternal HIV infection and mother to child transmission of HIV infection has an adverse effect on birth weight, survival and growth in infancy and childhood.

4.4 Interventions to improve dietary intake and nutritional status in women

Research studies in India and in other countries have shown that pregnant women with reduction in habitual dietary intake or excess energy expenditure or whose body weight is less than 40 kg are identified and given adequate continuous food supplementation and antenatal care and so there is substantial improvement in the outcome of pregnancy, birth weight and neonatal mortality. Encouraged by such data, India has included food supplementation for pregnant and lactating women under Integrated Child Development Services (ICDS) programme who come to *anganwadis.* The reported coverage is between 15% and 20% in most ICDS projects. Unfortunately, ICDS programme does not screen pregnant women for undernutrition or provide adequate, continuous supplements to those with energy gap or those with moderate/severe undernutrition. In ICDS programme, improvement in nutritional status and its impact on maternal nutrition and birth weight is very limited. Since food supplements are provided to pregnant and lactating women without screening, identifying undernourished women, and special efforts for ensuring continued supplementation and monitoring compliance.

One of the major problems is to ensure that food supplements reach the undernourished women. Even when the logistics of reaching the food to women is meticulously worked out and efficiently carried out, food sharing patterns within the family results in the 'target' women not getting significant quantities of the supplements. Obviously this is another important factor responsible for the demonstrated lack of beneficial effect. The lack of adequate antenatal care and continued physical work during pregnancy are two other factors responsible for the lack of impact.

The Tenth Five Year Plan of Government of India envisaged that efforts will be made to weigh all women as early as possible in pregnancy and monitor their weight gain. Well nourished women will be advised not to increase their dietary intake to prevent overnutrition and obesity. Pregnant women who weigh less than 40 kg will be identified and

- given food supplements consistently throughout pregnancy,
- given adequate antenatal care,
- monitored for weight gain during pregnancy and
- If weight gain is sub-optimal, efforts have to be made to identify the causes and attempt remedial measures.

Effective inter-sectoral coordination between auxiliary nurse midwives (ANMs), ASHAs and ICDS frontline workers (anganwadi workers or AWW) will enable the identification of undernourished pregnant and lactating women and provision of appropriate care to them. The *panchayti raj institutions* (PRIs) can play an important role by ensuring that these women receive food supplement throughout pregnancy.

During the Tenth Five Year Plan, a pilot project on food grain supplementation to under nourished, pregnant and lactating women was initiated in 51 backward districts in the country. Evaluation of this programme indicated that there was community acceptance of the idea that pregnant and lactating women should be weighed and undernourished persons identified on the basis of body weight should be given 6 kg of food grains free of cost every month until delivery or first year of lactation is completed. The AWWs were able to carry out weighing and identification of undernourished women. Families were able to have an access to grains in most cases. Inspite of food sharing most of these women gained weight.

The National Rural Health Mission (NRHM) envisages that on the village health and nutrition days, the ANM and AWW will work together and provide the required health and nutrition care. They will identify pregnant women with body weight less than 45 kg and lactating women with body weight less than 40 kg and give them food supplementation on priority. Prevention, detection and management of anemia will also receive the attention it deserves. It is expected that if effectively implemented, this strategy can bring about substantial improvement in maternal nutritional status in pregnancy and lactation.

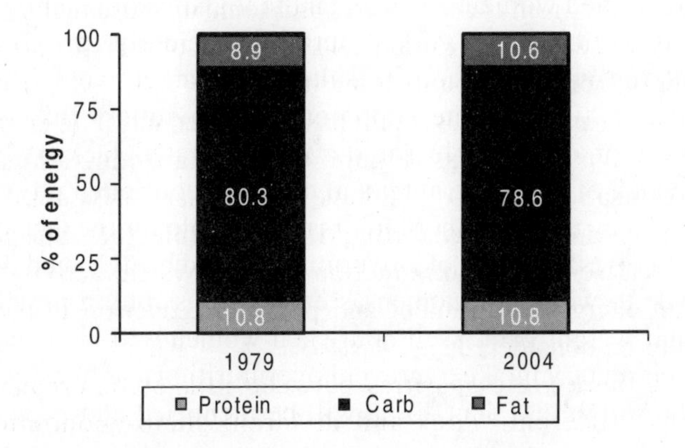

4.11 Contribution of nutrients to energy intake [1].

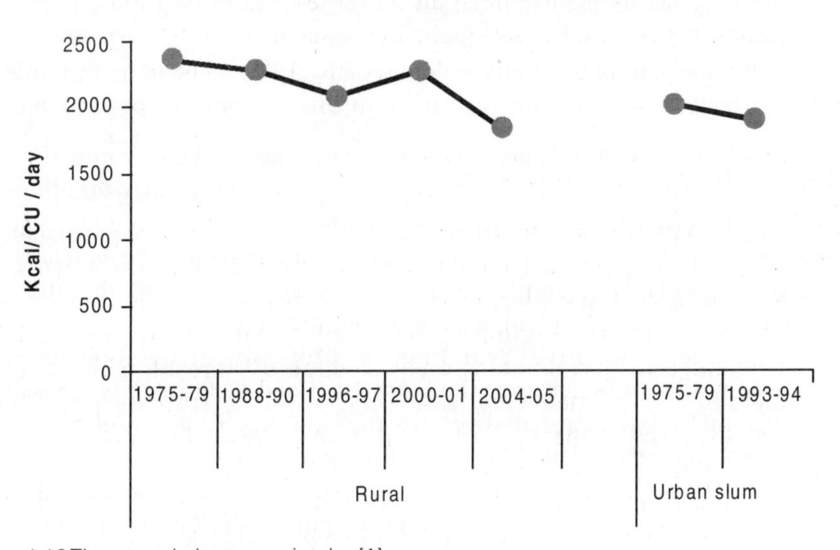

4.12 Time trends in energy intake [1].

4.5 Factors responsible for the emerging problem of overnutrition

4.5.1 Changes in dietary intake

Data on time trends in nutrient intake are available from surveys conducted by the NNMB [1] is presented in Figs. 4.11 and 4.12. There has been some decline in intake of most of the nutrients both in urban and rural areas over the last three decades. Energy intake is lower in urban areas in spite of higher intake of fats and oils because of lower cereal intake. Over the past three decades there have been a reduction in the percentage of total energy intake from carbohydrates and some increase in the percentage of dietary energy from fats (Figure 4.11). In spite of this, the proportion of dietary energy from fat remains lower than 15%.

Over the last three decades, there has been a reduction in energy intake both in urban and rural areas (Figure 4.12). Data from National Sample Survey Organisation (NSSO) [7] have shown that this is not due to lack of access to food or affordability. It is possible that the perceptive population realises that with reduction of the physical activity there is a reduction in energy requirement and possibly reduction in their energy intake has to be considered.

However, there are disparities between intakes of urban and rural populations, different states and different socio-economic groups. Among the affluent segments of population especially in urban and peri-urban areas, there has been an increase in the fast food and soft drink consumption and consequent increase in empty calorie intake. This coupled with increasingly sedentary life style has been responsible for the steep increase in overnutrition in this segment of population.

4.5.2 Physical activity

Physical activity is one of the major determinants of energy requirement. Physiologists recognize four domain of physical activity – work, domestic, transport and discretionary. Until two decades ago in most developing countries including India, physical activity in work, domestic and transport domains was very high. As a result majority of the population expended very little energy in discretionary physical activity. Because of the high physical activity level in daily chores, majority of the population were moderately active and hence their energy requirement was that of a moderately active population. They enjoyed the health benefits of moderate physical activity without any discretionary physical activity (Figure 4.13).

The last two decades witnessed significant changes in lifestyle. The availability of transport both personal and public has improved several folds (Figure 4.14) and energy expenditure in reaching places of study/work has become a fraction of what it was two decades ago. NSSO consumption expenditure surveys have shown steep increase in expenditure on transport confirming the trend of increasing use of mechanized transport. Better access to water and fuel both in urban and rural have resulted in substantial reduction in energy spent by women on collecting water and fuel.

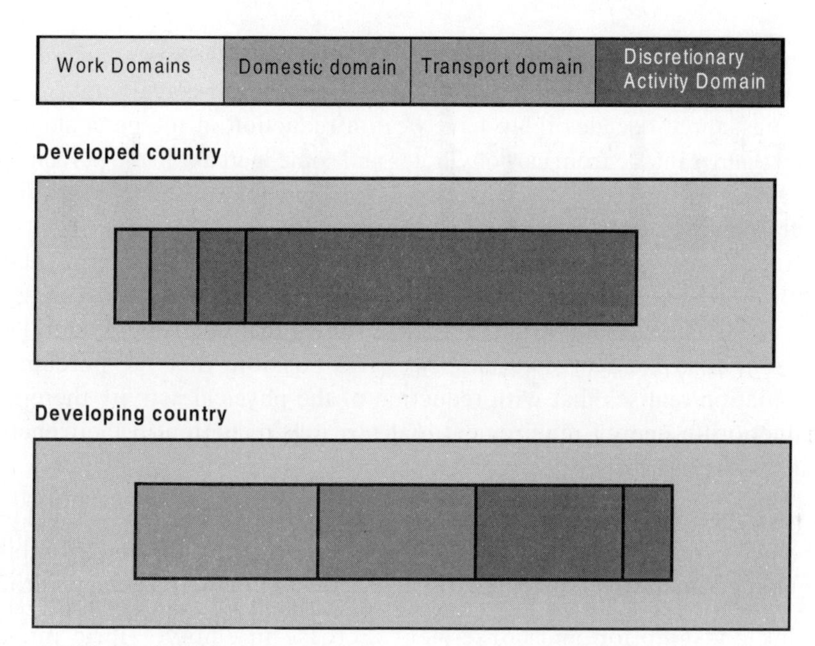

4.13 Physical activity: domain [13].

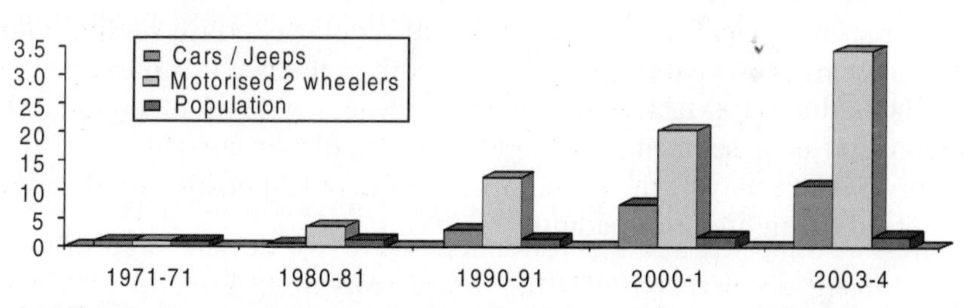

4.14 Relative increase in the production of vehicles and the population [8].

During the last decade some well-planned studies investigating physical activity pattern in urban and rural areas and in different income group have been initiated. The PURE India study documented level of mechanization for transport and domestic activities in urban and rural areas (Table 4.6). It is obvious that in urban areas, transport as well as household activity is highly mechanized. Majority of urban population are working in white or blue-collar jobs, where occupation related physical activity levels are low. As a result even though urban women spend time in domestic and occupation related activities, their energy expenditure for these activities is low (Figure 4.14). Their discretionary activities are TV viewing, computer games etc with very low energy expenditure. Unchanged dietary intake reduced physical activity and consequent energy requirement is responsible for positive energy balance and increase in overnutrition in the population.

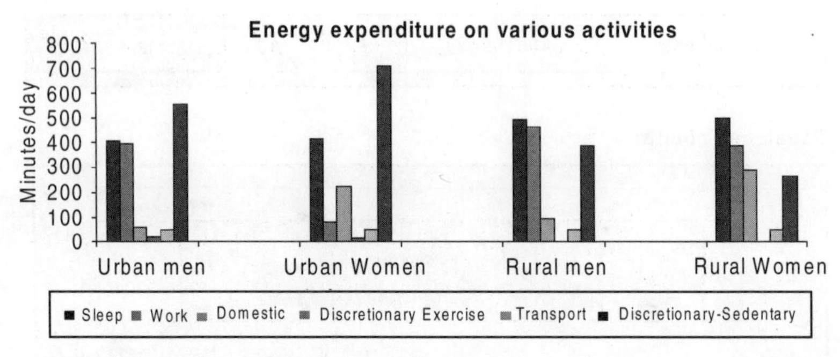

4.15 Energy expenditure on various activities [9].

4.5.3 Energy balance studies in urban-affluent population

Cross-sectional studies undertaken among affluent housewives [11] in the age group of 30–70 years in Delhi showed that their dietary intake remained unaltered between 2100 and 2300 kcal/day. In each age group the energy expenditure was lower by about 70–100 kcal/day [10]. This positive energy balance was associated with a weight gain of about 5 kg per decade (Table 4.7). These women did not make any conscious effort to increase physical activity nor take up regular exercise regime until they were over 60 years of age or had health problems. It is possible that similar situation exists among men in these segments of population. Among affluent segments of population, small but persistent positive energy balance may be the most important factor responsible for the slow but steady weight gain in adults.

Table 4.6 Level of mechanization in urban and rural populations (% household ownership) [9]

	Rural	Urban
Monthly household income (Rs)	1860	12674
Transport		
Motorized two-wheelers	7.9	78.2
Car	0.2	12.2
Household appliances		
Washing machine	0.1	41.4
Kitchen mixer/blender	4.5	95.2
Leisure		
Television	24.9	98.2

Table 4.7 Energy intake and expenditure in urban affluent housewives [10]

Groups	Weight (Kg)	BMI (kg/m²)	BF%	TDEI (kcal)	TDEE (Kcal/day)	Energy Balance (Kcal)	Measured RMR (kcal/day)	Parrmer (TDEE/ measured RMR)
D3 (30–39 years) [n=22]	59	24.8	32.8	2,134	2056±238.7 1724.5–2665.5)	+78	1562± 260 (1166–2059)	1.33±0.14 (1.12–1.59)
D4 (40–49 years) [n=20]	64	26.4	36.5	2,264	2191±306.6 (1785.4–2817.3)	+73	1779± 273 (1267–2304)	1.24±0.10 (1.10–1.49)
D5 (50–59 years) [n=20]	69	28.6	40.3	2,195	2146±173.1 (1849.4–2494.0)	+49	1752± 274 (1224–2203)	1.24±0.12 (1.06–1.51)
D6 (60–69 years) [n=14]	66	29.3	44.0	2,065	1971±118.4 (1770.0–2144.3)	+94	1457 ±154 (1224–1742)	1.36±0.14 (1.16–1.69)
D7 (70–88 years) [n=07]	56	24.5	38.5	1562	1736±162.8 (1553.0–2012.0)	?174	1292± 108 (1152–1454)	1.35±0.14 (1.15–1.52)

TDEI – Total Daily Energy Intake
TDEE – Total daily Energy Expenditure
BF – Body Fat
RMR – Resting Metabolic Rate

4.6 Undernutrition – overnutrition linkages

The seeds for obesity in adult life might be sown decades earlier. The thrifty gene hypothesis proposes that populations who had faced energy scarcity over millennia may evolve, so that majority has thrifty gene which conserves energy. If this population gets adequate or excess energy intake, they lay down fat, develop abdominal obesity, increased insulin resistance, which may progress to diabetes and incur risk of hypertension and CVD. Barker's thrifty phenotype hypothesis shifts the evolution of thriftiness to intrauterine period. Indians with one-third low birth weight rate can be deemed to have acquired the risk of metabolic syndrome in utero. Bhargava and co-workers [11] have shown that in urban Delhi during the nineties, even low middle-income adults who were undernourished in infancy, childhood and adolescence, develop obesity, both general and abdominal. About one-sixth of this cohort suffers from impaired glucose tolerance and hypertension at the age of 30 (Table 4.8 and 4.9).

Table 4.8 Time trends in nutritional status of Delhi cohort [11].

	Male		Female	
Age	No.	Weight (kg)	No.	Weight (kg)
At birth	803	2.89±0.44	561	2.79±0.38
2 yrs	834	10.3±1.3	609	9.8±1.2
12 yrs	867	30.9±5.9	625	32.2±6.7
30 yrs	886	71.8±14.0	640	59.2±13.4

Table 4.9 Current status of Delhi cohort [11]

Characteristic	Men		Women	
	No.	Value	No.	Value
Weight (Kg.)	886	71.8±14.0	640	59.2±13.4
Height (m)	886	1.70±0.06	638	1.55±0.06
BMI	886	24.9±4.3	638	24.6±5.1
Waist–hip ratio	886	0.92±0.06	639	0.82±0.07
BMI ≥ 25	886	47.4	638	45.5
BMI ≥ 23	886	66.0	638	61.8
Central Obesity (percent)	886	65.5	639	31
Impaired GTT	849	16	539	14

The lesson to be learnt from these data is that it is never too early for Indians to start practicing healthy lifestyle and dietary habits. Early detection and correction of undernutrition until children attain appropriate weight for their height is essential to promote linear growth. Adolescents and adults should consume balanced diet with just adequate energy intake. Exercise has to become a part of daily routine to promote muscle/bone health and prevent development of adiposity in all age groups.

4.6.1 Health consequences of overnutrition

It is well documented that Indians have higher body fat for the same BMI as compared to the Caucasians. Prevalence of abdominal obesity is higher in Indians. Both overnutrition and abdominal obesity are associated with increased risk of hypertension, diabetes and CVD. Nutrition Foundation of India carried out studies exploring relationship between overnutrition, hypertension and biochemical changes associated with increased risk of cardiovascular diseases in persons belonging to different income groups

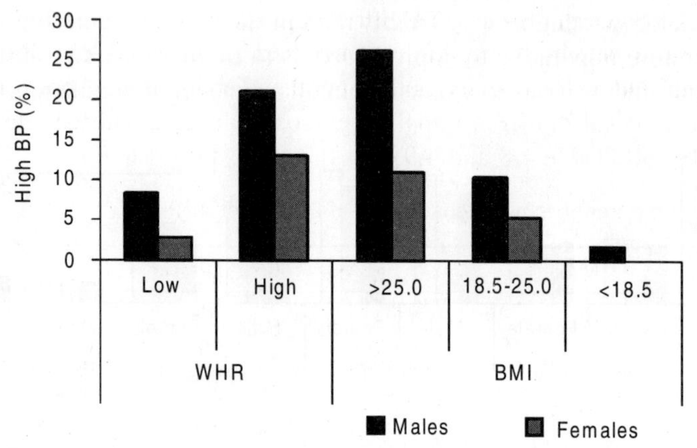

4.16 Overnutrition and hypertension High BP (%) [12].

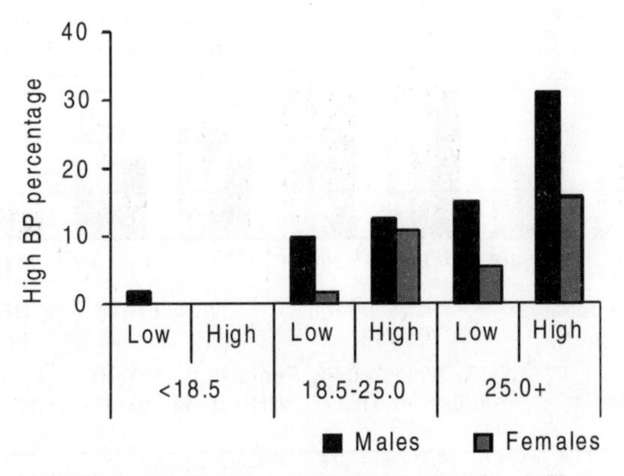

4.17 Abdominal adiposity and hypertension [12].

working in a government institution. Prevalence of abdominal adiposity (high waist–hip ratio (WHR)) was higher in subjects (50.3%) as compared to overnutrition (BMI>25; 30.8%). The higher the BMI and WHR, the higher were the prevalence rates of hypertension both in men and women (Figure 4.16). The prevalence of high blood pressure in the normal and overweight subjects was higher when WHR was high. Overweight/obese subjects of both sexes with abdominal adiposity had higher systolic and diastolic blood pressure as compared to those without abdominal obesity (Figure 4.16).

Blood glucose, serum cholesterol and triglycerides were significantly higher in subjects with BMI>25 (Figure 4.17) and higher WHR (Figure 4.18). A cluster of risk factors has been demonstrated to be associated with central obesity. These include glucose intolerance, obesity, hyperinsulinemia, hypertriglyceridemia, and hypertension, all of which are important risk factors for ischamic heart disease. Poor access to health care for non-communicable diseases among poorer segments of population (especially in women) might be associated with higher case fatality rates in all non-communicable diseases. It is therefore imperative to improve access to essential health care for non-communicable diseases to women from all segments of population.

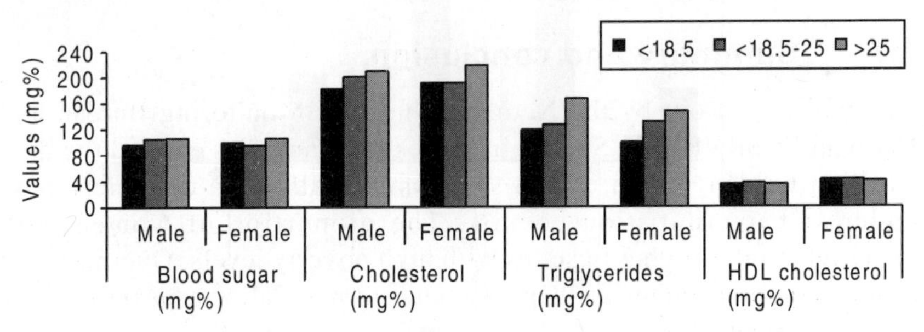

4.18 Effect of BMI on Biochemical Parameters [12].

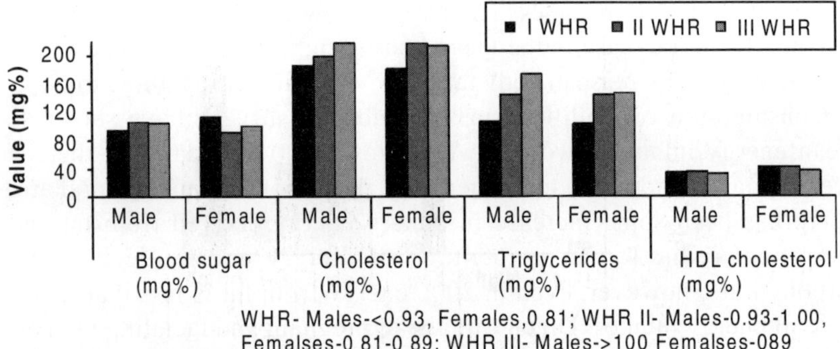

4.19 Effect of WHR on Biochemical Parameters [12].

4.6.2 Interventions to reduce overnutrition

Currently overnutrition rate in India is relatively low. It is imperative that vigorous efforts are made to ensure that further escalation in overnutrition does not occur. Sustained increase in physical activity especially discretionary physical activity is the major intervention required to combat emerging problem of overnutrition in women. The lifestyle changes that have led to steep reduction in physical activity have occurred mainly in the last decade. The urban elite among whom overnutrition rates are the highest have become aware of the need for increasing physical activity, it is likely that further escalation in overnutrition rates might be prevented. Currently, overnutrition rates in rural areas are low. Appropriate steps will have to be taken to generate awareness about the need for sustained high physical activity so that overnutrition rates continue to remain low.

Among the segments of population who are indulging in junk food eating, well directed nutrition education messages may help to bring about healthy eating habits. It is essential that these messages have to be repeated; efforts have to be made to provide to support them during the difficulties they experience in breaking the junk food habit.

4.7 Summary and conclusion

Surveys carried out by the National Nutrition Monitoring Bureau and National Family Health Survey indicates that India has entered the dual nutrition burden era. In all the states and in all strata of society both under and overnutrition coexist. The proportion of women with undernutrition is higher in states with high poverty levels. Overnutrition is more common among affluent segments of population especially those living in urban areas.

Over the last three decades there has been 2–4 cm increase in mean height and significant increase in the mean body weight. Increase in body weight is mostly due to increase in body fat as shown by increase fat fold thickness.

Consumption expenditure surveys and diet surveys have shown that mean energy intake in women well below 2000 kcal/day and there has been a small reduction in total energy intake in both urban and rural areas. There has been some increase in dietary energy derived from fat and a reciprocal reduction in percentage of dietary energy derived from carbohydrate; however, even in 2006 energy from fat is less than 15% of over all energy intakes. Dietary intake of pregnant and lactating women is similar to dietary intake of non-pregnant and non-lactating women. There is no deterioration in maternal nutrition with pregnancy and lactation provided inter pregnancy interval is over 2 years.

Reduction in dietary intake below habitual levels or increased workload above the habitual levels is associated with deterioration in maternal nutritional status and reduction in birth weight. Some readily identifiable situations associated with deterioration in maternal nutritional status and reduction in birth weight are

- reduction in habitual dietary intake (during drought and the pre-harvest season),
- increase in work (e.g., newly inducted manual laborers),
- combination of both the above (food for work programmes) during drought,
- adolescent pregnancy,
- pregnancy in lactating women,
- short inter-pregnancy interval, and
- infections during pregnancy.

In all states of India undernutrition continues to be a major problem in women. Maternal undernutrition is associated with low birth weight; leading to poor growth during infancy, childhood, adolescence and small stature in adults. Identification of pregnant women below 45 kg and special effort to provide food supplements and monitor for adequate weight gain in these women under the ICDS or NRHM Programme, would contribute to reduction in incidence of low birth weight.

Major factor responsible for emerging problem of overnutrition is substantial reduction in physical activity levels in all segments of population. In some segments of population junk food eating is a contributory factor.

Over the last two decades there has been

- reduction in the number of the persons engaged in manual work,
- substantial improvement in mechanical aids in agriculture, industry and allied activities,

- improvement in access to water and fuel near households both in urban and rural areas,
- availability of mechanized transport at affordable cost has resulted in fewer people walking or cycling to work place, school or market,
- kitchen aids have reduced physical activity during cooking and household chores, and
- among urban affluent class, TV and computers contributed to steep reduction in physical activity.

As a result of these lifestyle changes, there has been a reduction in energy requirements. Unchanged energy intake and reduced energy requirement is associated with positive energy balance, fat deposition and weight gain. Overnutrition and abdominal adiposity are associated with increased risk of non-communicable diseases.

Recent studies from Delhi have shown undernutrition in childhood may be a predisposing factor for overnutrition and increased risk of non-communicable diseases in adult life.

Indian women appear to have a predisposition for adiposity (especially abdominal), insulin resistance, diabetes, hyper-triglyceridaemia and cardiovascular diseases. It is essential that the dual nutrition and health burden is combated through efficient implementation of time tested, effective and inexpensive interventions to achieve significant reduction in both over and undernutrition and their adverse health consequences.

References

1. National Nutrition Monitoring Bureau (NNMB) (1979–2002).NNMB Reports. National Institute of Nutrition, Hyderabad.
2. IIPS National Family Health Survey (NFHS-2): http://www.nfhsindia.org/india2.html; last accessed on 24/09/07.
3. IIPS National Family Health Survey (NFHS-3): http://mohfw.nic.in/nfhsfactsheet.htm; last accessed on 24/09/07.
4. IIPS National Family Health Survey (NFHS-1) http://www.nfhsindia.org/anfhs1.html.
5. Department of Women and Child Development India Nutrition Profile 1 (1995–96), Government of India, New Delhi.
6. RAMACHANDRAN P (1989). Nutrition in pregnancy. In "Women and nutrition in India" GOPALAN C. and KAUR S. (eds). *Nutrition Foundation of India, Special Publication* (No.5), pp. 153.
7. National Sample Survey Organization: Reports of NSSO surveys 1973–2000. NSSO, New Delhi.
8. Economic Survey of India 2003–04; http://indiabudgetnic.in/es2006-07/esmain.htm last accessed on 24/09/07.
9. PURE Prospective Urban and Rural Epidemiological Study: http://www.ccc.mcmaster.ca/pure/index.html; last accessed on 24/09/07.

10. WASUJA M, SIDDHU A (2003). Decade wise alterations in energy expenditure and energy status of affluent women (30–88 years) – A cross-sectional study. Delhi University, New Delhi. (Ph.D. Thesis).
11. BHARGAVA SK, SACHDEV HP, FALL HD, OSMOND C, LAKSHMY R, BARKER DJP, BISWAS SKD, RAMJI S, PRABHAKARAN D, REDDY KS. Relation of serial changes in childhood Body Mass Index to impaired glucose tolerance in young adulthood. *New Eng J Med* vol. 350, pp. 865–875.
12. Nutrition Foundation of India (2005). Twenty Five Years Report 1980–2005. New Delhi.
13. KURPAD AV. Changing energy requirements of Indians. In: Proceedings of Nutrition Foundation of India (NFI)—WHO symposium on "Nutrition Development Transition in India", July 2010.

5

Measuring undernutrition and overnutrition in children

Dheeraj Shah and *H.P.S. Sachdev*

Dheeraj Shah MD, DNB, MNAMS is an Associate Professor in Pediatrics at University College of Medical Sciences, Delhi. He is also the Associate Editor of *Indian Pediatrics*. Dr. Shah has served as a visiting fellow at The Royal college of Pediatrics and Child Health, London, UK and was an Associate Professor at the Department of Pediatrics and Adolescent Medicine, B.P. Koirala Institute of Health Sciences, Dharan, Nepal.

H.P.S. Sachdev MD, FIAP, FAMS is a senior consultant in Pediatrics and Clinical Epidemiology at Sitaram Bhartia Institute of Science and Research, New Delhi. He is also an adjunct professor at St. John's Research Institute, Bangalore and visiting professor at MRC Epidemiology Resource Centre, Southampton. Dr. Sachdev has served as a professor in the Department of Pediatrics, Maulana Azad Medical College, National President of Indian Academy of Pediatrics, Secretary of Nutrition Society of India and Editor-in Chief of *Indian Pediatrics*.

5.1 Introduction

Nutritional status of the individuals and populations can be assessed by various methods such as measurement of food intake, biochemical parameters (e.g. serum proteins, lipid profile, iron studies, etc.) and nutritional anthropometry. Moreover in recent years, sophisticated methods such as magnetic resonance imaging (MRI), dual energy X-ray absorptiometry and Dexa-scan have been used to estimate various nutritional parameters. Anthropometry is the most commonly used method to assess nutritional status of individuals and populations as it is inexpensive, convenient and non-invasive. Depending on the anthropometric indicators selected, it can be used for various purposes such as screening at-risk children and measuring short-term or long-term changes in nutritional status. However, there are inherent limitations in using anthropometry as a tool for nutritional assessment [1]. One aspect of this is that changes in anthropometry may take some time after nutritional deprivation to set in and the deprivation may be fairly long standing for linear growth retardation. Also, simple anthropometry in the context of overnutrition may cause difficulty in distinguishing lean from adipose tissue thus failing to distinguish well-built (e.g. athletes) from obese people. Despite these limitations, anthropometry is the most practical way of measuring nutritional status of individuals or populations.

5.2 Anthropometric techniques

For anthropometry to be valid, it is necessary that the data are collected in a proper way and the recommended measurement technique is followed. The child's accurate age is required and any error in recording or interpreting child's age makes the whole process of anthropometry fruitless. In communities, it is common to state the age as the year of life the child has now entered. For example, if the child has completed 5 years of age in September 2007, parents might start telling his/her age as 6 years from as early as October 2007. If possible, the exact date of birth of the child should be asked or examined from a document (such as birth certificate or horoscope) and the exact age on the day of measurement should be calculated by the evaluator him/herself and measured to the nearest month. If dates cannot be recalled, use of a local calendar or recollection of important events may assist mothers in recalling the date of birth.

Accurate anthropometric measurement is a skill requiring specific instruments and training. Whatever equipment is chosen, staff needs training to ensure its proper use. The training of personnel on specific measurement and recording techniques should include not only theoretical explanations and demonstrations, but also provide an opportunity for participants to practice the measurement techniques, as well as reading and recording the results. Once all personnel have adequately practiced the measurement and recording techniques, and feel comfortable with their performance, standardization exercises should be carried out to ensure that all interviewers acquire the skills necessary to collect high quality data [2].

5.2.1 Measuring length/height

Length/height boards should be designed to measure children under 2 years of age lying down (recumbent) and older children standing up. The board should be able to measure up to 0.1 cm. A measuring board should be lightweight, durable and have few moving parts.

Length (for infants and children upto the age of 23 months) (Figure 5.1)

Place the measuring board on a hard flat surface, i.e. ground, floor, or steady table. Kneel/stand on the right side of the child so that you can hold the foot piece with your right hand. With the mother's help, lay the child on the board by supporting the back of the child's head with one hand and the trunk of the body with the other hand. Gradually lower the child onto the board. An assistant should cup his/her hands over the child's ears and place the child's head against the base of the board so that the child is looking straight up. The child's line of sight should be perpendicular to the ground. Make sure the child is lying flat and in the center of the board. Press the child's shins and knees firmly against the board and with your right hand place the foot piece firmly against the child's heels. When the child's position is correct, read the measurement to the nearest 0.1 cm, release the child carefully and record the value [2, 3].

Height (for children aged 24 months and older) (Figure 5.2)

Place the measuring board or stadiometer on a hard flat surface against a wall, table, tree, etc. Make sure the board/stadiometer is not moving. Ask the mother to remove the child's shoes and unbraid any hair that would interfere with the height measurement. Make sure the child's legs are straight and the heels and calves are against the board/wall. Tell the child to look straight ahead at the mother who should stand in front of the child. Make sure the child's line of sight is level with the ground and the shoulders are level. The hands of the child should be at the child's side and the head, shoulder blades and buttocks are against the board/wall. Place your open left hand under the child's chin and with your right hand lower the headpiece on top of the child's head making you push through the child's hair. When the child's position is correct, read the measurement to the nearest 0.1 cm, remove the headpiece from the child's head and your left hand from the child's chin. Record the measurement immediately to avoid any recall errors [2, 3].

5.2.2 Measuring weight

Weighing scales used should be portable, durable and sensitive. Spring scales are commonly used in field-studies. There are several different attachments that can be used to help weigh children with spring scales. The size of the child will determine which attachment should be used. For weighing infants, a sling or basket is usually attached to the spring scale. For children, weighing trousers are used to suspend them. These are small pants with straps that the child steps into. The trousers are then hung from the scale by the straps. Whatever is used to suspend the child, the scale should be zeroed to ensure that the weight of the trousers, sling or basket is not added to the child's weight.

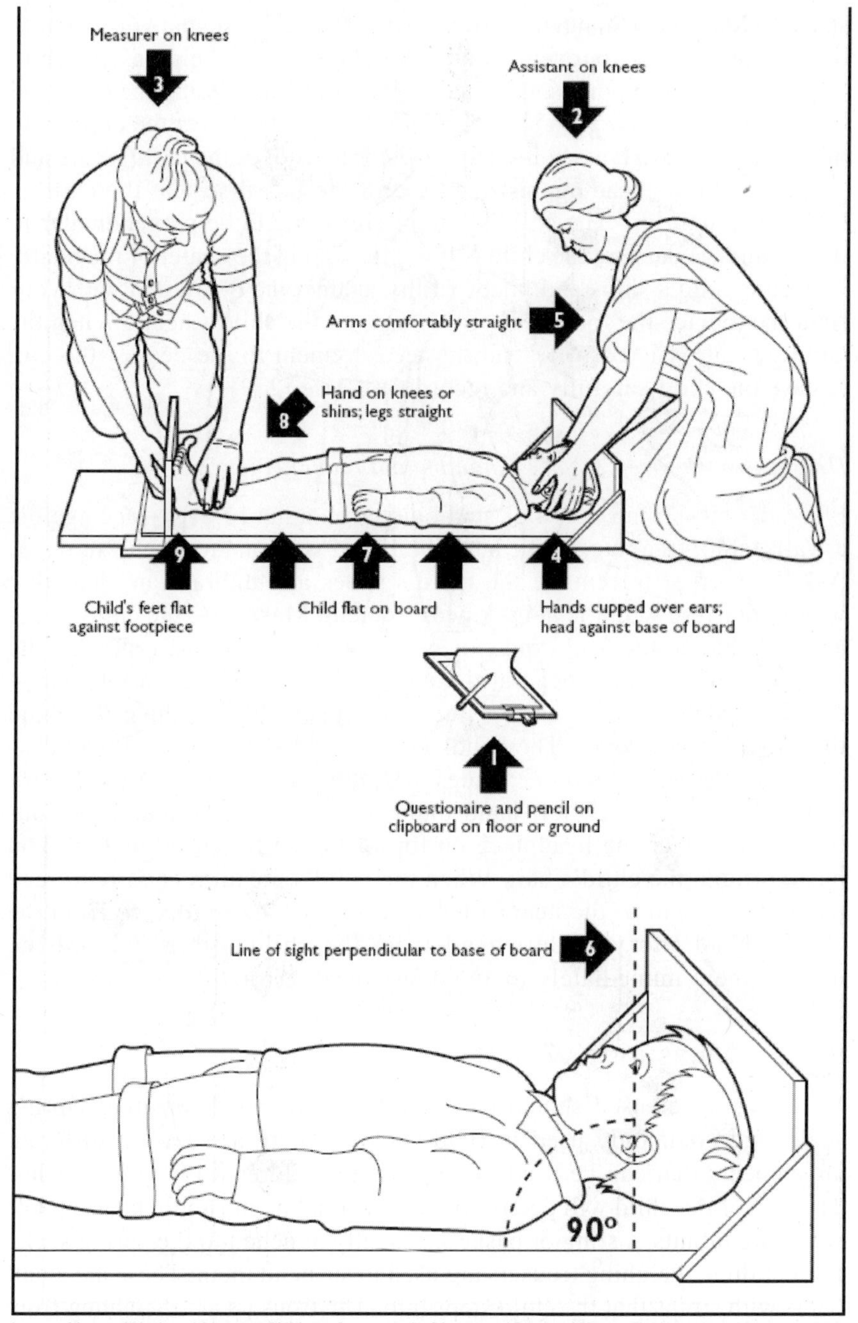

Source: How to Weigh and Measure Children: Assessing the Nutritional Status of Young Children, United Nations, 1986.

5.1 Technique for measuring length (for children 0–23 months)

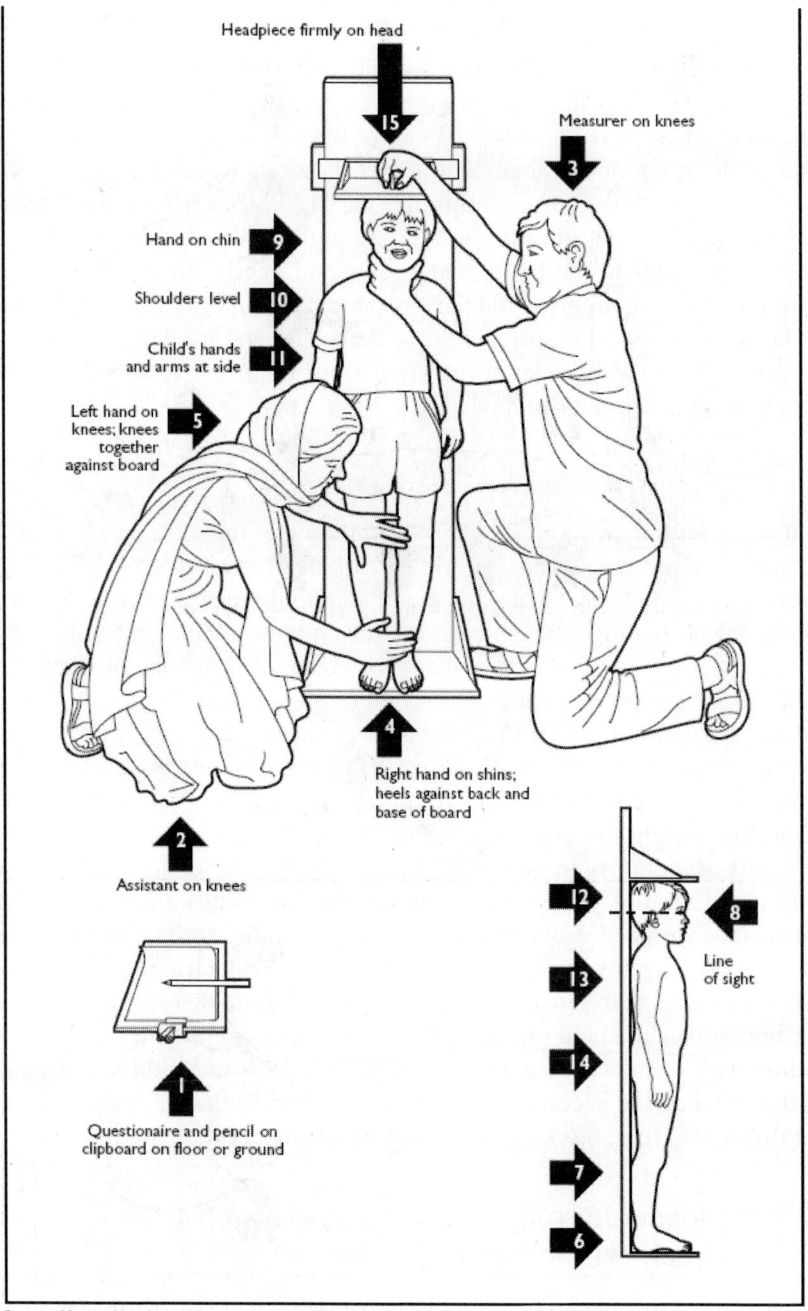

Source: How to Weigh and Measure Children: Assessing the Nutritional Status of Young Children, United Nations, 1986.

5.2 Technique for measuring height (for children >24 months)

Using a hanging scale (Salter-type or spring balance) (Figure 5.3)

Hang the scale from a secure place like the ceiling beam. You may need a piece of rope to hang the scale at eye level. Ask the mother to undress the child as much as possible. Attach a pair of the empty weighing trousers or sling to the hook of the scale and adjust the scale to zero, then remove from the scale. Put your arms through the leg holes of the trousers and grasp the child's feet pulling the legs through the leg holes. Attach the strap of the pants to the hook of the scale and gently lower the child to allow him/her hang freely. Hold the scale and read the weight to the nearest 0.1 kg when the child is still and the scale needle is stationary. Gently lift the child by the body, release the strap from the hook of the scale and record the measurement immediately.

Using an electronic or mechanical weighing scale

Remove or minimize the clothing on the child. Place the scale on a hard and flat surface. Correct any zero error in case of mechanical type of scales and ensure zero reading (by taring) in case of electronic scales. In case of older child using a standing type of scale, ask the child to stand on the middle of the scale and record the reading when the needle stops moving or when the numbers stop changing (in case of electronic scales). While weighing a young child on a lying-down type of scale, place a clean sheet of paper or warm cloth on the surface of the scale. Bring the reading to zero by adjusting the needle (in mechanical scales) or by taring (in case of electronic scales). Record the weight to the nearest accuracy possible on that scale.

If only standing type of scale is available and the child is unable to stand (as in case of young, sick or uncooperative child), the mother and child can be weighed simultaneously. However, the sensitivity of the scale should be 0.1 kg for this purpose (as in UNICEF electronic scale). The bathroom scales with sensitivity of 0.5 kg are not suitable for this purpose. Ask the mother to stand on the scale. Record the weight and include the reading with one decimal point (e.g. 57.4 kgs). Pass the child to a person nearby. Record the second reading with just the mother (e.g. 50.8 kgs). The difference (e.g. 6.6 kgs) is the weight of the child.

5.2.3 Measuring mid-arm/mid-upper arm (MUAC) circumference (Figure 5.4)

Very young children can be held by their mother during this procedure. Ask the mother to remove clothing that may cover the child's left arm. Calculate the midpoint of the child's left upper arm by first locating the tip of the child's shoulder with your finger tips. Bend the

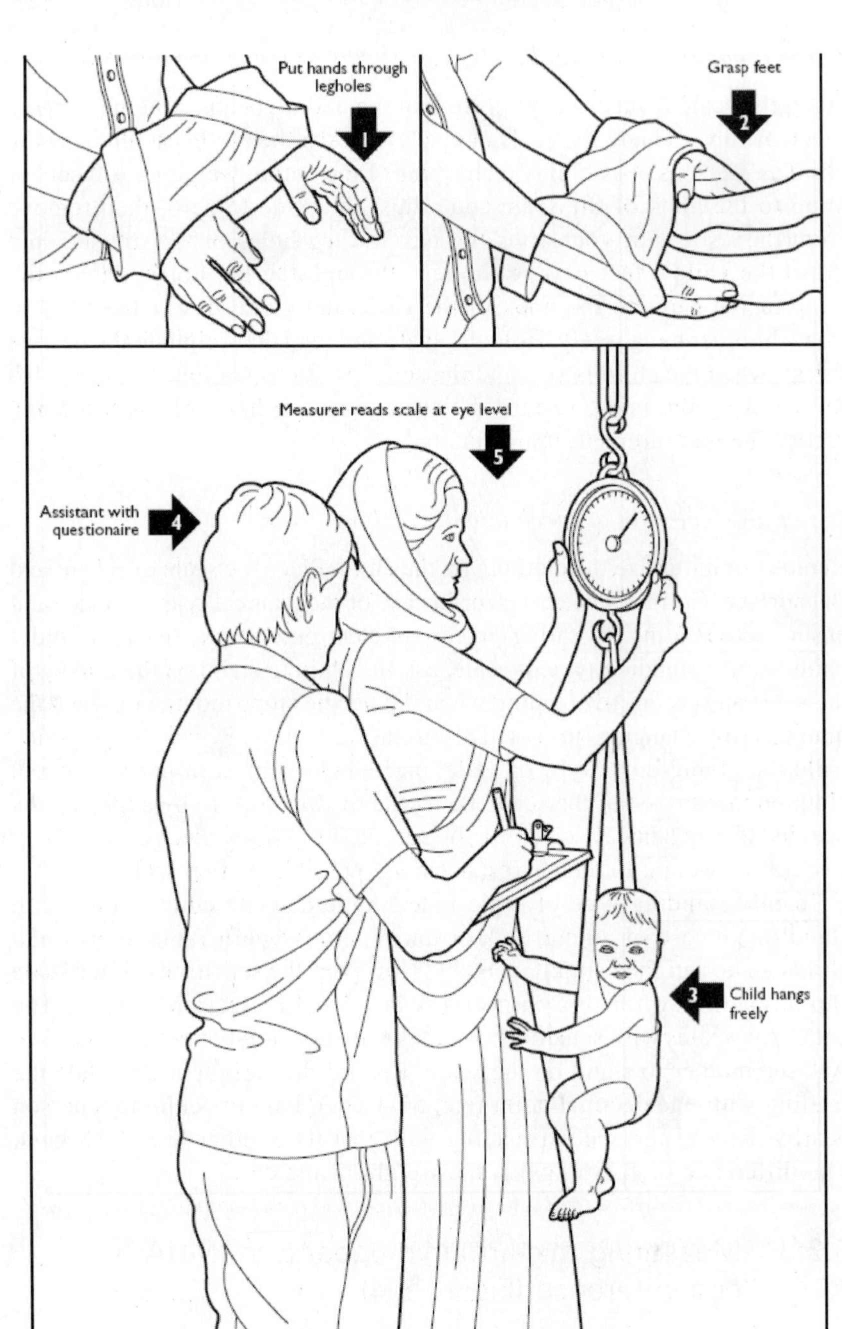

Source: How to Weigh and Measure Children: Assessing the Nutritional Status of Young Children, United Nations, 1986.

5.3 Measuring weight of a child using hanging scale

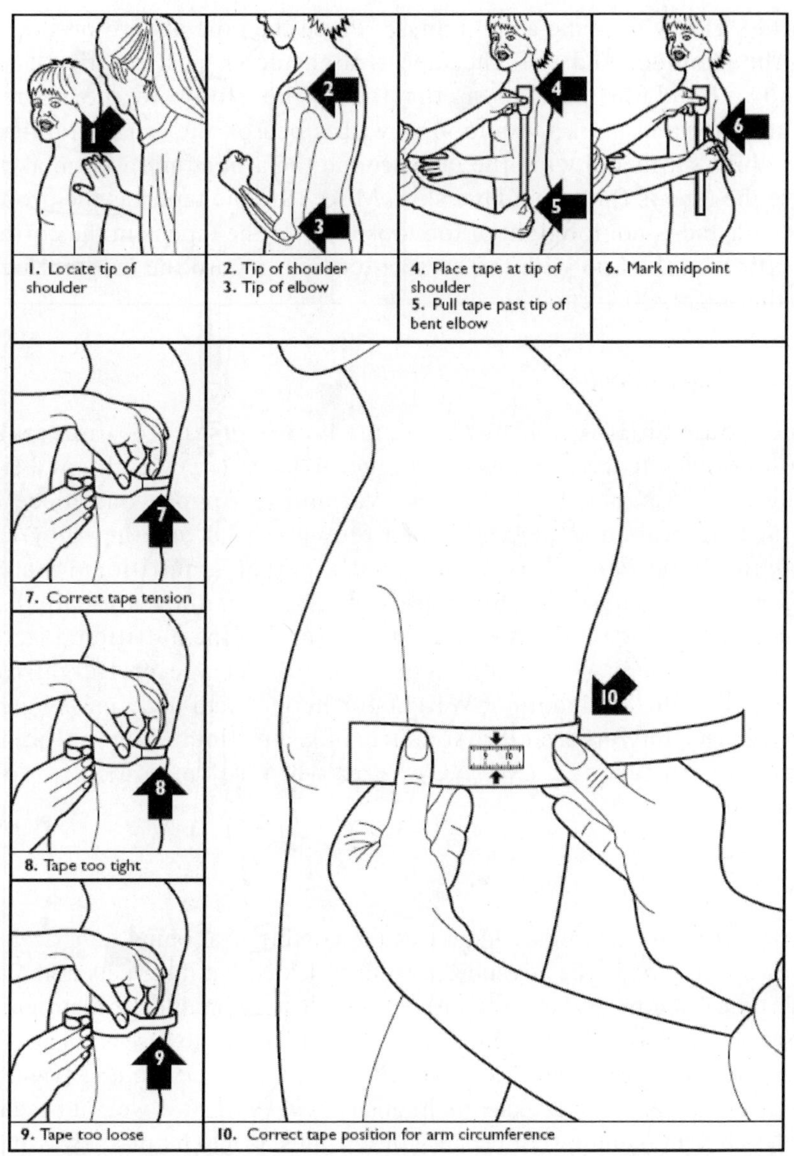

Source: How to Weigh and Measure Children: Assessing the Nutritional Status of Young Children, United Nations, 1986.

5.4 Measuring mid-upper arm circumference

child's elbow to make a right angle. Place the tape at zero on the tip of the shoulder and pull the tape straight down past the tip of the elbow. Read the number at the tip of the elbow to the nearest centimeter and mark the midpoint with a pen on the arm. Straighten the child's arm and wrap the tape around the arm at midpoint making sure the tape is flat around the skin. Make sure the tape has the proper tension and is not too tight or too loose. When the tape is in the correct position on the arm with the correct tension, record the measurement to the nearest 0.1 cm.

Anthropometric indices

The four building blocks or measures used to undertake anthropometric assessment are (i) age, (ii) sex, (iii) weight, and (iv) length (or height). Each of these variables provides one piece of information about a person. When they are used together they can provide important information about a person's nutritional status. When two of these variables are used together they are called an index. The indices commonly used in assessing the nutritional status of children are "Weight-for-age", "Length-for-age or Height-for-age", "Weight-for-length or Weight-for-height" and body mass index. There are many other anthropometric measures including mid-upper arm circumference (MUAC), waist-hip ratio and skin-fold thicknesses.

Weight-for-age

Low weight-for-age index identifies the condition of being underweight for a specific age. The advantage of this index is that it reflects both past (chronic) and/or present (acute), although it is unable to distinguish between the two and is recommended as the indicator to assess changes in the magnitude of malnutrition over time [4]. However, the disadvantage of this index is that it fails to distinguish between the low weight because of less height (stunting) or because of low muscle and fat mass (wasting). Another disadvantage is that this parameter may not detect or classify malnutrition accurately when there is a presence of increased extravascular fluid (as in edema or serous effusions) or tumor load as in cancer patients. In these conditions, any weight-based index is likely to underdiagnose malnutrition. Table 5.1 presents the weight for age index for boys and girls [5].

Table 5.1 WHO Growth Standards Weight-for-Age – boys and girls birth to 5 years (Z scores) [5]

Year :	Month	Boys							Girls						
Months		–3SD	–2SD	–1SD	Median	1 SD	2SD	3SD	–3SD	–2SD	–1SD	Median	1 SD	2SD	3SD
0:0	0	2.1	2.5	2.9	3.3	3.9	4.4	5.0	2.0	2.4	2.8	3.2	3.7	4.2	4.8
0:1	1	2.9	3.4	3.9	4.5	5.1	5.8	6.6	2.7	3.2	3.6	4.2	4.8	5.5	6.2
0:2	2	3.8	4.3	4.9	5.6	6.3	7.1	8.0	3.4	3.9	4.5	5.1	5.8	6.6	7.5
0:3	3	4.4	5.0	5.7	6.4	7.2	8.0	9.0	4.0	4.5	5.2	5.8	6.6	7.5	8.5
0:4	4	4.9	5.6	6.2	7.0	7.8	8.7	9.7	4.4	5.0	5.7	6.4	7.3	8.2	9.3
0:5	5	5.3	6.0	6.7	7.5	8.4	9.3	10.4	4.8	5.4	6.1	6.9	7.8	8.8	10.0
0:6	6	5.7	6.4	7.1	7.9	8.8	9.8	10.9	5.1	5.7	6.5	7.3	8.2	9.3	10.6
0:7	7	5.9	6.7	7.4	8.3	9.2	10.3	11.4	5.3	6.0	6.8	7.6	8.6	9.8	11.1
0:8	8	6.2	6.9	7.7	8.6	9.6	10.7	11.9	5.6	6.3	7.0	7.9	9.0	10.2	11.6
0:9	9	6.4	7.1	8.0	8.9	9.9	11.0	12.3	5.8	6.5	7.3	8.2	9.3	10.5	12.0
0:10	10	6.6	7.4	8.2	9.2	10.2	11.4	12.7	5.9	6.7	7.5	8.5	9.6	10.9	12.4
0:11	11	6.8	7.6	8.4	9.4	10.5	11.7	13.0	6.1	6.9	7.7	8.7	9.9	11.2	12.8
1:0	12	6.9	7.7	8.6	9.6	10.8	12.0	13.3	6.3	7.0	7.9	8.9	10.1	11.5	13.1
1:1	13	7.1	7.9	8.8	9.9	11.0	12.3	13.7	6.4	7.2	8.1	9.2	10.4	11.8	13.5
1:2	14	7.2	8.1	9.0	10.1	11.3	12.6	14.0	6.6	7.4	8.3	9.4	10.6	12.1	13.8
1:3	15	7.4	8.3	9.2	10.3	11.5	12.8	14.3	6.7	7.6	8.5	9.6	10.9	12.4	14.1
1:4	16	7.5	8.4	9.4	10.5	11.7	13.1	14.6	6.9	7.7	8.7	9.8	11.1	12.6	14.5
1:5	17	7.7	8.6	9.6	10.7	12.0	13.4	14.9	7.0	7.9	8.9	10.0	11.4	12.9	14.8
1:6	18	7.8	8.8	9.8	10.9	12.2	13.7	15.3	7.2	8.1	9.1	10.2	11.6	13.2	15.1
1:7	19	8.0	8.9	10.0	11.1	12.5	13.9	15.6	7.3	8.2	9.2	10.4	11.8	13.5	15.4
1:8	20	8.1	9.1	10.1	11.3	12.7	14.2	15.9	7.5	8.4	9.4	10.6	12.1	13.7	15.7
1:9	21	8.2	9.2	10.3	11.5	12.9	14.5	16.2	7.6	8.6	9.6	10.9	12.3	14.0	16.0
1:10	22	8.4	9.4	10.5	11.8	13.2	14.7	16.5	7.8	8.7	9.8	11.1	12.5	14.3	16.4
1:11	23	8.5	9.5	10.7	12.0	13.4	15.0	16.8	7.9	8.9	10.0	11.3	12.8	14.6	16.7
2:0	24	8.6	9.7	10.8	12.2	13.6	15.3	17.1	8.1	9.0	10.2	11.5	13.0	14.8	17.0
2:1	25	8.8	9.8	11.0	12.4	13.9	15.5	17.5	8.2	9.2	10.3	11.7	13.3	15.1	17.3
2:2	26	8.9	10.0	11.2	12.5	14.1	15.8	17.8	8.4	9.4	10.5	11.9	13.5	15.4	17.7
2:3	27	9.0	10.1	11.3	12.7	14.3	16.1	18.1	8.5	9.5	10.7	12.1	13.7	15.7	18.0
2:4	28	9.1	10.2	11.5	12.9	14.5	16.3	18.4	8.6	9.7	10.9	12.3	14.0	16.0	18.3
2:5	29	9.2	10.4	11.7	13.1	14.8	16.6	18.7	8.8	9.8	11.1	12.5	14.2	16.2	18.7
2:6	30	9.4	10.5	11.8	13.3	15.0	16.9	19.0	8.9	10.0	11.2	12.7	14.4	16.5	19.0

Year : Months	Month	Boys							Girls						
		–3SD	–2SD	–1SD	Median	1 SD	2SD	3SD	–3SD	–2SD	–1SD	Median	1 SD	2SD	3SD
2:7	31	9.5	10.7	12.0	13.5	15.2	17.1	19.3	9.0	10.1	11.4	12.9	14.7	16.8	19.3
2:8	32	9.6	10.8	12.1	13.7	15.4	17.4	19.6	9.1	10.3	11.6	13.1	14.9	17.1	19.6
2:9	33	9.7	10.9	12.3	13.8	15.6	17.6	19.9	9.3	10.4	11.7	13.3	15.1	17.3	20.0
2:10	34	9.8	11.0	12.4	14.0	15.8	17.8	20.2	9.4	10.5	11.9	13.5	15.4	17.6	20.3
2:11	35	9.9	11.2	12.6	14.2	16.0	18.1	20.4	9.5	10.7	12.0	13.7	15.6	17.9	20.6
3:0	36	10.0	11.3	12.7	14.3	16.2	18.3	20.7	9.6	10.8	12.2	13.9	15.8	18.1	20.9
3:1	37	10.1	11.4	12.9	14.5	16.4	18.6	21.0	9.7	10.9	12.4	14.0	16.0	18.4	21.3
3:2	38	10.2	11.5	13.0	14.7	16.6	18.8	21.3	9.8	11.1	12.5	14.2	16.3	18.7	21.6
3:3	39	10.3	11.6	13.1	14.8	16.8	19.0	21.6	9.9	11.2	12.7	14.4	16.5	19.0	22.0
3:4	40	10.4	11.8	13.3	15.0	17.0	19.3	21.9	10.1	11.3	12.8	14.6	16.7	19.2	22.3
3:5	41	10.5	11.9	13.4	15.2	17.2	19.5	22.1	10.2	11.5	13.0	14.8	16.9	19.5	22.7
3;6	42	10.6	12.0	13.6	15.3	17.4	19.7	22.4	10.3	11.6	13.1	15.0	17.2	19.8	23.0
3:7	43	10.7	12.1	13.7	15.5	17.6	20.0	22.7	10.4	11.7	13.3	15.2	17.4	20.1	23.4
3:8	44	10.8	12.2	13.8	15.7	17.8	20.2	23.0	10.5	11.8	13.4	15.3	17.6	20.4	23.7
3:9	45	10.9	12.4	14.0	15.8	18.0	20.5	23.3	10.6	12.0	13.6	15.5	17.8	20.7	24.1
3:10	46	11.0	12.5	14.1	16.0	18.2	20.7	23.6	10.7	12.1	13.7	15.7	18.1	20.9	24.5
3:11	47	11.1	12.6	14.3	16.2	18.4	20.9	23.9	10.8	12.2	13.9	15.9	18.3	21.2	24.8
4:0	48	11.2	12.7	14.4	16.3	18.6	21.2	24.2	10.9	12.3	14.0	16.1	18.5	21.5	25.2
4:1	49	11.3	12.8	14.5	16.5	18.8	21.4	24.5	11.0	12.4	14.2	16.3	18.8	21.8	25.5
4:2	50	11.4	12.9	14.7	16.7	19.0	21.7	24.8	11.1	12.6	14.3	16.4	19.0	22.1	25.9
4:3	51	11.5	13.1	14.8	16.8	19.2	21.9	25.1	11.2	12.7	14.5	16.6	19.2	22.4	26.3
4:4	52	11.6	13.2	15.0	17.0	19.4	22.2	25.4	11.3	12.8	14.6	16.8	19.4	22.6	26.6
4:5	53	11.7	13.3	15.1	17.2	19.6	22.4	25.7	11.4	12.9	14.8	17.0	19.7	22.9	27.0
4:6	54	11.8	13.4	15.2	17.3	19.8	22.7	26.0	11.5	13.0	14.9	17.2	19.9	23.2	27.4
4:7	55	11.9	13.5	15.4	17.5	20.0	22.9	26.3	11.6	13.2	15.1	17.3	20.1	23.5	27.7
4:8	56	12.0	13.6	15.5	17.7	20.2	23.2	26.6	11.7	13.3	15.2	17.5	20.3	23.8	28.1
4:9	57	12.1	13.7	15.6	17.8	20.4	23.4	26.9	11.8	13.4	15.3	17.7	20.6	24.1	28.5
4:10	58	12.2	13.8	15.8	18.0	20.6	23.7	27.2	11.9	13.5	15.5	17.9	20.8	24.4	28.8
4:11	59	12.3	14.0	15.9	18.2	20.8	23.9	27.6	12.0	13.6	15.6	18.0	21.0	24.6	29.2
5:0	60	12.4	14.1	16.0	18.3	21.0	24.2	27.9	12.1	13.7	15.8	18.2	21.2	24.9	29.5

Source: http://www.who.int/childgrowth/standards/en/

Height-for-age

For children below 2 years of age, the term is length-for-age and for above 2 years of age, the index is referred to as height-for-age. Low length or height-for-age index (stunting) identifies past undernutrition or chronic malnutrition. It is associated with a number of long-term factors including chronic insufficient protein and energy intake, frequent infection, sustained inappropriate feeding practices and poverty. This index cannot measure short term changes in malnutrition. Data on prevalence of stunting in a community may be used in problem analysis in designing interventions. Information on stunting for individual children is useful clinically as an aid to diagnosis. Stunting, based on height for-age, can be used for evaluation purposes but is not recommended for monitoring as it does not change in the short term such as 6–12 months [2, 4]. Another disadvantage of this index is that it fails to distinguish between short stature due to true nutritional cause or because of other problems such as genetic or hormonal. Tables 5.2 and 5.3 present the length-for-age and height-for-age index for age group birth to 2 years and 2 to 5 years.

Weight-for-height

It is calculated as the weight of each child in relation to the weight of a well-nourished reference child of the same sex and stature using the appropriate reference charts. Weight-for-height is expressed either using Z-scores (standard deviations from the reference median) or percentage of the reference median. Reporting using Z-score is preferred for assessments and surveys and weight-for-height percent of the median is preferred for admission into treatment [4, 5]. Tables 5.4 and 5.5 present weight-for-length and weight-for-length index for boys and girls birth to 2 years and 2 to 5 years respectively [5].

Low weight-for-height (weight-for-length in children under 2 years of age) is a measure of wasting. Wasting is the result of a weight falling significantly below the weight expected of a child of the same length or height. Wasting indicates current or acute malnutrition resulting from failure to gain weight or actual weight loss. Causes include inadequate food intake, incorrect feeding practices, disease, and infection or, more frequently, a combination of these factors. It is a very useful index when exact ages are difficult to determine. It is appropriate for examining short-term effects such as seasonal changes in food supply or short-term nutritional stress brought about by illness. Wasting in individual children and population groups can change rapidly and thus used for screening or targeting purposes in emergency settings and is sometimes used for annual reporting. As with weight-for-age, this index also carries the limitation of

Table 5.2 WHO Growth Standards Length-for-Age – boys and girls birth to 2 years (Z scores)* [5]

Year :	Month	Boys							Girls						
Months		–3SD	–2SD	–1SD	Median	1 SD	2SD	3SD	–3SD	–2SD	–1SD	Median	1 SD	2SD	3SD
0:0	0	44.2	46.1	48.0	49.9	51.8	53.7	55.6	43.6	45.4	47.3	49.1	51.0	52.9	54.7
0:1	1	48.9	50.8	52.8	54.7	56.7	58.6	60.6	47.8	49.8	51.7	53.7	55.6	57.6	59.5
0:2	2	52.4	54.4	56.4	58.4	60.4	62.4	64.4	51.0	53.0	55.0	57.1	59.1	61.1	63.2
0:3	3	55.3	57.3	59.4	61.4	63.5	65.5	67.6	53.5	55.6	57.7	59.8	61.9	64.0	66.1
0:4	4	57.6	59.7	61.8	63.9	66.0	68.0	70.1	55.6	57.8	59.9	62.1	64.3	66.4	68.6
0:5	5	59.6	61.7	63.8	65.9	68.0	70.1	72.2	57.4	59.6	61.8	64.0	66.2	68.5	70.7
0:6	6	61.2	63.3	65.5	67.6	69.8	71.9	74.0	58.9	61.2	63.5	65.7	68.0	70.3	72.5
0:7	7	62.7	64.8	67.0	69.2	71.3	73.5	75.7	60.3	62.7	65.0	67.3	69.6	71.9	74.2
0:8	8	64.0	66.2	68.4	70.6	72.8	75.0	77.2	61.7	64.0	66.4	68.7	71.1	73.5	75.8
0:9	9	65.2	67.5	69.7	72.0	74.2	76.5	78.7	62.9	65.3	67.7	70.1	72.6	75.0	77.4
0:10	10	66.4	68.7	71.0	73.3	75.6	77.9	80.1	64.1	66.5	69.0	71.5	73.9	76.4	78.9
0:11	11	67.6	69.9	72.2	74.5	76.9	79.2	81.5	65.2	67.7	70.3	72.8	75.3	77.8	80.3
1:0	12	68.6	71.0	73.4	75.7	78.1	80.5	82.9	66.3	68.9	71.4	74.0	76.6	79.2	81.7
1.1	13	69.6	72.1	74.5	76.9	79.3	81.8	84.2	67.3	70.0	72.6	75.2	77.8	80.5	83.1
1:2	14	70.6	73.1	75.6	78.0	80.5	83.0	85.5	68.3	71.0	73.7	76.4	79.1	81.7	84.4
1:3	15	71.6	74.1	76.6	79.1	81.7	84.2	86.7	69.3	72.0	74.8	77.5	80.2	83.0	85.7
1:4	16	72.5	75.0	77.6	80.2	82.8	85.4	88.0	70.2	73.0	75.8	78.6	81.4	84.2	87.0
1:5	17	73.3	76.0	78.6	81.2	83.9	86.5	89.2	71.1	74.0	76.8	79.7	82.5	85.4	88.2
1:6	18	74.2	76.9	79.6	82.3	85.0	87.7	90.4	72.0	74.9	77.8	80.7	83.6	86.5	89.4
1:7	19	75.0	77.7	80.5	83.2	86.0	88.8	91.5	72.8	75.8	78.8	81.7	84.7	87.6	90.6
1:8	20	75.8	78.6	81.4	84.2	87.0	89.8	92.6	73.7	76.7	79.7	82.7	85.7	88.7	91.7
1:9	21	76.5	79.4	82.3	85.1	88.0	90.9	93.8	74.5	77.5	80.6	83.7	86.7	89.8	92.9
1:10	22	77.2	80.2	83.1	86.0	89.0	91.9	94.9	75.2	78.4	81.5	84.6	87.7	90.8	94.0
1:11	23	78.0	81.0	83.9	86.9	89.9	92.9	95.9	76.0	79.2	82.3	85.5	88.7	91.9	95.0
2:0	24	78.7	81.7	84.8	87.8	90.9	93.9	97.0	76.7	80.0	83.2	86.4	89.6	92.9	96.1

*The standard for linear growth has a part based on length (length-for-age, 0 to 24 months) and another on height (height-for-age, 2 to 5 years). The two parts were constructed using the same model but the final curves reflect the average difference between recumbent length and standing height. By design, children between 18 and 30 months in the cross-sectional component of the MGRS had both length and height measurements taken. The resulting disjunction between the two standards thus in essence reflects the 0.7 cm difference between length and height.

Table 5.3: WHO Growth Standards Height-for-Age – boys and girls 2 and 5 years (Z scores)* [5]

Year :	Month	Boys							Girls						
Months		–3SD	–2SD	–1SD	Median	1 SD	2SD	3SD	–3SD	–2SD	–1SD	Median	1 SD	2SD	3SD
2.0	24	78.0	81.0	84.1	87.1	90.2	93.2	96.3	76.0	79.3	82.5	85.7	88.9	92.2	95.4
2:1	25	78.6	81.7	84.9	88.0	91.1	94.2	97.3	76.8	80.0	83.3	86.6	89.9	93.1	96.4
2:2	26	79.3	82.5	85.6	88.8	92.0	95.2	98.3	77.5	80.8	84.1	87.4	90.8	94.1	97.4
2:3	27	79.9	83.1	86.4	89.6	92.9	96.1	99.3	78.1	81.5	84.9	88.3	91.7	95.0	98.4
2:4	28	80.5	83.8	87.1	90.4	93.7	97.0	100.3	78.8	82.2	85.7	89.1	92.5	96.0	99.4
2:5	29	81.1	84.5	87.8	91.2	94.5	97.9	101.2	79.5	82.9	86.4	89.9	93.4	96.9	100.3
2:6	30	81.7	85.1	88.5	91.9	95.3	98.7	102.1	80.1	83.6	87.1	90.7	94.2	97.7	101.3
2:7	31	82.3	85.7	89.2	92.7	96.1	99.6	103.0	80.7	84.3	87.9	91.4	95.0	98.6	102.2
2:8	32	82.8	86.4	89.9	93.4	96.9	100.4	103.9	81.3	84.9	88.6	92.2	95.8	99.4	103.1
2:9	33	83.4	86.9	90.5	94.1	97.6	101.2	104.8	81.9	85.6	89.3	92.9	96.6	100.3	103.9
2:10	34	83.9	87.5	91.1	94.8	98.4	102.0	105.6	82.5	86.2	89.9	93.6	97.4	101.1	104.8
2:11	35	84.4	88.1	91.8	95.4	99.1	102.7	106.4	83.1	86.8	90.6	94.4	98.1	101.9	105.6
3:0	36	85.0	88.7	92.4	96.1	99.8	103.5	107.2	83.6	87.4	91.2	95.1	98.9	102.7	106.5
3:1	37	85.5	89.2	93.0	96.7	100.5	104.2	108.0	84.2	88.0	91.9	95.7	99.6	103.4	107.3
3:2	38	86.0	89.8	93.6	97.4	101.2	105.0	108.8	84.7	88.6	92.5	96.4	100.3	104.2	108.1
3:3	39	86.5	90.3	94.2	98.0	101.8	105.7	109.5	85.3	89.2	93.1	97.1	101.0	105.0	108.9
3:4	40	87.0	90.9	94.7	98.6	102.5	106.4	110.3	85.8	89.8	93.8	97.7	101.7	105.7	109.7
3:5	41	87.5	91.4	95.3	99.2	103.2	107.1	111.0	86.3	90.4	94.4	98.4	102.4	106.4	110.5
3;6	42	88.0	91.9	95.9	99.9	103.8	107.8	111.7	86.8	90.9	95.0	99.0	103.1	107.2	111.2
3:7	43	88.4	92.4	96.4	100.4	104.5	108.5	112.5	87.4	91.5	95.6	99.7	103.8	107.9	112.0
3:8	44	88.9	93.0	97.0	101.0	105.1	109.1	113.2	87.9	92.0	96.2	100.3	104.5	108.6	112.7
3:9	45	89.4	93.5	97.5	101.6	105.7	109.8	113.9	88.4	92.5	96.7	100.9	105.1	109.3	113.5
3:10	46	89.8	94.0	98.1	102.2	106.3	110.4	114.6	88.9	93.1	97.3	101.5	105.8	110.0	114.2
3:11	47	90.3	94.4	98.6	102.8	106.9	111.1	115.2	89.3	93.6	97.9	102.1	106.4	110.7	114.9
4:0	48	90.7	94.9	99.1	103.3	107.5	111.7	115.9	89.8	94.1	98.4	102.7	107.0	111.3	115.7
4:1	49	91.2	95.4	99.7	103.9	108.1	112.4	116.6	90.3	94.6	99.0	103.3	107.7	112.0	116.4
4:2	50	91.6	95.9	100.2	104.4	108.7	113.0	117.3	90.7	95.1	99.5	103.9	108.3	112.7	117.1
4:3	51	92.1	96.4	100.7	105.0	109.3	113.6	117.9	91.2	95.6	100.1	104.5	108.9	113.3	117.7

Year : Months	Month	Boys							Girls						
		–3SD	–2SD	–1SD	Median	1 SD	2SD	3SD	–3SD	–2SD	–1SD	Median	1 SD	2SD	3SD
4:4	52	92.5	96.9	101.2	105.6	109.9	114.2	118.6	91.7	96.1	100.6	105.0	109.5	114.0	118.4
4:5	53	93.0	97.4	101.7	106.1	110.5	114.9	119.2	92.1	96.6	101.1	105.6	110.1	114.6	119.1
4:6	54	93.4	97.8	102.3	106.7	111.1	115.5	119.9	92.6	97.1	101.6	106.2	110.7	115.2	119.8
4:7	55	93.9	98.3	102.8	107.2	111.7	116.1	120.6	93.0	97.6	102.2	106.7	111.3	115.9	120.4
4:8	56	94.3	98.8	103.3	107.8	112.3	116.7	121.2	93.4	98.1	102.7	107.3	111.9	116.5	121.1
4:9	57	94.7	99.3	103.8	108.3	112.8	117.4	121.9	93.9	98.5	103.2	107.8	112.5	117.1	121.8
4:10	58	95.2	99.7	104.3	108.9	113.4	118.0	122.6	94.3	99.0	103.7	108.4	113.0	117.7	122.4
4:11	59	95.6	100.2	104.8	109.4	114.0	118.6	123.2	94.7	99.5	104.2	108.9	113.6	118.3	123.1
5:0	60	96.1	100.7	105.3	110.0	114.6	119.2	123.9	95.2	99.9	104.7	109.4	114.2	118.9	123.7

Source: http://www.who.int/childgrowth/standards/en/ [5].

Table 5.4 WHO Growth Standards Weight-for-Length – boys and girls birth to 2 years (Z scores) [5]

Length		Boys						Length	Girls						
(cm)	–3SD	–2SD	–1SD	Median	1 SD	2SD	3SD	(cm)	–3SD	–2SD	–1SD	Median	1 SD	2SD	3SD
45.0	1.9	2.0	2.2	2.4	2.7	3.0	3.3	45.0	1.9	2.1	2.3	2.5	2.7	3.0	3.3
45.5	1.9	2.1	2.3	2.5	2.8	3.1	3.4	45.5	2.0	2.1	2.3	2.5	2.8	3.1	3.4
46.0	2.0	2.2	2.4	2.6	2.9	3.1	3.5	46.0	2.0	2.2	2.4	2.6	2.9	3.2	3.5
46.5	2.1	2.3	2.5	2.7	3.0	3.2	3.6	46.5	2.1	2.3	2.5	2.7	3.0	3.3	3.6
47.0	2.1	2.3	2.5	2.8	3.0	3.3	3.7	47.0	2.2	2.4	2.6	2.8	3.1	3.4	3.7
47.5	2.2	2.4	2.6	2.9	3.1	3.4	3.8	47.5	2.2	2.4	2.6	2.9	3.2	3.5	3.8
48.0	2.3	2.5	2.7	2.9	3.2	3.6	3.9	48.0	2.3	2.5	2.7	3.0	3.3	3.6	4.0
48.5	2.3	2.6	2.8	3.0	3.3	3.7	4.0	48.5	2.4	2.6	2.8	3.1	3.4	3.7	4.1
49.0	2.4	2.6	2.9	3.1	3.4	3.8	4.2	49.0	2.4	2.6	2.9	3.2	3.5	3.8	4.2
49.5	2.5	2.7	3.0	3.2	3.5	3.9	4.3	49.5	2.5	2.7	3.0	3.3	3.6	3.9	4.3
50.0	2.6	2.8	3.0	3.3	3.6	4.0	4.4	50.0	2.6	2.8	3.1	3.4	3.7	4.0	4.5
50.5	2.7	2.9	3.1	3.4	3.8	4.1	4.5	50.5	2.7	2.9	3.2	3.5	3.8	4.2	4.6
51.0	2.7	3.0	3.2	3.5	3.9	4.2	4.7	51.0	2.8	3.0	3.3	3.6	3.9	4.3	4.8
51.5	2.8	3.1	3.3	3.6	4.0	4.4	4.8	51.5	2.8	3.1	3.4	3.7	4.0	4.4	4.9
52.0	2.9	3.2	3.5	3.8	4.1	4.5	5.0	52.0	2.9	3.2	3.5	3.8	4.2	4.6	5.1
52.5	3.0	3.3	3.6	3.9	4.2	4.6	5.1	52.5	3.0	3.3	3.6	3.9	4.3	4.7	5.2
53.0	3.1	3.4	3.7	4.0	4.4	4.8	5.3	53.0	3.1	3.4	3.7	4.0	4.4	4.9	5.4
53.5	3.2	3.5	3.8	4.1	4.5	4.9	5.4	53.5	3.2	3.5	3.8	4.2	4.6	5.0	5.5
54.0	3.3	3.6	3.9	4.3	4.7	5.1	5.6	54.0	3.3	3.6	3.9	4.3	4.7	5.2	5.7
54.5	3.4	3.7	4.0	4.4	4.8	5.3	5.8	54.5	3.4	3.7	4.0	4.4	4.8	5.3	5.9
55.0	3.6	3.8	4.2	4.5	5.0	5.4	6.0	55.0	3.5	3.8	4.2	4.5	5.0	5.5	6.1
55.5	3.7	4.0	4.3	4.7	5.1	5.6	6.1	55.5	3.6	3.9	4.3	4.7	5.1	5.7	6.3
56.0	3.8	4.1	4.4	4.8	5.3	5.8	6.3	56.0	3.7	4.0	4.4	4.8	5.3	5.8	6.4
56.5	3.9	4.2	4.6	5.0	5.4	5.9	6.5	56.5	3.8	4.1	4.5	5.0	5.4	6.0	6.6
57.0	4.0	4.3	4.7	5.1	5.6	6.1	6.7	57.0	3.9	4.3	4.6	5.1	5.6	6.1	6.8
57.5	4.1	4.5	4.9	5.3	5.7	6.3	6.9	57.5	4.0	4.4	4.8	5.2	5.7	6.3	7.0
58.0	4.3	4.6	5.0	5.4	5.9	6.4	7.1	58.0	4.1	4.5	4.9	5.4	5.9	6.5	7.1
58.5	4.4	4.7	5.1	5.6	6.1	6.6	7.2	58.5	4.2	4.6	5.0	5.5	6.0	6.6	7.3
59.0	4.5	4.8	5.3	5.7	6.2	6.8	7.4	59.0	4.3	4.7	5.1	5.6	6.2	6.8	7.5
59.5	4.6	5.0	5.4	5.9	6.4	7.0	7.6	59.5	4.4	4.8	5.3	5.7	6.3	6.9	7.7
60.0	4.7	5.1	5.5	6.0	6.5	7.1	7.8	60.0	4.5	4.9	5.4	5.9	6.4	7.1	7.8

Length	Boys							Length	Girls						
(cm)	−3SD	−2SD	−1SD	Median	1 SD	2SD	3SD	(cm)	−3SD	−2SD	−1SD	Median	1 SD	2SD	3SD
60.5	4.8	5.2	5.6	6.1	6.7	7.3	8.0	60.5	4.6	5.0	5.5	6.0	6.6	7.3	8.0
61.0	4.9	5.3	5.8	6.3	6.8	7.4	8.1	61.0	4.7	5.1	5.6	6.1	6.7	7.4	8.2
61.5	5.0	5.4	5.9	6.4	7.0	7.6	8.3	61.5	4.8	5.2	5.7	6.3	6.9	7.6	8.4
62.0	5.1	5.6	6.0	6.5	7.1	7.7	8.5	62.0	4.9	5.3	5.8	6.4	7.0	7.7	8.5
62.5	5.2	5.7	6.1	6.7	7.2	7.9	8.6	62.5	5.0	5.4	5.9	6.5	7.1	7.8	8.7
63.0	5.3	5.8	6.2	6.8	7.4	8.0	8.8	63.0	5.1	5.5	6.0	6.6	7.3	8.0	8.8
63.5	5.4	5.9	6.4	6.9	7.5	8.2	8.9	63.5	5.2	5.6	6.2	6.7	7.4	8.1	9.0
64.0	5.5	6.0	6.5	7.0	7.6	8.3	9.1	64.0	5.3	5.7	6.3	6.9	7.5	8.3	9.1
64.5	5.6	6.1	6.6	7.1	7.8	8.5	9.3	64.5	5.4	5.8	6.4	7.0	7.6	8.4	9.3
65.0	5.7	6.2	6.7	7.3	7.9	8.6	9.4	65.0	5.5	5.9	6.5	7.1	7.8	8.6	9.5
65.5	5.8	6.3	6.8	7.4	8.0	8.7	9.6	65.5	5.5	6.0	6.6	7.2	7.9	8.7	9.6
66.0	5.9	6.4	6.9	7.5	8.2	8.9	9.7	66.0	5.6	6.1	6.7	7.3	8.0	8.8	9.8
66.5	6.0	6.5	7.0	7.6	8.3	9.0	9.9	66.5	5.7	6.2	6.8	7.4	8.1	9.0	9.9
67.0	6.1	6.6	7.1	7.8	8.4	9.2	10.0	67.0	5.8	6.3	6.9	7.5	8.3	9.1	10.0
67.5	6.2	6.7	7.2	7.9	8.5	9.3	10.2	67.5	5.9	6.4	7.0	7.6	8.4	9.2	10.2
68.0	6.3	6.8	7.3	8.0	8.7	9.4	10.3	68.0	6.0	6.5	7.1	7.7	8.5	9.4	10.3
68.5	6.4	6.9	7.5	8.1	8.8	9.6	10.5	68.5	6.1	6.6	7.2	7.9	8.6	9.5	10.5
69.0	6.5	7.0	7.6	8.2	8.9	9.7	10.6	69.0	6.1	6.7	7.3	8.0	8.7	9.6	10.6
69.5	6.6	7.1	7.7	8.3	9.0	9.8	10.8	69.5	6.2	6.8	7.4	8.1	8.8	9.7	10.7
70.0	6.6	7.2	7.8	8.4	9.2	10.0	10.9	70.0	6.3	6.9	7.5	8.2	9.0	9.9	10.9
70.5	6.7	7.3	7.9	8.5	9.3	10.1	11.1	70.5	6.4	6.9	7.6	8.3	9.1	10.0	11.0
71.0	6.8	7.4	8.0	8.6	9.4	10.2	11.2	71.0	6.5	7.0	7.7	8.4	9.2	10.1	11.1
71.5	6.9	7.5	8.1	8.8	9.5	10.4	11.3	71.5	6.5	7.1	7.7	8.5	9.3	10.2	11.3
72.0	7.0	7.6	8.2	8.9	9.6	10.5	11.5	72.0	6.6	7.2	7.8	8.6	9.4	10.3	11.4
72.5	7.1	7.6	8.3	9.0	9.8	10.6	11.6	72.5	6.7	7.3	7.9	8.7	9.5	10.5	11.5
73.0	7.2	7.7	8.4	9.1	9.9	10.8	11.8	73.0	6.8	7.4	8.0	8.8	9.6	10.6	11.7
73.5	7.2	7.8	8.5	9.2	10.0	10.9	11.9	73.5	6.9	7.4	8.1	8.9	9.7	10.7	11.8
74.0	7.3	7.9	8.6	9.3	10.1	11.0	12.1	74.0	6.9	7.5	8.2	9.0	9.8	10.8	11.9
74.5	7.4	8.0	8.7	9.4	10.2	11.2	12.2	74.5	7.0	7.6	8.3	9.1	9.9	10.9	12.0
75.0	7.5	8.1	8.8	9.5	10.3	11.3	12.3	75.0	7.1	7.7	8.4	9.1	10.0	11.0	12.2
75.5	7.6	8.2	8.8	9.6	10.4	11.4	12.5	75.5	7.1	7.8	8.5	9.2	10.1	11.1	12.3
76.0	7.6	8.3	8.9	9.7	10.6	11.5	12.6	76.0	7.2	7.8	8.5	9.3	10.2	11.2	12.4
76.5	7.7	8.3	9.0	9.8	10.7	11.6	12.7	76.5	7.3	7.9	8.6	9.4	10.3	11.4	12.5

Length		Boys						Length		Girls					
(cm)	–3SD	–2SD	–1SD	Median	1 SD	2SD	3SD	(cm)	–3SD	–2SD	–1SD	Median	1 SD	2SD	3SD
77.0	7.8	8.4	9.1	9.9	10.8	11.7	12.8	77.0	7.4	8.0	8.7	9.5	10.4	11.5	12.6
77.5	7.9	8.5	9.2	10.0	10.9	11.9	13.0	77.5	7.4	8.1	8.8	9.6	10.5	11.6	12.8
78.0	7.9	8.6	9.3	10.1	11.0	12.0	13.1	78.0	7.5	8.2	8.9	9.7	10.6	11.7	12.9
78.5	8.0	8.7	9.4	10.2	11.1	12.1	13.2	78.5	7.6	8.2	9.0	9.8	10.7	11.8	13.0
79.0	8.1	8.7	9.5	10.3	11.2	12.2	13.3	79.0	7.7	8.3	9.1	9.9	10.8	11.9	13.1
79.5	8.2	8.8	9.5	10.4	11.3	12.3	13.4	79.5	7.7	8.4	9.1	10.0	10.9	12.0	13.3
80.0	8.2	8.9	9.6	10.4	11.4	12.4	13.6	80.0	7.8	8.5	9.2	10.1	11.0	12.1	13.4
80.5	8.3	9.0	9.7	10.5	11.5	12.5	13.7	80.5	7.9	8.6	9.3	10.2	11.2	12.3	13.5
81.0	8.4	9.1	9.8	10.6	11.6	12.6	13.8	81.0	8.0	8.7	9.4	10.3	11.3	12.4	13.7
81.5	8.5	9.1	9.9	10.7	11.7	12.7	13.9	81.5	8.1	8.8	9.5	10.4	11.4	12.5	13.8
82.0	8.5	9.2	10.0	10.8	11.8	12.8	14.0	82.0	8.1	8.8	9.6	10.5	11.5	12.6	13.9
82.5	8.6	9.3	10.1	10.9	11.9	13.0	14.2	82.5	8.2	8.9	9.7	10.6	11.6	12.8	14.1
83.0	8.7	9.4	10.2	11.0	12.0	13.1	14.3	83.0	8.3	9.0	9.8	10.7	11.8	12.9	14.2
83.5	8.8	9.5	10.3	11.2	12.1	13.2	14.4	83.5	8.4	9.1	9.9	10.9	11.9	13.1	14.4
84.0	8.9	9.6	10.4	11.3	12.2	13.3	14.6	84.0	8.5	9.2	10.1	11.0	12.0	13.2	14.5
84.5	9.0	9.7	10.5	11.4	12.4	13.5	14.7	84.5	8.6	9.3	10.2	11.1	12.1	13.3	14.7
85.0	9.1	9.8	10.6	11.5	12.5	13.6	14.9	85.0	8.7	9.4	10.3	11.2	12.3	13.5	14.9
85.5	9.2	9.9	10.7	11.6	12.6	13.7	15.0	85.5	8.8	9.5	10.4	11.3	12.4	13.6	15.0
86.0	9.3	10.0	10.8	11.7	12.8	13.9	15.2	86.0	8.9	9.7	10.5	11.5	12.6	13.8	15.2
86.5	9.4	10.1	11.0	11.9	12.9	14.0	15.3	86.5	9.0	9.8	10.6	11.6	12.7	13.9	15.4
87.0	9.5	10.2	11.1	12.0	13.0	14.2	15.5	87.0	9.1	9.9	10.7	11.7	12.8	14.1	15.5
87.5	9.6	10.4	11.2	12.1	13.2	14.3	15.6	87.5	9.2	10.0	10.9	11.8	13.0	14.2	15.7
88.0	9.7	10.5	11.3	12.2	13.3	14.5	15.8	88.0	9.3	10.1	11.0	12.0	13.1	14.4	15.9
88.5	9.8	10.6	11.4	12.4	13.4	14.6	15.9	88.5	9.4	10.2	11.1	12.1	13.2	14.5	16.0
89.0	9.9	10.7	11.5	12.5	13.5	14.7	16.1	89.0	9.5	10.3	11.2	12.2	13.4	14.7	16.2
89.5	10.0	10.8	11.6	12.6	13.7	14.9	16.2	89.5	9.6	10.4	11.3	12.3	13.5	14.8	16.4
90.0	10.1	10.9	11.8	12.7	13.8	15.0	16.4	90.0	9.7	10.5	11.4	12.5	13.7	15.0	16.5
90.5	10.2	11.0	11.9	12.8	13.9	15.1	16.5	90.5	9.8	10.6	11.5	12.6	13.8	15.1	16.7
91.0	10.3	11.1	12.0	13.0	14.1	15.3	16.7	91.0	9.9	10.7	11.7	12.7	13.9	15.3	16.9
91.5	10.4	11.2	12.1	13.1	14.2	15.4	16.8	91.5	10.0	10.8	11.8	12.8	14.1	15.5	17.0
92.0	10.5	11.3	12.2	13.2	14.3	15.6	17.0	92.0	10.1	10.9	11.9	13.0	14.2	15.6	17.2
92.5	10.6	11.4	12.3	13.3	14.4	15.7	17.1	92.5	10.1	11.0	12.0	13.1	14.3	15.8	17.4
93.0	10.7	11.5	12.4	13.4	14.6	15.8	17.3	93.0	10.2	11.1	12.1	13.2	14.5	15.9	17.5
93.5	10.7	11.6	12.5	13.5	14.7	16.0	17.4	93.5	10.3	11.2	12.2	13.3	14.6	16.1	17.7

Length	Boys							Length	Girls						
(cm)	−3SD	−2SD	−1SD	Median	1 SD	2SD	3SD	(cm)	−3SD	−2SD	−1SD	Median	1 SD	2SD	3SD
94.0	10.8	11.7	12.6	13.7	14.8	16.1	17.6	94.0	10.4	11.3	12.3	13.5	14.7	16.2	17.9
94.5	10.9	11.8	12.7	13.8	14.9	16.3	17.7	94.5	10.5	11.4	12.4	13.6	14.9	16.4	18.0
95.0	11.0	11.9	12.8	13.9	15.1	16.4	17.9	95.0	10.6	11.5	12.6	13.7	15.0	16.5	18.2
95.5	11.1	12.0	12.9	14.0	15.2	16.5	18.0	95.5	10.7	11.6	12.7	13.8	15.2	16.7	18.4
96.0	11.2	12.1	13.1	14.1	15.3	16.7	18.2	96.0	10.8	11.7	12.8	14.0	15.3	16.8	18.6
96.5	11.3	12.2	13.2	14.3	15.5	16.8	18.4	96.5	10.9	11.8	12.9	14.1	15.4	17.0	18.7
97.0	11.4	12.3	13.3	14.4	15.6	17.0	18.5	97.0	11.0	12.0	13.0	14.2	15.6	17.1	18.9
97.5	11.5	12.4	13.4	14.5	15.7	17.1	18.7	97.5	11.1	12.1	13.1	14.4	15.7	17.3	19.1
98.0	11.6	12.5	13.5	14.6	15.9	17.3	18.9	98.0	11.2	12.2	13.3	14.5	15.9	17.5	19.3
98.5	11.7	12.6	13.6	14.8	16.0	17.5	19.1	98.5	11.3	12.3	13.4	14.6	16.0	17.6	19.5
99.0	11.8	12.7	13.7	14.9	16.2	17.6	19.2	99.0	11.4	12.4	13.5	14.8	16.2	17.8	19.6
99.5	11.9	12.8	13.9	15.0	16.3	17.8	19.4	99.5	11.5	12.5	13.6	14.9	16.3	18.0	19.8
100.0	12.0	12.9	14.0	15.2	16.5	18.0	19.6	100.0	11.6	12.6	13.7	15.0	16.5	18.1	20.0
100.5	12.1	13.0	14.1	15.3	16.6	18.1	19.8	100.5	11.7	12.7	13.9	15.2	16.6	18.3	20.2
101.0	12.2	13.2	14.2	15.4	16.8	18.3	20.0	101.0	11.8	12.8	14.0	15.3	16.8	18.5	20.4
101.5	12.3	13.3	14.4	15.6	16.9	18.5	20.2	101.5	11.9	13.0	14.1	15.5	17.0	18.7	20.6
102.0	12.4	13.4	14.5	15.7	17.1	18.7	20.4	102.0	12.0	13.1	14.3	15.6	17.1	18.9	20.8
102.5	12.5	13.5	14.6	15.9	17.3	18.8	20.6	102.5	12.1	13.2	14.4	15.8	17.3	19.0	21.0
103.0	12.6	13.6	14.8	16.0	17.4	19.0	20.8	103.0	12.3	13.3	14.5	15.9	17.5	19.2	21.3
103.5	12.7	13.7	14.9	16.2	17.6	19.2	21.0	103.5	12.4	13.5	14.7	16.1	17.6	19.4	21.5
104.0	12.8	13.9	15.0	16.3	17.8	19.4	21.2	104.0	12.5	13.6	14.8	16.2	17.8	19.6	21.7
104.5	12.9	14.0	15.2	16.5	17.9	19.6	21.5	104.5	12.6	13.7	15.0	16.4	18.0	19.8	21.9
105.0	13.0	14.1	15.3	16.6	18.1	19.8	21.7	105.0	12.7	13.8	15.1	16.5	18.2	20.0	22.2
105.5	13.2	14.2	15.4	16.8	18.3	20.0	21.9	105.5	12.8	14.0	15.3	16.7	18.4	20.2	22.4
106.0	13.3	14.4	15.6	16.9	18.5	20.2	22.1	106.0	13.0	14.1	15.4	16.9	18.5	20.5	22.6
106.5	13.4	14.5	15.7	17.1	18.6	20.4	22.4	106.5	13.1	14.3	15.6	17.1	18.7	20.7	22.9
107.0	13.5	14.6	15.9	17.3	18.8	20.6	22.6	107.0	13.2	14.4	15.7	17.2	18.9	20.9	23.1
107.5	13.6	14.7	16.0	17.4	19.0	20.8	22.8	107.5	13.3	14.5	15.9	17.4	19.1	21.1	23.4
108.0	13.7	14.9	16.2	17.6	19.2	21.0	23.1	108.0	13.5	14.7	16.0	17.6	19.3	21.3	23.6
108.5	13.8	15.0	16.3	17.8	19.4	21.2	23.3	108.5	13.6	14.8	16.2	17.8	19.5	21.6	23.9
109.0	14.0	15.1	16.5	17.9	19.6	21.4	23.6	109.0	13.7	15.0	16.4	18.0	19.7	21.8	24.2
109.5	14.1	15.3	16.6	18.1	19.8	21.7	23.8	109.5	13.9	15.1	16.5	18.1	20.0	22.0	24.4
110.0	14.2	15.4	16.8	18.3	20.0	21.9	24.1	110.0	14.0	15.3	16.7	18.3	20.2	22.3	24.7

Table 5.5 WHO Growth Standards Weight-for-Height – boys and girls over 2 to 5 years (Z scores) [5]

Length	Boys							Length	Girls						
(cm)	–3SD	–2SD	–1SD	Median	1 SD	2SD	3SD	(cm)	–3SD	–2SD	–1SD	Median	1 SD	2SD	3SD
65.0	5.9	6.3	6.9	7.4	8.1	8.8	9.6	65.0	5.6	6.1	6.6	7.2	7.9	8.7	9.7
65.5	6.0	6.4	7.0	7.6	8.2	8.9	9.8	65.5	5.7	6.2	6.7	7.4	8.1	8.9	9.8
66.0	6.1	6.5	7.1	7.7	8.3	9.1	9.9	66.0	5.8	6.3	6.8	7.5	8.2	9.0	10.0
66.5	6.1	6.6	7.2	7.8	8.5	9.2	10.1	66.5	5.8	6.4	6.9	7.6	8.3	9.1	10.1
67.0	6.2	6.7	7.3	7.9	8.6	9.4	10.2	67.0	5.9	6.4	7.0	7.7	8.4	9.3	10.2
67.5	6.3	6.8	7.4	8.0	8.7	9.5	10.4	67.5	6.0	6.5	7.1	7.8	8.5	9.4	10.4
68.0	6.4	6.9	7.5	8.1	8.8	9.6	10.5	68.0	6.1	6.6	7.2	7.9	8.7	9.5	10.5
68.5	6.5	7.0	7.6	8.2	9.0	9.8	10.7	68.5	6.2	6.7	7.3	8.0	8.8	9.7	10.7
69.0	6.6	7.1	7.7	8.4	9.1	9.9	10.8	69.0	6.3	6.8	7.4	8.1	8.9	9.8	10.8
69.5	6.7	7.2	7.8	8.5	9.2	10.0	11.0	69.5	6.3	6.9	7.5	8.2	9.0	9.9	10.9
70.0	6.8	7.3	7.9	8.6	9.3	10.2	11.1	70.0	6.4	7.0	7.6	8.3	9.1	10.0	11.1
70.5	6.9	7.4	8.0	8.7	9.5	10.3	11.3	70.5	6.5	7.1	7.7	8.4	9.2	10.1	11.2
71.0	6.9	7.5	8.1	8.8	9.6	10.4	11.4	71.0	6.6	7.1	7.8	8.5	9.3	10.3	11.3
71.5	7.0	7.6	8.2	8.9	9.7	10.6	11.6	71.5	6.7	7.2	7.9	8.6	9.4	10.4	11.5
72.0	7.1	7.7	8.3	9.0	9.8	10.7	11.7	72.0	6.7	7.3	8.0	8.7	9.5	10.5	11.6
72.5	7.2	7.8	8.4	9.1	9.9	10.8	11.8	72.5	6.8	7.4	8.1	8.8	9.7	10.6	11.7
73.0	7.3	7.9	8.5	9.2	10.0	11.0	12.0	73.0	6.9	7.5	8.1	8.9	9.8	10.7	11.8
73.5	7.4	7.9	8.6	9.3	10.2	11.1	12.1	73.5	7.0	7.6	8.2	9.0	9.9	10.8	12.0
74.0	7.4	8.0	8.7	9.4	10.3	11.2	12.2	74.0	7.0	7.6	8.3	9.1	10.0	11.0	12.1
74.5	7.5	8.1	8.8	9.5	10.4	11.3	12.4	74.5	7.1	7.7	8.4	9.2	10.1	11.1	12.2
75.0	7.6	8.2	8.9	9.6	10.5	11.4	12.5	75.0	7.2	7.8	8.5	9.3	10.2	11.2	12.3
75.5	7.7	8.3	9.0	9.7	10.6	11.6	12.6	75.5	7.2	7.9	8.6	9.4	10.3	11.3	12.5
76.0	7.7	8.4	9.1	9.8	10.7	11.7	12.8	76.0	7.3	8.0	8.7	9.5	10.4	11.4	12.6
76.5	7.8	8.5	9.2	9.9	10.8	11.8	12.9	76.5	7.4	8.0	8.7	9.6	10.5	11.5	12.7
77.0	7.9	8.5	9.2	10.0	10.9	11.9	13.0	77.0	7.5	8.1	8.8	9.6	10.6	11.6	12.8
77.5	8.0	8.6	9.3	10.1	11.0	12.0	13.1	77.5	7.5	8.2	8.9	9.7	10.7	11.7	12.9
78.0	8.0	8.7	9.4	10.2	11.1	12.1	13.3	78.0	7.6	8.3	9.0	9.8	10.8	11.8	13.1
78.5	8.1	8.8	9.5	10.3	11.2	12.2	13.4	78.5	7.7	8.4	9.1	9.9	10.9	12.0	13.2

Length		Boys						Length		Girls					
(cm)	–3SD	–2SD	–1SD	Median	1 SD	2SD	3SD	(cm)	–3SD	–2SD	–1SD	Median	1 SD	2SD	3SD
79.0	8.2	8.8	9.6	10.4	11.3	12.3	13.5	79.0	7.8	8.4	9.2	10.0	11.0	12.1	13.3
79.5	8.3	8.9	9.7	10.5	11.4	12.4	13.6	79.5	7.8	8.5	9.3	10.1	11.1	12.2	13.4
80.0	8.3	9.0	9.7	10.6	11.5	12.6	13.7	80.0	7.9	8.6	9.4	10.2	11.2	12.3	13.6
80.5	8.4	9.1	9.8	10.7	11.6	12.7	13.8	80.5	8.0	8.7	9.5	10.3	11.3	12.4	13.7
81.0	8.5	9.2	9.9	10.8	11.7	12.8	14.0	81.0	8.1	8.8	9.6	10.4	11.4	12.6	13.9
81.5	8.6	9.3	10.0	10.9	11.8	12.9	14.1	81.5	8.2	8.9	9.7	10.6	11.6	12.7	14.0
82.0	8.7	9.3	10.1	11.0	11.9	13.0	14.2	82.0	8.3	9.0	9.8	10.7	11.7	12.8	14.1
82.5	8.7	9.4	10.2	11.1	12.1	13.1	14.4	82.5	8.4	9.1	9.9	10.8	11.8	13.0	14.3
83.0	8.8	9.5	10.3	11.2	12.2	13.3	14.5	83.0	8.5	9.2	10.0	10.9	11.9	13.1	14.5
83.5	8.9	9.6	10.4	11.3	12.3	13.4	14.6	83.5	8.5	9.3	10.1	11.0	12.1	13.3	14.6
84.0	9.0	9.7	10.5	11.4	12.4	13.5	14.8	84.0	8.6	9.4	10.2	11.1	12.2	13.4	14.8
84.5	9.1	9.9	10.7	11.5	12.5	13.7	14.9	84.5	8.7	9.5	10.3	11.3	12.3	13.5	14.9
85.0	9.2	10.0	10.8	11.7	12.7	13.8	15.1	85.0	8.8	9.6	10.4	11.4	12.5	13.7	15.1
85.5	9.3	10.1	10.9	11.8	12.8	13.9	15.2	85.5	8.9	9.7	10.6	11.5	12.6	13.8	15.3
86.0	9.4	10.2	11.0	11.9	12.9	14.1	15.4	86.0	9.0	9.8	10.7	11.6	12.7	14.0	15.4
86.5	9.5	10.3	11.1	12.0	13.1	14.2	15.5	86.5	9.1	9.9	10.8	11.8	12.9	14.2	15.6
87.0	9.6	10.4	11.2	12.2	13.2	14.4	15.7	87.0	9.2	10.0	10.9	11.9	13.0	14.3	15.8
87.5	9.7	10.5	11.3	12.3	13.3	14.5	15.8	87.5	9.3	10.1	11.0	12.0	13.2	14.5	15.9
88.0	9.8	10.6	11.5	12.4	13.5	14.7	16.0	88.0	9.4	10.2	11.1	12.1	13.3	14.6	16.1
88.5	9.9	10.7	11.6	12.5	13.6	14.8	16.1	88.5	9.5	10.3	11.2	12.3	13.4	14.8	16.3
89.0	10.0	10.8	11.7	12.6	13.7	14.9	16.3	89.0	9.6	10.4	11.4	12.4	13.6	14.9	16.4
89.5	10.1	10.9	11.8	12.8	13.9	15.1	16.4	89.5	9.7	10.5	11.5	12.5	13.7	15.1	16.6
90.0	10.2	11.0	11.9	12.9	14.0	15.2	16.6	90.0	9.8	10.6	11.6	12.6	13.8	15.2	16.8
90.5	10.3	11.1	12.0	13.0	14.1	15.3	16.7	90.5	9.9	10.7	11.7	12.8	14.0	15.4	16.9
91.0	10.4	11.2	12.1	13.1	14.2	15.5	16.9	91.0	10.0	10.9	11.8	12.9	14.1	15.5	17.1
91.5	10.5	11.3	12.2	13.2	14.4	15.6	17.0	91.5	10.1	11.0	11.9	13.0	14.3	15.7	17.3
92.0	10.6	11.4	12.3	13.4	14.5	15.8	17.2	92.0	10.2	11.1	12.0	13.1	14.4	15.8	17.4
92.5	10.7	11.5	12.4	13.5	14.6	15.9	17.3	92.5	10.3	11.2	12.1	13.3	14.5	16.0	17.6
93.0	10.8	11.6	12.6	13.6	14.7	16.0	17.5	93.0	10.4	11.3	12.3	13.4	14.7	16.1	17.8
93.5	10.9	11.7	12.7	13.7	14.9	16.2	17.6	93.5	10.5	11.4	12.4	13.5	14.8	16.3	17.9

Length		Boys						Length		Girls					
(cm)	–3SD	–2SD	–1SD	Median	1 SD	2SD	3SD	(cm)	–3SD	–2SD	–1SD	Median	1 SD	2SD	3SD
94.0	11.0	11.8	12.8	13.8	15.0	16.3	17.8	94.0	10.6	11.5	12.5	13.6	14.9	16.4	18.1
94.5	11.1	11.9	12.9	13.9	15.1	16.5	17.9	94.5	10.7	11.6	12.6	13.8	15.1	16.6	18.3
95.0	11.1	12.0	13.0	14.1	15.3	16.6	18.1	95.0	10.8	11.7	12.7	13.9	15.2	16.7	18.5
95.5	11.2	12.1	13.1	14.2	15.4	16.7	18.3	95.5	10.8	11.8	12.8	14.0	15.4	16.9	18.6
96.0	11.3	12.2	13.2	14.3	15.5	16.9	18.4	96.0	10.9	11.9	12.9	14.1	15.5	17.0	18.8
96.5	11.4	12.3	13.3	14.4	15.7	17.0	18.6	96.5	11.0	12.0	13.1	14.3	15.6	17.2	19.0
97.0	11.5	12.4	13.4	14.6	15.8	17.2	18.8	97.0	11.1	12.1	13.2	14.4	15.8	17.4	19.2
97.5	11.6	12.5	13.6	14.7	15.9	17.4	18.9	97.5	11.2	12.2	13.3	14.5	15.9	17.5	19.3
98.0	11.7	12.6	13.7	14.8	16.1	17.5	19.1	98.0	11.3	12.3	13.4	14.7	16.1	17.7	19.5
98.5	11.8	12.8	13.8	14.9	16.2	17.7	19.3	98.5	11.4	12.4	13.5	14.8	16.2	17.9	19.7
99.0	11.9	12.9	13.9	15.1	16.4	17.9	19.5	99.0	11.5	12.5	13.7	14.9	16.4	18.0	19.9
99.5	12.0	13.0	14.0	15.2	16.5	18.0	19.7	99.5	11.6	12.7	13.8	15.1	16.5	18.2	20.1
100.0	12.1	13.1	14.2	15.4	16.7	18.2	19.9	100.0	11.7	12.8	13.9	15.2	16.7	18.4	20.3
100.5	12.2	13.2	14.3	15.5	16.9	18.4	20.1	100.5	11.9	12.9	14.1	15.4	16.9	18.6	20.5
101.0	12.3	13.3	14.4	15.6	17.0	18.5	20.3	101.0	12.0	13.0	14.2	15.5	17.0	18.7	20.7
101.5	12.4	13.4	14.5	15.8	17.2	18.7	20.5	101.5	12.1	13.1	14.3	15.7	17.2	18.9	20.9
102.0	12.5	13.6	14.7	15.9	17.3	18.9	20.7	102.0	12.2	13.3	14.5	15.8	17.4	19.1	21.1
102.5	12.6	13.7	14.8	16.1	17.5	19.1	20.9	102.5	12.3	13.4	14.6	16.0	17.5	19.3	21.4
103.0	12.8	13.8	14.9	16.2	17.7	19.3	21.1	103.0	12.4	13.5	14.7	16.1	17.7	19.5	21.6
103.5	12.9	13.9	15.1	16.4	17.8	19.5	21.3	103.5	12.5	13.6	14.9	16.3	17.9	19.7	21.8
104.0	13.0	14.0	15.2	16.5	18.0	19.7	21.6	104.0	12.6	13.8	15.0	16.4	18.1	19.9	22.0
104.5	13.1	14.2	15.4	16.7	18.2	19.9	21.8	104.5	12.8	13.9	15.2	16.6	18.2	20.1	22.3
105.0	13.2	14.3	15.5	16.8	18.4	20.1	22.0	105.0	12.9	14.0	15.3	16.8	18.4	20.3	22.5
105.5	13.3	14.4	15.6	17.0	18.5	20.3	22.2	105.5	13.0	14.2	15.5	16.9	18.6	20.5	22.7
106.0	13.4	14.5	15.8	17.2	18.7	20.5	22.5	106.0	13.1	14.3	15.6	17.1	18.8	20.8	23.0
106.5	13.5	14.7	15.9	17.3	18.9	20.7	22.7	106.5	13.3	14.5	15.8	17.3	19.0	21.0	23.2
107.0	13.7	14.8	16.1	17.5	19.1	20.9	22.9	107.0	13.4	14.6	15.9	17.5	19.2	21.2	23.5
107.5	13.8	14.9	16.2	17.7	19.3	21.1	23.2	107.5	13.5	14.7	16.1	17.7	19.4	21.4	23.7
108.0	13.9	15.1	16.4	17.8	19.5	21.3	23.4	108.0	13.7	14.9	16.3	17.8	19.6	21.7	24.0
108.5	14.0	15.2	16.5	18.0	19.7	21.5	23.7	108.5	13.8	15.0	16.4	18.0	19.8	21.9	24.3

Length	Boys							Length	Girls						
(cm)	–3SD	–2SD	–1SD	Median	1 SD	2SD	3SD	(cm)	–3SD	–2SD	–1SD	Median	1 SD	2SD	3SD
109.0	14.1	15.3	16.7	18.2	19.8	21.8	23.9	109.0	13.9	15.2	16.6	18.2	20.0	22.1	24.5
109.5	14.3	15.5	16.8	18.3	20.0	22.0	24.2	109.5	14.1	15.4	16.8	18.4	20.3	22.4	24.8
110.0	14.4	15.6	17.0	18.5	20.2	22.2	24.4	110.0	14.2	15.5	17.0	18.6	20.5	22.6	25.1
110.5	14.5	15.8	17.1	18.7	20.4	22.4	24.7	110.5	14.4	15.7	17.1	18.8	20.7	22.9	25.4
111.0	14.6	15.9	17.3	18.9	20.7	22.7	25.0	111.0	14.5	15.8	17.3	19.0	20.9	23.1	25.7
111.5	14.8	16.0	17.5	19.1	20.9	22.9	25.2	111.5	14.7	16.0	17.5	19.2	21.2	23.4	26.0
112.0	14.9	16.2	17.6	19.2	21.1	23.1	25.5	112.0	14.8	16.2	17.7	19.4	21.4	23.6	26.2
112.5	15.0	16.3	17.8	19.4	21.3	23.4	25.8	112.5	15.0	16.3	17.9	19.6	21.6	23.9	26.5
113.0	15.2	16.5	18.0	19.6	21.5	23.6	26.0	113.0	15.1	16.5	18.0	19.8	21.8	24.2	26.8
113.5	15.3	16.6	18.1	19.8	21.7	23.9	26.3	113.5	15.3	16.7	18.2	20.0	22.1	24.4	27.1
114.0	15.4	16.8	18.3	20.0	21.9	24.1	26.6	114.0	15.4	16.8	18.4	20.2	22.3	24.7	27.4
114.5	15.6	16.9	18.5	20.2	22.1	24.4	26.9	114.5	15.6	17.0	18.6	20.5	22.6	25.0	27.8
115.0	15.7	17.1	18.6	20.4	22.4	24.6	27.2	115.0	15.7	17.2	18.8	20.7	22.8	25.2	28.1
115.5	15.8	17.2	18.8	20.6	22.6	24.9	27.5	115.5	15.9	17.3	19.0	20.9	23.0	25.5	28.4
116.0	16.0	17.4	19.0	20.8	22.8	25.1	27.8	116.0	16.0	17.5	19.2	21.1	23.3	25.8	28.7
116.5	16.1	17.5	19.2	21.0	23.0	25.4	28.0	116.5	16.2	17.7	19.4	21.3	23.5	26.1	29.0
117.0	16.2	17.7	19.3	21.2	23.3	25.6	28.3	117.0	16.3	17.8	19.6	21.5	23.8	26.3	29.3
117.5	16.4	17.9	19.5	21.4	23.5	25.9	28.6	117.5	16.5	18.0	19.8	21.7	24.0	26.6	29.6
118.0	16.5	18.0	19.7	21.6	23.7	26.1	28.9	118.0	16.6	18.2	19.9	22.0	24.2	26.9	29.9
118.5	16.7	18.2	19.9	21.8	23.9	26.4	29.2	118.5	16.8	18.4	20.1	22.2	24.5	27.2	30.3
119.0	16.8	18.3	20.0	22.0	24.1	26.6	29.5	119.0	16.9	18.5	20.3	22.4	24.7	27.4	30.6
119.5	16.9	18.5	20.2	22.2	24.4	26.9	29.8	119.5	17.1	18.7	20.5	22.6	25.0	27.7	30.9
120.0	17.1	18.6	20.4	22.4	24.6	27.2	30.1	120.0	17.3	18.9	20.7	22.8	25.2	28.0	31.2

being insensitive in the presence of edema or in cancer patients with large tumor load. Edema can be diagnosed by applying moderate thumb pressure to the back of the foot or ankle. The impression of the thumb will remain for some time when edema is present. The presence of edema in individuals should be recorded when using any weight-based index.

When a child has edema, it is automatically included with children counted as severely malnourished, independently of its wasting, stunting, or underweight status. This is due to the strong association between edema and mortality.

Body mass index (BMI)

BMI is measured as weight (in kg) divided by height^2 (in meters^2). Body mass index is known to track significantly from childhood to adolescence and then to adulthood. However, both sex and pubertal development are associated with dramatic changes in body composition and the values may require adjustment as per the sexual maturity. BMI has been used since the 1960s to assess obesity in adults and more recently in children. With the availability of BMI cut-offs for children and WHO BMI reference charts from 0–19 years, the use of BMI can be extended for assessing thinness in children and adolescence [7]. Table 5.6 presents BMI for age index for both boys and girls from birth to 5 years.

Mid-upper arm circumference (MUAC)

It is relatively easy to measure and a good predictor of immediate risk of death. It is used for rapid screening of acute malnutrition in the age group of 1–5 years. MUAC can be used for screening in emergency situations and for estimating the prevalence of malnutrition in the populations but is not typically used for evaluation purposes. Though grossly mid-arm circumference may be considered an age independent index in children between 1 and 5 years of age, recently age specific cut-offs for mid-arm circumference have been released by WHO [5]. MUAC is also recommended for rapid identification of severe acute malnutrition (SAM) in a community – MUAC of less than 115 mm being indicative of SAM.

5.3 Comparison of indices with references

Once value of any index is obtained or calculated, it has to be compared with the expected value and interpretation is to be made. References are used to standardize a child's measurement by comparing the child's measurement with the average measure for healthy children of the same

Table 5.6 WHO Growth Standards BMI-for-Age – boys and girls birth to 5 years (Z scores) [5]*

Year:	Months	Boys							Girls						
Month		–3SD	–2SD	–1SD	Median	1 SD	2SD	3SD	–3SD	–2SD	–1SD	Median	1 SD	2SD	3SD
0:0	0	10.2	11.1	12.2	13.4	14.8	16.3	18.1	10.1	11.1	12.2	13.3	14.6	16.1	17.7
0:1	1	11.3	12.4	13.6	14.9	16.3	17.8	19.4	10.8	12.0	13.2	14.6	16.0	17.5	19.1
0:2	2	12.5	13.7	15.0	16.3	17.8	19.4	21.1	11.8	13.0	14.3	15.8	17.3	19.0	20.7
0:3	3	13.1	14.3	15.5	16.9	18.4	20.0	21.8	12.4	13.6	14.9	16.4	17.9	19.7	21.5
0:4	4	13.4	14.5	15.8	17.2	18.7	20.3	22.1	12.7	13.9	15.2	16.7	18.3	20.0	22.0
0:5	5	13.5	14.7	15.9	17.3	18.8	20.5	22.3	12.9	14.1	15.4	16.8	18.4	20.2	22.2
0:6	6	13.6	14.7	16.0	17.3	18.8	20.5	22.3	13.0	14.1	15.5	16.9	18.5	20.3	22.3
0:7	7	13.7	14.8	16.0	17.3	18.8	20.5	22.3	13.0	14.2	15.5	16.9	18.5	20.3	22.3
0:8	8	13.6	14.7	15.9	17.3	18.7	20.4	22.2	13.0	14.1	15.4	16.8	18.4	20.2	22.2
0:9	9	13.6	14.7	15.8	17.2	18.6	20.3	22.1	12.9	14.1	15.3	16.7	18.3	20.1	22.1
0:10	10	13.5	14.6	15.7	17.0	18.5	20.1	22.0	12.9	14.0	15.2	16.6	18.2	19.9	21.9
0:11	11	13.4	14.5	15.6	16.9	18.4	20.0	21.8	12.8	13.9	15.1	16.5	18.0	19.8	21.8
1:0	12	13.4	14.4	15.5	16.8	18.2	19.8	21.6	12.7	13.8	15.0	16.4	17.9	19.6	21.6
1.1	13	13.3	14.3	15.4	16.7	18.1	19.7	21.5	12.6	13.7	14.9	16.2	17.7	19.5	21.4
1:2	14	13.2	14.2	15.3	16.6	18.0	19.5	21.3	12.6	13.6	14.8	16.1	17.6	19.3	21.3
1:3	15	13.1	14.1	15.2	16.4	17.8	19.4	21.2	12.5	13.5	14.7	16.0	17.5	19.2	21.1
1:4	16	13.1	14.0	15.1	16.3	17.7	19.3	21.0	12.4	13.5	14.6	15.9	17.4	19.1	21.0
1:5	17	13.0	13.9	15.0	16.2	17.6	19.1	20.9	12.4	13.4	14.5	15.8	17.3	18.9	20.9
1:6	18	12.9	13.9	14.9	16.1	17.5	19.0	20.8	12.3	13.3	14.4	15.7	17.2	18.8	20.8
1:7	19	12.9	13.8	14.9	16.1	17.4	18.9	20.7	12.3	13.3	14.4	15.7	17.1	18.8	20.7
1:8	20	12.8	13.7	14.8	16.0	17.3	18.8	20.6	12.2	13.2	14.3	15.6	17.0	18.7	20.6
1:9	21	12.8	13.7	14.7	15.9	17.2	18.7	20.5	12.2	13.2	14.3	15.5	17.0	18.6	20.6
1:10	22	12.7	13.6	14.7	15.8	17.2	18.7	20.4	12.2	13.1	14.2	15.5	16.9	18.5	20.4
1:11	23	12.7	13.6	14.6	15.8	17.1	18.6	20.3	12.2	13.1	14.2	15.4	16.9	18.5	20.4
2:0	24	12.7	13.6	14.6	15.7	17.0	18.5	20.3	12.1	13.1	14.2	15.4	16.8	18.4	20.3
2.0	24	12.9	13.8	14.8	16.0	17.3	18.9	20.6	12.4	13.3	14.4	15.7	17.1	18.7	20.6
2:1	25	12.8	13.8	14.8	16.0	17.3	18.8	20.5	12.4	13.3	14.4	15.7	17.1	18.7	20.5
2:2	26	12.8	13.7	14.8	15.9	17.3	18.8	20.5	12.3	13.3	14.4	15.6	17.0	18.7	20.6
2:3	27	12.7	13.7	14.7	15.9	17.2	18.7	20.4	12.3	13.3	14.4	15.6	17.0	18.6	20.5
2:4	28	12.7	13.6	14.7	15.9	17.2	18.7	20.4	12.3	13.3	14.3	15.6	17.0	18.6	20.5
2:5	29	12.7	13.6	14.7	15.8	17.1	18.6	20.3	12.3	13.2	14.3	15.6	17.0	18.6	20.4

Year: Month	Months	Boys							Girls						
		–3SD	–2SD	–1SD	Median	1 SD	2SD	3SD	–3SD	–2SD	–1SD	Median	1 SD	2SD	3SD
2:6	30	12.6	13.6	14.6	15.8	17.1	18.6	20.2	12.3	13.2	14.3	15.5	16.9	18.5	20.4
2:7	31	12.6	13.5	14.6	15.8	17.1	18.5	20.2	12.2	13.2	14.3	15.5	16.9	18.5	20.4
2:8	32	12.5	13.5	14.6	15.7	17.0	18.5	20.1	12.2	13.2	14.3	15.5	16.9	18.5	20.4
2:9	33	12.5	13.5	14.5	15.7	17.0	18.5	20.1	12.2	13.1	14.2	15.5	16.9	18.5	20.3
2:10	34	12.5	13.4	14.5	15.7	17.0	18.4	20.0	12.2	13.1	14.2	15.4	16.8	18.5	20.3
2:11	35	12.4	13.4	14.5	15.6	16.9	18.4	20.0	12.1	13.1	14.2	15.4	16.8	18.4	20.3
3:0	36	12.4	13.4	14.4	15.6	16.9	18.4	20.0	12.1	13.1	14.2	15.4	16.8	18.4	20.3
3:1	37	12.4	13.3	14.4	15.6	16.9	18.3	19.9	12.1	13.1	14.1	15.4	16.8	18.4	20.3
3:2	38	12.3	13.3	14.4	15.5	16.8	18.3	19.9	12.1	13.0	14.1	15.4	16.8	18.4	20.3
3:3	39	12.3	13.3	14.3	15.5	16.8	18.3	19.9	12.0	13.0	14.1	15.3	16.8	18.4	20.3
3:4	40	12.3	13.2	14.3	15.5	16.8	18.2	19.9	12.0	13.0	14.1	15.3	16.8	18.4	20.3
3:5	41	12.2	13.2	14.3	15.5	16.8	18.2	19.9	12.0	13.0	14.1	15.3	16.8	18.4	20.4
3:6	42	12.2	13.2	14.3	15.4	16.8	18.2	19.8	12.0	12.9	14.0	15.3	16.8	18.4	20.4
3:7	43	12.2	13.2	14.2	15.4	16.7	18.2	19.8	11.9	12.9	14.0	15.3	16.8	18.4	20.4
3:8	44	12.2	13.1	14.2	15.4	16.7	18.2	19.8	11.9	12.9	14.0	15.3	16.8	18.5	20.4
3:9	45	12.2	13.1	14.2	15.4	16.7	18.2	19.8	11.9	12.9	14.0	15.3	16.8	18.5	20.5
3:10	46	12.1	13.1	14.2	15.4	16.7	18.2	19.8	11.9	12.9	14.0	15.3	16.8	18.5	20.5
3:11	47	12.1	13.1	14.2	15.3	16.7	18.2	19.9	11.8	12.8	14.0	15.3	16.8	18.5	20.5
4:0	48	12.1	13.1	14.1	15.3	16.7	18.2	19.9	11.8	12.8	14.0	15.3	16.8	18.5	20.6
4:1	49	12.1	13.0	14.1	15.3	16.7	18.2	19.9	11.8	12.8	13.9	15.3	16.8	18.5	20.6
4:2	50	12.1	13.0	14.1	15.3	16.7	18.2	19.9	11.8	12.8	13.9	15.3	16.8	18.6	20.7
4:3	51	12.1	13.0	14.1	15.3	16.6	18.2	19.9	11.8	12.8	13.9	15.3	16.8	18.6	20.7
4:4	52	12.0	13.0	14.1	15.3	16.6	18.2	19.9	11.7	12.8	13.9	15.2	16.8	18.6	20.7
4:5	53	12.0	13.0	14.1	15.3	16.6	18.2	20.0	11.7	12.7	13.9	15.3	16.8	18.6	20.8
4:6	54	12.0	13.0	14.0	15.3	16.6	18.2	20.0	11.7	12.7	13.9	15.3	16.8	18.7	20.8
4:7	55	12.0	13.0	14.0	15.2	16.6	18.2	20.0	11.7	12.7	13.9	15.3	16.8	18.7	20.9
4:8	56	12.0	12.9	14.0	15.2	16.6	18.2	20.1	11.7	12.7	13.9	15.3	16.8	18.7	20.9
4:9	57	12.0	12.9	14.0	15.2	16.6	18.2	20.1	11.7	12.7	13.9	15.3	16.9	18.7	21.0
4:10	58	12.0	12.9	14.0	15.2	16.6	18.3	20.2	11.7	12.7	13.9	15.3	16.9	18.8	21.0
4:11	59	12.0	12.9	14.0	15.2	16.6	18.3	20.2	11.6	12.7	13.9	15.3	16.9	18.8	21.0
5:0	60	12.0	12.9	14.0	15.2	16.6	18.3	20.3	11.6	12.7	13.9	15.3	16.9	18.8	21.1

*The WHO length- and height-based BMI-for-age standards do not overlap, i.e. the length-based interval ends at 730 days and the height-based interval starts at 731 days.

age and sex [8]. Taking age and sex into consideration, differences in measurements can be expressed in a number of ways:

- Percentage of the median
- Standard deviation units, or Z-scores
- Percentiles

Percentage of the median

The percentage of the median is defined as the ratio of a measured or observed value of the individual to the median value of the reference data for the same age or height for the specific sex, expressed as a percentage. The median is the average or 50th percentile value. If a child's measurement is exactly the same as the median of the reference population we say that it is 100% of the median. This can be calculated as:

$$\text{Percent of median} = \frac{\text{Observed value} \times 100}{\text{Median value of reference population}}$$

Z-Scores

The Z-score or standard deviation unit (SD) is defined as the difference between the value for an individual and the median value of the reference population for the same age or height, divided by the standard deviation of the reference population [9]. This can be written in equation form as:

$$\text{Z-score (or SD Score)} = \frac{\text{(Observed value)} - \text{(Median reference value)}}{\text{Standard deviation of reference population}}$$

Z-scores are more commonly used by the international nutrition community because they offer two major advantages. First, using Z-scores allows us to identify a fixed point in the distributions of different indices and across different ages. For all indices for all ages, 2.28% of the reference population lies below a cut-off of –2 Z-scores. The percent of the median does not have this characteristic. For example, because weight and height have different distributions (variances), –2 Z-scores on the weight-for-age distribution is about 80% of the median, and –2 Z-scores on the height-for-age distribution is about 90% of the median. Further, the proportion of the population identified by a particular percentage of the median varies at different ages on the same index. The second major advantage of using Z-scores is that useful summary statistics can be calculated from them. The approach allows the mean and standard deviation to be calculated for the Z-scores for a group of children. The Z-score application is considered the simplest way of describing the reference population and making comparisons to it. It is the statistic recommended for use when reporting results of nutritional assessments. The distribution of Z-scores follows a normal (bell-shaped or Gaussian) distribution.

Percentiles

The percentile is the rank position of an individual on a given reference distribution, stated in terms of what percentage of the group the individual equals or exceeds. The percentiles can be thought of as the percentage of children in the reference population below the equivalent cut-off. For example, 10 percent of children would be expected to be below 10th percentile in a normally distributed population. The commonly used cut-offs of –3, –2, and –1 Z-scores are respectively, the 0.13th, 2.28th, and 15.8th percentiles.

5.4 Cut-offs

Cut-offs are used for identifying children who are at higher risk of adverse outcomes either due to undernutrition or overnutrition. The most commonly used cut-off with Z-scores is "–2 standard deviations" irrespective of the indicator used. This means children with a Z-score below -2 SD for weight-for-age, height-for-age or weight-for-height are considered underweight, stunted and wasted, respectively. (Tables 5.1, 5.2, 5.3, 5.4 and 5.5). Children having Z-scores below –3 SD are considered to be having severe forms of these conditions. For example, a child with a Z-score for weight-for-height of –2.5 is classified as being wasted whereas a child with a Z-score of –1.9 is not considered wasted. In the reference population, by definition, 2.3% of the children would be below -2 SD and 0.13% would be below -3 SD. *WHO Classification of Undernutrition* is based on this currently accepted nomenclature. This classification is used for assessing the magnitude of malnutrition amongst under-five children in national health programs (Table 5.1). In some classifications, the cut-off for defining malnutrition used is –1 SD. The use of –1 SD as cut-off over-estimates malnutrition as a significant proportion (15.8%) of healthy children normally would fall below this cut-off.

Using the percentile method, the cut-offs of –3, –2, and –1 Z-scores are, respectively the 0.13th, 2.28th, and 15.8th percentiles [2]. For practical purpose, the cut-off for defining malnutrition (wasting or stunting) of –2 SD (Z-score) is taken as less than 3rd percentile. The percentile method of classification also retains the advantage of Z-score in terms of uniformity in classifications for all indicators (underweight, wasting or stunting). However, this method is less useful for classifying the extreme forms (e.g. < 3 SD or >3 SD) of malnutrition as the equivalent percentile values become extremely small and difficult to calculate or represent.

The cut-offs can also decided by percentage of reference median. This carries the advantage of ease of calculation as the only parameter required for this is observed value and the expected (median reference) value. However, the disadvantage is that the cut-off would be different for different parameters depending on the variability of the parameter in the population. Also, these derivations are approximate and there might be few subjects who are wrongly classified as being or not being malnourished by percentage method in comparison to Z-score technique. A comparison of cut-offs for percent of median and Z-scores illustrates the following:

80% for weight-for-age = –2 Z-score (Underweight)
90% for height-for-age = –2 Z-score (Stunting)
85% for height-for-age = –3 Z-score (Severe stunting)
80% for weight-for-height = –2 Z-score (Wasting)
70% for weight-for-height = –3 Z-score (Severe wasting)

For BMI cut-offs, adult values of overweight and obesity in childhood have been used to construct statistical models for children [10]. The choice of cut-off is fundamentally important to identify correctly those children at risk and ideally should be related to known outcomes for morbidity and mortality. Yet while adult body mass index values of 25 (overweight) and 30 (obesity) are related to morbidity, evidence on morbidity related to cut-offs for thinness, particularly in children, is less clear. Recently, this work has been extended to provide cut-offs for body mass index to define "thinness" in children and adolescents [11, 12].

5.5 Growth references

When the comparisons of the anthropometric indices are to be made using percentile, percentage or Z-score method, reference tables/charts/curves are required. It is important that the reference chosen is reflective of a good nutritional status and thus should be based on the growth of children who had optimum nutrition and not having any adverse health constraints. The growth charts obtained from such reference population are called growth references.

Local (country-specific) references

Growth charts are widely used throughout the world for assessing the nutritional status of young children. When these began to be widely disseminated in the 1970s, there was considerable debate as to whether separate growth references should be developed for each country or whether a single international reference would suffice. Some argued that the growth of children of high socio-economic status was very similar throughout the world, irrespective of ethnic background. Others believed that although international references were useful for comparing across populations, country-specific references were essential for assessing the growth of individual children. Country-specific and sometimes even geographic-specific references are available for many settings. For India, locally derived references are available but require frequent updating as India is still experiencing secular trends of increasing weight and height because of continuous improvement in nutritional and socio-economic structure of the country.

NCHS growth references for children

The NCHS reference was developed in the United States in 1975 by pooling four different sources of data [13]. The reference for 2–18 year olds was based on three representative surveys conducted in the US between 1960 and 1975. For children less than 2 years of age the data came from the Fels Longitudinal Study carried out in Yellow Springs, Ohio, from 1929 to 1975. The group was of homogeneous genetic, geographic, and socio-economic backgrounds. For older children, the data came from nationally representative cross-sectional surveys of children in the United States and include all ethnic groups and social classes. These growth references have been used for decades all over the world to assess the growth of individual children and for comparisons across populations. However, recently concerns have been raised about validity of these references for healthy breastfed children as these reflect the growth of children who were fed primarily infant formula and in whom complementary feeding often was initiated before 4 months [14, 15].

WHO child growth references

A comprehensive review of the uses and interpretation of anthropometric undertaken by WHO in the 1990s concluded that new growth curves were needed to replace the existing international reference [16]. To develop new references, a multi-country study was carried out to collect primary growth data and related information from 8440 healthy breastfed infants and young children from diverse ethnic backgrounds and cultural settings (Brazil, Ghana, India, Norway, Oman and the USA). The growth references represent the description of physiological growth for children under-5 years of age, under optimal environmental conditions [17]. The children included in the study were raised in environments that minimized constraints to growth such as poor diets and infection. In addition, their mothers followed health practices such as breastfeeding their children and not smoking during and after pregnancy.

These growth charts were released in 2006 [5]. Based on these simplified field tables were developed. These are presented in Tables 5.1, 5.2, 5.3, 5.4, 5.5, 5.6 and 5.7, (length/height-for-age, weight-for-age, weight-for-length, weight-for-height, body mass index-for-age, Recently, WHO proceeded to reconstruct the 1977 NCHS/WHO growth reference from 5 to 19 years, using the original sample (a non-obese sample with expected heights) supplemented with data from the WHO Child Growth References (to facilitate a smooth transition at 5 years) and applying complex statistical methods [6]. The 2007 height-for-age and BMI-for-age charts extend to 19 years, which is the upper age limit of adolescence as defined by WHO. The weight-for-age charts extend to 10 years for the benefit of countries that routinely measure only weight and would like to monitor growth throughout childhood. Weight-for-age is inadequate for monitoring growth beyond childhood due to its inability to distinguish between relative height and body mass, hence, the provision here of BMI-for-age to complement height-for-age in the assessment of thinness (low BMI-for-age), overweight and obesity (high BMI-for-age) and stunting (low height-for-age) in school-aged children and adolescents.

The new WHO growth charts are likely to change the current estimates of undernutrition and overnutrition in children [18]. A notable effect is that stunting (low height-for-age) will be greater throughout childhood when assessed using the new WHO references compared to the previous international reference. There will be a substantial increase in underweight rates during the first half of infancy (i.e., 0–6 months) and a decrease thereafter. For wasting (low weight-for-length/height), the main difference between the new references and the old reference is during infancy (i.e., up to about 70 cm length) when wasting rates will be substantially higher using the new WHO references. With respect to overweight, use of the new WHO references will result in a greater prevalence that will vary by age, sex and nutritional status of the index population.

Table 5.7 WHO Growth Standards BMI for Age boys and girls over 5 to 19 years (Z scores) [5]

Year:	Months	Boys							Girls						
Month		–3SD	–2SD	–1SD	Median	1 SD	2SD	3SD	–3SD	–2SD	–1SD	Median	1 SD	2SD	3SD
5:1	61	12.1	13.0	14.1	15.3	16.6	18.3	20.2	11.8	12.7	13.9	15.2	16.9	18.9	21.3
5:2	62	12.1	13.0	14.1	15.3	16.6	18.3	20.2	11.8	12.7	13.9	15.2	16.9	18.9	21.4
5:3	63	12.1	13.0	14.1	15.3	16.7	18.3	20.2	11.8	12.7	13.9	15.2	16.9	18.9	21.5
5:4	64	12.1	13.0	14.1	15.3	16.7	18.3	20.3	11.8	12.7	13.9	15.2	16.9	18.9	21.5
5:5	65	12.1	13.0	14.1	15.3	16.7	18.3	20.3	11.7	12.7	13.9	15.2	16.9	19.0	21.6
5:6	66	12.1	13.0	14.1	15.3	16.7	18.4	20.4	11.7	12.7	13.9	15.2	16.9	19.0	21.7
5:7	67	12.1	13.0	14.1	15.3	16.7	18.4	20.4	11.7	12.7	13.9	15.2	16.9	19.0	21.7
5:8	68	12.1	13.0	14.1	15.3	16.7	18.4	20.5	11.7	12.7	13.9	15.3	17.0	19.1	21.8
5:9	69	12.1	13.0	14.1	15.3	16.7	18.4	20.5	11.7	12.7	13.9	15.3	17.0	19.1	21.9
5:10	70	12.1	13.0	14.1	15.3	16.7	18.5	20.6	11.7	12.7	13.9	15.3	17.0	19.1	22.0
5:11	71	12.1	13.0	14.1	15.3	16.7	18.5	20.6	11.7	12.7	13.9	15.3	17.0	19.2	22.1
6:0	72	12.1	13.0	14.1	15.3	16.8	18.5	20.7	11.7	12.7	13.9	15.3	17.0	19.2	22.1
6:1	73	12.1	13.0	14.1	15.3	16.8	18.6	20.8	11.7	12.7	13.9	15.3	17.0	19.3	22.2
6:2	74	12.2	13.1	14.1	15.3	16.8	18.6	20.8	11.7	12.7	13.9	15.3	17.0	19.3	22.3
6:3	75	12.2	13.1	14.1	15.3	16.8	18.6	20.9	11.7	12.7	13.9	15.3	17.1	19.3	22.4
6:4	76	12.2	13.1	14.1	15.4	16.8	18.7	21.0	11.7	12.7	13.9	15.3	17.1	19.4	22.5
6:5	77	12.2	13.1	14.1	15.4	16.9	18.7	21.0	11.7	12.7	13.9	15.3	17.1	19.4	22.6
6:6	78	12.2	13.1	14.1	15.4	16.9	18.7	21.1	11.7	12.7	13.9	15.3	17.1	19.5	22.7
6:7	79	12.2	13.1	14.1	15.4	16.9	18.8	21.2	11.7	12.7	13.9	15.3	17.2	19.5	22.8
6:8	80	12.2	13.1	14.2	15.4	16.9	18.8	21.3	11.7	12.7	13.9	15.3	17.2	19.6	22.9
6:9	81	12.2	13.1	14.2	15.4	17.0	18.9	21.3	11.7	12.7	13.9	15.4	17.2	19.6	23.0
6:10	82	12.2	13.1	14.2	15.4	17.0	18.9	21.4	11.7	12.7	13.9	15.4	17.2	19.7	23.1
6:11	83	12.2	13.1	14.2	15.5	17.0	19.0	21.5	11.7	12.7	13.9	15.4	17.3	19.7	23.2
7:0	84	12.3	13.1	14.2	15.5	17.0	19.0	21.6	11.8	12.7	13.9	15.4	17.3	19.8	23.3
7:1	85	12.3	13.2	14.2	15.5	17.1	19.1	21.7	11.8	12.7	13.9	15.4	17.3	19.8	23.4
7:2	86	12.3	13.2	14.2	15.5	17.1	19.1	21.8	11.8	12.8	14.0	15.4	17.4	19.9	23.5
7:3	87	12.3	13.2	14.3	15.5	17.1	19.2	21.9	11.8	12.8	14.0	15.5	17.4	20.0	23.6
7:4	88	12.3	13.2	14.3	15.6	17.2	19.2	22.0	11.8	12.8	14.0	15.5	17.4	20.0	23.7

Year:	Months	Boys							Girls						
Month		–3SD	–2SD	–1SD	Median	1 SD	2SD	3SD	–3SD	–2SD	–1SD	Median	1 SD	2SD	3SD
7:5	89	12.3	13.2	14.3	15.6	17.2	19.3	22.0	11.8	12.8	14.0	15.5	17.5	20.1	23.9
7:6	90	12.3	13.2	14.3	15.6	17.2	19.3	22.1	11.8	12.8	14.0	15.5	17.5	20.1	24.0
7:7	91	12.3	13.2	14.3	15.6	17.3	19.4	22.2	11.8	12.8	14.0	15.5	17.5	20.2	24.1
7:8	92	12.3	13.2	14.3	15.6	17.3	19.4	22.4	11.8	12.8	14.0	15.6	17.6	20.3	24.2
7:9	93	12.4	13.3	14.3	15.7	17.3	19.5	22.5	11.8	12.8	14.1	15.6	17.6	20.3	24.4
7:10	94	12.4	13.3	14.4	15.7	17.4	19.6	22.6	11.9	12.9	14.1	15.6	17.6	20.4	24.5
7:11	95	12.4	13.3	14.4	15.7	17.4	19.6	22.7	11.9	12.9	14.1	15.7	17.7	20.5	24.6
8:0	96	12.4	13.3	14.4	15.7	17.4	19.7	22.8	11.9	12.9	14.1	15.7	17.7	20.6	24.8
8:1	97	12.4	13.3	14.4	15.8	17.5	19.7	22.9	11.9	12.9	14.1	15.7	17.8	20.6	24.9
8:2	98	12.4	13.3	14.4	15.8	17.5	19.8	23.0	11.9	12.9	14.2	15.7	17.8	20.7	25.1
8:3	99	12.4	13.3	14.4	15.8	17.5	19.9	23.1	11.9	12.9	14.2	15.8	17.9	20.8	25.2
8:4	100	12.4	13.4	14.5	15.8	17.6	19.9	23.3	11.9	13.0	14.2	15.8	17.9	20.9	25.3
8:5	101	12.5	13.4	14.5	15.9	17.6	20.0	23.4	12.0	13.0	14.2	15.8	18.0	20.9	25.5
8:6	102	12.5	13.4	14.5	15.9	17.7	20.1	23.5	12.0	13.0	14.3	15.9	18.0	21.0	25.6
8:7	103	12.5	13.4	14.5	15.9	17.7	20.1	23.6	12.0	13.0	14.3	15.9	18.1	21.1	25.8
8:8	104	12.5	13.4	14.5	15.9	17.7	20.2	23.8	12.0	13.0	14.3	15.9	18.1	21.2	25.9
8:9	105	12.5	13.4	14.6	16.0	17.8	20.3	23.9	12.0	13.1	14.3	16.0	18.2	21.3	26.1
8:10	106	12.5	13.5	14.6	16.0	17.8	20.3	24.0	12.1	13.1	14.4	16.0	18.2	21.3	26.2
8:11	107	12.5	13.5	14.6	16.0	17.9	20.4	24.2	12.1	13.1	14.4	16.1	18.3	21.4	26.4
9:0	108	12.6	13.5	14.6	16.0	17.9	20.5	24.3	12.1	13.1	14.4	16.1	18.3	21.5	26.5
9:1	109	12.6	13.5	14.6	16.1	18.0	20.5	24.4	12.1	13.2	14.5	16.1	18.4	21.6	26.7
9:2	110	12.6	13.5	14.7	16.1	18.0	20.6	24.6	12.1	13.2	14.5	16.2	18.4	21.7	26.8
9:3	111	12.6	13.5	14.7	16.1	18.0	20.7	24.7	12.2	13.2	14.5	16.2	18.5	21.8	27.0
9:4	112	12.6	13.6	14.7	16.2	18.1	20.8	24.9	12.2	13.2	14.6	16.3	18.6	21.9	27.2
9:5	113	12.6	13.6	14.7	16.2	18.1	20.8	25.0	12.2	13.3	14.6	16.3	18.6	21.9	27.3
9:6	114	12.7	13.6	14.8	16.2	18.2	20.9	25.1	12.2	13.3	14.6	16.3	18.7	22.0	27.5
9:7	115	12.7	13.6	14.8	16.3	18.2	21.0	25.3	12.3	13.3	14.7	16.4	18.7	22.1	27.6
9:8	116	12.7	13.6	14.8	16.3	18.3	21.1	25.5	12.3	13.4	14.7	16.4	18.8	22.2	27.8
9:9	117	12.7	13.7	14.8	16.3	18.3	21.2	25.6	12.3	13.4	14.7	16.5	18.8	22.3	27.9
9:10	118	12.7	13.7	14.9	16.4	18.4	21.2	25.8	12.3	13.4	14.8	16.5	18.9	22.4	28.1

Year:	Months	Boys							Girls						
Month		–3SD	–2SD	–1SD	Median	1 SD	2SD	3SD	–3SD	–2SD	–1SD	Median	1 SD	2SD	3SD
9:11	119	12.8	13.7	14.9	16.4	18.4	21.3	25.9	12.4	13.4	14.8	16.6	19.0	22.5	28.2
10:0	120	12.8	13.7	14.9	16.4	18.5	21.4	26.1	12.4	13.5	14.8	16.6	19.0	22.6	28.4
10:1	121	12.8	13.8	15.0	16.5	18.5	21.5	26.2	12.4	13.5	14.9	16.7	19.1	22.7	28.5
10:2	122	12.8	13.8	15.0	16.5	18.6	21.6	26.4	12.4	13.5	14.9	16.7	19.2	22.8	28.7
10:3	123	12.8	13.8	15.0	16.6	18.6	21.7	26.6	12.5	13.6	15.0	16.8	19.2	22.8	28.8
10:4	124	12.9	13.8	15.0	16.6	18.7	21.7	26.7	12.5	13.6	15.0	16.8	19.3	22.9	29.0
10:5	125	12.9	13.9	15.1	16.6	18.8	21.8	26.9	12.5	13.6	15.0	16.9	19.4	23.0	29.1
10:6	126	12.9	13.9	15.1	16.7	18.8	21.9	27.0	12.5	13.7	15.1	16.9	19.4	23.1	29.3
10:7	127	12.9	13.9	15.1	16.7	18.9	22.0	27.2	12.6	13.7	15.1	17.0	19.5	23.2	29.4
10:8	128	13.0	13.9	15.2	16.8	18.9	22.1	27.4	12.6	13.7	15.2	17.0	19.6	23.3	29.6
10:9	129	13.0	14.0	15.2	16.8	19.0	22.2	27.5	12.6	13.8	15.2	17.1	19.6	23.4	29.7
10:10	130	13.0	14.0	15.2	16.9	19.0	22.3	25.7	12.7	13.8	15.3	17.1	19.7	23.5	29.9
10:11	131	13.0	14.0	15.3	16.9	19.1	22.4	25.9	12.7	13.8	15.3	17.2	19.8	23.6	30.0
11:0	132	13.1	14.1	15.3	16.9	19.2	22.5	28.0	12.7	13.9	15.3	17.2	19.9	23.7	30.2
11:1	133	13.1	14.1	15.3	17.0	19.2	22.5	28.2	12.8	13.9	15.4	17.3	19.9	23.8	30.3
11:2	134	13.1	14.1	15.4	17.0	19.3	22.6	28.4	12.8	14.0	15.4	17.4	20.0	23.9	30.5
11:3	135	13.1	14.1	15.4	17.1	19.3	22.7	28.5	12.8	14.0	15.5	17.4	20.1	24.0	30.6
11:4	136	13.2	14.2	15.5	17.1	19.4	22.8	28.7	12.9	14.0	15.5	17.5	20.2	24.1	30.8
11:5	137	13.2	14.2	15.5	17.2	19.5	22.9	28.8	12.9	14.1	15.6	17.5	20.2	24.2	30.9
11:6	138	13.2	14.2	15.5	17.2	19.5	23.0	29.0	12.9	14.1	15.6	17.6	20.3	24.3	31.1
11:7	139	13.2	14.3	15.6	17.3	19.6	23.1	29.2	13.0	14.2	15.7	17.7	20.4	24.4	31.2
11:8	140	13.3	14.3	15.6	17.3	19.7	23.2	29.3	13.0	14.2	15.7	17.7	20.5	24.5	31.4
11:9	141	13.3	14.3	15.7	17.4	19.7	23.3	29.5	13.0	14.3	15.8	17.8	20.6	25.7	31.5
11:10	142	13.3	14.4	15.7	17.4	19.8	23.4	29.6	13.1	14.3	15.8	17.9	20.6	24.8	31.6
11:11	143	13.4	14.4	15.7	17.5	19.9	23.5	29.8	13.1	14.3	15.9	17.9	20.7	24.9	31.8
12:0	144	13.4	14.5	15.8	17.5	19.9	23.6	30.0	13.2	14.4	16.0	18.0	20.8	25.0	31.9
12:1	145	13.4	14.5	15.8	17.6	20.0	23.7	30.1	13.2	14.4	16.0	18.1	20.9	25.1	32.0
12:2	146	13.5	14.5	15.9	17.6	20.1	23.8	30.3	13.2	14.5	16.1	18.1	21.0	25.2	32.2
12:3	147	13.5	14.6	15.9	17.7	20.2	23.9	30.4	13.3	14.5	16.1	18.2	21.1	25.3	32.3
12:4	148	13.5	14.6	16.0	17.8	20.2	24.0	30.6	13.3	14.6	16.2	18.3	21.1	25.4	32.4

Year:	Months	Boys							Girls						
Month		–3SD	–2SD	–1SD	Median	1 SD	2SD	3SD	–3SD	–2SD	–1SD	Median	1 SD	2SD	3SD
12:5	149	13.6	14.6	16.0	17.8	20.3	24.1	30.7	13.3	14.6	16.2	18.3	21.2	25.5	32.6
12:6	150	13.6	14.7	16.1	17.9	20.4	24.2	30.9	13.4	14.7	16.3	18.4	21.3	25.6	32.7
12:7	151	13.6	14.7	16.1	17.9	20.4	24.3	31.0	13.4	14.7	16.3	18.5	21.4	25.7	32.8
12:8	152	13.7	14.8	16.2	18.0	20.5	24.4	31.1	13.5	14.8	16.4	18.5	21.5	25.8	33.0
12:9	153	13.7	14.8	16.2	18.0	20.6	24.5	31.3	13.5	14.8	16.4	18.6	21.6	25.9	33.1
12:10	154	13.7	14.8	16.3	18.1	20.7	24.6	31.4	13.5	14.8	16.5	18.7	21.6	26.0	33.2
12:11	155	13.8	14.9	16.3	18.2	20.8	24.7	31.6	13.6	14.9	16.6	18.7	21.7	26.1	33.3
13:0	156	13.8	14.9	16.4	18.2	20.8	24.8	31.7	13.6	14.9	16.6	18.8	21.8	26.2	33.4
13:1	157	13.8	15.0	16.4	18.3	20.9	24.9	31.8	13.6	15.0	16.7	18.9	21.9	26.3	33.6
13:2	158	13.9	15.0	16.5	18.4	21.0	25.0	31.9	13.7	15.0	16.7	18.9	22.0	26.4	33.7
13:3	159	13.9	15.1	16.5	18.4	21.1	25.1	32.1	13.7	15.1	16.8	19.0	22.0	26.5	33.8
13:4	160	14.0	15.1	16.6	18.5	21.1	25.2	32.2	13.8	15.1	16.8	19.1	22.1	26.6	33.9
13:5	161	14.0	15.2	16.6	18.6	21.2	25.2	32.3	13.8	15.2	16.9	19.1	22.2	26.7	34.0
13:6	162	14.0	15.2	16.7	18.6	21.3	25.3	32.4	13.8	15.2	16.9	19.2	22.3	26.8	34.1
13:7	163	14.1	15.2	16.7	18.7	21.4	25.4	32.6	13.9	15.2	17.0	19.3	22.4	26.9	34.2
13:8	164	14.1	15.3	16.8	18.7	21.5	25.5	32.7	13.9	15.3	17.0	19.3	22.4	27.0	34.3
13:9	165	14.1	15.3	16.8	18.8	21.5	25.6	32.8	13.9	15.3	17.1	19.4	22.5	27.1	34.4
13:10	166	14.2	15.4	16.9	18.9	21.6	25.7	32.9	14.0	15.4	17.1	19.4	22.6	27.1	34.5
13:11	167	14.2	15.4	17.0	18.9	21.7	25.8	33.0	14.0	15.4	17.2	19.5	22.7	27.2	34.6
14:0	168	14.3	15.5	17.0	19.0	21.8	25.9	33.1	14.0	15.4	17.2	19.6	22.7	27.3	34.7
14:1	169	14.3	15.5	17.1	19.1	21.8	26.0	33.2	14.1	15.5	17.3	19.6	22.8	27.4	34.7
14:2	170	14.3	15.6	17.1	19.1	21.9	26.1	33.3	14.1	15.5	17.3	19.7	22.9	27.5	34.8
14:3	171	14.4	15.6	17.2	19.2	22.0	26.2	33.4	14.1	15.6	17.4	19.7	22.9	27.6	34.9
14:4	172	14.4	15.7	17.2	19.3	22.1	26.3	33.5	14.1	15.6	17.4	19.8	23.0	27.7	35.0
14:5	173	14.5	15.7	17.3	19.3	22.2	26.4	33.5	14.2	15.6	17.5	19.9	23.1	27.7	35.1
14:6	174	14.5	15.7	17.3	19.4	22.2	26.5	33.6	14.2	15.7	17.5	19.9	23.1	27.8	35.1
14:7	175	14.5	15.8	17.4	19.5	22.3	26.5	33.7	14.2	15.7	17.6	20.0	23.2	27.9	35.2
14:8	176	14.6	15.8	17.4	19.5	22.4	26.6	33.8	14.3	15.7	17.6	20.0	23.3	28.0	35.3
14:9	177	14.6	15.9	17.5	19.6	22.5	26.7	33.9	14.3	15.8	17.6	20.1	23.3	28.0	35.4
14:10	178	14.6	15.9	17.5	19.6	22.5	26.8	33.9	14.3	15.8	17.7	20.1	23.4	28.1	35.4

Year:	Months	Boys							Girls						
Month		–3SD	–2SD	–1SD	Median	1 SD	2SD	3SD	–3SD	–2SD	–1SD	Median	1 SD	2SD	3SD
14:11	179	14.7	16.0	17.6	19.7	22.6	26.9	34.0	14.3	15.8	17.7	20.2	23.5	28.2	35.5
15:0	180	14.7	16.0	17.6	19.8	22.7	27.0	34.1	14.4	15.9	17.8	20.2	23.5	28.2	35.5
15:1	181	14.7	16.1	17.7	19.8	22.8	27.1	34.1	14.4	15.9	17.8	20.3	23.6	28.3	35.6
15:2	182	14.8	16.1	17.8	19.9	22.8	27.1	34.2	14.4	15.9	17.8	20.3	23.6	28.4	35.7
15:3	183	14.8	16.1	17.8	20.0	22.9	27.2	34.3	14.4	16.0	17.9	20.4	23.7	28.4	35.7
15:4	184	14.8	16.2	17.9	20.0	23.0	27.3	34.3	14.5	16.0	17.9	20.4	23.7	28.5	35.8
15:5	185	14.9	16.2	17.9	20.1	23.0	27.4	34.4	14.5	16.0	17.9	20.4	23.8	28.5	35.8
15:6	186	14.9	16.3	18.0	20.1	23.1	27.4	34.5	14.5	16.0	18.0	20.5	23.8	28.6	35.8
15:7	187	15.0	16.3	18.0	20.2	23.2	27.5	34.5	14.5	16.1	18.0	20.5	23.9	28.6	35.9
15:8	188	15.0	16.3	18.1	20.3	23.3	27.6	34.6	14.5	16.1	18.0	20.6	23.9	28.7	35.9
15:9	189	15.0	16.4	18.1	20.3	23.3	27.7	34.6	14.5	16.1	18.1	20.6	24.0	28.7	36.0
15:10	190	15.0	16.4	18.2	20.4	23.4	27.7	34.7	14.6	16.1	18.1	20.6	24.0	28.8	36.0
15:11	191	15.1	16.5	18.2	20.4	23.5	27.8	34.7	14.6	16.2	18.1	20.7	24.1	28.8	36.0
16:0	192	15.1	16.5	18.2	20.5	23.5	27.9	34.8	14.6	16.2	18.2	20.7	24.1	28.9	36.1
16:1	193	15.1	16.5	18.3	20.6	23.6	27.9	34.8	14.6	16.2	18.2	20.7	24.1	28.9	36.1
16:2	194	15.2	16.6	18.3	20.6	23.7	28.0	34.8	14.6	16.2	18.2	20.8	24.2	29.0	36.1
16:3	195	15.2	16.6	18.4	20.7	23.7	28.1	34.9	14.6	16.2	18.2	20.8	24.2	29.0	36.1
16:4	196	15.2	16.7	18.4	20.7	23.8	28.1	34.9	14.6	16.2	18.3	20.8	24.3	29.0	36.2
16:5	197	15.3	16.7	18.5	20.8	23.8	28.2	35.0	14.6	16.3	18.3	20.9	24.3	29.1	36.2
16:6	198	15.3	16.7	18.5	20.8	23.9	28.3	35.0	14.7	16.3	18.3	20.9	24.3	29.1	36.2
16:7	199	15.3	16.8	18.6	20.9	24.0	28.3	35.0	14.7	16.3	18.3	20.9	24.4	29.1	36.2
16:8	200	15.3	16.8	18.6	20.9	24.0	28.4	35.1	14.7	16.3	18.3	20.9	24.4	29.2	36.2
16:9	201	15.4	16.8	18.7	21.0	24.1	28.5	35.1	14.7	16.3	18.4	21.0	24.4	29.2	36.3
16:10	202	15.4	16.9	18.7	21.0	24.2	28.5	35.1	14.7	16.3	18.4	21.0	24.4	29.2	36.3
16:11	203	15.4	16.9	18.7	21.1	24.2	28.6	35.2	14.7	16.3	18.4	21.0	24.5	29.3	36.3
17:0	204	15.4	16.9	18.8	21.1	24.3	28.6	35.2	14.7	16.4	18.4	21.0	24.5	29.3	36.3
17:1	205	15.5	17.0	18.8	21.2	24.3	28.7	35.2	14.7	16.4	18.4	21.1	24.5	29.3	36.3
17:2	206	15.5	17.0	18.9	21.2	24.4	28.7	35.2	14.7	16.4	18.4	21.1	24.6	29.3	36.3
17:3	207	15.5	17.0	18.9	21.3	24.4	28.8	35.3	14.7	16.4	18.5	21.1	24.6	29.4	36.3
17:4	208	15.5	17.1	18.9	21.3	24.5	28.9	35.3	14.7	16.4	18.5	21.1	24.6	29.4	36.3

Year: Month	Months	Boys							Girls						
		−3SD	−2SD	−1SD	Median	1 SD	2SD	3SD	−3SD	−2SD	−1SD	Median	1 SD	2SD	3SD
17:5	209	15.6	17.1	19.0	21.4	24.5	28.9	35.3	14.7	16.4	18.5	21.1	24.6	29.4	36.3
17:6	210	15.6	17.1	19.0	21.4	24.6	29.0	35.3	14.7	16.4	18.5	21.2	24.6	29.4	36.3
17:7	211	15.6	17.1	19.1	21.5	24.7	29.0	35.4	14.7	16.4	18.5	21.2	24.7	29.4	36.3
17:8	212	15.6	17.2	19.1	21.5	24.7	29.1	35.4	14.7	16.4	18.5	21.2	24.7	29.5	36.3
17:9	213	15.6	17.2	19.1	21.6	24.8	29.1	35.4	14.7	16.4	18.5	21.2	24.7	29.5	36.3
17:10	214	15.7	17.2	19.2	21.6	24.8	29.2	35.4	14.7	16.4	18.5	21.2	24.7	29.5	36.3
17:11	215	15.7	17.3	19.2	21.7	24.9	29.2	35.4	14.7	16.4	18.6	21.2	24.8	29.5	36.3
18:0	216	15.7	17.3	19.2	21.7	24.9	29.2	35.4	14.7	16.4	18.6	21.3	24.8	29.5	36.3
18:1	217	15.7	17.3	19.3	21.8	25.0	29.3	35.4	14.7	16.5	18.6	21.3	24.8	29.5	36.3
18:2	218	15.7	17.3	19.3	21.8	25.0	29.3	35.5	14.7	16.5	18.6	21.3	24.8	29.6	36.3
18:3	219	15.7	17.4	19.3	21.8	25.1	29.4	35.5	14.7	16.5	18.6	21.3	24.8	29.6	36.3
18:4	220	15.8	17.4	19.4	21.9	25.1	29.4	35.5	14.7	16.5	18.6	21.3	24.8	29.6	36.3
18:5	221	15.8	17.4	19.4	21.9	25.1	29.5	35.5	14.7	16.5	18.6	21.3	24.9	29.6	36.2
18:6	222	15.8	17.4	19.4	22.0	25.2	29.5	35.5	14.7	16.5	18.6	21.3	24.9	29.6	36.2
18:7	223	15.8	17.5	19.5	22.0	25.2	29.5	35.5	14.7	16.5	18.6	21.4	24.9	29.6	36.2
18:8	224	15.8	17.5	19.5	22.0	25.3	29.6	35.5	14.7	16.5	18.6	21.4	24.9	29.6	36.2
18:9	225	15.8	17.5	19.5	22.1	25.3	29.6	35.5	14.7	16.5	18.7	21.4	24.9	29.6	36.2
18:10	226	15.8	17.5	19.6	22.1	25.4	29.6	35.5	14.7	16.5	18.7	21.4	24.9	29.6	36.2
18:11	227	15.8	17.5	19.6	22.2	25.4	29.7	35.5	14.7	16.5	18.7	21.4	25.0	29.7	36.2
19:0	228	15.9	17.6	19.6	22.2	25.4	29.7	35.5	14.7	16.5	18.7	21.4	25.0	29.7	36.2

5.6 Undernutrition

Undernutrition is the most widely prevalent form of malnutrition among children. Nutritional status of children is an indicator of nutritional profile of the entire community. Protein energy malnutrition (PEM) affects every fourth child world-wide. About 129 million are underweight while 195 million are stunted [19]. Despite an overall decrease of stunting in developing countries, child malnutrition still remains a major public health problem in developing countries. In India, there has been a significant decline in extreme forms of protein energy malnutrition (classical kwashiorkor and extreme forms of marasmus) over the past few decades but the decline has been only modest for anthropometrically measured undernutrition. The proportion of children under-5 years of age who were underweight decreased from 53 percent in National Family Health Survey-1 (NFHS-1) conducted in 1992–93 to 47 percent in NFHS-2 (1998–99) and 46 percent in NFHS-3 (2005–2006). Similarly, prevalence of stunting decreased from 52% in NFHS-1 to 45% in NFHS-2 and 38% in NFHS-3 [20].

Classification

Undernutrition is the result of food intake that is continuously insufficient to meet dietary energy requirements, poor absorption and/or poor biological use of nutrients consumed. This usually results in loss of body weight. Contrary to common usage, the term "malnutrition" correctly includes both undernutrition and overnutrition. Several systems are used for classifying undernutrition. Mild, moderate and severe are different in each of the classification systems. Thus, it is important to use the same system to analyze and present data while making the comparisons or describing trends. PEM may be classified according to the severity, course and the relative contributions of energy or protein deficit. Some classifications based on anthropometric measurements, mainly weight and height are described below:

(i) *Indian Academy of Pediatrics (IAP) classification based on weight-for-age.* IAP takes a weight of more than 80% of the expected weight-for-age as normal. Grades of malnutrition are Grade I (71–80%), II (61–70%), III (51–60%) and IV ($\leq$50%) of the expected weight for that age. Alphabet *K* is post-fixed in presence of edema. For example, a male child weighing 8 kg at 2 years of age with pedal edema (50th percentile for 2 years is 12.3 kg) is classified as PEM Grade II (k) as per IAP classification.

IAP classification is simple and the cut-offs are suitable for Indian population. However, the disadvantage is that it does not take in account the child's height. The weight is also dependent on height besides the built; thus children who are short statured (not necessarily because of nutritional deprivation) are also misclassified as PEM by this classification.

(ii) *Welcome Trust Classification* is also based on deficit in body weight for age and presence or absence of edema. Children weighing between 60% and 80% of their expected weight-for-age with edema are classified as *kwashiorkor*. Those weighing between 60% and 80% of the expected weight without edema are known as having undernutrition. Those without edema and weighing less than 60 per cent of their expected weight-for-age are considered to be having marasmus. Marasmic kwashiorkor is applied to children with edema and body weight less than 60% of the expected.

(iii) *WHO classification.* The above referred classifications measure undernutrition and are based on weight-for-age alone. However, it is important to distinguish undernutrition from wasting (deficits in weight-for-height) and stunting (deficits in height-for-age). WHO Classification of malnutrition is based on the statistical cut-offs for defining wasting and stunting as those below –2 SD (Table 5.2, 5.3, 5.4, 5.5). Severe wasting and stunting are defined when the weight-for-height and height-for-age, respectively are less than 3 SD scores. Severe wasting (weight-for-height <3 SD or < 70% of median) is used as an admission criteria to identify individual children for inpatient management of severe malnutrition (Table 5.8).

(iv) *Age-independent anthropometric indices.* Some anthropometric indices which are ratios of weight or height and are based on circumference such as Dugale's, Rao's and Kanawati do not require consideration of age. These serve as useful one time indicators to assess nutritional status in clinical practice, where exact age of the child is not known (e.g., orphanages, street children, etc.). However, most of these indices are no longer used now as these are difficult to calculate and interpret. Also, these are not truly age independent but the effect of age on these indices is less pronounced especially in under-5 children.

Overnutrition (overweight and obesity)

Overnutrition refers to a chronic condition where intake of food is in excess of dietary energy requirements, resulting in overweight and/or obesity. Obesity may be defined as an excessive storage of energy as fat relative to the lean body mass. Body fat expressed as a percentage of body weight

Table 5.8 WHO Classification for Undernutrition

	Moderate undernutrition	Severe *undernutrition*
Symmetrical edema	No	Yes[a] Edematous malnutrition
Weight for height *(measure of wasting)*	SD score -2 to –3 (70–79% of expected[b]) Wasting	SD score < -3 (<70% of expected) Severe wasting
Height for age *(measure of stunting)*	SD score -2 to –3 (85–89% of expected[b]) Stunting	SD score < -3 (<85% of expected) Severe stunting

[a]This includes kwashiorkar and marasmic kwashiorkar
[b]Median (50th percentile of NCHS references)

(% body fat) is the most relevant measure against which all anthropometric measures is correlated. Estimates of body composition can be made by dual energy X-ray absorbiometry (DEXA). The complex nature, high cost and difficult methodology of direct estimation of body fat content has ensured that this is limited to research purpose only. This led to the search for other measurements which can be easily performed and correlate satisfactorily with the percentage of body fat. Skin-fold thickness provides a reliable estimate of body fat and its distribution. It can be measured at several sites including triceps, biceps, axilla, mid-abdominal, subscapular and suprailiac. The biceps and the triceps skin-fold thickness estimate the peripheral body fat, whereas subscapular and suprailiac skin-folds reflect the central adiposity. Skin-fold thicknesses above the 85th percentile for age and sex suggest obesity and above the 95th percentile suggest super-obesity. Triceps skin-fold thickness is the most common site of measurement. Although accurate under research settings, the use of this method for epidemiologic assessment of obesity is hindered by methodological problems. In contrast, the high reliability of measurement of weight and height suggests that an anthropometric parameter based on these indices would provide a more useful measure of adiposity for comparison within and between populations. Traditionally, obesity in children has been defined as a weight-for-height above the 90th percentile on the growth charts from the National Centre of Heath Statistics or weight in excess of 120% of the median weight for a given height. Super-obesity is defined as a weight for height above the 95th percentile and weight in excess of 140% of the median weight for a given height.

Body mass index [weight (kg)/height^2 (meter^2)] is widely accepted as a convenient measure of a person's fatness. It is a rather robust index which is extremely useful for large-scale epidemiological work. For adults the BMI categories are underweight <18.5, ideal 18.5–24.9, preobese 25.0–

29.9, obese class I 30.0–34.9, obese class II 35.0–39.9 and obese class III >40 kg/m^2 (Table 5.9). The risk for medical complications in adults has a direct correlation with the BMI. In recent years, there was a growing debate on whether there are possible needs for developing lower BMI cut-off points for Asian populations due to their different body composition. The proportion of Asian people with a high risk of type 2 diabetes and cardiovascular disease is substantial at BMI's lower than the existing WHO cut-off point for overweight i.e. 25 kg/m^2. However, the cut-off point for observed risk varies from 22 to 25 kg/m^2 in different Asian populations, and for high risk it varies from 26 to 31 kg/m^2. The current WHO BMI cut-off points (Table 5.9) is the international classification. However, the cut-off points of 23, 27.5, 32.5 and 37.5 kg/m^2 are important and need to be considered as points for public health action. It means that the public health action for prevention of overweight and obesity in Indian populations should start at BMI >23 kg/m^2 despite the person being defined as normal as per the International classification.

BMI in children changes substantially with age. It is obvious that a single cut-off point for defining obesity cannot be used. The 85th and the 95th percentiles of BMI for age and sex have been recommended to identify overweight and obesity. Given the relative ease of measurement and its accuracy vis-à-vis other parameters, BMI is the most acceptable indicator of body fatness. International BMI cut-offs for child overweight and obesity, based on data from six countries, have been developed. The international BMI cut-offs for child overweight and obesity cover the age

Table 5.9 The International classification of nutritional status in adults according to BMI [21]

Classification	BMI (kg/m^2)	
	Principal cut-off points	Additional cut-off points[a]
Underweight	<18.50	<18.50
Severe thinness	<16.00	<16.00
Moderate thinness	16.00–16.99	16.00–16.99
Mild thinness	17.00–18.49	17.00–18.49
Normal range	18.50–24.99	18.50–22.99
		23.00–24.99
Overweight	≥ 25.00	≥ 25.00
Pre-obese	25.00–29.99	25.00–27.49
		27.50–29.99
Obese	≥ 30.00	≥ 30.00
Obese class I	30.00–34.99	30.00–32.49
		32.50–34.99
Obese class II	35.00–39.99	35.00–37.49
		37.50–39.99
Obese class III	≥ 40.00	≥ 40.00

[a] The additional cut-off points in these categories are important for public health action in Asian populations.

range 2–18 years and are based on the adult cut-offs of 25 and 30 at 18 years. BMI charts developed by WHO for children and adolescents up to the ages of 19 years are presented in the chapter.

Types of obesity: android and gynecoid

Obesity should also be evaluated in terms of distribution of body fat. Adipose tissue accumulates in two main sites – intra-abdominal and subcutaneous. Intra-abdominal fat comprises fat surrounding the omentum and mesentery with the retroperitoneal fat whereas subcutaneous fat is distributed all over the body. In males both kinds of fat accumulation is more prominent in the upper segment of the body, visible as an apple shaped distribution. In females the tissue is more subcutaneous and over the thighs in a pear shaped distribution. This is important because it has been demonstrated that in comparison to obese individuals with pelvic or "gynecoid" fat distribution, equally obese individuals with central or 'android obesity' are more likely to develop obesity related disorders including insulin resistance, Non Insulin Dependent Diabetes Mellitus (NIDDM), hypertension and hyperlipidemias. The distribution of body fat can be estimated using the *waist–hip ratio (WHR).* WHR>0.8 is the cut-off point associated with above listed clinical problems. However in children no correlation has been shown between WHR and visceral fat. The visceral subcutaneous fat ratio (VSR) measured with the help of the CT scan has been shown to be a better index of fat distribution. There is no controversy with respect to the importance of visceral fat as a determinant of adult health. Unfortunately, there is a paucity of similar data for pediatric population largely because of absence of a method other than radiological for its measurement.

References

1. WHO Working Group (1986). Use and interpretation of anthropometric indicators of nutritional status. *Bull WHO* vol. 64, pp. 929–941.
2. COGILL B (2003). Anthropometric Indicators Measurement Guide. Food and Nutrition Technical Assistance Project, Academy for Educational Development, Washington, D.C.
3. How to Weigh and Measure Children: Assessing the Nutritional Status of Young Children in Household Surveys, United Nations Department of Technical Cooperation for Development and Statistical Office, 1986.
4. GORSTEIN J, SULLIVAN K, YIP R, DE ONIS M, TROWBRIDGE F, FAJANS P, CLUGSTON G (1994). Issues in the assessment of nutritional status using anthropometry. *Bull WHO* vol. 72, pp. 273–283.
5. World Health Organization. Growth standards (2006). Available at http://www.who.int/childgrowth/standards.

6. Physical Status: the Use and Interpretation of Anthropometry. Report of a WHO Expert Committee. Geneva, World Health Organization, 1995 (WHO Technical Report Series, No. 854).
7. DE ONIS M, ONYANGO AW, BORGHI E, SIYAM A, NISHIDAA C, SIEKMANNA J (2007). Development of a WHO growth reference for school-aged children and adolescents. *Bull WHO* vol. 85, pp. 660–667.
8. DIBLEY MJ et al (1987). Development of normalized curves for the international growth reference: historical and technical considerations. *Am J Clin Nutr* vol. 46, pp. 736–748.
9. DIBLEY MJ et al (1987). Interpretation of z-score anthropometric indicators derived from the international growth reference. *Am J Clin Nutr* vol. 46, pp. 749–762.
10. COLE TJ, BELLIZZI MC, FLEGAL KM, DIETZ WH (2000). Establishing a standard definition for child overweight and obesity: international survey. *BMJ* vol. 320, pp. 1240–1243.
11. COLE TJ, FLEGAL KM, NICHOLLS D, JACKSON AA (2007). Body mass index cut-offs to define thinness in children and adolescents: international survey. *BMJ* vol. 335, p. 194.
12. CAMERON N (2007). Body mass index cut offs to define thinness in children and adolescents. *BMJ* vol. 335, pp. 166–167.
13. National Center for Health Statistics (1977). In: Hamill, PVV et al., (eds) Growth curves for children birth-18 years United States. Washington, DC, National Center for Health Statistics (Vital and health statistics. Series 11: No. 165 (DHEW publication (PHS) #78-1650)), 1977.
14. DE ONIS M (1997). Time for a new growth reference. *Pediatrics* vol. 100, p. e8.
15. VICTORA CG, MORRIS SS, BARROS FC, DE ONIS M, YIP R (1998). The NCHS reference and the growth of breast- and bottle-fed infants. *J Nutr* vol. 128, pp. 1134–1138.
16. DE ONIS M, GARZA C, VICTORA CG, BHAN MK, NORUM KR (2004). The WHO Multicentre Growth Reference Study (MGRS): rationale, planning and implementation. *Food Nutr Bull* vol. 25 (Suppl. 1).
17. WHO Multicentre Growth Reference Study Group (2006). Enrolment and baseline characteristics in the WHO Multicentre Growth Reference Study. *Acta Paediatrica* Suppl 450, pp. 7–15.
18. DE ONIS M, ONYANGO AW, BORGHI E, GARZA C, YANG H, for the WHO Multicentre Growth Reference Study Group. Comparison of the WHO Child Growth Standards and the NCHS growth reference: implications for child health programs. (In press)
19. UNICEF (2009). Tracking progress on child and maternal nutrition. www.unicef.org
20. National Family Health Survey (NFHS-3), India, 2005–2006. Mumbai, International Institute for Population Sciences and ORC Macro, 2007.
21. WHO. Global database on Body Mass Index: http://apps.who.int/bmi/index.jsp?introPage=intro_3html

6

Essential new-born care and child survival

Richa Singh Pandey and *Sheila C. Vir*

Richa Singh Pandey, MD, has several years of experience in the field of public health and nutrition. Dr. Singh is currently a nutrition specialist with UNICEF (India). Prior to joining UNICEF, Dr. Pandey worked on an important newborn care project with Saksham Study Group of Johns Hopkins–King George Medical College Collaborative Centre and as a consultant with UNICEF on maternal & child health and nutrition issues.

Sheila C Vir, MSc, PhD, is a senior nutrition consultant and Director of Public Health Nutrition and Development Centre, New Delhi. Following MSc (Food and Nutrition) from University of Delhi, Dr Vir was awarded PhD by the Queen's University of Belfast, United Kingdom. Dr. Vir, a past secretary of the Nutrition Society of India, is a recipient of the fellowship of the Department of Health and Social Services, UK, and Commonwealth Van den Bergh Nutrition Award. Dr Vir worked briefly with the Aga Khan Foundation (India) and later with UNICEF. As a Nutrition Programme Officer with UNICEF for twenty years, Dr. Vir provided strategic and technical leadership for policy formulation and implementation of nutrition programmes in India.

6.1 Neonatal period – a risky start to childhood

The greatest risk to life is in its beginning. A good start in life begins well before birth, however it is just before, during and in the very first hours and days that life is most at risk [1].

A newborn is known a "neonate" during the first 28 days of life and this period is referred to as the neonatal period. On the basis of survival, the neonatal period is further classified into early neonatal period 0–7 days and late neonatal period 8–28 days (Figure 6.1). The probability of dying in first month of life is known as neonatal mortality [2] and when expressed as "deaths within the first twenty eight days per 1000 live births" the term is known as neonatal mortality rate.

The neonatal period is only 28 days and yet accounts for 38% of all deaths in children younger than age 5 years in age. The remaining 62% of deaths in under five arise over a period of 1800 days, i.e. 59 months [3].

Thus, the average daily mortality rate during the neonatal period nearly 30-fold higher than during the post-neonatal period. Within the neonatal period, early neonatal period is more risky with 50–70% of fatal and life threatening illnesses occur during the first 7 days [1, 4].

6.1.1 Neonatal mortality – global magnitude

Globally, more than 4 million newborns die within the first 28 days of coming into this world. Amongst the developing nations, countries of Africa

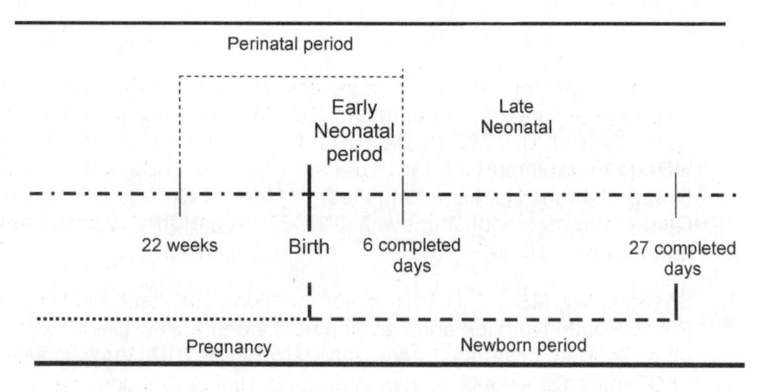

6.1 Neonatal period [5].

(28%) and South East Asia (36%) account for two-thirds of total neonatal deaths, with rates being highest in Africa (Figure 6.2) and numbers in Asia [3, 6]. Ten countries account for two-thirds of neonatal deaths [3].

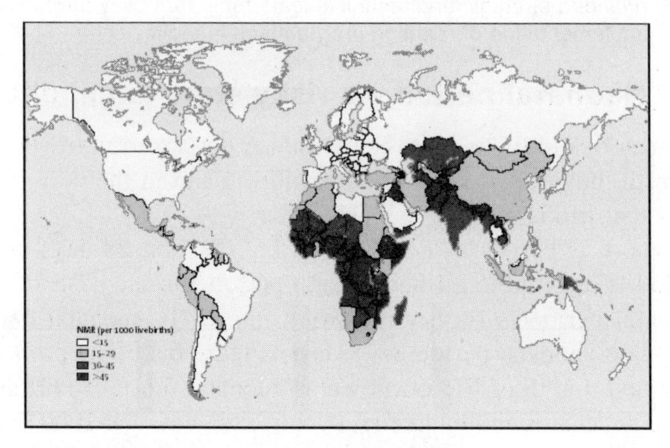

6.2 Variations between countries in NMR [3].

Owing to its large population size, India's contribution to neonatal mortality is highest in terms of numbers (Table 6.1).

Table 6.1 Countries with largest number of neonatal deaths worldwide (2000) [3]

Countries	Number of neonatal deaths (1000s)	Percentage of global neonatal deaths	NMR (per 1000 live births)
India	1098	27%	43
China	416	10%	21
Pakistan	298	7%	57
Nigeria	247	6%	53
Bangladesh	153	4%	36
Ethiopia	147	4%	51
Democratic Republic of Congo	116	3%	47
Indonesia	82	2%	18
Afghanistan	63	2%	60
United Republic of Tanzania	62	2%	43
Total	2682	67%	

6.2 Millennium development goal 4 (MDG-4) and neonatal mortality

The fourth goal (MDG-4) commits the international community to reducing child mortality (under five mortality rate) by two-thirds between 1990 and 2015. Inherent in this goal is reduction in neonatal mortality rates. Available data shows that decline in neonatal mortality rates is not commensurate with decline in IMR or child mortality rates Between 1980 and 2000, child mortality after the first month of life – i.e. from month 2 to age 5 years – fell by a third, whereas the neonatal mortality rate (NMR) was reduced by only about a quarter [3] (Figure 6.3). Even in neonatal mortality, the visible reduction was primarily due to reduction in late neonatal mortality with almost no change in the early neonatal mortality (Figure 6.3).

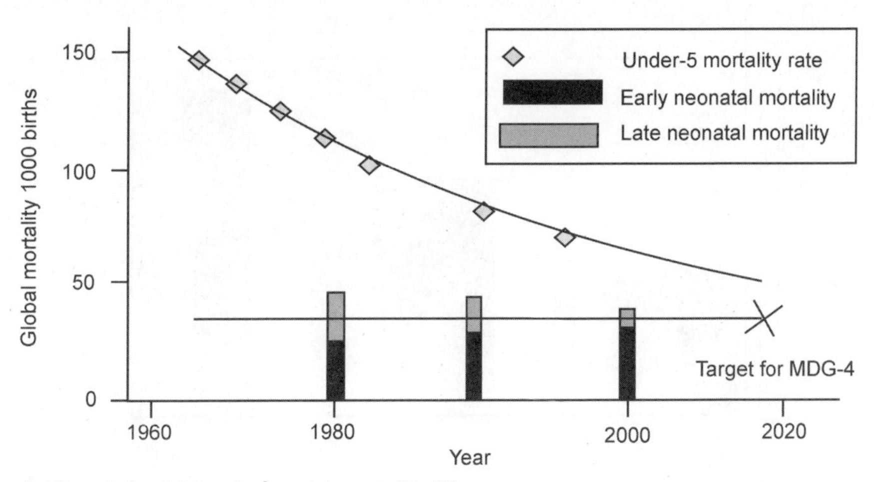

6.3 Trends in child and neonatal mortality [3].

Public health experts predict that MDG-4 cannot be met unless neonatal mortality is at least halved [7]. Concerted efforts, with focus on reducing

NMR in high mortality countries of South East Asia which constitute 25% of global population but have more than 36% share in global neonatal burden [8], are critical to success; Indian subcontinent has a key role achieving the success.

6.3 Neonatal mortality – an Indian perspective

The Indian subcontinent accounts for nearly 27–30% of global burden of neonatal deaths [9]. The Government of India has set a target of reducing the infant mortality rate from 64 to 30 per 1000 live births by the year 2010, which can only be possible if neonatal mortality is reduced by 54%, i.e. from 44/1000 live births to 20/1000 live births in this period. However, there has been only a 15% decline in neonatal mortality during the 1990s which has plateaued in recent years [10]. A Lancet study of 2005 puts this reduction further lower at just 11% [3]. The modest drop in neonatal mortality rate (NMR) is largely the result of late neonatal mortality reductions (deaths after the first week of life), in part due to a fall in deaths from tetanus [3]. The country has not been able to reduce early neonatal deaths. Moreover, the burden of neonatal deaths continues to be primarily from with five northern states (Bihar, Madhya Pradesh, Uttar Pradesh, Rajasthan) of the country contributing to more than half of all neonatal deaths [9].

The recent National Family Health Survey(NFHS) data confirms that India is also following global trend of rapid fall in U5MR (from 109 to 74) and Infant mortality (from 79 to 57) rate but has stagnant NMR which has reduced marginally from 49 to only 39 [11] (from 49 to 39) (Figure 6.4).

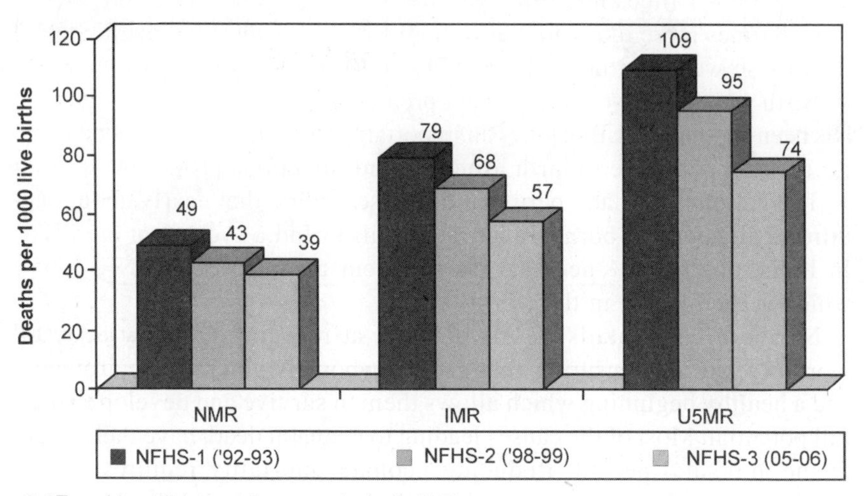

6.4 Trend in child mortality rates in India [12].

6.4 Neonatal mortality - direct and underlying determinants

The distribution of causes of neonatal death varies between countries and correlates closely with the degree of neonatal mortality [3]. Based on the data of 193 countries, the major causes of neonatal death globally are estimated to be infections (35%) – this includes (sepsis/pneumonia, tetanus, and diarrhea), preterm birth (28%), and asphyxia (23%) [13]. In India, a study conducted in Gadhchiroli, a small district in Maharashtra ascribed sepsis/pneumonia (52.5%), asphyxia (20%), prematurity <32 weeks (15%), hypothermia (2.5%), and other/not known (10%) as the primary cause of neonatal deaths in India.

6.4.1 Low birth weight – an important contributor to neonatal mortality

On the basis of birth weight, newborn is categorized into normal (≥2500 g), low birth weight (<2500 g), very low birth weight (<1500 g), and extremely low birth weight (<1000 g) groups [14]. Low birth weight can be an outcome of pre-term delivery (gestational age <37 completed weeks) or prematurity (intrauterine growth retardation or IUGR), or both. Prematurity or IUGR is a greater risk with fifty percent of the 4 million neonatal deaths per year occurring in babies who are small for their age [15].

The lower the birth weight, higher the chances of mortality. The Lancet malnutrition series 2008 observes that infants born at term weighing 1500–1999 g are 8.1 times more likely to die and those weighing 2000–2499 g are 2.8 times more likely to die from all causes during the neonatal period than those weighing more than 2499 g at birth.

Birth weight is also an important predictor of clinical complications. It has been shown that LBW plays an important role in almost 60% of neonatal deaths occurring due to birth asphyxia and infections [16].

The national neonatal perinatal database reports that nearly about one-third of all neonates born in major hospitals of India every year are LBW. In India, nearly 82% neonatal deaths occur among LBW (NNF, 1995), which is the highest in the world [17].

Newborn care entails efforts directed at reducing not only neonatal mortality but also ensuring that each newborn is given an environment and a healthy beginning which allows them to survive and develop to their full potential. Most of the causes leading to neonatal death have their origin in the antenatal period. Reducing neonatal mortality requires efforts directed throughout pregnancy, through delivery and after birth, that is, care along the continuum.

6.5 Continuum of care – a comprehensive approach to saving newborn lives

Neonatal health is intrinsically linked to the health and nutrition of the mother and the care she receives before, during and immediately after giving birth [1]. Cost-effective prenatal and delivery interventions that improve maternal health and nutrition and save mothers' lives can save most newborns too [18]. This principle of care which extends and links two or more phases (maternal health and child health) is often termed as continuum of care.

The continuum of care has recently been highlighted as a core principle of programmes for maternal, newborn, and child health, and as a means to reduce the burden of half a million maternal deaths, 4 million neonatal deaths, and 6 million children [19]. According to World Health Report 2005, the term "continuum of care" encompasses both person and place, i.e. care provided as a continuum throughout the lifecycle, including adolescence, pregnancy, childbirth and childhood and secondly care provided in a continuum that spans the home, the community, the health center and the hospital – Figs. 6.5a and 6.5b. The interventions for saving newborn lives "Essential newborn care" is based on the principles of continuum of care.

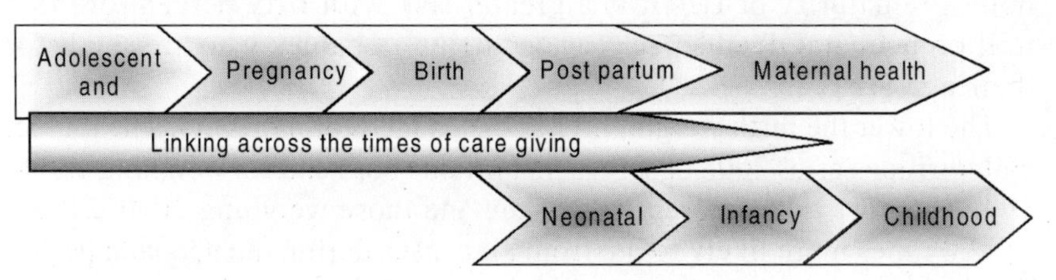

6.5a Connecting care giving across the continuum for maternal, newborn and child health.

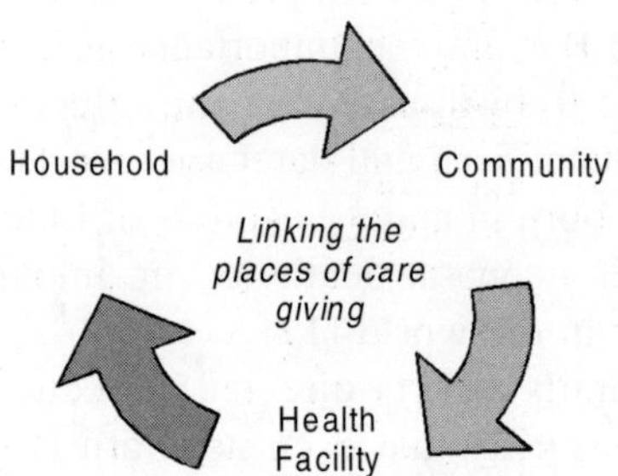

6.5b Connecting care giving across the continuum between households and health facilities to reduce maternal, newborn and child deaths.

6.6 Essential newborn care interventions

Essential newborn care is a comprehensive strategy designed to improve the health of newborns through interventions before conception, during pregnancy, at and soon after birth, and in the postnatal period [20]. On the basis of birth weight and gestational age, WHO proposes two types of essential newborn care: basic care and special care.

Basic care means interventions for all infants to meet their physiological needs. Basic newborn care assures survival of those that are born well-equipped to survive (term, well-grown newborns without malformations) and give good start for preterm and small newborns. Simple, effective, low cost interventions notably, tetanus toxoid vaccination, exclusive breastfeeding, kangaroo mother care come under basic interventions.

Special care is required for a small group of newborns because of diseases acquired before, during or after birth and/or because they were born too soon and/or too small.

Figure 6.6 given below shows the package of interventions (both basic and special) which have a proven role in promoting health and preventing deaths in newborns, the linkages between the physiological stage and subsequent outcome and the type of care provider needed for providing the care.

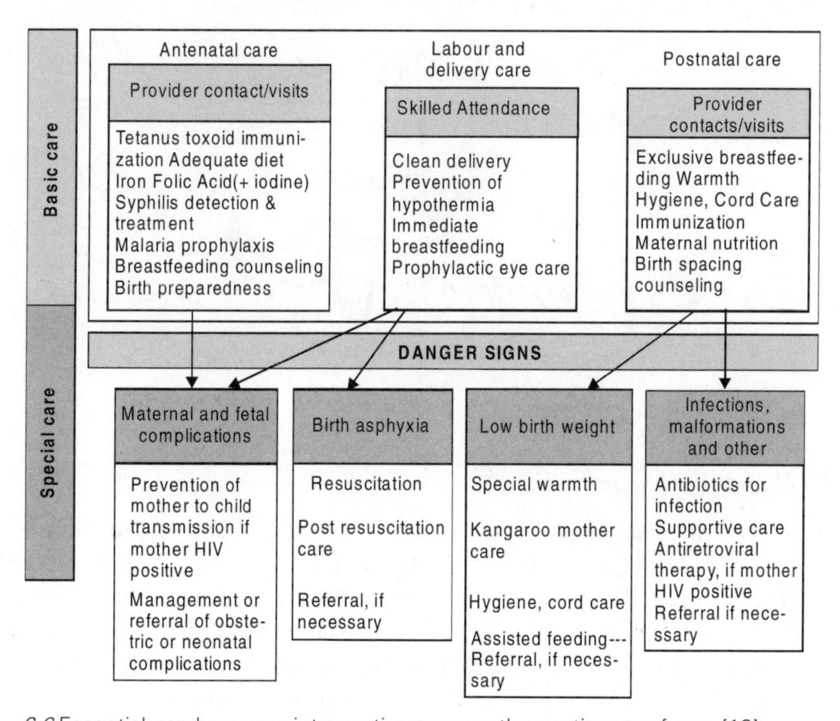

6.6 Essential newborn care interventions across the continuum of care [18].

Following sections give a brief insight into selected basic essential newborn care interventions as recommended by WHO.

Basic care

(a) Protecting newborn against infections

Almost 75% deliveries in India occur at home in presence of unskilled birth attendants/family members thereby exposing the mother and the newborn to the risk of infection, inappropriate management of pregnancy complications and poor hygiene during the delivery. Tetanus and sepsis are the commonest infection during the early neonatal period and are a manifestation of unhygienic delivery practices. Ensuring clean delivery and clean cord is essential for minimizing the risk of neonatal tetanus and sepsis.

Clean delivery – The hands of the birth attendant should be clean (washed with water and soap) and the delivery surface should be sterile.

Clean cord – The cord should be cut with a new blade, stump should be short (length approximately 1.5–2.0 cm) to prevent soiling from urine (Figure 6.7) and nothing should be applied on the cut surface of umbilical cord. The cut surface should be inspected for bleeding within 2–4 hours after birth. The shriveled dry cord normally falls within 5–10 days.

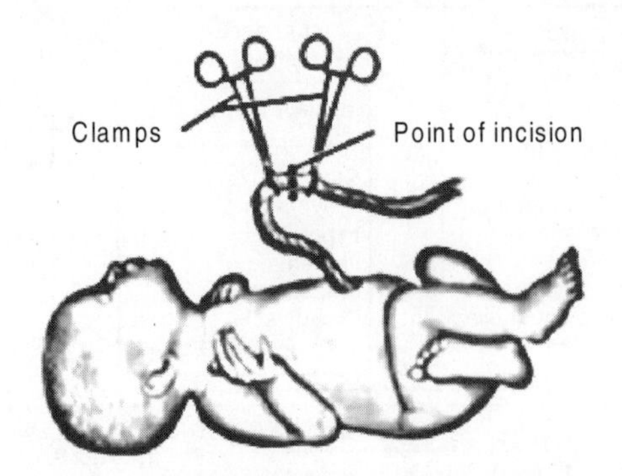

6.7 Clamping and cutting umbilical cord [21].

(b) Thermal protection

Newborn's vulnerability to hypothermia – The normal body temperature of the newborn infant is 36.5–37.5°C. Hypothermia occurs when the body temperature drops below 36.5°C. Relatively large surface area, poor thermal insulation, small body mass to produce and conserve heat, little ability to conserve heat by changing posture and no ability to adjust its own clothing in response to thermal stress put a newborn at risk to hypothermia.

Hypothermia can easily occur in a cold environment, if newborn is left wet, naked and unprotected from cold while waiting for the placenta to be delivered or cord to be cut. Hypothermia can also occur if the newborn is bathed soon after birth.

Preventing hypothermia – Ensuring delivery of the baby in a warm room, drying the head, body and face (preferably in that order) thoroughly after birth, wrapping it in layers of clean, dry warm cloth taking care to cover the head and the feet and giving it to the mother as soon as possible are the simplest measures for preventing hypothermia. Early skin-to-skin contact (kangaroo mother care – Box 6.1) for the first few hours after birth is the simplest and most effective way for providing warmth. The newborn should be kept away from draft and should be bathed only after temperature stabilizes, preferably after 24 hours.

Box 6.1 Kangaroo mother care [22, 23]

Kangaroo care is a method of holding a baby that involves skin-to-skin contact. The baby, who is naked except for a diaper and a piece of cloth covering his or her back (either a receiving blanket or the parent's clothing), is placed in an upright position against a parent's bare chest. This snuggling of the infant inside the pouch of their parent's shirt, much like a kangaroo's pouch, led to the creation of the term "kangaroo care.

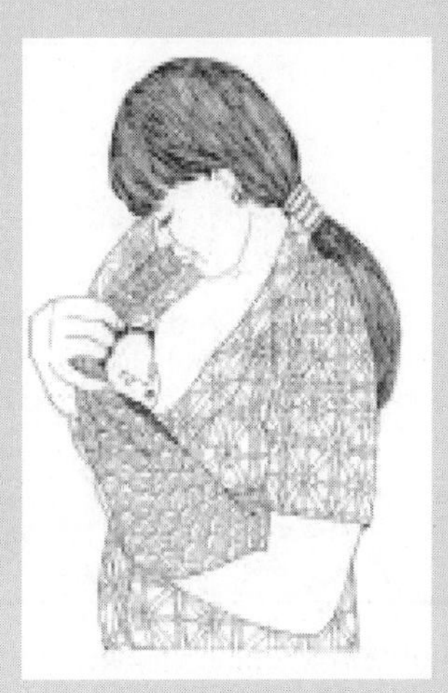

Kangaroo Mother Care *was designed to reduce hypothermia by keeping mother and newborn together but it has other benefits too.* Kangaroo Care *also encourages mother and child to bond emotionally and enables the baby to breastfeed at will, giving the baby the energy to produce its own body heat. The action reduces the need for incubators, which are prohibitively expensive in developing countries.*

Kangaroo mother Care is a universally available and biologically sound method of care for all newborns, but in particular for premature babies

(c) Early, exclusive breastfeeding and newborn nutrition

Intrauterine growth and gestational age are important determinants of nutritional status of a newborn. The transition from fetal to extra fetal life poses a serious challenge for a term normal newborn. The goal of neonatal nutrition is to meet the metabolic requirements of developing organ systems, satisfy normal growth requirements and avoid deficiency or excess states without imposing detrimental stress on developing metabolic or excretory systems [24].

Just as the nutritional requirements of an infant are different from those of an adult, the nutritional requirements of the term neonate differ from those of the preterm neonate. Babies born after less than 37 weeks in the womb (preterm) have different nutritional needs than babies born at term (38–42 weeks). Preterm babies because of their short gestational age do not have enough stored up nutrients and they usually need supplements. Most neonates need 100–120 calories per kilogram of weight per day (cal/kg/d) in order to grow properly. Infants who have health problems may need extra nutrition – up to 160–180 cal/kg/d. Table 6.2 compares daily requirement of selected nutrients in healthy versus preterm neonate.

Table 6.2 Daily requirements of selected nutrients in healthy term and preterm infants [25]

Nutrient	Normal requirement Term[(a)]	 Preterm
Energy		
Total (kcal/kg)	100	120
Carbohydrate (g/kg)	10	12.0–14.0
Fat (g/kg)	3.3–6.0	4.0–7.0
Protein (g/kg)	1.5–2.2	3.0–4.0
Mineral and Trace elements		
Sodium (mEq/kg)	1 to 3	2 to 4
Potassium (mEq/kg)	1 to 2	2 to 4
Calcium (mg/kg)	45 to 60	120 to 230
Orthophosphate (mg/kg)	25 to 40	60 to 140
Magnesium (mg/kg)	6 to 8	7.9 to 15
Iron (mg/kg)	1[(b)]	2 to 4[(b)]
Vitamins		
A (IU/kg)	333	700 to 1500
E (IU)	3 to 25	5 to 25

(a) Based on infants fed human milk.
(b) Iron supplementation starts at 2 weeks postnatal age.

(1) Principles of feeding a newborn

The neonate's gastric capacity ranges from 40 to 60 ml during the first 24 hours after delivery. Nutrient needs must be met through frequent, small-volume feedings. Gastric emptying time – typically 2 to 4 hours – varies with feeding volume and the neonate's age. As the newborn gains weight, the stomach capacity also increases and so does the daily intake of feeds. The given feed must meet the special nutrient requirements of the neonate with organ systems that are still developing and must not exceed the limited concentrations that these same premature organ systems can tolerate [14]. In institutional settings, preterm newborns are kept in the neonatal intensive care unit (NICU), where they are carefully monitored to make sure they are getting the right balance of fluids, minerals such as sodium and potassium (electrolytes), and nutrition until their bodies mature and they are able to suckle breast milk. The NICU is equipped with careful temperature control, often with an incubator or special warmer which helps to reduce excess calorie needs. Humidified (moistened) air helps maintain body temperature and avoid fluid loss. Table 6.3 summarizes the usual principles adopted while feeding newborns with different gestational ages

Early exclusive breastfeeding is dealt in another chapter in this book.

(2) Benefits of breastfeeding in context of neonatal health

- In the first week of life, breastfeeding can help prevent hypothermia and hypoglycemia in newborns, which are contributory causes of death. Suckling increases body temperature, and the nearness to the mother that breastfeeding provides is beneficial in reducing hypothermia. Delaying first feed leads to starvation which increases the risk of hypoglycemia. Recent research evidence from Ghana (Box 6.2) highlights that neonatal deaths will be reduced by 22%, if all newborns are exclusively breastfed within an hour of their birth. WHO recommends that infants should be put to breast within one hour after birth and should not go without breastfeeding for more than 3 hours between feeds.
- Studies in Brazil and Philippines have shown that breastfeeding has a greater role in preventing late neonatal deaths (from 8 to 28 days) – deaths that are primarily due to infections such as sepsis, pneumonia, meningitis, umbilical infection, and diarrhea. A study in Brazil has shown that there are substantial benefits of exclusive breastfeeding over partial breastfeeding. The relative risk of death found to be 24.7 for infants not breastfed, and 3.1 for infants partially breastfed, compared to 1 for those exclusively breastfed [27].

(d) Initiation of breathing, resuscitation

During the intrauterine life, the fetal lungs are filled with fluid and they do not serve ventilatory purpose since placenta supplies oxygen to the fetus. Most babies have a smooth transition from fetal to neonatal life and establish spontaneous breathing without any active assistance. About 3.5–7.5% of babies are likely to experience difficulty in breathing termed as "birth asphyxia" and need active resuscitation. The operational definition of birth asphyxia is a delay in initiating breathing at birth. If a newborn infant does not cry after initial stimulation by drying, it must be assessed for breathing. If the infant is not breathing or the breathing is poor, it needs active resuscitation.

Table 6.3 Feeding guidelines for neonates with different gestational ages [26]

	Pre-term/Premature <34 weeks	34–37 weeks	Term 38–42 weeks
Problem	Can't feed from a bottle or breast because of immature reflexes and trouble coordinating sucking, breathing, and swallowing. Also they may have accompanying medical problems like breathing problems, very low oxygen levels, gagging, circulatory problems, blood infection, or other illnesses might not be able to feed through a nipple (orally).		
Process and type of nutrition	Very premature babies get nutrition and fluids through a vein (intravenously)—parenteral nutrition. As they get bigger and their systems mature, they can be given breast milk or formula through a small tube inserted through the nose or mouth into the stomach (gavage feeding). Premature babies are fed very slowly to reduce the risk of getting an intestinal infection	Often can be fed from a bottle or the mother's breast. Sometimes it's easier for a premature baby to drink expressed breast milk from a bottle with a large hole in the nipple than from the breast. Babies who are breastfed may need a supplement called human milk fortifier added to the breast milk. This supplement contains the extra protein, calories, iron, calcium, and vitamins that premature babies need. If it is not possible for the baby to take breast milk, special preterm formulas can be used. Those fed formula may need to take added supplements of certain nutrients, including vitamins A, C, and D and folic acid. These formulas have a higher amount of fat and protein to meet the special growth needs of premature babies. Once babies reach 34–36 weeks gestation, they can be switched to regular formula.	Exclusive breastfeeding

Box 6.2 The Ghana study [28]

Objective – The primary objective was to evaluate the association between the timing of initiation of breastfeeding and neonatal mortality. The secondary objective was to assess whether the different types of breastfeeding (exclusive, predominant, and partial breastfeeding) were associated with substantially different risks of neonatal death.

Methodology – The study took advantage of the 4-weekly surveillance system from a large ongoing maternal vitamin A supplementation trial in rural Ghana involving all women of childbearing age and their infants.

The analysis was based on 10,947 breastfed singleton infants born between July 2003 and June 2004 who survived to day 2 and whose mothers were visited in the neonatal period. Women were visited once every 4 weeks by a network of trained village-based fieldworkers to distribute vitamin A capsules and collect data on morbidity and mortality. When a birth was reported, the fieldworker administered a "birth" questionnaire, which included details on delivery and newborn care practices including early breastfeeding practices.

The mother was asked when she initiated breastfeeding and was prompted for the exact timing (within 1 hour, after 1 hour but first day, day 2, day 3, day 4–7, or after day 7). She was then asked what she offered her child to eat or drink in the 24 hours before the interview. After noting the unprompted response, the mother was asked if she offered her own breast milk, breast milk from a wet nurse, animal milk, infant formula, milk-based fluids, water-based fluids, or solid foods. The mother was also asked about the infant's health on the day of birth and in the previous 24 hours. At the next 4-week visit, an "infant" questionnaire was administered to obtain additional outcome data (infant morbidity and mortality) and information about infant feeding practices. Infants were followed up at subsequent visits every 4 weeks until they reached 12 months of age.

Results – Breastfeeding was initiated within the first day of birth in 71% of the infants and by the end of day 3 in all but 1.3% of them; 70% of the infants were exclusively breastfed during the neonatal period. The risk of neonatal death was fourfold higher in children given milk-based fluids or solids in addition to breast milk. Late initiation (after day 1) was associated with a 2.4-fold increase in risk. The study concluded that 16 % of neonatal deaths could be saved if all infants were breastfed from day 1 and 22% if breastfeeding started within the first hour. The risk of neonatal death increased approximately fourfold if milk-based fluids or solids were provided.

Birth asphyxia should be recognized promptly and management should follow the basic principles of resuscitation: open airway (aspiration of mouth and nostrils), initiating breathing (by tactile stimulation and or end ventilation with positive pressure) and maintaining circulation through external cardiac massage. As asphyxia management entails involvement of a trained person, it should be preferably done in institutional setting. Asphyxia should ideally be managed in institutional settings. If done at home, presence of a trained attendant is important.

(e) Immunization

At birth BCG, OPV-0 and Hepatitis B vaccines are recommended by WHO as a part of overall immunization. BCG should be given as soon after birth as possible in all populations at high risk of tuberculosis infection. A single dose of OPV at birth or in the two weeks after birth is recommended to increase early protection.

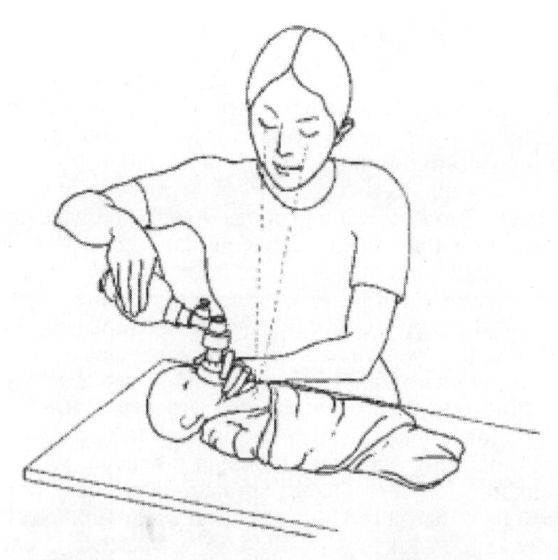

6.8 Resuscitating a newborn using bag and mask ventilation.

Where perinatal infections of Hepatitis B are common it is important to administer the first dose as soon as possible after birth.

(f) Management of newborn illness

Danger signs in the newborn period are non-specific and can be a manifestation of almost any newborn disease. The most common initial presentation of illness in an infant who has been doing well after birth is that it stops feeding well, is irritable and is cold to the touch. The initial signs may advance to fast and difficult breathing sometimes accompanied with grunting and intercostal retractions; the infant become lethargic, hypotonic and may or may not wake for feeds. Alternatively, the newborn may vomit; have diarrhoea and a distended abdomen. Pus draining from red swollen eyes or from the umbilicus is a sure indication of underlying infection. Jaundice on the first day and convulsions are always a sign of a serious illness. The danger signs of newborn illnesses need to be recognized early by family members and grass-root health functionaries for speedy referral. The underlying pathological condition needs management by a clinical specialist.

(g) Care of the preterm and/or low birth weight newborn

The World Health Organization (WHO), on the basis of world wide data, recommends that newborns with birth weight (b wt) less than 2500 g may be considered to fall in the low birth weight (LBW) category.

Globally, more than 20 million infants are born with low birth weight (Table 6.4). The number of low birth weight babies is concentrated in two

Table 6.4 Percentage of LBW by UN regions [30]

World	15.5
Africa	14.3
Asia	18.3
Europe	6.4
Latin America and Caribbean	10
North America	7.7
Oceania	10.5

regions of the developing world: Asia and Africa. Seventy-two per cent of low birth weight infants in developing countries are born in Asia where most births also take place and 22 per cent are born in Africa. India with 30% LBW alone accounts for 40 per cent of low birth weight births in the developing world and more than half of those in Asia. It is estimated there are more than 8 million newborns born every year in India with LBW [29].

LBW is governed by two major processes: a short gestational period, i.e. the infant is born too soon and is qualified as premature (birth weight <2500 g and gestational age <37 weeks), or a retarded intrauterine growth rate (IUGR), i.e. the infant is small for gestational age (birth weight <2500 g and gestation age >37 weeks) [31].

In the developed countries, the overwhelming majority of LBW infants are pre-terms, whereas in the developing nations, including South Asia, majority of LBW are IUGR [32]. Two-third LBW neonates born in India fall in IUGR category [31].

IUGR is caused predominately by maternal malnutrition, either before conception or during pregnancy [33]. Three factors have maximum impact: poor maternal nutritional status before conception, short stature (due mostly to undernutrition and infections during childhood or onset of pregnancy during adolescence which interferes with the normal growth velocity), and poor nutrition during pregnancy. LBW especially IUGR babies, carry relatively greater risks of perinatal and neonatal morbidity and mortality, and substandard growth and development in later life [33, 34]. Additionally, there is now increasing evidence (Box 6.3 Barker's hypothesis) that LBW is associated with an increased prevalence of diseases such as diabetes, hypertension, ischaemic heart disease and stroke in adult life. The latter is often known as fetal origin of adult disease.

Reduced weight, poor immunity and a poor insulation because of lack of fat as the source of energy makes low birth weight babies susceptible to the risk of frequent infection, hypothermia and poor growth, impact of which is maximum during the neonatal period. Given below are few elements of care which should essentially be provided to all LBW newborns:

Prevention of hypothermia – Skin-to-skin contact, adequately clothing the baby, provision of additional heat and regularly recording the temperature will help prevent hypothermia.

Box 6.3 Barker's hypothesis [35]

Barker's Hypothesis is named after David J. P. Barker a researcher at the University of Southampton who published the theory in 1997 (Ref). The theory states that reduced fetal growth is strongly associated with a number of chronic conditions later in life. This increased susceptibility results from adaptations made by the fetus in an environment limited in its supply of nutrients. These chronic conditions include coronary heart disease, stroke, diabetes, and hypertension.

Barker hypothesis explains that malnutrition in utero has a far-reaching impact on the future health of the newborn. The undernourished fetus (mainly IUGR) adapts to its nutrition deficient environment by undergoing changes in the body's structure, metabolism, hormonal sensitivity and physiology to ensure its continual survival and growth, but in the process compromising development of certain organs or processes.

IUGR infants, having failed to attain full growth potential are at greater risks of suffering from the consequences of chronic diseases.

Barker's hypothesis asserts the need of a public health strategy which targets women in different point of their life cycle-starting before birth, infancy, adolescence, to adulthood, i.e. a preventive strategy having focus on continuum of care.

Traditional practice of giving both soon after birth needs to be avoided to prevent hypothermia.

Provision of early and exclusive breastfeeding – In a low birth weight baby nutrient stores at birth are low, feeding, digestion and absorption systems are immature and there are high requirements for rapid growth. Concomitant illnesses may interfere with growth potential ,add to organ dysfunction and further increase the demand for energy and nutrients [24]. The window of tolerance of nutrient intake is extremely narrow for these infants. LBW babies must be frequently fed (preferably 2 hours or more frequently) because initially most of them suck briefly and consume small quantities of milk with each feed. Some LBW babies suck poorly during the first few days even though they are active. Expressed milk stored in a clean vessel and fed with a spoon could be practiced where acceptable. Early initiation of breastfeeding helps in averting hypoglycemia. It is important that bottle feeding is completely avoided as it increases the risk of infection.

Prevention of infection – Because of low immunity, LBW are especially vulnerable to infection. Adoption of clean hygienic feeding practices, restriction of entry of family members suffering from infection like seasonal cold, avoiding pre lacteal feeds and water and wrapping the baby in a clean cloth are some of the precautions that need to be taken.

6.7 Delivering essential newborn care (ENBC) interventions through public health systems – opportunities and challenges

Despite the public health significance, few programs target neonatal health in developing countries. Interventions to reduce neonatal deaths have been traditionally covered by two health system programmes namely maternal health as well as child health. Maternal health programmes focus on pregnancy, childbirth and immediate care of the newborn while the child health programmes concentrates on late neonatal period, infancy and childhood. Much too often neonatal care "falls between the cracks" in maternal and child health programmes [7]. Though Essential Newborn Care (ENBC) has been acknowledged and incorporated in most of the maternal child health programmes across the countries but lack of integration and implementation bottlenecks have resulted in very little impact.

Additionally, countries have continued to spend millions on provision of institution based care for maternal and newborn complications with little efforts and funds directed at providing services along the continuum, i.e. from household, community to health facility. This has created two parallel levels of care – a community governed family based care and an institution based clinical care. Both the levels work independently with little synergy between the two. The picture is especially true for low resource settings countries like India where almost 80% of deliveries are conducted at home with assistance from unskilled family members or community approved person. The services received by a newborn delivered at home are often those that are approved by community and practiced by majority. The "essentials" of newborn care like drying and wrapping the baby, immediate initiation of breastfeeding and resuscitation are severely compromised in home settings.

An understanding of community practices throughout the continuum of care, i.e. from maternal through neonate and from home to outreach to facility (care seeking behaviour—recognition, labeling and seeking treatment for an illness) is critical for success of ENBC. Factors contributing to poor care seeking like poverty, illiteracy, poor maternal health, traditional barriers, harmful traditional practices and inadequate health care facilities and transport need to be studied and taken into consideration before introducing interventions which do not conform to their traditional beliefs and customs.

In recent years, renewed global interest and generation of large body of evidence regarding neonatal health has seen a revival and the belief is taking ground that neonatal mortality is, in fact, amenable to simple effective public health initiatives including community-based interventions [8]. The importance of community involvement and participation in impacting neonatal health has also been demonstrated through successful community trials such as (Shivgarh study and Warmi project [35, 36]). These projects have provided the needed evidence that family/Community engagement can avoid many deaths by ensuring that families are equipped with appropriate healthcare messages on danger signs and care-seeking. Boxes 6.4 and 6.5 give a brief account of successful projects undertaken with support of people residing within the community.

Box 6.4 The Warmi project [36]

Background – The Warmi, conducted from July 1990 to June 1993, attempted to improve maternal and child health through involving communities in health care. An intervention to improve maternal and child health was conducted in a remote Bolivian province of Inquivisi with limited access to modern medical facilities.

Methodology – Fifty communities in Inquivisi Province participated in the Warmi project.

The total population in the demonstration area is 15 000. There were a variety of types of women's groups in the Inquivisi area, including women's organizations, cooperatives, mothers' clubs, and agrarian unions. The groups' functions varied together with their degrees of effectiveness. The project staff considered women's organizations best able to organize women around health issues. Consequently, the staff focused on these groups, initiating or strengthening 50 women's organizations. Study personnel included five to six teams, each consisting of two auxiliary nurses Monthly or more frequently, each team met individually with all women's organizations,

At these meetings, attended by approximately 10–30 group members, a technique called "autodiagnosis" was employed to address community problems. Autodiagnosis consists of the following four steps: (a) identification and prioritization of problems, (b) group development of a formal action plan, (c) implementation of the plan, and (d) evaluation. Each community identified a different set of problems and approaches, and accordingly, specific interventions varied by community. However, certain objectives were addressed by all the women's groups: to (a) increase knowledge of reproduction, contraceptive use, danger signs of complications, and self-care, (b) improve immediate newborn care, and (c) increase the percentage of women who receive delivery care from trained birth attendants.

Intervention – The intervention focused on initiating and strengthening women's organizations, developing women's skills in problem identification and prioritization, and training community members in safe birthing techniques.

Results – The impact was evaluated by comparing perinatal mortality rates and obstetric behavior among 409 women before and after the intervention. Perinatal mortality decreased from 117 deaths per 1 000 births before the intervention to 43.8 deaths per 1 000 births after. There was a significant increase in the number of women participating in women's organizations following the intervention, as well as in the number of organizations. The proportion of women receiving prenatal care and initiating breast-feeding on the first day after birth was also significantly larger. The number of infants attended to immediately after delivery likewise increased, but the change was not statistically significant. One of the greatest changes observed in this study was a doubling of participation in women's organizations.

6.8 Addressing neonatal health in India – initiatives by Government of India

Over a period of three decades, a review of strategy and approach of maternal and child health programmes initiated by Government of India (GoI) shows that the maternal and child health programmes in India have retained their focus on provision of antenatal care and prevention of post neonatal deaths through diarrhea, pneumonia and immunization programmes (Box 6.6).

Box 6.5 Shivgarh trial [37]

Background – In rural India, most births take place in the home, where high-risk care practices are common. In Shivgarh trial the intervention developed was behavior change management, with a focus on prevention of hypothermia, aimed at modifying practices and reducing neonatal mortality.

Methods – Cluster-randomised controlled efficacy trial in Shivgarh, a rural area in Uttar Pradesh. Thirty-nine village-administrative units (population 104, 123) were allocated to one of three groups: a control group, which received the usual services of governmental and non-governmental organizations in the area; an intervention group, which received a preventive package of interventions for essential newborn care (birth preparedness, clean delivery and cord care, thermal care (including skin-to-skin care), breastfeeding promotion, and danger sign recognition) and another intervention group, which received the package of essential newborn care plus use of a liquid crystal hypothermia indicator (ThermoSpot). In the intervention clusters, community health workers delivered the packages via collective meetings and two antenatal and two postnatal household visitations. Outcome measures included changes in newborn-care practices and neonatal mortality rate compared with the control group.

Results – Improvements in birth preparedness, hygienic delivery, thermal care (including skin-to-skin care), umbilical cord care, skin care, and breastfeeding were seen in intervention arms. There was little change in care-seeking. Compared with controls, neonatal mortality rate was reduced by 54% in the essential newborn-care intervention and by 52% in the essential newborn care plus Thermo Spot arm.

Interpretation – A socio-culturally contextualized, community-based intervention, targeted at high-risk newborn-care practices, can lead to substantial behavioural modification and reduction in neonatal mortality. This approach can be applied to behaviour change along the continuum of care, harmonise vertical interventions and build community capacity for sustained development.

Box 6.6 – Child health programmes in India

1977 – Family Planning changed to Family Welfare Programme
1978 – Diarrhoeal Disease Control programme launched
1985 – Universal Immunization programme (UIP) launched
1990 – Acute Respiratory Infection Control Programme
1992 – Child Survival and Safe Mother (CSSM) Programme launched
1997 – Reproductive and Child Health (RCH) Programme – Phase I/RCH I
2002 – Reproductive and Child Health Programme (Phase II)
2005 – National Rural Health Mission (NRHM)

It is interesting to note that though reduction of neonatal mortality rate was one of the objectives of National health policy drafted in 1983, and essential newborn care was included as one of the components in Child Survival and Safe Motherhood Programmes (CSSM) launched in 1992, apart from neonatal tetanus immunization of pregnant mother, other activities failed to achieve any success in improving neonatal health due in part to lack of reliable information on the magnitude and causes of neonatal deaths.

Being one of the signatory countries to United Nations Millennium Development Goals (MDGs), India has lately initiated several measures toward improving the neonatal health scenario in the country towards achieving MDG 4 and MDG 5. In addition to giving renewed thrust to ENBC through ongoing RCH II programme (being implemented under the umbrella of National Rural Health Mission) across the entire country, Government of India has also launched "Integrated Management of Childhood Illnesses (IMCI)" strategy in selected districts of the country, added "newborn" to it and renamed it as "Integrated Management of Neonatal and Childhood Illnesses" or IMNCI which is a key strategy within the RCH-II programme.

Additionally, several governmental and non-governmental agencies, both national and international, have joined hands to support a nationwide Neonatal Health Research Initiative (NHRI) [8]. This has been under the auspices of the India Clinical Epidemiology Network (IndiaCLEN) with the active support of National Neonatology Forum, Ministry of Health-Government of India, Saving Newborn Lives, Johns Hopkins University and USAID. Under NHRI several multi-centric studies for identifying simple and better ways for promoting newborn health in community settings are being undertaken in various centers representing the entire country.

6.9 Integrated Management of Childhood Illnesses (IMCI) – the global strategy

IMCI is an integrated approach to child health that focuses on the well-being of the whole child. IMCI includes both preventive and curative elements that are implemented by families and communities as well as by health facilities. The success of IMCI in reducing childhood mortality depends on improvements of overall health systems as well as improvement of family and community health care practices [38].

Developed in mid-nineties by WHO and UNICEF, the global IMCI strategy focused primarily on the most common causes of child mortality like – diarrhea, pneumonia, measles, malaria and malnutrition, illnesses affecting children aged 1 week to 2 months and 2 months to 5 years, including both preventive and curative elements to be implemented by families and communities as well as by health facilities [39]. It promotes all the essential new born components except safe delivery. IMCI acknowledges contribution of malnutrition to child morbidity and mortality and includes nutrition assessment and counseling for all sick infants and children.

The health workers are trained to follow an algorithmic systematic approach health to assess a sick child and address several medical conditions that often co-exist rather than only the main presenting symptom [39]. IMCI helps workers broaden their approach to consider and respond to the child and manage the different factors that could be contributing to child's sickness [40]. For instance, all children, during an IMCI consultation are screened for malnutrition and assessed for immunization status, and given age appropriate feeding advice and immunization services.

6.10 Integrated Management of Neonatal Care and Childhood Illnesses (IMNCI)

The Indian adaptation gives thrust to neonatal component, the most critical period affecting infant and child mortality. A community-component for routine care of all newborn children has been added to the initiative. Box 6.6 gives information on such changes made in the IMNCI strategy in Indian adaptation.

Box 6.7 Differences between generic IMCI and Indian IMNCI [41]

	Features	Generic IMCI	India's IMNCI
1	*Scope* Includes birth to 7 d of life (early newborn period)	No	Yes
2	*Target providers* Facility-based providers such as physicians	Yes	Yes
3	Community-based providers (auxiliary nurse midwives/ Anganwadi workers)	No	Yes
4	Training program Training time – newborn and young infant	~20% (2 of 11 days)	50% (4 of 8 days)
5	Sequence of training	First, the child (2 months to 5 years) module, followed by young infant (7 days to 2 months)	First, the newborn and young infant (0–2 months) module; then the child (2 months to 5 years)
6	Training for home visits for postnatal care of newborn	No	Yes
7	Implementation – facility-based application	yes	Yes
8	Community-based application (3 home contacts within first 10 days)	No	Yes
9	Implement only young infant or older child package	No	Yes

The incorporation of home visits in India's adaptation of IMNCI is an effort to ensure continuum of care from home to outreach to facility. Trained front-line workers extend quality inputs of the health system to household; helping to prevent illness and ensuring timely referral to a health facility for severe cases. During home visits, all newborns are assessed, any problems are identified and referred if necessary. In addition, and mother are taught ways to prevent illnesses and counseling to practice exclusive breastfeeding, keeping baby warm, and other essential newborn care. During these visits, mothers are also taught to keys signs of illnesses – when and where to seek timely care.

Outreach health workers (the auxiliary nurse-midwives and ASHAs) and community nutrition and child development workers (grass-root workers or anganwadi workers of Integrated Child Development Services or ICDS) are mandated to visit all neonates at home three times (within 24 hours, 3–4 days and 7–10 days) within the first 10 days, starting soon after birth, to provide home-based preventive care/health promotion and to detect neonates with sickness requiring referral. For ensuring appropriate growth and feeding of low birth weight babies, nutritional counseling through extra contacts are also proposed in IMNCI on day 14, day 21 and day 28. These visits will also be used to provide post-partum care to the mother [42].

The specific newborn components that have been added to IMNCI include early and exclusive breastfeeding, warmth, care-seeking for severe illness, LBW care and treatment of umbilical sepsis.

6.11 Conclusion

Translating knowledge on effective interventions into a successful public health programme which integrates the continuum of care is a daunting task for countries struggling to achieve MDGs. The challenge becomes more in context of developing countries where incidence of low birth weight is high, service delivery structures are poor and utilization of health services is determined by care-seeking behavior of families and communities. In case of newborns, care seeking is more an outcome of prevalent and accepted cultural practices and traditions. Changing behaviours or developing a health care system responsive to newborns requires an understanding and appreciation of community practices, health education, dedicated health professionals, proper channeling of human and financial resources as well as political will, all of which continue to remain a challenge in developing countries. Identifying simple, acceptable and practiced by communities, require little modification should be introduced and promoted first These selected interventions should be such that these can be delivered by the primary care system and the community health care provider. The acceptability of other complex interventions will increase when communities start perceiving benefits of these simple interventions thereby contributing to reduced neonatal mortality rates in developing countries.

References

1. WHO (2005). World Health Report: Newborns: no longer going unnoticed; Chapter 5, in Make every Mother and Child Count.
2. IIPS, National Family Health Survey (1998–1999), p. 181.
3. LAWN JE, COUSENS A, and ZUPAN J (2005). Neonatal Survival 1; 4 million neonatal deaths: When? Where? Why? *Lancet* pp. 891–900.
4. DARMSTADT GL and BLACK RE (2000). Research priorities and postpartum care strategies for the prevention and optimal management of neonatal infections in less developed countries. *Pediatr Infec Dis J* vol. 19, no. 6, pp. 739–750.
5. NARAYANAN I, et al. (2004). The components of essential newborn care. Perinatal/Neonatal brief: Basics II, USAID.
6. SINES E, SYED U, WALL S, WORLEY H. Postnatal Care: A Critical Opportunity to Save Mothers and Newborns: Save the Children; Population Reference Bureau, 2007.
7. SEARO (2006). Operationalizing the Neonatal Health Care Strategy in South-East Asia Region. In 11th Meeting of Health Secretaries of Member States of SEAR. New Delhi, India.
8. WHO (2002). Improving Neonatal Health in South-East Asia Region: Report of a Regional Consultation New Delhi, India, 1–5 April 2002.
9. THACKER N (2007). Improving status of neonatal health in India. *Indian Pediatrics* vol. 44, pp. 891–892.
10. MKC NAIR, JANA A and NISWADE A (2005). Neonatal Survival and Beyond (editorial). *Indian Pediatrics* vol. 42, pp. 985–988.
11. KAUSHAL M, AGGARWAL R, SINGHAL A, SHUKLA H, PAUL VK. Breastfeeding practices and health seeking behaviour for neonatal sickness in a rural community. *Journal of Tropical Paediatrics* 2005; **51**(6)**:**366–376.
12. IIPS, National Family Health Survey (NFHS-3) (2005–2006).
13. LAWN JE, WILCZYNSKA-KETENDE K and COUSENS SN (2006). Estimating the causes of 4 million neonatal deaths in the year 2000. *Int J Epidemiol* vol. 35, pp. 706–718.
14. BORUM PR (1993). Use of the colostrum-deprived piglet to evaluate parenteral feeding formulas symposium: animal models in neonatal and infant nutrition research. *The Journal of Nutrition*, pp. 392–394.
15. SHERIF NA (2004). Postgraduate Training Course in Reproductive Health 2004 Balanced protein energy supplementation during pregnancy for the prevention of IUGR in Geneva Foundation for Medical Education and Research.
16. BLACK RR, ALLEN LH, BHUTTA ZA, et al. Maternal and child undernutrition: global and regional exposures and health consequences. *Lancet: Maternal and Child Undernutrition Study Group* 2008; **371:**243–260.
17. BISAI S, SEN A, MAHALANABIS D, DATTA N and BOSE K; The Effect of Maternal Age and Parity on Birth Weight Among Bengalees of Kolkata, India. *Human Ecology*, 2006(14):139–143.
18. Essential newborn care: at a glance (2001). In: Save the children.
19. KERBER KJ, et al (2007). Continuum of care for maternal, newborn, and child health: from slogan to service delivery. *Lancet* vol. 370, pp. 1358–1369.
20. NARAYANAN I, ROSE M and CORDERO D (2004). The Components of Essential Newborn Care, in Perinatal/Neonatal Brief 2004, BASICS II.
21. www.umn.edu/pregnancy/100159/html.
22. WHO (2003). Kangaroo Mother Care: A Practical Guide.

23. Essential Newborn nursing for small hospitals. In resource restricted countries, Learner's guide. Department of Paediatrics, WHO collaborating Centre for training and Research in Newborn Care. All India Institute of Medical Sciences, New Delhi.
24. WINN HN and HOBBINS JC (2000). Clinical Maternal-Fetal Medicine. Parthenon Publishing, p. 877.
25. PREMER DM and GEORGIEFF MK (1990). Nutrition for Ill Neonates. *Pediatrics in Review* vol. 20, pp. e56–e62.
26. GREENE A (2007). Neonatal weight gain and nutrition. Medline Plus: A service of U.S. National Library of Medicine and the National Institutes of Health: Adam.
27. Reducing perinatal and neonatal mortality. Child Health Research Project. Report of a Meeting Baltimore, Maryland May 10–12, 1999, vol. 3, no. 1.
28. EDMOND KM, et al. (2006). Delayed breastfeeding initiation increases risk of neonatal mortality. *Pediatrics* vol. 117, no. 3.
29. Saving newborn lives and national neonatology forum; State of India's Newborn.
30. UNICEF and WHO, Low birth weight: Country Regional and Global Estimates. 2004.
31. NORTON R. Maternal nutrition during pregnancy as it affects infant growth, development and health. [Available from: http://www.unsystem.org/scn/archives/scnnews11/ch06].
32. SACHDEV HPS (2001). Low birth weight in South Asia. *Int I of Diab Dev Countries* vol. 21, pp. 13–31.
33. GALLOWAY R. Pre-pregnancy nutritional status and its impact on birth weight. [Available from: http://www.unsystem.org/scn/archives/scnnews11/ch06].
34. TOMKINS A, MURRAY S,RONDO P, FILTEAU S; *Impact of Maternal Infection on Foetal Growth and Nutrition.* [cited; Available from: http://www.unsystem.org/scn/archives/scnnews11/ch08
35. BARKER DJP (1997). Maternal nutrition, fetal nutrition, and disease in later life. *Nutrition* vol. 13, p. 807.
36. O'ROURKE K, HOWARD-GRABMAN L and SEOANE G (1998). Impact of community organization of women on perinatal outcomes in rural Bolivia. *Pan Am J Public Health* vol. 3, no. 1, pp. 9–14.
37. KUMAR V, MOHANTY S, KUMAR A et al (2008). Effect of community-based behaviour change management on neonatal mortality in Shivgarh, Uttar Pradesh, India: a cluster-randomised controlled trial. *The Lancet* vol. 372, pp. 1151–1162.
38. Funding Research Activities [Publications]. Available from: Funding Research, Child Health and Nutrition Research Initiatives.
39. THACKER N (2007). Integrated management of neonatal and childhood illnesses: a new hope for child survival. *Indian Pediatrics* vol. 44, pp. 169–171.
40. INGLE GK and MALHOTRA C (2007). Integrated management of neonatal and childhood illness: an overview. *Indian J of Comm Medicine* vol. 32, no. 2, pp. 108–110.
41. BHANDARI N, MAZUMDAR S and DUBE B. Evaluation of the Impact of Integrated Management of Neonatal and Childhood Illness (IMNCI) Strategy on Neonatal and Infant Mortality in Haryana, India, Society for Applied Studies, New Delhi.
42. MARTINES J, PAUL VK, BHUTTA ZA, KOBLINSKY M, SOUCAT A, WALKER N, BAHL R, FOGSTAD H, COSTELLO A, for the Lancet Neonatal Survival Steering Team (2005); Neonatal Survival 4 Neonatal survival: a call for action; *Lancet* vol. 365 pp. 43–51.

7

Integrating breastfeeding in public health programming – scientific facts, current status and future directions

Kajali Paintal

Kajali Paintal, MSc, PhD, is a Nutrition Specialist (Infant and Young Child Nutrition) at UNICEF, New Delhi. Formely, she was a nutritionist at PATH India working for the Ultra Rice and Sure Start programmes. She was rewarded Senior Research Fellowship by the Indian Council of Medical Research (ICMR) for research projects on pediatric health and nutrition. Dr. Paintal has research and field experience in the area of breastfeeding and reproductive child health issues and has worked on short-/long-term projects with CARE (Delhi), Indian Social Science Institute (Delhi) and Breast Feeding Promotion Network of India (BPNI).

7.1 Introduction

The future potential of human societies largely depends on children's optimal physical growth and psycho-social development.

For a decent start in life, meeting the nutritional needs of infants and providing adequate care in the early years is fundamental for physical, motor, cognitive, social and emotional development. At this critical stage of life, a neonate is extremely vulnerable and primarily dependant on the mother for nourishment that is provided through breastfeeding [1]. Optimal nourishment at this stage of life has not only short-term effect on growth, body composition/functions, but also long-term effect on morbidity and mortality risks in adulthood. If not managed in time, malnutrition disturbs the foundation of life, growth and development and its ill effects become virtually irreversible after 2 years of age.

"Malnutrition has been responsible, directly or indirectly, for 35% of the 8.7 million deaths that occur annually among under-5 children; over two-thirds of these deaths are often associated with inappropriate feeding practices in first year of life" [2, 3].

Box 7.1 WHO/UNICEF definitions of breastfeeding practices

- **Early initiation of breastfeeding** – Proportion of children born in the last 24 months who were put to the breast within one hour of birth.
- **Exclusive breastfeeding under 6 months** – Proportion of infants (0 to <6 months) fed with only breast milk (including milk expressed or from a wet nurse) including ORS, drops, syrup (vitamins, minerals, medicines) in the previous 24 hours.
- **Predominant breastfeeding** – Proportion of infants predominantly fed with breast milk (including milk expressed or from a wet nurse) as the main source of nourishment in the previous 24 hours.
- **Breastfeeding** – Proportion of infants being fed with breast milk (including milk expressed or from a wet nurse) in the previous 24 hours [4].

In developing countries, breastfeeding is a cultural norm and most children are breast-fed during the first year of life; yet the irony is that malnutrition owing to faulty feeding practices is associated with 35% of the young child deaths. The *Lancet 2008* series indicate that sub-optimal breastfeeding increases the risk of poor nutrient intake, illness and malnutrition due to poor feeding practices. It is estimated that sub-optimum breastfeeding, especially non-exclusive breastfeeding in the first six months of life is responsible for 1.4 million child deaths and 44 million global childhood DALYs[1] (10% of the disease burden in children younger than 5 years) [5].

In India, alone 2.4 million child deaths occur annually; two thirds of which are attributed to inappropriate infant feeding practices. The *Lancet 2003* series on child survival identified breastfeeding interventions to have the potential to prevent 13% of all under-5 deaths in developing areas of the world, ranking it as the most important preventive approach for saving child lives, more than any other preventive intervention. Presently in Asia, only about one third of babies (<6 months) are exclusively breast fed; in order to achieve a reasonable reduction in the prevalence of child morbidity, malnutrition and mortality, ideally the exclusive breastfeeding rates should be 90–100% [6]. *Lancet 2008* estimates that a universal coverage in breastfeeding promotion and support can reduce infant mortality by nearly 12% and that the benefits from exclusive breastfeeding would be much more [7].

Standing Committee on Nutrition of the United Nations Working Group on Breastfeeding and Complementary Feeding (2003), in its endeavour to reach the Millennium Development Goals (MDGs) has stated that governments should keep in mind that "Inappropriate feeding practices and their consequences are major obstacles to sustainable socio-economic development and poverty reduction. Governments will be unsuccessful in their efforts to accelerate significant long term economic development until optimal child growth and development, especially through appropriate feeding practices are ensured" [8, 9].

---

1 DALYs i.e., Disability Adjusted Life Years is a measure of overall disease burden.

Optimal infant and young child feeding practices rank among the most effective interventions to improve child health. It has been estimated that optimal breastfeeding of children under two years of age has the potential to prevent 1.4 million deaths in children under five in the developing world annually [5]. In developing countries, less than 40% of the 136 million babies born each year benefit from early initiation of breastfeeding and similarly, 37% are exclusively breastfed in the first six months of life. Early cessation of breastfeeding in favour of commercial breast milk substitutes, giving water and other liquids along with breast milk, needless supplementation and poorly timed introduction of solid, semi-solid and soft foods, often of poor quality, are far too common. Professional and commercial influences combine to discourage breastfeeding, as do continued gaps in maternity legislation. To improve this situation, mothers and families need support to initiate and sustain appropriate infant and young child feeding practices. Overall, increasing the rates of early initiation of breastfeeding and of exclusive breastfeeding is critical in improving young child survival and development [5, 6].

Child health in general, and infant and young child feeding more specifically is often not well addressed in the basic training of doctors, nurses and other allied health professionals. Because of lack of adequate knowledge and skills, health professionals are often barriers to improved feeding practices. For example, they may not know how to assist a mother to initiate and sustain exclusive breastfeeding; they may recommend too-early introduction of supplements when there are feeding problems, and they may overtly or covertly promote breast-milk substitutes. Other socio-cultural constraints to improving infant feeding practices include lack of counseling and support in the community; poor awareness of populations on benefits of breastfeeding, early initiation and exclusive breastfeeding; absence of effective and ongoing communication strategies; lack of workplace support; lack of effective legislation on marketing of breastmilk substitutes; poor empowerment of women; exposure to domestic violence, financial independence; autonomy in decision-making, etc.

Health care professionals can play a critical role in providing that support, through influencing decisions about feeding practices among mothers and families. Therefore, it is critical for health professionals to have basic knowledge and skills to give appropriate advice. This scientific knowledge needs to be integrated into health and nutrition programmes to enable health professionals and service providers to counsel and help solve feeding difficulties, and know when and where to refer a mother who experiences more complex feeding problems [10].

7.2 Breastfeeding – the science for integrating scientific facts into programming

The high mortality and disease burden resulting from nutrition related factors make a compelling case for the urgent implementation of proven interventions. Breastfeeding promotion has been identified to be one of the most effective interventions for reducing child deaths and future disease burden. Countries should focus resources on proven interventions and scale them up as quickly as possible [5, 11, 12].

7.2.1 Breastfeeding – foundation of infant care

Breastfeeding is much more than providing food to a baby; it is the foundation of infant care that goes a long way in protecting against the early onset of malnutrition. Caring for women and children for survival, growth and development has gained significant importance only in the last one to two decades.

Breastfeeding is one of the most important caring activities that has a positive influence on the infant's nutritional status and also increases chances of survival even under extreme conditions of poverty and food insecurity. Box 7.2 highlights how breastfeeding can support the baby in the transition from fetal life to the external environment.

Inadequate care has been identified as one of the underlying causes of malnutrition amongst children. In addition, a mother's health status, quality of care provided is closely interlinked to the baby's health, growth and survival. A caregiver plays a critical role in providing the physical and emotional environment in which the infant can balance and regulate both internal and external stimuli as well as achieve their full growth potential [13].

Box 7.2 Breastfeeding supports the transition from fetal life to the external environment

Before birth, the foetus in a sterile, protected, moist and warm environment of the womb and gets all necessary nutrients/ oxygen for its metabolic, digestive and sensory functions through the umbilical cord. After birth, the placental-uterine metabolic inter-relationship between the mother and her infant continues through breastfeeding. Mother's milk is a part of the naturally ordained system uniquely adapted to meet the metabolic requirements of the new-born. It is intended to help the infant adapt to the sudden change(s) from fully dependant and secure intrauterine existence to an independent way of life in hostile extero-gestate environment. Breast milk provides the necessary nutrients and protective factors to the neonate to facilitate this transition [14, 15].

7.2.2 Benefits of breastfeeding

Breastfeeding protects the infant not only from disastrous consequences of malnutrition but also from degenerative diseases later in life. It has been well documented that breast milk is thus a natural resource of tremendous value, with medical and nutritional benefits. In addition to individual benefits, breastfeeding provides significant social and economic benefits to the family and nation. At the family level, breastfeeding results in reduced health care costs and abated absenteeism for care attributable to child's illness. The significantly lower incidence of illness in the breast fed infants allows parents more time for attention to siblings and other family responsibilities. Thus, it provides direct economic benefits to the family by reducing work absenteeism and loss in earnings. The economic benefits of breastfeeding is evident from the fact that the estimated cost of purchasing breastmilk substitutes is double than the cost of increased maternal food intake [16].

Successful lactation is a complex interaction between the mother and her new born which is not entirely instinctive but is based on learned behaviour that helps to build a close psychological relationship between the mother-infant dyad during early months of life. Optimum quantity and quality of breast milk coupled with adequate care helps in the healthy growth and psycho-social development of a child.

7.2.3 Lactation process: anatomy and physiology

Lactation cycle begins with growth of the breast (mammogenesis), initiation of milk synthesis and secretion (lactogenesis 1 and lactogenesis 2), established lactation (galactopoiesis), regression of the breast during and after weaning (involution) [17]. Figure 7.1 presents different stages in the lactation cycle starting from Mammogenesis (getting ready for lactation) to lactogenesis (initiation and establishment of lactation) to galactopoiesis (maintenance of lactation).

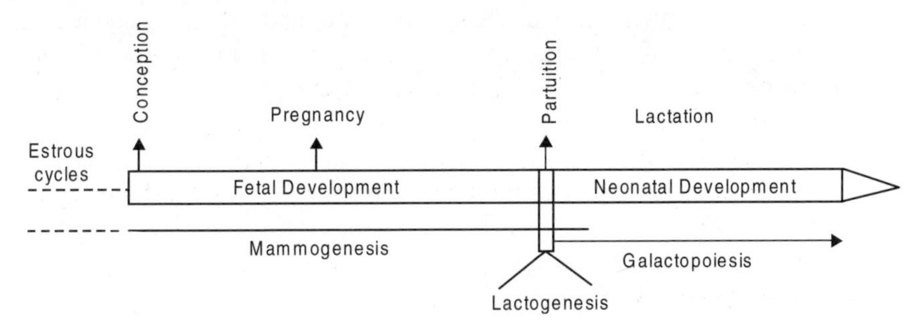

7.1 Lactational cycle.

(i) *Mammogenesis* is a stage when the mammary gland develops its histological and bio-chemical capacity to synthesize milk. This stage is characterized by increase in number and size of the alveoli, where milk is secreted and stored [18, 19].

(ii) *Lactogenesis* is a stage where the body secretes and produces milk for the baby. In humans, lactogenesis (referred to as the time when milk '*comes in*') starts about 40 hours before the infant's birth and is largely complete within five days. During this stage, a profound and rapid series of changes in the activity of differentiated mamary epithelial cells from a quiescent state to a fully active secretory state occurs. Lactogenesis has 2 stages: the first stage, lactogenesis 1 occurs by mid pregnancy, when the mammary gland becomes competent to secrete milk. The secretion of milk, however, is held in check by high circulating levels of progesterone and estrogen [18]. The second stage, lactogenesis 2 occurs around the time of delivery and is defined as the onset of copious milk secretion. The hormonal changes during parturition and the subsequent removal of the placenta act as a lactogenic trigger which is necessary for initiation of milk secretion [20]. For the ongoing synthesis and secretion of human milk, continuous hormonal signals received by the mammary gland (due to stimulation of nipple and areola), relayed to the central nervous system are essential to induce milk secretion [21]. Milk is secreted more or less continuously into alveolar lumens and stored until the let-down reflex induces milk ejection where it exits through ducts into small sinuses near the areola and then opens directly on the nipple [22]. *Hence, an infant's mouth placement during breastfeeding is important so that these sinuses are not blocked and ensure free milk secretion.*

Breastfeeding initiation is a commonly used term which is used when a neonate is put to the breast. When the infant starts suckling at the breast, it causes the stimulation of touch receptors that are densely located around the nipple and areola (Box 7.3). Tactile sensations (created by infant's suckling) create impulses that ascend the spinal cord, creating a neuronal pathway between the hypothalamus and pituitary gland which release oxytocin resulting in the expulsion of stored milk from alveoli into the sinuses through the nipple pore. Once milk secretion has started, suckling by the neonate influences subsequent functioning of the mammary that is jointly controlled by the nervous/endocrine systems through the release of appropriate hormones as well as transfer of nerve impulses [23].

Box 7.3 Suckling reflex

Immediately after birth, the sucking reflex is strongest and babies are more active and alert during the first 30-60 minutes. If a baby is put to the mother's breast within this period, exclusive breastfeeding and establishment of optimal breastfeeding is more likely. Early initiation of breastfeeding also ensures the intake of colostrum which is considered to be the *first immunization for the baby.*

Findings from the Ghana study also demonstrated ensuring initiation of breastfeeding within 1 hour could reduce 22% of all neonatal mortality [24].

Milk 'coming in', which is sensed by mothers as a sudden heaviness of their breasts with milk, is an event that occurs 2–3 days after delivery [25]. The physiological significance of this sensation of 'milk coming in' can perhaps be explained by the transition from an endocrine promoted lactogenesis to established lactation. Over the first few days post-partum, the maternal plasma levels of progesterone and estrogen fall by 3–5 times, while oxytocin and prolactin increase; these hormonal changes release the mammary cells from the inhibition. However, milk ejection reflex is also sensitive to minor emotional and psychological disturbances which may influence breast milk availability to the baby [26, 27].

Box 7.4 Prelacteal feeding and its harmful effects

Honey is one of the most commonly used prelacteals in South Asia. Honey is primarily given because it is believed to be a laxative to help clean the meconium or as means to "bless and welcome the baby at birth". However, modern science has found that honey is a known source of the heat resistant organism *Clostridium botulinum,* which can lead to infant botulism. With ingestion of honey, colonization may occur in the gut, especially in babies under six months as (i) they have immature immune systems, (ii) gut lacks the clostridium inhibiting bile acids and (iii) their gut flora has not been sufficiently well established to prevent colonization. Once colonized the bacterial spores release a fatal neurotoxin resulting in severe constipation (=3 days). Over the next few weeks, infants with botulism get lethargic, are afebrile, have a weak cry, droopy eyelids, listlessness, diminished appetite or activity, have either absent or diminished spontaneous movements, decreased suckling, floppy head and decreased motor response to stimuli. If untreated, these symptoms may progress to cause paralysis of the arms, legs, trunk and respiratory muscles. Botulism can even result in death due to respiratory failure. The symptoms of botulism appear around 8 to 36 hours after consuming the honey or other contaminated food.

Further, antibiotic treatment is not recommended as killing the bacteria may increase the amount of toxin released into the body. Hence, the best recommendation is to avoid feeding honey to infants less than 1 year of age.

Microbiologic surveys of honey products in USA have reported the presence of clostridial spores in up to 25% of honey products. However, no published information is available from India [28, 29].

Prelacteal feeding is a harmful practice that adversely effects on the establishment of breastfeeding, increases susceptibility to infections and increase the likelihood of early termination of exclusive breastfeeding (Box 7.4).

(iii) *Galactopoiesis* is the maintenance of lactation. Once lactation has been established, prolactin is the primary hormone involved in maintenance of milk production. In the first few weeks post partum, maternal serum prolactin levels are continuously high and undergo further elevation (5- to 10-fold) with each nursing episode. Once breast enzyme systems are activated, lactation can continue with normal prolactin levels (essential to maintain lactation).

However, suckling, i.e. actual removal of milk, is required to maintain lactation. Without frequent emptying of the mammary gland, milk synthesis will not continue in spite of adequate hormonal status. Hence, intense suckling by the infant, milk removal, autocrine control of lactation, milk secretion rate, milking interval, and milking frequency all contribute towards maintenance of lactation.

Breastfeeding the baby in the first few days of life is important for establishment of lactation.

Frequent feeding in the early days increases the number of prolactin receptor sites within the breast, indicating that these receptors could have a greater control in breast milk output rather than serum prolactin levels [17].

Successful establishment of lactation depends on the proper development of adequate prolactin receptors (laid down in the first 3 months post-partum) which in turn appears to be correlated with frequency of feedings – with more frequent breastfeeds, the stimulation for receptor development is greater [30, 31, 32].

Increase in milk volume is perceived by the parturient woman as 'coming in' of milk. This phenomenon is brought about by a substantial increase in the rates of synthesis and/or secretion of almost all the components of mature milk, which result in the increase in milk volume [33, 34]. Amongst the other nutrients, concentration of secretory immunoglobulin A and lactoferrin (protective proteins) increase dramatically and remain high for approximately 48 hours after birth; however, as the milk volume increases, their concentration falls rapidly, indicating that breastfeeding is an extension of maternal protection that helps the infant to transition [35].

(iv) *Involution* is a transitional phase of the mammary gland from lactating to non-lactating state. If milk is not removed from the breasts, the glands become distended. After termination of breastfeeding, milk continues to accumulate for 48 hours before the rate of milk synthesis and its secretion begin to decrease rapidly and dries out.

One of the most serious problems leading to termination of breastfeeding is m*aternal perception of breast milk insufficiency*.

In addition, psychological factors like maternal self-confidence and her attitude are the strongest predictors perceived breast milk inadequacy. An anxious mother may suckle her infant less often, which may result in impaired milk volume [36]. Further, insecurity about the adequacy of her milk may cause the mother to wean her infant completely/introduce supplementary foods, which may reduce suckling frequency and impair milk synthesis leading to milk stasis.

Regular removal of milk, adequate maternal diet, positive psychological attitude towards nursing and an intact hypothalamic pituitary axis are key factors to successful nursing. Failure to remove milk adequately results in the reduction of milk synthesis because the 'milk dilated alveoli' obstruct the mammary capillary blood flow. Initially, the intraductal pressure rises due to milk stasis (a plugged duct/breast engorgement – precursor of mastitis); with consequent flattening of alveolar cells and development of spaces between these cells some components (mainly immuno-proteins and sodium) cross from plasma into the milk and from milk into the interstitial tissue through this space, inducing an inflammatory response. The accumulated milk, the inflammatory response, and the resulting tissue damage facilitate the establishment of the infection, usually by Staphylococcus (aureus and albus), occasionally by Escherichia coli or Streptococcus [37]. Moreover, in the absence of suckling stimulus, secretion of prolactin or oxytocin is adversely affected, resulting in cessation of lactation [38, 39, 40, 41, 42]. Box 7.5 further elaborates upon the phenomenon during failed lactogenesis.

Box 7.5 Failed lactogenesis

After childbirth and expulsion of the placenta, the maternal serum levels of progesterone decrease drastically, the consequent prolactin secretion by the anterior pituitary gland stimulates lactogenesis phase II and the milk secretion begins. Oxytocin secreted from the posterior pituitary gland causes contraction of the myoepithelial cells allowing milk to be secreted. Breast milk synthesis in the initial phase is controlled by hormonal action and '*it comes in*,' by the third to fourth day after delivery even without the infant's suckling). After that, lactogenesis phase III (galactopoiesis) begins lasting up to the end of lactation; it is controlled by autocrine mechanisms and basically depends on emptying of the breast. Therefore at this stage, the quality (vigorousness) and quantity (frequency and duration) of suckling by the infant regulate the synthesis of breast milk. With the degree of suckling and transfer of milk to the infant, the hypothalamus inhibits dopamine secretion (prolactin inhibitory factor); the decreased dopamine levels stimulate prolactin secretion, which in turn promotes milk secretion. The integrity of hypothalamic-pituitary axis (which regulates prolactin and oxytocin levels) is essential to trigger and maintain the synthesis of breast milk.

An elevated breast milk sodium concentration is a reflection of failed lactogenesis, which may be a marker of poor interaction between the baby and breast resulting in low consumption of breast milk. Lowered breast milk consumption / high breast milk sodium concentrations on or before day 3 were observed in cases where the infant failed to *latch on* properly [44, 45]. High sodium concentration was found to be statistically related to impending lactation failure and could be reversed by effective milk removal, suggesting that milk removal and/or effective suckling are necessary to increase in milk volume secretion [46].

Studies have reported that on one hand oxytocin secretion can occur in response to conditioned stimuli such as thought, sight, vision, smell, infant's cry as well as emotional factors such as motivation, self-confidence and tranquility; while on the other hand, pain, discomfort, stress, anxiety, fear and lack of self-confidence may inhibit the let-down reflex; thus hampering lactation. Acute maternal stress can also temporarily reduce the flow of breast milk, which the mother may perceive that the milk has 'dried up'; however with adequate support the mother can resume breastfeeding [43].

A mother needs to be counseled and assured that her milk is sufficient for the baby. She also needs to be supported during the breastfeeding episodes so that lactation is re-established. WHO has guidelines for counseling and extending support to mothers with perceived breast milk insufficiency.

7.2.4 Composition of human milk – quality and quantity

Breast milk volume and composition is not uniform; concentration of many of its constituents varies not only inter and intra-individually as well as during the course of lactation. Further, there are variations during the course of the day as well as during the course of suckling (differences between fore and hind milk). These changes are the greatest and occur rapidly during the first week post partum after which the levels stabilize [47, 48, 38, 49]. Maternal age, parity, diet/nutritional status, regional differences and, in some situations season also influence breast milk composition.

Human milk evolves to meet the changing needs of baby during growth and maturation; depending upon the stage of lactation, breast milk is designated as colostrum (3–5 days post partum), transitional milk (5–15 days) and mature milk (>15 days).

(i) *Colostrum* – The volume of colostrum in the first 12 hours post partum is reported to be 44 ± 4.83 mL; while in the first 24 hours, the volume ranges from 7 mL to 123 mL [17, 50, 51]. With the infants' suckling, the volume increases by nearly ten fold by 36 hours after birth and levels off to 500 mL by the 4th day; the dramatic changes in volume in the 0–72 hours period can be attributed to a fall in sodium and chloride concentration coupled with an increase in lactose [52]. This stage is known as the "coming in" of milk. In this stage, breast milk starts to be produced in larger amounts between the 2 and 4 days after delivery, making the breasts feel full; the milk is then said to have 'come-in'. On the 3rd day, an infant is normally takes about 300–400 ml of milk in 24 hours and on the 5th day it is 500–800 ml. Human colostrum is rich in protein, fat-soluble vitamins and minerals essentially for meeting the need for rapid cellular growth as well as protecting the newborn against infections. It is thick and sticky due to high lactose content in the milk.

- The comparatively higher protein content of colostrum (than mature milk) aids in the development of certain digestive enzymes. Its high levels non-specific anti-microbial factors such as lactoferrin (inhibits proliferation of iron binding micro-organisms in the gut).

- Colostrum contains bifidus factor that promotes the removal of intestinal meconium and facilitates the establishment of bifidus flora in digestive tract of the new born. The bifidus factor provides resistance against pathogenic bacteria and also influenza virus activities [27, 42].
- It has been observed that the epidermal growth factor and insulin are high in colostrum (as compared to mature milk) especially in the 1–3 days post partum indicating that their important role in the proliferation and differentiation of infant tissues [53].
- Most immune bodies directed against various pathogens are provided transplacentally to the foetus; however, after birth, it is completed via a postnatal transfer of through the colostrum (passive immunization); this is critical for child survival in the first few months of life [46].
- The yellowish colour of colostrum is due to the presence of â-carotene and therefore is the major source of vitamin A for the infants. Carotenoids have an important role to play in immuno-enhancement and are found to be upto five times greater in colostrum ($p<0.05$) than the mature breast milk [54].

Hence, colostrum provides the important immune protection to a neonate who is newly been exposed to the micro-organisms in the environment and because of its immense beneficial properties it is called the first natural vaccination for the infant.

Factors such as nutritional status of the mothers have an influence on the colostrum composition of breast milk. Garg et al (1988) found lower fat concentrations in the colostrum of undernourished as compared to the well-nourished Indian mothers [55].

Table 7.1 Nutrient composition of colostrum [60]

Protein	5.36 g/dL
Triglycerides	5.4 g/dL
Cholesterol	67.5 mg/dL
Phospholipid	36.36 mg/dL
Vitamin A	61.2 IU/dL
Vitamin E	1180 μg/dL
Calcium	0.996 g/dL
Zinc	3.9 mg/dL
Iron	0.42 μg/dL

Studies indicate that although maternal nutritional status did not influence the serum immunoglobulin concentrations during pregnancy, but IgA, IgG and lysozyme concentrations in both colostrum and mature milk of malnourished mothers were only half as compared to the well-nourished ones [56–58]. No significant relationship has been demonstrated between maternal age, income, BMI, parity and the micronutrient contents of colostrum [59].

(ii) *Transitional milk* – Transitional milk can appear as early as twelve hours after delivery and may continue for 7–14 days. It retains some of the yellow color of colostrum. The concentration of immunoglobulins and total protein decreases, while lactose, fat as well as the total calorific value increases. There is also an increase in the water-soluble vitamins. By the 14th day, a white colour (due to emulsified lipids and presence of calcium caseinate) emerges.

(iii) *Mature milk* – Breast milk secreted after approx 15 days post partum is the mature milk. At this stage, the composition of most milk constituents become stable and their levels remain more or less similar. Not only are there variations in the composition of colostrum, transitional and mature milk but there are following variations in the nutrient composition of mature milk itself.

- *Variations in nutrient concentration during the course of lactation.* During the first six months of lactation, a significant increase in lactose, glucose, pH and ionized calcium (for growing bones); while decrease in protein, sodium, potassium, chloride and calcium concentrations has been observed.
- *Daily variations in nutrient composition in breast milk.* There are day-to-day fluctuations observed in certain breast milk constituents like fat and water soluble vitamins.
- *Within feed variations in breast milk.* The fore milk has a lower fat content, appears thin and bluish in colour. Over the next several minutes of breastfeeding, fat content increases (hind milk) and the milk attains a light cream colour, appears comparatively thicker and helps in satiating the infant. Studies show that although total lipid content rises during individual feeds, diurnally and with the length of nursing; the fat composition of milk remains relatively constant [61, 62]. In a research study, it was observed that the fat content of milk increased from 3.0 g/100mL to 5.0 g/100mL in the course of feeds lasting 7 minutes; hind milk may contain almost twice as much fat as fore milk [63]. DaCunha et al (2005) reported that the fat content of milk varies with the duration and intensity of suckling; hind milk has three-fold fat content than foremilk. Diurnally, the fat rises from 2- to 5-folds early morning to a plateau at about mid-day [64].

7.2.5 Quantity of breast milk

The vital stimulants to milk production are infants' size, health status and activity which determine the frequency/length of feeding, strength of their suckling as well as appetite. Further, time of introduction, type and amount of complementary feeds are as important as mother's emotional state and physical health can influence both the milk production and let-down reflex [65]. In order to stimulate the prolactin and oxytocin secretion, it is necessary to put the infant to mother's breast within a few hours post partum, preferably within the first hour when the baby is alert and the suckling reflex is the strongest. In the first few days post partum, 3 minutes of suckling at each breast at 3–4 hourly intervals is sufficient for the milk flow; thereafter the suckling period can be increased by 1 minute every day [42].

Theoretically, WHO/FAO recommended that the breast milk requirement for a 50th centile male child at 3 months is 900 mL/day and at 6 months 1,250 mL/day [66]. In Indian studies, average milk yield of mothers from the low socio-economic group was reported to be 450–600 g/day in the first 6 months of lactation; the average yield being lower than the reported values of 700–800 g for developed countries [67]. However, in a 2006 study, carried out in rural and urban India, the infants were reported to consume slightly higher amounts of breast milk in the first six months – 679.2±209.8 g/day [691.8±212.2 g (rural), 623.5±163.8 g (urban poor) and 709.8±241.6 g (urban elite)] [68].

Volume of breast milk secreted is according to the infant's requirement and is related to the degree of emptiness or fullness of the breast. The emptier breast produces milk faster than the fuller one. It has been noted that there are individual differences in the breast milk intake of babies. Some babies drink large volumes of milk at a single feed and smaller number of feeds in a day, while others drink smaller volumes of milk but feed more frequently. Day-to-day differences have also been noted in the breast milk intakes of a baby [69].

The breast milk consumption of an exclusively breast fed infant was found to be positively correlated to the infant's current weight and negatively with the amount of other liquids given in the early days post partum; it was also found to be related to the number of breast feeds given and child rearing practices [38, 70].

7.3 Trends in exclusive breastfeeding practices

Poor breastfeeding and complementary feeding practices are widespread. Worldwide, it is estimated that only 37% of infants are exclusively breastfed for the first 6 months of life, the majority receiving some other food or fluid in the early months [2].

WHO/UNICEF (2008) defines exclusive breastfeeding means the infant receives only breast milk and no other liquids, not even water or complementary foods with the exception of undiluted vitamin/mineral drops or syrups, ORS and medicines for the first 6 months of life (see Box 7.1) [4]. There are limitations in the existing definition of the indicator has been described in Box 7.6.

Box 7.6 Limitation of the exclusive breastfeeding indicator

A limitation of the exclusive breastfeeding indicator is that it does not reflect the exclusive breastfeeding status of an infant for the entire six months period. At the time of survey, the data collected on exclusive breastfeeding denotes the status in the previous 24 hour period, whereas reality is that even if a woman has practiced exclusive breastfeeding for the last 24 hours it does not necessarily imply that she has exclusively breastfed her baby in the entire six month period. This issue still needs to be addressed in the new WHO publication which defines breastfeeding status of infants [4].

(a) Exclusive breastfeeding for 6 months

The advantages of exclusive breastfeeding compared to partial breastfeeding were recognized in 1984, when a review of available studies found that the risk of death from diarrhoea of partially breastfed infants 0–6 months of age was 8.6 times the risk for exclusively breastfed children. For those who received no breast milk the risk was 25 times that of those who were exclusively breastfed. A study in Brazil in 1987 found that compared with exclusive breastfeeding, partial breastfeeding was associated with 4.2 times the risk of death, while no breastfeeding had 14.2 times the risk. More recently, a study in Dhaka, Bangladesh found that deaths from diarrhoea and pneumonia could be reduced by one third if infants were exclusively instead of partially breastfed for the first 4 months of life. Exclusive breastfeeding for 6 months has been found to reduce the risk of diarrhoea and respiratory illness compared with exclusive breastfeeding for 3 and 4 months respectively.

If the breastfeeding technique is satisfactory, exclusive breastfeeding for the first 6 months of life meets the energy and nutrient needs of the vast majority of infants. No other foods or fluids are necessary. Several studies have shown that healthy infants do not need additional water during the first 6 months if they are exclusively breastfed, even in a hot climate. Breast milk itself is 88% water, and is enough to satisfy a baby's thirst. Extra fluids displace breast milk, and do not increase overall intake. Water supplementation is unnecessary as it reduces the baby's desire to suckle and could also be a potential source of contamination. Even in the hot summers, an infant does not need water supplementation. Very often in newborn babies, water and teas are commonly given in the first week of life. This practice has also been associated with a two-fold increased risk of diarrhoea.

For the mother, exclusive breastfeeding can delay the return of fertility and accelerate recovery of pre-pregnancy weight. Mothers who breastfeed exclusively and frequently have less than a 2% risk of becoming pregnant in the first 6 months postpartum, provided that they still have amenorrhoea [71].

Recent data from 64 countries covering 69% of births in the developing world suggest that there have been improvements in this situation. Between 1996 and 2006 the rate of exclusive breastfeeding at global level for the first 6 months of life increased from 33% to 37%. Significant increases were made in Sub-Saharan Africa, where rates increased from 22% to 30%; and Europe, with rates increasing from 10% to 19% (Figure 7.2). In Latin America and the Caribbean, excluding Brazil and Mexico, the percentage of infants exclusively breastfed increased from 30% in around 1996 to 45% in around 2006 [72]. Even though the global data over the last decade show that although exclusive breastfeeding rates have increased with time, worldwide, it is estimated that only 34.8% of infants are exclusively breastfed for the first 6 months of life and that the majority receiving some other food or fluid in the early months [71].

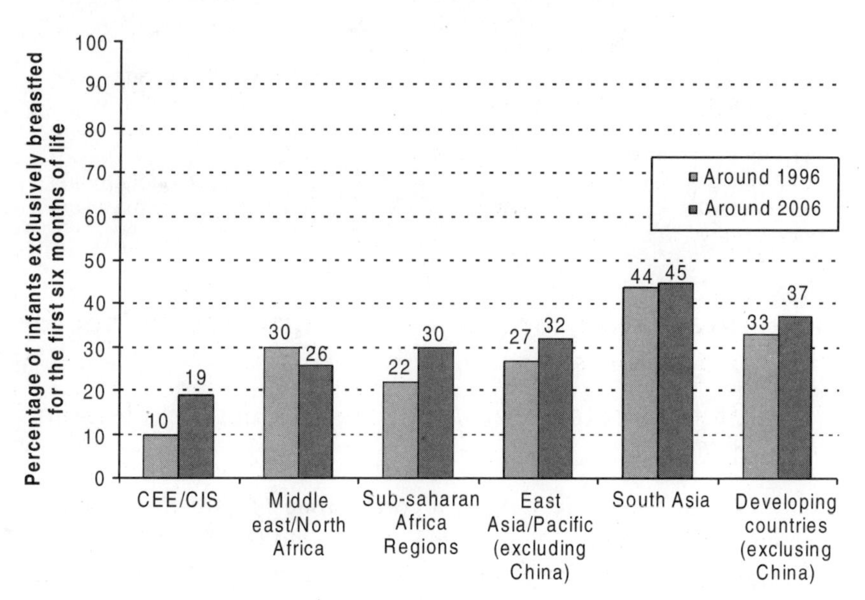

7.2 Trends in exclusive breastfeeding rates in the first 6 months of life (1996–2006) [72].

Box 7.7 Assessment and analysis of the situation reveals the following facts regarding why so many babies not breastfed exclusively

- Mothers, health professionals, family and community members do not understand what exclusive breastfeeding is or that it makes a difference. They do not know enough about how breastfeeding works best, how to start it and what to do when a mother has difficulties. Therefore they are not able to provide the advice and support that is required.
- Mothers, health professionals, family and community members do not believe that exclusive breastfeeding for six months is possible, is convenient or that mothers have enough milk. They do not appreciate that any additional foods or fluids can actually be harmful to the baby.
- Mothers have to return to work before six months, either in or out of the home.
- Commercial advertising conveys the message that breast plus formula is even better than just breast milk.
- Mothers or caregivers "perceive" milk secreted is insufficient and introduce diluted animal milk.
- Water is introduced to quench thirst since mothers are not aware that no water is required to be given to exclusively breastfed infant.

Box 7.8 Exclusive breastfeeding in India

The latest NFHS-3 figures indicate that less than half of the children are exclusively breastfed during the first six months of life. In most cases, along with mothers' milk, foods such as water, cow/goats milk, honey, sugar water, ghutti, etc, are given to the baby. It is a well-established fact that introduction of other foods before six months displaces breastfeeding, which potentially marks the beginning of malnutrition and increased vulnerability to illnesses.

In India, though infants are being breast-fed, only 69% babies are being exclusively breastfed at 2 months of life, between 2 and 3 months of age about half of the babies are being exclusively breastfed while at 3–4 months of age barely quarter of the babies in the country are being exclusively breast; indicating that exclusive breastfeeding is virtually nonexistent [73].

India is still far from achieving universal exclusive breastfeeding for the first six months of life which will help to achieve a substantial reduction in infant mortality indicators.

7.4 Integrating breastfeeding into public sector programmes

7.4.1 Global strategy for Infant and Young Child Feeding (IYCF)

Infant and young child feeding is a cornerstone of care for childhood development. In resource poor settings, improved feeding practices can lead to improved intakes of energy and nutrients, leading to better nutritional status. At present, there is ample amount of scientific data explaining the benefits of breastfeeding. Much has been learnt about effective interventions during the past few decades. These interventions

Box 7.9 Breastfeeding patterns in India

In India, breastfeeding is a traditional norm and is universal, yet there are many customs that are not conducive to health of the child. Systematic review of a large number of Indian studies indicate that usually, initiation of breast-feeding is often delayed being, nearly around 48–72 hours after birth while only a small proportion started within 24 hours. Early initiation of breastfeeding is relatively high among urban women, those with middle school education, from households with a high standard of living; women from several tribes have also been found to initiate timely breastfeeding. Circumstances surrounding child birth can have an important effect on early initiation of breastfeeding. Studies have noted that in rural and urban settings, cases where delivery was assisted by trained health professional or an institutional delivery, breastfeeding was initiated earlier than others.

The policy on Infant and Young Child feeding (GoI) 2006 recommends that initiation of breastfeeding should begin immediately after childbirth, preferably within one hour. In India, only 23.4% newborns across the country are being breastfed in the first hour of birth. In other words, the early initiation of breastfeeding is not being practiced as desired. The NFHS data in the last 15 years indicates that there has been an improvement, but the rate has been extremely slow at nearly 1% per year [73]. Given the state of infant health and mortality indicators and the proven benefits of initiating breastfeeding in the first hour of life, timely initiation of breastfeeding surely needs to catch up pace [8]. The NFHS 3 data indicates that even in the better performing states, like the Northeastern states and the Southern states of the country, the early breastfeeding initiation rates are between 55% and 65%; the rates in the northern and central part of the country is between 4% and 19%, indicating that early breastfeeding initiation rates are far below the goal of universal follow up of this practice. Health care providers both at the facility and community level need to address this issue aggressively in order to make a substantial improvement [73].

Local customs/beliefs and socio-educational level of a population influence the feeding of prelacteals. Literature has indicated that the administration of prelacteals is quite rampant and has not changed much in the last four to five decades, especially among the low socio-economic groups. The infants are generally administered boiled water, tea, sugar, honey, jaggery or glucose with plain water or the diluted animal milk; the mode of feeding is often unhygienic and generally practiced by the illiterate women from lower socioeconomic background [74, 75] The latest NFHS – III data indicate that over half the mothers (57%) still gave their new born child prelacteals [73].

Presently, the benefits of colostrum feeding have been globally acknowledged. Unfortunately in India, ancient physicians did not recommend colostrum feeding; instead honey with clarified butter and gold ash was recommended to facilitate the discharge of meconium [76] have pointed out that colostrum rejection too is a traditional practice as it was considered to be "dirty" / blocked milk that needed to be discarded before the "real/pure" milk was secreted [77]. Various researches carried out till the 1990s reveal that a majority of mothers discarded colostrum because of the traditional beliefs regarding colostrum; however, since the last three decades, the situation has noted to have improved considerably [77, 78]. Many studies carried out at this time reported that 30–40% of Indian mothers discard colostrum; however, it is not clear whether they totally discarded the breast milk continuously over 3 days or emptied out the breast once or merely discarded a few drops before initiating breastfeeding. Bhale et al (1999) noted that the amount of breast milk discarded for first two days varied largely from few drops to few spoons. In some communities, the mother's breast fed their babies after two days without discarding the initial milk, which actually means that initiation of breast feed was delayed, but colostrum was not really discarded [79]. This indicates that a large majority of the neonates are deprived of the valuable immunoglobulins, vitamins and proteins which help to protect the baby from infections and support to adapt to the external environment.

indicate that mothers need support to initiate and sustain breastfeeding within the family, community, workplace and health system. Organizations like WHO and UNICEF have been pioneers in laying down infant feeding policies and creating supportive environments for mothers to breast feed [80, 81].

Evidence from a variety of countries indicates that marked improvements in exclusive breastfeeding are possible if supported by effective regulatory frameworks and guidelines and when comprehensive programmatic approaches are at scale [2].

The *Global Strategy for Infant and Young Child Feeding*, endorsed by WHO Member States and the UNICEF Executive Board in 2002, aims to revitalize efforts to protect, promote and support appropriate infant and young child feeding. The Strategy is a guiding framework to provide technical support to countries for implementation of child feeding programmes. According to the Global Strategy for Infant and Young Child Feeding, "Inappropriate feeding practices and their consequences is a major obstacle to sustainable socio-economic development and poverty reduction. Governments will be unsuccessful in the efforts to accelerate economic development in any significant long-term sense until optimal child growth and development, especially through appropriate feeding practices, is ensured." According to WHO/UNICEF, supporting, protecting and promoting optimal breastfeeding practices is the single most effective intervention against child survival [8].

The strategy calls on the member states to act urgently. It urges all national policymakers, public health authorities, professional bodies, UN agencies, technical programme managers and NGOs to promote breastfeeding for the survival, growth and development of their children and societies. The strategy specifies not only responsibilities of governments, but also engages all relevant stakeholders and provides a framework for accelerated action, linking relevant intervention areas and using resources available in a variety of sectors [8].

At present, many countries need plans of action to protect, promote, and support exclusive breastfeeding at the national, health centre and community levels.

- At the national level, creation of appropriate structures that ensure the adoption and implementation of appropriate policies and legislation is vital. This includes the development and carrying out of national infant and young child feeding policies and strategy frameworks as well as the development and enforcement of legislation that relates to the International Code of Marketing of Breast-milk Substitutes and maternity protection.
- At the health systems level, this includes improving breastfeeding practices in maternity facilities, including through the implementation of the 'Baby-Friendly Hospital Initiative' (BFHI) as well as implementation of IYCF counseling and support at all relevant maternal and child health contacts, for which capacity-building and mentoring of health workers on topics such as breastfeeding counselling is essential.
- At the community level, mother support activities involving community health workers, lay counsellors and mother-to-mother support groups are crucial.
- Implementation of an evidence-based comprehensive communication strategy using multiple channels, which ties efforts at the three levels together, is also vital for the successful protection, promotion and support of breastfeeding. Governments are in fact obliged, under Article 24 of the Convention on the Rights of the Child, to ensure that all sectors of society know about the benefits of breastfeeding.

In the developed countries, programmes like the Baby Friendly Hospital Initiative (BFHI) have been instrumental in directing necessary resources to improve the care quality of feeding care in maternity services. These programmes contributed significantly towards not only increasing early breastfeeding initiation rates but also extended skilled services to the mother in case she encountered a problem. However, this initiative has helped to improve breastfeeding trends only in some countries. In addition, communities were also mobilized (i) to create breastfeeding friendly environments and (ii) community-based resource persons in providing this support to mothers. Although BFHI includes a community component, its implementation for instance in India, has been particularly weak. The initiative started off with a great amount of fervor in the early 1990s, however, towards the latter half of the decade it became weak. In many countries, the BFHI has not been implemented as a vertical project and has not been well institutionalized within the standard operating and quality assurance procedures for all maternity facilities. Even those institutions that received BFHI training, support was only available to the mothers during a short period before and after delivery. Post partum follow-ups to ensure that the mothers followed exclusive breastfeeding or counseling (in case the mothers encountered any problems) were virtually nonexistent.

Box 7.10 Ten steps to successful breastfeeding [10, 86]

1. Have a written breastfeeding policy that is routinely communicated to all health care staff.
2. Train all health care staff in skills necessary to implement this policy.
3. Inform all pregnant women about the benefits and management of breastfeeding.
4. Help mothers initiate breastfeeding within one half-hour of birth.
5. Show mothers how to breastfeed and maintain lactation, even if they should be separated from their infants.
6. Give newborn infants no food or drink other than breast milk, unless medically indicated.
7. Practice rooming in - that is, allow mothers and infants to remain together 24 hours a day.
8. Encourage breastfeeding on demand.
9. Give no artificial teats or pacifiers (also called dummies or soothers) to breastfeeding infants.
10. Foster the establishment of breastfeeding support groups and refer mothers to them on discharge from the hospital or clinic.

Since in many developing countries including India, a large number of women in rural areas still deliver at home, interventions at the community level continue to be extremely important for supporting and promoting early and exclusive breastfeeding. Much needs to be done to scale up promotion of and integrate breastfeeding into the national maternal and child health programmes at both health service and community level. Synthesis of lessons learnt, especially with reference to effective trials conducted in population-based programmes which promote timely initiation and exclusive breastfeeding is critical for effective programme designing and moving forward. The next step is to identify proficient and well proven interventions into child health programmes [87].

7.4.2 Scaling-up breastfeeding interventions into national programmes

The key processes required for exclusive breastfeeding scale-up are

(1) An evidence-based policy and science-driven technical guidelines; and
- This includes political will, strong advocacy, enabling policies and legal framework that makes it possible for mothers to exclusively breast feed.
- Well-defined short- and long-term programme implementation strategy, sustained financial support, clear definition of roles of multiple stakeholders and emphasis on delivery at the community level. A set of approaches that ensure programmatic success include [82].

- Formative research for designing programmes, its interventions and delivery.
- Effective use of antenatal, birth and post-natal contacts at homes through community mobilization efforts.
- Strong communication strategy and support.
- Committed good quality trainers and training.
- Monitoring and evaluation with feedback systems that allow for periodic programme corrections and continued innovation.
- Legal framework such as maternity leave that facilitate mothers to exclusively breastfeed for at least 4 months.
- Strong national- and state-level leadership.

In addition to these it is essential for sustained programme efforts to achieve high coverage.

Figure 7.3 highlights the components needed at the policy, health services and community level for a comprehensive breastfeeding programme.

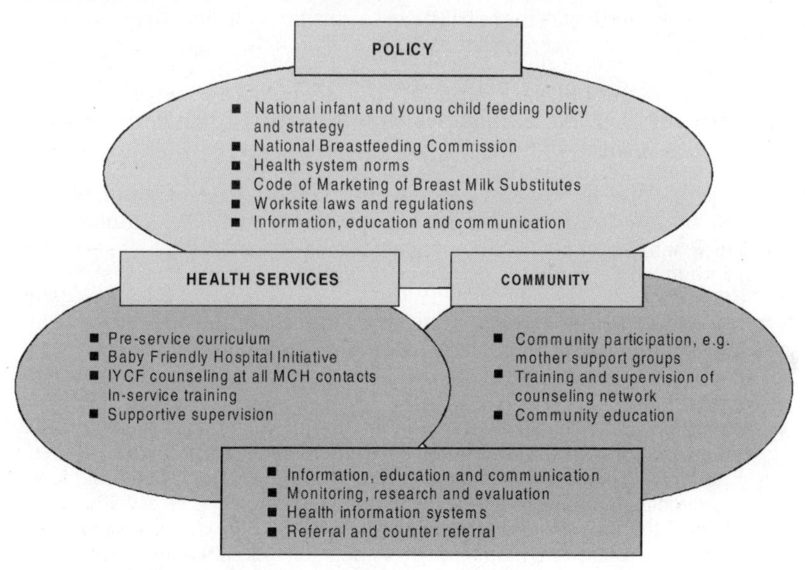

POLICY
National infant and young child feeding policy and strategy
National Breastfeeding Commission
Health system norms
Code of Marketing of Breast Milk Substitutes
Worksite laws and regulations
Information, education and communication
HEALTH SERVICES
Pre-service curriculum
Baby Friendly Hospital Initiative
IYCF counseling at all MCH contacts
In-service training
Supportive supervision
COMMUNITY
Community participation, e.g. mother support groups
Training and supervision of counseling network
Community education
Information, education and communication
Monitoring, research and evaluation
Health information systems
Referral and counter referral

7.3 Elements of a comprehensive breastfeeding programme.

(i) Policy framework

Creation of a policy framework to promote the formation of supportive systems for exclusive breastfeeding is the first step towards designing an effective breastfeeding programme. These frameworks have started at have started at the international level and need to be adopted at the national, state and district till the village level.

Breastfeeding can only be promoted and protected if the environment is conducive. In order to make the environment facilitating and supportive so that mothers are motivated to breastfeed their babies, a number of worldwide efforts are constantly being made by various governments, INGOs UN bodies to protect and promote breastfeeding (Box 7.10–7.12).

Box 7.11 Breastfeeding promotion, protection and support

The various global and Indian policies to promote, protect and support breastfeeding include:

- International Code of Marketing of Breast Milk Substitutes (1981) aims to curb marketing practices of baby food manufacturers and protect the nursing mothers from misinformation. Infant Milk Substitutes, Feeding Bottles, and Infant Foods Regulation of Production, Supply and Distribution Amendment Bill, 2003 (IMSAB) bans all forms of promotion of infant feeding products, including offering benefits to any person. Funding of seminars, meetings, research or any sponsorship is also prohibited [83].
- Innocenti Declaration (1990) aimed to create a global environment that protects, promotes and supports breastfeeding; empowers women to breastfeed exclusively for 4 – 6 months and continue to breastfeed for 2 years or more. Building on the previous one, the 2005 Innocenti Declaration highlights roles and responsibilities of key players to be met so that mothers, families and other caregivers can make informed decisions about optimal infant feeding. [84, 85].
- Infant Milk Substitutes, Feeding Bottles and Infant Foods (Regulation of Production, Supply and Distribution) Act (IMS) indicates that in case of infants requiring artificially feeds, the feeding decisions should be untainted by commercial influences [83].
- The Baby Friendly Hospital Initiative (BFHI) (1991, updated materials 2009) aims to encourage hospitals and maternity services to promote the health and well-being of babies born in hospitals by (i) increasing breast-feeding, (ii) counselling mothers, (iii) promoting early initiation of breast-feeding through rooming-in, and (iv) establishing support groups for mothers [86].
- The World Health Assembly in May 2001 resolved the confusion on appropriate time of introducing complementary feeding and stated that exclusive breast-feeding for the first six months (180 days) is most appropriate.
- WHO/UNICEF's Global Strategy on infant and young child feeding (2003) based on Innocenti Declaration is reflective of rights-based, lifecycle programming, recognition of gender needs, supportive of mother and family and directly improving early childhood survival, growth and development. It emphasizes that exclusive breastfeeding for first six months significantly reduces morbidity and mortality, while continued breastfeeding together with nutrient-dense complementary feeding into the 2nd year is advisable [8].

(ii) Making an effective implementation plan

Once the decision to scale up a programme for exclusive breastfeeding is made in a region or state or country, the logical starting point is to review the relevant, existing national policies and to assess whether these address varying circumstances and are able to provide supporting environment(s) under which women deliver and live (such as urban or rural residence, working women and place of delivery).

Box 7.12 Indian policy scenario on promoting breastfeeding programmes

In the Indian context, the National Guidelines on Infant and Young Child Feeding (2006) recognize clearly that poor feeding practices in infancy and early childhood, result in malnutrition, contribute to impaired cognitive and social development, poor school performance and reduced productivity in later life. The Ministry of Women and Child Development and Ministry of Health and Family Welfare hold special responsibility to contribute to optimal infant and young child nutrition by making National Guidelines on infant and young child feeding an integral part of nation-wide Integrated Child Development services (ICDS) and Reproductive and Child Health (RCH) programme or National Rural Health Mission (NRHM). To effectively operationalise these guidelines, field functionaries of these ongoing programmes need to provide assistance to all mothers starting at antenatal stage for influencing feeding at the first hour of birth. These field functionaries need to have the training for providing regular skilled support for early initiation of breastfeeding, exclusive and continued breastfeeding as well as appropriate complementary feeding after six months. However, at present, the recommended patterns of breastfeeding are far from the optimal levels [73].

Subsequent to a national policy being in place, a policy framework for implementation needs to be developed prior to scale-up. This framework should include a vision, consensus on technical issues, on programme strategy, roles, relationships and responsibilities of implementing partners, measurable goals within defined time lines and predictable adequate funding to achieve these outcomes. The framework needs to also address the capacity of all implementing partners as well as emphasize breastfeeding promotion through community-based programmes. Further, political commitment and ownership by relevant government departments at national, state and district levels is critical for effective scale-up and any lacunae in the system needs to be addressed [88].

The next step is designing a potentially effective programme implementation strategy which would help in achieving high coverage, quality and sustaining service delivery combined with capacity building and effective programme management is good [88]. Breastfeeding scale-up programmes when integrated into ongoing activities are more likely to be more sustainable. Further, emphasis needs to be laid on delivery of interventions at the community level so that mothers have easy access to support.

(iii) Programme delivery

Following formulation of broad strategy for implementing the programme, attention must then shift to the operationalization of the strategy. Programmes can be delivered through existing health systems either through institutions or through communities based systems.

Box 7.13 International code of marketing of breast-milk substitutes

In 1981, Member States of the World Health Organization adopted the International Code of Marketing of Breast-milk Substitutes, with the aim to protect, promote and support appropriate infant and young child feeding practices. The adoption of the Code was a key milestone in global efforts to improve breastfeeding, and countries have taken action to implement and monitor the Code.

In the 1970s, a general decline in breastfeeding was noted in many parts of world due to soc-cultural reasons and increased promotion of breast milk substitutes. It is recognized that the encouragement and protection of breast-feeding is an important part of the health and nutrition and other social measures are required to promote healthy growth and development of infants and young children; and that breastfeeding is an important aspect of primary health care. It is highlighted that the governments should develop social support systems to protect, facilitate and encourage breastfeeding, and that they should create an environment that fosters breast-feeding, provides appropriate family and community support, and protects mothers from factors that inhibit breast-feeding.

The infant formula should not be marketed or distributed in ways that may interfere with the protection and promotion of breastfeeding and that improper practices in the marketing of breast-milk substitutes and related products can contribute to these major public health problems. In view of the vulnerability of infants in the early months of life and the risks involved in inappropriate feeding practices, including the unnecessary and improper use of breast-milk substitutes, the marketing of breast-milk substitutes requires special treatment, which makes usual marketing practices unsuitable for these products. Governments are called upon to take action appropriate to their social and legislative framework and their overall development objectives to give effect to the principles and aim of this Code, including the enactment of legislation, regulations or other suitable measures. The Code has 11 articles which highlight the aim of the code, specify the definition of breast milk substitutes, responsibility of the governments in the marketing of breast milk substitutes, increasing awareness and providing consistent information on infant and young child feeding through various medium. These articles also highlight quality specifications for production of the breast milk substitutes so that the health of infants is protected, advertisement, labelling of the product and marketing restrictions of breast milk substitutes. Role and responsibilities of health care systems, health workers at the community level has been specified. Lastly, for implementation and monitoring of the Code, social and legislative framework, regulations or other suitable measures to be undertaken by government to protect, promote and support breastfeeding has also been described [83].

Experiences from regions where hospital deliveries are the norm, scale-up efforts through BFHI has been successful and the strategy has helped increase rates of exclusive breastfeeding [89, 90]. However, in many countries, after initial years of enthusiasm, the scale-up effort seems to have reached a plateau. Programmatic experience has shown that in communities with higher number of hospital deliveries, the initial high rate of exclusive breastfeeding was not sustained after mothers were discharged from facilities [91]. The challenge, therefore, is to continue support that was available in institutes in the post-delivery phase at home and community levels and in all subsequent child health contacts. This could be given through public and private providers to sustain exclusive breastfeeding [92]. Countries have addressed this issue of home level support in different ways. In the last few decades, in most developed countries, a cadre of breastfeeding counsellors has been created.

Developing countries, recognizing that facility-based interventions are insufficient, are expanding the community-based strategies. At the community level, multiple platforms can be used to give the same advice for a specific behavioural change. In some instances, routine activities in regular health programmes have been modified to incorporate exclusive breastfeeding counselling. In India, immunization sessions could be used as a platform for counseling in the presence of another local worker during the session. Another illustration is the adaptation of Integrated Management of Childhood Illness (IMCI) programme of the WHO/ UNICEF (2002) to the Integrated Management of Neonatal and Childhood Illness (IMNCI) by India. The IMNCI includes three home visits for all births in the first 7 days of life by an existing community worker, the Anganwadi worker to promote essential newborn care elements and one of these is promotion of exclusive breastfeeding. Further in regions where coverage through other channels is low or not feasible and a cadre of community workers exists, home visits are particularly important. Pilot programmes in India have shown that exclusive breastfeeding can be promoted through health worker's home visits, at immunization clinics, growth monitoring sessions and at sick-child contacts [82].

Effectiveness trials with a variety of local workers such as peer counsellors (Bangladesh), lady health workers (Pakistan) and the 'Accredited Social Health Activists' (ASHA) worker (India) to promote exclusive breastfeeding by itself or as a part of essential newborn care have been tried and found to be effective before being scaled up and integrated in the national programmes. In addition, these peer counselors / lay counselors can be linked with the auxiliary nurse midwife (ANM) or other professional person in the existing primary health care system. This is because these frontline workers may not be able to resolve complex breastfeeding problems as the management of breastfeeding problems is too technical and beyond the capacity of a grassroots level functionary to solve. Another alternative to address this problem at the grassroots level could be to train frontline service providers and PHC staff for atleast 6–8 days in addressing breastfeeding problems; however, this strategy is cost intensive [82]. Box 7.13 describes the various contact points to reach out to the community to promote breastfeeding.

Box 7.14 Contact points that can be used for community outreach and support

Potential contact points	IYCF topics for discussion
Maternity services, Health centres	Early initiation of breast feeding and exclusive breastfeeding
Growth monitoring and promotion programmes, immunization clinics or campaigns	Exclusive breastfeeding and complementary feeding
Mother support groups	Exclusive breastfeeding and complementary feeding
Women's groups	Exclusive breastfeeding and complementary feeding
Home visits	Exclusive breastfeeding and complementary feeding
Workplaces, community meetings, Schools	Early initiation of breast feeding, Exclusive breastfeeding and complementary feeding
Health fairs, agricultural extension programmes, credit or micro-enterprise programmes	Exclusive breastfeeding and complementary feeding
Family planning programmes	Early initiation breast feeding and exclusive breast feeding

Channels that can be used for community outreach and support

- Health service personnel, home birth attendants, traditional healers, staff or volunteers from NGOs, lay or peer counselors, teachers, agricultural extension agents, family planning staff

Some activities for infant and young child feeding community outreach and support

- Individual counseling, group counseling, community education, cooking demonstrations, promotion of production of food that can fill gaps in the local diets, micronutrient campaigns mother-to-mother support, trials of new infant or young child feeding practices, baby shows or contests featuring infant and young child feeding, organization of workplace nurseries for breastfeeding infants, breastfeeding rooms or areas, social mobilization activities – planned actions that reach, influence and involve all relevant segments of society like world breastfeeding week activities, world walk for breastfeeding.

Community support strategies should focus on protection, promotion and support of both breastfeeding and complementary feeding [93].

Programmes that used multiple channels reported broader coverage [94, 95]. In India, formative research showed that immunization sessions and private providers were the channels to which a majority of infants and their mothers could be addressed. Following constitution of a breastfeeding-promotion programme, caregivers most often received exclusive breastfeeding counseling at immunization sessions (~40%), weighing sessions (~25%) and home visits (25–30%). In reality, through the government physicians or private providers were supposed to carry out periodic counseling, however in reality, despite being trained, these counseling sessions rarely (~2%) took place. When all the opportunities were considered together, 55–60% of caregivers had been counselled at least once, by at least one of the channels in the last 3 months, indicating that multiple channels reached more families [94]. The frequency of contact with caregivers or the intensity of counseling influences the cumulative benefit of the counselling; for example, six contacts with mothers resulted in higher adoption rates for exclusive breastfeeding as compared with three [96]. In India, the number of channels at which caregivers were counselled was positively associated with the rates of exclusive breastfeeding at 3 months of age [97].

There is a growing recognition that progammes which reach beyond the walls of health care facilities and which involve community as partners have a great potential for reducing child mortality rates at minimal cost. Community based health programmes have the potential to accelerate progress in reaching the MDGs in health [98].

Box 7.15 presents an overview of efforts made by various developing countries in improving exclusive breastfeeding rates through community based health workers and volunteers.

(iv) Capacity building

Prior to scale-up, it is critical that the training needs are assessed and defined for developing the training strategy. Use could be made of the extensive experiences such as the adapted versions of the UNICEF/WHO Breastfeeding Counseling Course for a wide range trainees including health workers, counselors etc [109, 110].

From global experience, it is evident that the duration of training is from 3 full days to 10 part days for different cadre of workers. Experience has shown that the training strategies were effective when designs were '*concise and action oriented*' and aimed to equip trainers with practical skills and confidence to counsel appropriately. The recommended courses indicate a wide variation in focus e.g. for frontline workers training needs to be an integrated course on infant and young child counseling while for the midwives, the course content needs to address specific problems like feeding problems in young infants, feeding low birth weight babies etc. It is critical that health professionals, both from the private and government sector, are trained in infant and young child feeding so that there is uniform information on management of breastfeeding in community and institutional set up. Further, basic course in counseling could be organized for programme managers, trainers, supervisors, district managers and administrators using the WHO decision maker's course module [8].

Box 7.15 Experiences from other developing countries in improving breastfeeding rates through frontline workers

Developing countries around the world have sought support from the community, peer counselors and have empowered primary care workers and health workers in hospitals in different ways to provide conducive environments that have helped more mothers to breastfeed exclusively. Findings from projects and community based studies indicate the following:

- In Gambia, Village Support Groups, for example parent-to-parent support groups were trained to give accurate information and help with correct breastfeeding technique. More mothers started to breastfeed within an hour of delivery, and 99.5% breastfed exclusively for 4 months instead of only 1.3% at baseline. Over 200 communities in the Gambia are now Baby-Friendly Communities [99].
- In Ghana, several different methods of communication, workshops, and training were used to reach the wider community (including grandmothers, fathers, and the media) and mother support groups were formed. Within 2 years, the number of mother's breastfeeding exclusively at 5 months had increased from 44% to 78% [100].
- In Ghana, Village Banks made small loans to women to help them to become economically active. The women were also given education on health and child feeding. The average duration of exclusive breastfeeding increased from 1.7 months to 4.2 months, and the nutrition of the children at one year improved [101].
- In India, health and nutrition workers learned to counsel mothers on breastfeeding while they were doing their other primary care work. At six months, 42% of mothers who were counselled breastfed exclusively, but only 4% of the mothers who were not counselled did so [97].
- In Bangladesh, mothers from the community were trained as peer counsellors for breastfeeding. They visited women during pregnancy and for five months after delivery, making a total of 15 visits. Counselled mothers started breastfeeding earlier, and 70% of them breastfed exclusively for 5 months, compared with only 6% of the other mothers [102].
- In Mexico, mothers from the community were trained to counsel about breastfeeding during home visits. 12% of mothers who were not visited breastfed exclusively; and the rate increased to 50% for mothers who were visited 3 times, and 67% for mothers who were visited six times (Morrow, 1999).
- In Belarus, 43% of the mothers who delivered in the 16 baby-friendly hospitals breastfed exclusively at three months, but only 6% of mothers who delivered in the 15 hospitals which are not baby-friendly [103].
- In Bolivia, Guinea, India and Nicaragua, NGOs such as Save the Children and CARE mobilized the community by training health and community workers, involving grandmothers and fathers, men's groups and mother support groups. Exclusive breastfeeding rates increased from 11% to 44% in Guinea; 41% to 71% in India and 10% to 50% in Nicaragua. In Bolivia, diarrhoea rates were halved and exclusive breastfeeding of infants under six months increased to over 75% when support groups were integrated into community activities in low-income neighborhoods in La Paz [104]. In India, Dular and MCHN programmes also indicated failure to promote exclusive breastfeeding despite counseling by community volunteers [105,106].
- In Philippines baby-friendly crèches were formed to cater to working women. Mothers can drop in anytime to breastfeed, leave their expressed breastmilk, or avail themselves of the services of a wet nurse. Solid foods to complement breastmilk for babies above six months were made of natural and indigenous ingredients [107].

Successful strategy adopted in developed countries such as in Norway and Sweden, demonstrates that breastfeeding rates are much higher than in other parts of Europe. This is partly because health authorities consulted mothers' organizations. Their advice and criticisms are listened to, respected and followed more than in most countries [108].

(v) Behaviour change and communications approach

A comprehensive communication strategy is critical for improving the breastfeeding behaviours of mothers. This would involve a mix of following communication channels which are directed to mothers as well as to family members, community leaders and other social, religious and political influences for influencing individual behaviours and social norms. These communication channels include

- mass, electronic and print media (e.g., radio, TV, newspapers, flyers)
- community advocacy and events (e.g., theater, fairs, community gatherings, religious institutions)
- interpersonal communication (e.g., community groups, individual counseling, mother-to-mother support groups, home visits)

In addition to mass media, interpersonal and group counseling are two approaches which have the potential in bringing about the desired behavioural modifications. Effective counseling involves not only building on assessment of existing feeding practices, but also recognition of problems and negotiation with the mother in choosing improved "do-able" practices [110]. The messages and negotiation strategies with caregivers should be simple, action oriented and based on evidence of the context-specific barriers to optimal practices. Generic, empirical messages (e.g. "breast is best"; "breastfeeding your baby exclusively for six months gives a baby the best start in life" etc) usually don't motivate behavior change.

Both one-on-one counselling during opportunities in which more time is available such as home visits have been found to be effective. Group counselling can be carried out in communities where there are fewer opportunities for one to one communication and the health workers have lesser available time [94]. Peer counsellors can be employed for counseling mothers/caregivers during home visits [96, 102]. The more diverse the functions of the local worker, lesser will be the emphasis on a single component such as exclusive breastfeeding.

Community mobilization programmes, such as street plays, rallies, radio programmes and songs, helped disseminate messages and increase community involvement [94, 95].

Figure 7.4 describes the direct/ proximate factors that influence infant feeding practices of mothers and caregivers. The intermediate determinants influence these direct factors while the underlying determinants have an influence on both intermediate and proximate determinants. Programmes seek to address all these factors to improve infant feeding behaviours through different communication channels or combination of different approaches.

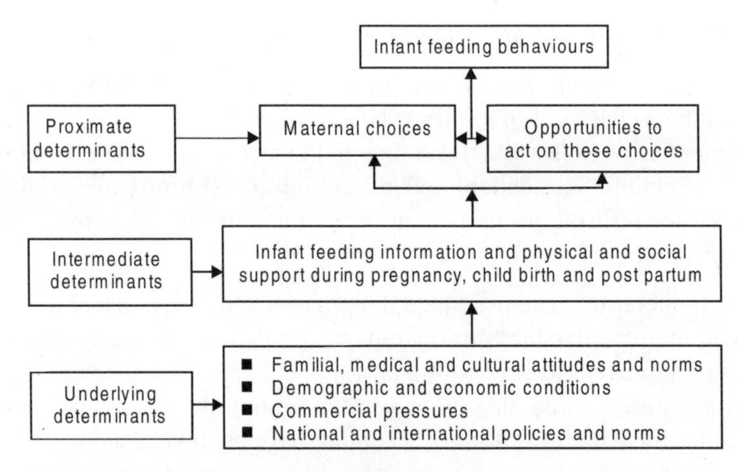

7.4 Model of determinants of breastfeeding behaviour [111].

Box 7.16 presents the stages through which an individual or communities undergo before there is a change in knowledge and attitudes. The change model also highlights the different communication approaches that need to be applied at each stage. The communication approach needs to be modified when the community/individual moves from one stage to another.

Box 7.16 Stages of change and communication approaches [112]

Stages of change	Level of knowledge and attitude toward or experience with the new practice	Purpose of appropriate communication interventions to move individual to next stage
Pre-awareness	Has not heard of new practice	Provide information
Awareness	Has heard of new practice	Provide more information and begin to focus on persuasion
Contemplation	Considers the resources and tasks needed to actually perform the practice	Provide encouragement that practice is "do-able" and introduce role playing, role modeling
Intention	Intends to try new practice	Focus on appreciating benefits and overcomeing obstacles; introduce negotiation of trying new practice; home visits are very appropriate
Trial of new practice	Tries new practice to experience benefits and overcome obstacles	Reinforce benefits and overcoming obstacles with family and community influentials; provide additional support mothers through home visits and support groups
Adoption of new practice	Appreciates benefits and has overcome obstacles during the trial of new practice; adopts practice	Continue to reinforce and support practice, including praise from influentials
Maintenance	Decides to continue new practice	Continue to reinforce and support practice, including praise from influentials
Telling others	Believes in new practice and wants to tell others	Provide opportunities for practitioners to communicate their messages to other women widely (mass electronic and print media) or within the comm.-unity (comm.-unity events and advocacy; interpersonal communication)

(vi) Enhancing programme coverage

In addition, to engaging workers from within the community, other interventions which mobilize and involve communities are also critical in improving child health. Interventions like participatory women's groups for empowerment and education about maternal health and infant health issues, micro-credit programmes for women, conditional cash transfers to women (in which poor women receive cash transfers with the condition that they obtain certain health services) have found to be effective.

Programmes with a strong community outreach component which include home visits to all households, involving the local leaders, programme managers and strong partnerships with the community have also appeared to be beneficial

Experience has shown that stronger the community outreach services of a community based programme, it is more likely that such a programme will reach (i) those who need child survival interventions and (ii) those who belong to the lowest wealth quintile.

(vii) Monitoring and evaluation

Monitoring and evaluation is a critical area to support programme implementation. Designing of programme strategy needs to include systems for monitoring and evaluation of the programme implementation. A number of tools are already available for monitoring progress within the context of BFHI, IMCI and routine health reporting systems in some countries [112] Simple, valid and reliable indicators are crucial for tracking progress and guiding investment to improve nutrition and health during the first two years of life. These indicators have been issued by the WHO / UNICEF / AED / USAID, 2008 for assessing breastfeeding practices and have been valuable in informing programme efforts in many countries. Examples of facility based indicators include – percentage of children less than two years assessed for feeding problems, feeding counseling received by parents of malnourished children, percentage of pregnant women provided breastfeeding counseling in health facilities, percentage of mothers provided breastfeeding counseling post partum. The outcome indicators that can be used for both monitoring and evaluation are outlined in the table below [87] Evaluations need to be carried out periodically and ideally results of evaluation surveys would help to make programme adjustments for improving infant and young child feeding. This will help to maintain the effectiveness of the programme as the scale of implementation expands. The possible process indicators could include the availability of infant and young child feeding counseling, IYCF pre-service education for service providers and frontline workers, worker performance during programme intervention, referral and action etc. On the other hand, process indicators could include information on other indicators to be included are for national actions and adequacy of resources etc.

Box 7.17 Indicators for monitoring and evaluation of breastfeeding practices

Feeding practice	Requires that infants receive	Allows the infant to receive	Does not allow the infant to receive
Exclusive breastfeeding	Breast milk (including milk expressed or from a wet nurse)	ORS, drops, syrup (vitamins, minerals, medicines)	Anything else
Predominant breastfeeding	Breast milk (including milk expressed or from a wet nurse) as the predominant source of nourishment	Certain liquids (water and water-based drinks, fruit juice), ritual fluids and ORS, drops or syrups (vitamins, minerals, medicines)	Anything else (in particular, non-human milk, food based fluids)
Complementary feeding[(a)]	Breast milk (including milk expressed or from a wet nurse) and solid or semi-solid foods	Anything else; any food or liquid including non-human milk and formula	NA
Breastfeeding	Breast milk (including milk expressed or from a wet nurse)	Anything else; any food or liquid including non	NA
Bottle feeding	Any liquid (including breast milk or semi-solid food from a bottle with a nipple/teat)	Anything else; any food or liquid including non	NA

(a) The term complementary feeding, reserved to describe appropriate feeding in breast fed children 6 months of age or beyond, is no longer used in the indicators to assess infant and young child feeding practices. The previously used indicator "Timely complementary feeding rate" which combined continued breastfeeding with consumption of solid, semi-solid or soft foods, was difficult to interpret. This indicator has therefore been replaced by the indicator "Introduction of solid, semi-solid or soft foods", which is a measure of a single feeding practice. Nevertheless the term complementary feeding is still very useful to describe appropriate feeding practices in breastfed children 6–23 months of age and will continue to be used in programmatic efforts to improve infant and young child feeding as guided by the Global Strategy on Infant and Young Child Feeding. The timely complementary feeding rate can also be calculated using the data generated for measuring the new and updated indicators [4].

Monitoring and evaluation when integrated and built into the existing health programmes and system is more sustainable. Some ways in which monitoring and evaluation could be built into the system include

- Recording information on infant and young child feeding practices in the mother child health cards that are kept by caregivers;
- Inclusion of infant and young child feeding indicators into the routine monitoring system;
- Incorporation of key infant and young child feeding activities in

the monitoring system of other sectors (i.e., maternity entitlements in the Labour Ministry, adoption and compliance with the code and reference to Codex standards in food laws regulating trade and industry).

The most important use of the monitoring and evaluation process is to ensure that the service providers who are stakeholders are fully involved in the analysis and/or interpretation of emerging information. Such efforts are critical for ongoing system strengthening and serve as a catalyst for improving programmes, workers skills and performance [112].

(viii) Programme management and working towards sustainability

Programme management involves periodic assessment of barriers and revising programme strategy to address the barriers and improve the programme outcomes. It is crucial that with reference to breastfeeding programmes the assessment of programme barriers is undertaken at all levels through a good monitoring system i.e., from national right down to the district and village levels. Feedback at all levels from periodic assessments is essential for improving the programme implementation and interventions. Most developing countries are progressing towards this approach and are going through a process of decentralization with increasing responsibility for planning, implementation and evaluation being delegated to lower levels of the health-care system. This principle applies towards building long term sustainability into the various health programmes including promoting infant and young child feeding. However, building local capacity at the local level requires time, resources and patience [89].

7.5 Programme design – community based

7.5.1 Significance of community-based programmme approaches

For sustained improvements in child health, experience has shown that community-based programes are beneficial. There is growing scientific evidence that community based programmes can improve the health of children at scale at an affordable cost. This means that even the most impoverished societies have a powerful incentive to expand community based programs; however, high-quality field research and monitoring of mortality impact are fundamental. This will ensure progress in improving the health of children and the achievement of the Millennium Development Goal for children in the future.

Community based systems can make its greatest contribution when health systems are weak and under-5 mortality is high. When health systems are strong (as in case of many developed countries), strengthening community based systems may not provide additional health benefits. In many developing countries where health systems are often weak, establishing a strong community based programme would prove to be beneficial. In addition, areas where primary health care facilities are burdened with more patients (than can be adequately managed at the facilities), strong community based activities can also support to reduce the patient load, thereby actually saving money for the health system as well as for the patient and their families. In other settings, community based programmes can also increase the utilization of services, making health care system more efficient and effective. To build strong community based activities, it is important to engage communities in programmes, build upon their trust and develop strong community participation and partnerships. Community-based services can be integrated at all levels of health services.

It is crucial that community based programme models are designed with a vision of scale, as all too often they remain small-scale NGO-supported initiatives without national Government ownership that are never taken to scale and are not sustained beyond the life of the NGO project. Their design is often not amenable to scale-up and too resource and support intensive to be taken to scale.

The processes required to develop and maintain effective partnerships between health intervention delivery systems and communities vary greatly, mainly, because of the marked variations in conditions encountered from one locale to another. Populations with the most limited access to formal health care are typically in the most un-reached areas/socially excluded areas where mortality is the highest and impact can be greatest.

Training community health workers, promoting partnerships between communities and health programs, drawing on local resources for program support, and promoting community and women's empowerment were common features of successful community based programs.

7.5.2 Community-based programme and IYCF

(1) Community-based approaches are particularly relevant for interventions which involve behavior change at the household level. Examples of such interventions are improving neonatal care practices, infant feeding practices, etc, all of which have great importance for child health. Many of these behaviors are based on ingrained cultural beliefs and practices, and health systems have been ineffective in changing them.

Behaviour change communication interventions need active community involvement (in planning, implementation and assessment of the programme). Successful promotion of these kinds of behaviors requires stronger linkages between health systems and community than 'simple' outreach activities as is in the case of immunization or vitamin A coverage.

(2) Promoting community empowerment can increase intervention effectiveness. Activities through which communities can contribute to improving effectiveness of child health interventions and at the same time can be sustained include

- Involving local leadership in mobilizing a partnership between communities and programme managers at the local level for planning and managing program activities and resources.
- Clarifying respective value systems to help both health care workers and community members develop joint understanding and respect as they work together for benefits that are effective and equitable.
- Involving women's groups to provide peer-to-peer education and home-based care while also involving men and mothers-in-law in creative ways to encourage community action for healthy behavior and appropriate health care utilization.
- Adapting the health delivery system to local realities and culture, with integration of interventions and practices for maximizing acceptability and efficiency.
- Enabling communities to collaborate with the health system not just in the initial stages of implementation but in a continuing relationship so that families feel ownership of the process and together they can establish a long-term partnership for robust and sustainable improvements in child health.

Registering vital events registration, identifying newborns who need to be enrolled in community based services and programs, and tracking under-5 mortality rates at the local level.

Community-based approaches necessary for facilitating the effectiveness of community-based programmes are summarized below

(i) *Trust in the health system* – It is essential that the community trusts, respects and has confidence in the local health and community based system. Trust, respect, and confidence arise when people believe that the health system and community based system provides quality services and has basic medicines and supplies to solve some commonly occurring problems and health concerns.

(ii) *Strong outreach system* – Some of the interventions required to improve child health and nutrition require technical expertise and equipments not available within the community. Health systems need to provide these services for which coverage outreach sites readily available to the populations are required. These outreach service delivery points provide a key opportunity for strengthening other community-based services.

(iii) Experience has shown that stronger the outreach services of a community based programme, more likely the programme will reach those who really need them, especially those in the lowest wealth quintile. Programmes which are facility based with poor outreach services are inherently inequitable for 2 main reasons (i) utilization of health facilities decreases exponentially as one's distance from the facility increases (ii) health facility utilization involves pro-active decision that involves significant costs in terms of time, transport fees and other associated costs. As a result, the poorest household (those who are in greatest need of services) are less likely to use the facility based services. With a strong community outreach service component, these barriers are diminished. From this perspective, the community based approaches which provide services to all households can have a strongly positive equity impact.

(iv) *Community-based workers* – In order to implement interventions and to reach out to populations who need these services appropriately trained community based workers are an essential element of the programme. These workers can be employed by the health / community based system or other local Government structure or can be volunteers. If they are unpaid volunteers, they must have a limited set of tasks and not be expected to work more than a few hours a week; otherwise they tend to abandon their responsibilities.

(v) *Needs-based interventions* – Programme interventions targeted at child health and nutrition should be designed such that they (i) address the priority health needs of children in a population and (ii) reach out to those at greatest risk. This is because such children in such populations are at a higher risk of death. For e.g. if poor infant feeding practices is one of the leading cause of malnutrition among children less than 2 years, then promoting optimal infant and young child feeding practices should be prioritized in the programme interventions from both the public health point of view as well as from equity point of view.

(vi) *Increasing programme coverage* – A method of developing and maintaining contact with all homes and mothers is necessary in order to identify pregnant women and young children, to provide services in the home when possible, and to identify those in need of services which cannot be provided in the home. Routine systematic visitation of all homes by community-based workers is a common approach to achieving this. Maintaining a register of vital events, including births and deaths, and a register of all families facilitates tracking of children to ensure that all are reached with program services.

Emphasizing expanded coverage of interventions that require a trained provider near the home to respond to serious and urgent childhood issues, improving childhood nutrition through promotion of exclusive breastfeeding and appropriate complementary feeding (for which there are available proven interventions is important). Though these interventions have great potential for reducing mortality, but in reality they have particularly low coverage in priority countries.

Programme coverage can be improved through health programmes by making additional efforts to reach the unreached i.e., (i) the highly vulnerable groups (children <3 years; pregnant and lactating mothers); and (ii) reaching out to the geographically remote areas, (iii) the tribals, (iv) the socially excluded groups and (iv) the minorities.

(3) Referral care – Finally, high-quality curative and referral care, which can address the local health care needs and problems like basic hospital care, lends credibility to the community-based work and the workers that provide it [98].

7.6 Large scale community-based programmes – lessons learned

Quinn et al (2005) examined the strategies and successes of large-scale community-level, communication-centred programmes designed to improve breastfeeding practices rapidly at scale in Bolivia, Ghana, and Madagascar through the Linkages project (1996 to 2006) using a multi-faceted, communication-focused approach, tailored specifically to increase the timely initiation of breastfeeding (TIBF) – primarily among mothers with young infants in resource-poor settings. In each country programme, an overall monitoring and evaluation system was established to provide data to track progress and use in programme management [95].

Over 3–4 years, early breastfeeding initiation (within 1 hour of birth) increased from 56% to 74% ($P < 0.001$) in Bolivia, 32% to 40% ($P < 0.05$) in Ghana and 34% to 78% ($P < 0.001$) in Madagascar. Marked increases in exclusive breastfeeding of infants 0 to 6 months of age were also documented: from 54% to 65% ($P < 0.001$) in Bolivia, 68% to 79% ($P < 0.001$) in Ghana, and 46% to 68% ($P < 0.001$) in Madagascar. In Ghana and Madagascar, significant results were seen within 1 year of community interventions.

The strategies of these successful programmes were analysed to have been built on four core components: partnerships, training, behaviour change communication (BCC), and community activities.

- *Partnership-building* – collaborating with partners and carrying out participatory programme design, implementation, programme monitoring and evaluating activities. The partners were national government health workers collaborating with partner non-governmental organizations (in Bolivia), local radio announcers, journalists, university staff, members of the Food and Nutrition Security Network (Ghana). The government and other local groups, including donors were assisted to disseminate nutrition messages and share experiences.
- *Capacity-building* – In all these three countries, training materials were developed to meet the specific, short-term, and practical needs of service providers and community volunteers. Apart from strengthening the counseling skills of the service providers, frontline workers and community volunteers, negotiation skills necessary to convince mothers to change their infant-feeding behaviours were also fostered.
- *Behaviour change communication (BCC)* – The intention of BCC was to change individual behaviour while educating and engaging fathers and/or grandmothers, who influence the mother's choices. "Targeted, concise messages" were developed to promote "do-able" actions, and "edutainment" strategies dominated. These messages were disseminated through the mass media or at the local level. In some countries, the mass media was used to complement BCC change in the community level.
- *Community activities* – Women were reached through small- and large-group activities, one-on-one counselling in homes and at local health posts, breastfeeding promotion songs performed by women's groups and musical troupes, and community mobilization events such as local theatre, health fairs, and festivals celebrating breastfeeding and child health days. Celebrations of success through village festivals, healthy baby contests, and "nutrition certificates" for families with optimally fed babies were drawn upon to fuel enthusiasm in the communities. A key communication strategy highlighted here is the value of peer group support and interaction.

It is evident that a mix of activities, such as interpersonal counselling, community mobilization, and mass media, contributes to behaviour change when these activities deliver consistent messages. Further, linking health workers and community health promoters (particularly for referral) are useful strategies for ensuring that mothers receive consistent messages. In addition to harmonizing approaches and messages through partnership and community involvement, it is also important to have a positive policy environment for exclusive breastfeeding promotion for improving nutrition.

WHO/UNICEF/AED/USAID (2008) also conducted a 'lesson learnt' review of large scale community-based breastfeeding programmes in ten countries with diversity in the programmatic approaches and different rates of exclusive breastfeeding: Benin, Bolivia, Cambodia, Ethiopia, Ghana, Honduras, India, Madagascar, Mali and Nepal. These were large scale IYCF programmes (coverage of >1 million). In these countries, programme implementation was made effective by employing a combination of the following approaches:

- Integrating the IYCF interventions with the child survival, reproductive health or maternal and child health initiatives.
- Implementing a range of programme interventions which included facility based to community owned and led initiatives through multiple partners.
- Creating strong political commitment, a well developed advocacy framework, clear programme implementation plan in collaboration with the state and district level stakeholders for implementation and scale-up.
- *C*reating/strengthening linkages with the health systems, *community-based services* and also engaging communities.
- Developing and implementing a robust communication strategy with a clear-cut vision (engaging opinion leaders, policy makers and programme planners), simple, consistent, targeted messages which were delivered and reinforced through multiple and well-coordinated systems/platforms.
- Expanding nutrition contacts to multiple contact points during programme delivery with the help of community health workers and volunteers.
- Building capacity of service providers and nutritional promoters in inter personal communication (IPC) through single or cascade trainings and conducted periodic performance monitoring.
- Implementing proven interventions at the community level by local trained and well-supervised health workers so that coverage, impact, and equity were favorably affected.
- Mobilizing and engaging communities as well as supporting the building of strong community partnerships with the health delivery systems in improving the health of children.
- Monitoring, measuring progress and evaluating the interventions to identify successful and unsuccessful steps and making appropriate programme adjustments.

The story of their vision, innovations in programme delivery, partnerships, trials, errors and programmatic outcomes indicate that (1) The community offers indispensable resources for breastfeeding promotion and support, and these resources need continual mentoring and encouragement; (2) Multiple programme frameworks offer opportunities for community-based breastfeeding promotion and support; (3) Breastfeeding practices can change over a relatively short period and need continued reinforcement to be sustained; (4) Effective communication and advocacy are vital to set policy priorities, influence community norms, and improve household practices; (5) More attention needs to be given during training to interpersonal counselling skills; (6) Partnerships, leadership, proof of concept, and resources, facilitate programme scale up; and (7) Monitoring and evaluation is critical to measure progress, identify successful and unsuccessful strategies, and make appropriate programmes adjustments [87].

Conclusion

It is a well-known fact that the 0–2 years period in a child's life is critical for preventing malnutrition. Many developing countries are struggling to resolve this issue. Ensuring optimal infant and young child feeding during this period has its significant implications in reducing infant morbidity and mortality; but these practices need to be accelerated to achieve universal coverage before a noticeable improvement is seen in these indicators. To accomplish this, optimizing and improving breastfeeding practices has been identified to be the single most crucial indicator for improving child survival.

At present, there is sufficient scientific evidence on effective interventions to improve breastfeeding indicators and practical solutions on how to incorporate the proven interventions into a comprehensive approach for scale-up. Leveraging scientific knowledge and previous programming wisdom along with a strong political will; national and local leadership; and efficient governance will make programme delivery more efficient in order to make IYCF programmes effective. Such programming is feasible when adequate policies and regulatory frameworks are backed by strong management and functioning service delivery systems, and sufficient resources – it is also imperative to achieve a high coverage of service delivery and to effect widespread change in community and household behaviours and practices.

Over the past 5–10 years, 16 countries have recorded gains of 20 percentage points or more in exclusive breastfeeding rates. Many of these countries face serious development challenges as well as emergency situations. Experience has shown that the implementation of large scale programmes in these countries was based on national policies and often guided by the WHO–UNICEF Global Strategy for Infant and Young Child feeding. The country programmes included the adoption and implementation of national legislation on the International Code of marketing of breast-milk substitutes and subsequent World Health Assembly resolutions, as well as maternity protection for working women. Further actions included ensuring that breastfeeding was initiated in maternity facilities (and that no infant formulae were given in facilities). Community based strategies like strengthening of local capacity, building health worker capacity to offer counselling on infant and young child feeding, and mother-to-mother support groups in the community helped to provide integrated and effective package of key interventions. Further partnerships of health systems with communities were promoted for achieving sustainable health outcomes along with increasing the demand for health and nutrition, services at community level. These actions were also accompanied by communication strategies to promote breastfeeding using multiple channels and messages tailored to the local context [3].

References

1. BERNT KM and WALKER WA (1999). Human milk as a carrier of biochemical messages. *Acta Pediatr Suppl* **88**, no. 430, pp. 27–41.
2. UNICEF (2009a). The State of the World's Children (special edition) – Celebrating 20 years of the convention on the rights of the child. UNICEF November 2009, pp. 1–91.
3. UNICEF (2009b). Tracking the progress on Child and Maternal Nutrition – A survival and development priority. UNICEF November 2009, pp. 1–118.
4. WHO (2008a). Indicators for assessing infant and young child feeding practices; Part I (Definitions): Conclusions of a consensus meeting held 6–8 November 2007 in Washington DC, USA.
5. BLACK RE, ALLEN LH, BHUTTA ZA, CAULFIELD LE, DE ONIS M, EZZATI M, MATHERS C, RIVERA J (2008). Maternal and child undernutrition: global and regional exposures and health consequences. *The Lancet* **371**, no. 9608, pp. 243–260.
6. JONES G, STEKETEE R, BLACK RE, BHUTTA ZA, MORRIS S (2003). The Bellagio Child Survival Study Group. How Many child deaths can we prevent this year? *The Lancet* **362**, pp. 65–71.
7. BHUTTA ZA, AHMED T, BLACK RE, COUSENS S, DEWEY K, GIUGLIANI E, HAIDER BA, KIRKWOOD B (2008). What works? Interventions for maternal and child undernutrition and survival. *The Lancet* **2**, no. 9610, pp. 417–440.
8. WHO/UNICEF (2003). Global Strategy for Infant and Young Child Feeding, web document: http://who.int/child.adolescent-health.
9. GUPTA A (2004). Addressing child malnutrition – solutions lie during first 24 months. Paper presented at the Regional Ministerial Consultation on Maternal and child nutrition in Asian Countries, 2004.
10. WHO/UNICEF (2008b). Baby Friendly Hospital Initiative: Revised, updated and expanded for integrated care. Geneva: WHO.
11. VICTORIA CG, ADAIR L, FALL C, HALLAL PC, MARTORELL R, RICHTER L, SACHDEV HPS (2008). Maternal and child undernutrition: consequences for adult health and human capital. *The Lancet* **371**, no. 9609, pp. 340–357.

12. BRYCE J, COITINHO D, DARNTON-HILL I, PELLETIER D, PINSTRUP-ANDERSEN P (2008). Maternal and child under nutrition: effective action at national level. *The Lancet* **371**, no. 9611, pp. 510–526.
13. ESTRIK PV (1995). Care and caregivers. *Food and Nutrition Bulletin* **16**, no. 4, pp. 378–388.
14. HURLEY W (2003). Lactation Biology. Department of Animal Sciences, University of Illinois, Urbana–Champaign: http://classes.aces.uiuc.edu/AnSci308/.
15. JELLIFFE DB and JELLIFFE EFP (1978). The volume and composition of human milk in poorly nourished communities. A review. *American Journal of Clinical Nutrition* **31**, pp. 492–497.
16. American Academy of Pediatrics (AAP, 2005). AAP policy statement of breastfeeding and the use of human milk. *Pediatrics* **115**, no. 2, pp. 496–506.
17. RIORDAN J and AUERBACH KG (eds) (1993). Breastfeeding and Human Lactation, 2nd ed. Boston: Jones and Bartlett.
18. SALAZAR H, TOBON H (1974). Morphologic changes of the mammary gland during development, pregnancy and lactation. In. Josimovich JB, Reynolds M, Cobo E (eds). Lactogenic Hormones, Fetal Nutrition, and Lactation. New York: John Wiley and Sons, pp. 221–77.
19. HARTMANN PE, OWENS RA, COX DB and KENT JC (1996). Establishing lactation. Breast development and control of milk synthesis. *Food and Nutrition Bulletin* **17**, no. 4, pp. 292–301.
20. NEVILLE MC and MORTON J (2001). Physiology and Endocrine Changes Underlying Human Lactogenesis II. Symposium: Human Lactogenesis II: Mechanisms, Determinants and Consequences. *Journal of Nutrition* **131**, pp. 3005S–3008S.
21. MCNEILLY AS, GLASIER A, and HOWIE PW (1985). Endocrine control of lactational infertility. Maternal Nutrition and Lactational Infertility. Dobbing J (ed.). New York: Raven Press.
22. HAYWARD AR (1983). The immunology of breast milk. Lactation: Physiology, Nutrition and Breast-Feeding. NEVILLE MC and NEIFERT MA (eds). New York: Plenum Press, pp. 249–272.
23. TINDAL JS, KNAGGS GS, HART IC, BLAKE LA (1978). Release of growth hormone in lactating and non-lactating goats in relation to behaviour, stages of sleep, electroencephalograms, environmental stimuli and levels of prolactin, insulin, glucose and free fatty acids in the circulation. *Journal of Endocrinology* **76**, no. 2, pp. 333–346.
24. EDMOND KM, ZANDOH C, QUIGLEY MA, AMENGA-ETEGO S, OWUSU-AGYEI S, and KIRKWOOD BR (2006). Delayed breastfeeding initiation increases risk of neonatal mortality. *Pediatrics* **117**, pp. 380–386.
25. KULSKI JK, SMITH M, HARTMANN PE (1981). Normal and caesarean section delivery and the initiation of lactation in women. *Australian Journal of Experimental Biology and Medical Science* **59**, pp. 405–412.
26. MARTIN RH, GLASS MR, CHAPMAN C, WILSON GD, WOODS KL (1980). Human alpha-lactalbumin and hormonal factors in pregnancy and lactation. *Clin Endocrinol* **13**, pp. 223–230.
27. HARFOUCHE JK (1970). The importance of breast-feeding. *Journal of Tropical Pediatrics* **16**, no. 3, pp. 133–169.
28. NANTEL AJ (2002). Clostridium Botulinum. International Programme on Chemical Safety Poisons Information Monograph 858 Bacteria. WHO, pp. 1–32.
29. KRELL R (1996). Value added products from bee-keeping. FAO Agricultural Services Bulletin no. 124: http://www.fao.org/docrep/w0076E/w0076e00.htm/

30. HENNART PF, BRASSEUR DJ, DELOGNE-DESNOECK JB, DRAMAIX MM, ROBYN CE. Lysozyme, lactoferrin and secretory immunoglobulin A content of breast milk: influence of duration of lactation, nutrition status, prolactin status and parity of mother. *American Journal of Clinical Nutrition* **53**, no. 4, pp. 32–39.
31. DECARVALHO M, ROBERTSON S, FRIEDMAN A, KLAUS M (1983). Effect of frequent breastfeeding on early milk production and infant weight gain. *Pediatrics* **72**, no. 3, pp. 307–311.
32. PERRY HM and JACOBS LS(1978). Rabbit mammary prolactin receptors. *Journal of Biological Chemistry* **253**, pp. 15–60.
33. NEVILLE MC, KELLER R, SEACAT L, LUTES Y, NEIFERT, M (1988). Studies in human lactation: milk volumes in lactating women during the onset of lactation and full lactation. *American Journal of Clinical Nutrition* **48**, pp.1375–1386.
34. PATTON S, HUSTON GE, MONTGOMERY PA and JOSEPHSON RV (1986). Approaches to the study of colostrum – the onset of lactation. In Hamosh M. and Goldman AS (eds). Human Lactation 2: Maternal and Environmental Factors. New York: Plenum Press, pp. 231–240.
35. LEWIS-JONES DI, LEWIS-JONES MS, CONNOLLY RC, LLOYD DC and WEST CR (1985). Sequential changes in the anti-microbial protein concentrations in human milk during lactation and its relevance to banked human milk. *Pediatric Research* **19**, pp. 561–565.
36. WYLIE J, VERBER IJ (1994). Why do women fail to breast feed: a prospective study from booking to 25 days post partum. *International Journal of Human Nutrition and Dietetics* **7**, pp. 115–120.
37. GIULIANI ERJ (2004). Common problems during lactation and their management. *J PEDIATR (Rio J)* **80**, no. 5, pp. 147–154.
38. MICHAELSEN KF, LARSEN PS, THAMSEN BL and SAMUELSON G (1994). The Copenhagen Cohort Study on Infant Nutrition and Growth: breast milk intake, human milk macronutrient content and influencing factors. *American Journal of Clinical Nutrition* **59**, pp. 600–611.
39. MEPHAM TB (1987). Physiology of lactation. Milton Keynes, UK: Open University Press.
40. HURLEY WL, REJMAN JJ (1986). ß-Lactoglobulin and a-lactalbumin in mammary secretions during the dry period: parallelism of concentration changes. *Journal of Dairy Science* **69**, pp. 1642–1647.
41. HURLEY WL (1987). Mammary function during the non-lactating period; enzyme, lactose, protein concentrations, and pH of mammary secretions. *Journal of Dairy Science* **70**, pp. 20–28.
42. VORHERR H (1978). Human lactation and breastfeeding. In: LARSON BL (ed). Lactation – A Comprehensive Treatise IV. The Mammary Gland/Human Lactation/Milk Synthesis. New York: Academic Press, pp. 182–280.
43. World Health Organization (WHO) (1995). Not getting enough milk. *Division of Child Health and Development Update* **21**, no. 2, pp. 1–5.
44. MORTON JA (1994). The clinical usefulness of breast milk sodium in the assessment of lactogenesis. *Pediatrics* **93**, pp. 802–806.
45. APERIA A, BROBERGER O, HERIN P and ZETTERSTROEM R (1979). Salt content in human breast milk during the first three weeks after delivery. *Acta Paediatrica Scandanavia* **68**, pp. 441–442.

46. MCCLELLAND DBL, MCGRATH J, SAMSON RR (1978). Anti-microbial factors in human milk. Studies of concentration and transfer to the infant during the early stages of lactation. *Acta Pediatrica Scandanavia* **271**, pp. S1–S20.
47. DONANGELO CM, TRUGO NM, KOURY JC, BARRETO SILVA MI, FREITAS LA, FELDHEIM W, BARTH C (1989). Iron, zinc, folate and vitamin B_{12} nutritional status and milk composition of low-income Brazilian mothers. *Eur J Clin Nutr* **43**, no. 4, pp. 253 –266.
48. LAMOUNIER JA, DANELLUZZI JC, VANNUCHI H (1989). Zinc concentrations in human milk during lactation: a 6-month longitudinal study in southern Brazil. *Journal of Tropical Pediatrics* **35**, pp. 31–34.
49. NAGRA SA. Longitudinal study in biochemical composition of human milk during the first year of lactation *Journal of Tropical Pediatrics* **35**, pp. 126–128.
50. LÖNNERDAL B, FORSUM E and HAMBRAEUS L (1976a). A longitudinal study of the protein, nitrogen and lactose content of human milk from Swedish well-nourished mothers. *American Journal of Clinical Nutrition* **29**, no. 10, pp. 1127–1133.
51. LÖNNERDAL B, FORSUM E, GEBRE-MEDHIN M, HAMBRAEUS L (1976b). Breast milk composition in Ethiopian and Swedish mothers. II. Lactose, nitrogen and protein contents. *American Journal of Clinical Nutrition* **29**, no. 10, pp. 1134–1141.
52. NEVILLE MC, ALLEN JC, and WATTERS C (1991). The mechanisms of milk secretion. In: Lactation – Physiology, Nutrition and Breast-Feeding. NEVILLE MC and NIEFERT MR, eds (1983) NEVILLE MC, ALLEN JC, ARCHER P, SEACAT J, CASEY C, LUTES V, RASBACH J. AND NEIFERT M. STUDIES IN HUMAN LACTATION: Milk volume and nutrient composition during weaning and lactogenesis. *American Journal of Clinical Nutrition* **54**, pp. 81–93.
53. READ LC, UPTON FM, FRANCIS GL, WALLACE JC, DAHLENBERG GW and BALLARD FJ (1984). Changes in the growth-promoting activity of milk during lactation. *Pediatric Research* **18**, no. 2, pp. 133–139.
54. SOMMERBURG O, MEISSNER K, NELLE M, LENHARTZ H, LEICHSENRING M (2000). Carotenoid supply in breast fed and formula fed neonates. *European Journal of Pediatrics* **159**, pp. 86–90.
55. GARG M, THIRUPURAM S, SAHA K (1988). Colostrum composition, maternal diet and nutrition in North India. *Journal of Tropical Pediatrics* **34**, pp. 79–87.
56. CHANG SJ (1990). Anti-microbial proteins of maternal and cord sera and human milk in relation to maternal nutritional status. *American Journal of Clinical Nutrition* **51**, pp. 183–187.
57. HOUGHTON MR, GRACEY M, BURKE V, BOTTRELL C and SPARGO RM (1985). Breast milk lactoferrin levels in relation to maternal nutritional status. *Journal of Pediatric Gastroenterology and Nutrition* **4**, pp. 230–233.
58. MIRANDA R, SARAVIA NG, ACKERMAN R, MURPHY N, BERMAN S and MCMURRAY DN (1983). Effect of maternal nutritional status on immunological substances in human colostrum and milk. *American Journal of Clinical Nutrition* **37**, pp. 632–640.
59. AHMED L, NAZRUL ISLAM SK, KHAN MNI, HUQUE S and AHSANB M (2004). Antioxidant Micronutrient Profile (Vitamin E, C, A, Copper, Zinc and Iron) of Colostrum: Association with Maternal Characteristics. *Journal of Tropical Pediatrics* **50**, no. 6, pp. 357–358.
60. SAHA K and GARG M (1999). Studies on Colostrum – Nutrients and Immunologic Factors: http://www.nutritionfoundationin.org/ARCHIVES/OCT91C.HTM
61. JENSEN RG, HAGERTY MM and MCMAHON KE (1978). Lipids of human milk and infant formulas. A Review. *American Journal of Clinical Nutrition* **31**, pp. 990.

62. JENSEN RG (1989). Lipids in human milk – composition and fat soluble vitamins. In: Lebenthal E (ed). Textbook of gastroenterology and nutrition in infancy, 2nd edition. New York: Raven Press, pp. 157–208.
63. WOODWARD DR, REES B, BOON JA (1989). The fat content of suckled breast milk: a new approach to its assessment. *Early Human Development* **20**, no. 3–4, pp. 183–189.
64. DA CUNHA J, MACEDO DA COSTA TH, ITO MK (2005). Influences of maternal dietary intake and suckling on breast milk lipid and fatty acid composition in low-income women from Brasilia, Brazil. *Early Human Development* **81**, no. 3, pp. 303–311.
65. DELGADO H, MCNEILLY AS, HARTMANN PE (1983). Non-nutritional factors affecting milk production: maternal diet, breastfeeding capacity and lactational infertility. In: Maternal Diet, Breast-Feeding Capacity, and Lactational Infertility. Whitehead RG (ed). United Nations University, Tokyo.
66. WHITEHEAD RG and PAUL AA (1981). Infant growth and human milk requirements: A fresh approach. *Lancet* ii, pp. 161–163.
67. BELAVADY B (1999). Breastfeeding and human milk: a review of some aspects. *The Indian Journal of Nutrition and Dietetics* **36**, pp. 168–174.
68. PAINTAL K and PASSI SJ (2006). Lactational Performance: Quality/ Quantity of Milk Secreted and Breastfeeding/ Childcare Practices – A Study among the Rural, Urban Poor and Urban Elite Nursing Mothers in Delhi, PhD thesis. Department of Nutrition and Dietetics, University of Delhi, (Unpublished) 2006.
69. STUFF JE, GARZA C, BOUTTE C, FRALEY JK, SMITH EO, KLEIN ER and NICHOLS BL (1986). Sources of variance in milk and caloric intakes in breast fed infants: Implications for lactation study design and interpretation. *American Journal of Clinical Nutrition* **43**, pp. 361–366.
70. OMOLULU A (1982). Breastfeeding practice and breast milk intake in rural Nigeria. *Human Nutrition and Applied Nutrition* **36**, no. 6, pp. 445–451.
71. WHO (2009a). WHO Global Data Bank on Infant and Young Child Feeding, 2009 In. WHO (2009). Infant and young child feeding: model chapter for textbooks for medical students and allied health professionals. 2009: 1–78. http://whqlibdoc.who.int/publications/2009/9789241597494_eng.pdf accessed on October, 2009.
72. UNICEF (2007). Progress for children: a world fit for children. Statistical Review Number 6. New York, UNICEF, 2007. In: WHO (2009). Infant and young child feeding: model chapter for textbooks for medical students and allied health professionals. 2009: 1–78. http://whqlibdoc.who.int/publications/2009/9789241597494_eng.pdf accessed on October, 2009.
73. National Family Health Survey (NFHS–III), 2005–2006. International Institute for Population Sciences, Mumbai, & ORC Macro, Calverton; September 2007, pp. 274–284.
74. KHAN ME (1990). Breast-feeding and weaning practices in India. *Asia Pacific Population Journal* **5**, no. 1, pp. 71–88.
75. SRIVASTAVA SP, SHARMA VK, KUMAR V (1994). Breastfeeding pattern in neonates. *Indian Pediatrics* **31**, no. 9, pp. 1079–1082.
76. SINGHAL GD, GURU LV (1973). Anatomical and Obstetric considerations in Ancient Indian Surgery (based on Susruta) Varanasi: BHU Press, pp. 2–8.
77. AGARWAL DK, AGARWAL KH, TEWARI IC, SINGH R, YADAV KNS (1981). Breastfeeding practices in urban slum and rural area of Varanasi. *Journal of Environmental*

Child Health 1981 In: Agarwal KN, Agarwal DK. Infant feeding in India. *Indian Journal of Pediatrics* **49**, pp. 285–288.

78. CHANDRASEKHAR U and UMA NN (1990). Food habits and practices of infant feeding in certain rural and urban communities of Coimbatore district. *The Ind. J Nutr Dietet* **27**, no. 12, pp. 340–346.
79. BHALE P, JAIN S (1999). Is Colostrum Really Discarded by Indian Mothers? *Indian Pediatrics* **36**, no. 10, pp. 1069–1070.
80. WHO (2009b). Infant and young child feeding: model chapter for textbooks for medical students and allied health professionals. WHO 2009: 1–78. http://whqlibdoc.who.int/publications/2009/9789241597494_eng.pdf accessed on October, 2009.
81. WHO (2009c). Global strategy for infant and young child feeding. World Health Organization website. 2009. http://www.who.int/child_adolescent_health/topics/prevention_care/child/nutrition/global/en/index.html accessed in September 2009.
82. BHANDARI N, IQBAL KABIR AKM AND MOHAMMED AS (2008). Mainstreaming nutrition into maternal and child health programmes: scaling up of exclusive breastfeeding. *Maternal and Child Nutrition* **4**, pp. 5–23.
83. The Infant Milk Substitutes, Feeding Bottles and Infant Foods (Regulation of Production, Supply and Distribution) Amendment Act 2003. What has changed? *Indian Pediatrics* 2003, **40**, pp. 747–757.
84. Innocenti Declaration (1990). In: WHO/UNICEF: Innocenti declaration on the protection, promotion and support of breastfeeding. *Ecology of Food and Nutrition* **26**, pp. 271–273.
85. Innocenti Declaration (2005). In: http://www.unicef.org/nutrition/index_24806.html. Accessed on 6th January 2008.
86. UNICEF. Baby Friendly Hospital Initiative (1991). In: http://www.unicef.org/nutrition/index_24806.html. Accessed on 6th January 2008.
87. WHO/UNICEF/AED/USAID (2008). Learning from large-scale community-based programmes to improve breastfeeding practices, pp. 1–83.
88. The Core Group (2005). Scale and Scaling Up: A CORE Group Background Paper on 'Scaling-Up' Maternal, Newborn and Child Health Services. CORE Spring Membership Meeting, 2005. The Core Group: Washington, DC. Available at: http://www.coregroup.org/resources/meetings/april05/Scaling_Up_Background_Paper_7-13.pdf
89. WHO/UNICEF (1992). The global criteria for the WHO/UNICEF Baby-Friendly Hospital Initiative. In: *Baby-Friendly Hospital Initiative. Part II. Hospital Level Implementation*. World Health Organization: Geneva.
90. PEREZ-ESCAMILLA R (2007). Evidence based breast-feeding promotion: The Baby-Friendly Hospital Initiative. *Journal of Nutrition* **137**, pp. 484–487.
91. COUTINHO SB, DE LIRA PI, DE CARVALHO LM and ASHWORTH A (2005). Comparison of the effect of two systems for the promotion of exclusive breastfeeding. *Lancet* **366**, pp. 1094–1100.
92. DE OLIVEIRA LD, GIUGLIANI ER, DO ESPIRITO SLC, FRANCA MC, WEIGERT EM, KOHLER CV et al (2006). Effect of intervention to improve breastfeeding technique on the frequency of exclusive breastfeeding and lactation related problems. *Journal of Human Lactation* **22**, pp. 315–321.
93. World Health Organization/Linkages (2003). Infant and young child feeding: A tool for assessing national practices, policies and programmes. Geneva, 2003.

Available at: http://www.who.int/child-adolescent-health/New_Publications/NUTRITION/icyf.pdf accessed in September 2009.

94. BHANDARI N, MAZUMDER S, BAHL R, MARTINES J, BLACK RE, BHAN MK, and other members of the infant feeding study group (2005). Use of multiple opportunities for improving feeding practices in under-twos within child health programmes. *Health Policy Plan* **20**, pp. 328–336.
95. QUINN VJ, GUYON AB, SCHUBERT JW, STONE-JIMÉNEZ M, HAINSWORTH MD, MARTIN LH (2005). Improving breastfeeding practices on a broad scale at the community level: success stories from Africa and Latin America. *Journal of Human Lactation* **21**, no. 3, pp. 345–354.
96. MORROW AL, GUERRERO ML, SHULTS J, et al (1999). Efficacy of home-based peer counseling to promote exclusive breastfeeding: a randomized controlled trial. *Lancet* **353**, pp. 1226–1231.
97. BHANDARI N, BAHL R, MAZUMDAR S, MARTINES J, BLACK RE AND BHAN MK (2003). Effect of community based promotion of exclusive breastfeeding on diarrheal illnesses and growth: a cluster randomized controlled trial. *Lancet* **361**, pp. 1418–1423.
98. PERRY H, FREEMAN P, GUPTA S, RASSEKH MB (2009). How effective is community based primary health care in improving the health of children? Summary findings – Report to the expert review panel, pp. 1–45.
99. SEMEGA-JANNEH IJ, BOHLER E, HOLM H, MATHESON I, HOLMBOE-OTTESEN G (2001). Promoting breastfeeding in rural Gambia: combining traditional and modern knowledge. *Health Policy and Planning* **16**, no. 2, pp. 199–205.
100. Linkages (2000). World Linkages/Ghana. LINKAGES project (1997–2004). http://www.linkagesproject.org/media/publications/world%20linkages//worldghana.pdf. Accessed October, 2009.
101. MCNELLY B and DUNFORD C (1998). Impact of credit with education on mothers and their young children's nutrition: lower pra rural bank credit with education program in Ghana. *Freedom from Hunger* Research Paper No. 4. Davis, CA: Freedom from Hunger 1998.
102. HAIDER R, ASHWORTH A, KABIR I, HUTTLY SRA (2000). Effects of community based peer counselors on exclusive breastfeeding practices in Dhaka, Bangladesh: a randomized controlled trial. *Lancet* **356**, pp. 1643–1647.
103. KRAMER MS, CHALMERS B, HODNETT ED, SEVKOVSKAYA Z, DZIKOVICH I, SHAPIRO S, COLLET JP (2001). Promotion of breastfeeding intervention trials (PROBIT): a randomized trial in the Republic of Belarus. *Journal of the American Medical Association* **285**, pp. 413–420.
104. Save the Children final evaluation, Mandiana Prefecture, Guinea. CARE India, Nicaragua and Bolivia, Final Evaluation of Child Survival Projects, 2002 and 2003. In: Exclusive breastfeeding: A gold standard. Safe, sound and sustainable. World Breastfeeding Week action folder, 2004. http://www.waba.org.my/whatwedo/wbw/wbw04/WBW2004%20Action%20Folder%20(11May04).doc. Accessed in October, 2009.
105. DUBOWITZ T, LEVINSON D, PETERMAN JN, VERMA G, JACOB S and SCHULTINK W (2007). Intensifying efforts to reduce child malnutrition in India: An evaluation of the Dular program in Jharkhand, India. *Food and Nutrition Bulletin* **28**, no. 3, pp. 266–273.
106. VIR S, NANDAN D, MOHAPATRA SC, DWIVEDI S, GUPTA SB, SRIVASTAVA VK, SINGH R, JAIN R (2000). Addressing Child Malnutrition – Community Based Approach

Targeting "At Risk" Families in Rural Uttar Pradesh, India. MCHN report Government of UP and UNICEF.

107. WABA (2004). http://www.waba.org.my/womenwork/seedgrants/arugaan.htm) In: Exclusive breastfeeding: A gold standard. Safe, sound and sustainable. World Breastfeeding Week action folder, 2004. http://www.waba.org.my/whatwedo/wbw/wbw04/WBW2004%20Action%20Folder%20(11May04).doc. Accessed in October, 2009.
108. EIDE I, et al (2000). The breastfeeding investigation in the year 2000. Report submitted to the Board of Health, Norway, May 2003. In: Exclusive breastfeeding: A gold standard. Safe, sound and sustainable. World Breastfeeding Week action folder, 2004. http://www.waba.org.my/whatwedo/wbw/wbw04/WBW2004%20Action%20Folder%20(11May04).doc. Accessed in October, 2009.
109. UNICEF/ WHO (2007). The integrated IYCF Counseling Course: Available at: http://www.who.int/nutrition/iycf_intergrated_course/en/index.html
110. WHO (2009). The 20-hour lactation management course (WHO 2009): http://www.who.int/nutrition/publications/infantfeeding/9789241594950/en/index.html
111. LUTTER CK (2003). Breastfeeding promotion – Is its effectiveness supported by scientific evidence and global changes in breastfeeding behaviours? *Advances in Experimental Medicine and Biology* **478**, pp. 355–368. In: Community based strategies for breastfeeding promotion and support in developing countries. WHO, pp. 1–28.
112. WHO (2007). Planning Guide for national implementation of the Global Strategy for Infant and Young Child Feeding. World Health Organization, pp. 1–49.

8

Complementary feeding of infants and young children

Veenu Seth and *Aashima Garg*

Veenu Seth, MSc, PhD, is an Associate Professor at the Department of Food and Nutrition, Lady Irwin College, University of Delhi. Dr. Seth has extensive research experience in the area of infant and young child feeding, specifically on complementary feeding.

Aashima Garg is a Nutrition Specialist with UNICEF (India Country Office). Her PhD research is in the area of improving complementary feeding practices in rural Uttar Pradesh, India.

8.1 Complementary feeding practices – a critical determinant of undernutrition in young children

Appropriate infant and young child feeding practices constitute a critical determinant of child nutrition, survival, growth and development. The importance of nutrition as a foundation for optimal health is undisputable. On the other hand, poor nutrition leads to ill health and ill health can contribute to further deterioration of nutritional status. These effects are most evident in infants and young children, who bear the brunt of the onset of malnutrition [1].

Childhood malnutrition is a significant health problem in developing countries and one of the main causes of infant and young child morbidity and mortality [2]. Recent estimates on status of undernutrition in developing countries [3] report 112 million and 178 million children under 5 years to be underweight and stunted, respectively A vast majority of these malnourished children are from South-Central Asia and Sub-Saharan Africa. Of these, 90% (160 million) live in just 36 countries of the world, representing almost half (46%) of the 348 million children from these countries.

India is home to 40% of the World's malnourished children [4], where approximately about 50% of children under the age of 3 years are still malnourished and this figure has only marginally changed over the past almost 2 decades [5–8]. It has been documented that poor fetal growth or stunting in the first 2 years of life leads to irreversible damage, including shorter adult height, lower attained schooling, reduced adult income and decreased offspring birth weight [9].

In developing countries, the critical period when growth faltering occurs often with long term adverse consequences, has been shown to be around 6 months to 2 years, with the start of undernutrition at 6 months and peak between 18 and 24 months. This period of progressive increase in undernutrition coincides with inadequate breast milk to meet the growing child's nutritional needs and concurrent unsatisfactory and inadequate introduction of semi-solid foods other than breast milk, or complementary foods [10].The complementary foods, when delivered inappropriately, results in growth retardation from mid infancy onwards. Scientific research identifies sub-optimal complementary feeding is as a significant determinant of stunting and urges to focus improvements in feeding frequency and energy density of complementary foods fed to infants and young children [3].

For India, this pattern of onset of malnutrition in infants and young children has been reported in all the three national surveys of 1992–93 [5], 1997–98 [6] and in 2005–06 [8]. Figure 8.1 presents the data of national survey of 2005–06 [8]. This period of complementary feeding is especially vulnerable, as infants are just learning to eat and must be fed appropriate and adequate foods, patiently and frequently, while continuing with breast milk. The nutrition provided in this phase of life, lays the foundation of health and healthy feeding habits.

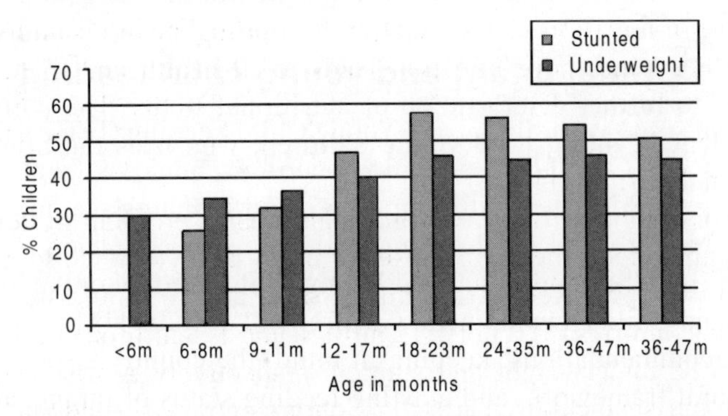

8.1 Pattern of onset of malnutrition in infants and young children in India [8].

This critical period between 6 and 24 months of age has thus, rightly been described as the *'window of opportunity'* for prevention of malnutrition, since the extent of undernutrition reaches its maximum level during this early and critical phase of life. It is well known that poor nutrition during this period contributes to significant morbidity and mortality, some of the long term consequences being reduced work capacity, impaired intellectual performance and increased risk of chronic diseases. Increase in number of brain cells is almost complete before birth, but most of the neuronal connections are established before the age of 3 years. Therefore if malnutrition persists during this period, consequences on physical growth and mental development can be long term and not amenable to management. The rate of growth, at this stage, is incomparable to that in later life. Birth weight doubles by 6 months and triples by 1 year with body length increasing by 1.5 times by first year. Most of the organs of the body also grow rapidly, both structurally and functionally, during the early years with a slower growth rate later on. Most of the growth in the nervous system and brain is complete in the first 2 years of life. Thus to achieve optimum growth and development, there is an increased demand of energy and essential nutrients. Breastfeeding alone is not able to meet the increased requirements for nutrients and needs to be complemented with feeding of food other than breast milk. This additional food is referred as "complementary food". Adequate complementary feeding from 6 months, with continued breastfeeding up to 2 years and beyond, is important for sustaining growth and development of the infant. Appropriate complementary feeding helps to promote growth, prevent stunting, and increase a child's chances for a healthy, productive life as an adult. The quality of infant and young child feeding, comprising breastfeeding and complementary feeding, thus becomes fundamental for improved nutritional status, achieving optimal growth and development.

8.2 Optimal infant and young child feeding

The global strategy for Infant and Young Child Feeding (IYCF), developed by WHO/UNICEF [10], provides a comprehensive framework for promoting appropriate feeding practices and reducing malnutrition. The strategy has been adopted by many developing countries. The Indian National Guidelines on Infant and Young Child Feeding of the Ministry of Women and Child Development, Government of India [11] conform to the global recommendations, keeping in mind, the country's socioeconomic and cultural framework, and existing feeding status of infants and young children. The strategy recommends exclusive breastfeeding for infants for the first 6 months of life and there after, safe and adequate complementary foods, while breastfeeding is continued for 2 years at least. The transition from exclusive breastfeeding to complementary feeding covers the period from 6 months to 2 years, the vulnerable period, when growth faltering begins in many children.

Pioneering studies carried out in India, in the sixties and seventies clearly showed that exclusive breastfeeding for the first six months and continued breastfeeding thereafter, coupled with adequate and appropriate foods available at home, promotes growth and is associated with lowering morbidity. According to the Lancet [12] Child Survival Series, exclusive breastfeeding for the first 6 months and continued breastfeeding along with complementary feeding for the next 6 months could cut down all child deaths by 13% and prove as the single most effective prevention intervention. Adequate complementary feeding between 6 and 24 months could prevent an additional 6% of all such deaths. The recent Lancet Maternal and Undernutrition Series [13] has reported revised mortality reduction attributable to optimization of infant feeding practices with improved breastfeeding practices contributing to the reduction of about 8% and appropriate complementary feeding strategies contributing to mortality reduction of another 1%. The difference in the rates of mortality reduction in the two Lancet series have been due to the difference in the outcome indicator, which in 2003 series was increase in weight-for-age Z scores (underweight) and in 2008 series was height-for-age Z scores (stunting).

This implies that extending coverage of exclusive breastfeeding to at least 2 years and introduction of appropriate complementary feeding at 6 months could save over 450,000 child deaths each year in India [14]. Thus, identifying approaches to reduce the prevalence of malnutrition particularly in the vulnerable first 2 years of life and focusing on infant feeding practices, is a priority for developing countries, appropriate Infant and Young Child Feeding (IYCF) could improve child survival, growth and development, with health benefits extending into adult years.

8.3 Complementary feeding – issues and guidelines

Complementary feeding refers to giving foods, in addition to breast milk or breast milk substitutes, in case of non breastfed infants. These complementary foods, of varying texture, locally prepared or manufactured, complement breast milk or infant formula, when either becomes insufficient to meet the needs of the baby. Historically, the period of transition from only breast milk to complementary foods for the infants has been referred to as *weaning period* and the foods other than breast milk are described as *weaning foods* [15]. The terminology "weaning" is discouraged since it is viewed to imply termination of breastmilk and weaning from breast. The term preferred is "complementary feeding", i.e. complementing breast milk with introduction of semi-solid food.

During the period of complementary feeding, a baby gradually becomes accustomed to eating family foods. By the end of this period, usually around 2 years, breast milk is entirely replaced by family foods, although some children may still be breastfed occasionally or allowed to suckle for comfort. The transition from exclusive breastfeeding to family and other foods, typically covering the period from 6 to 18–24 months of age, is critical, as eating patterns and habits developed in the first two years of life usually continue till later years [16]. Moreover infants during this period of accelerated growth also are increasingly exposed to infections such as diarrhea [17]. If this feeding is inappropriate, as discussed, malnutrition starts to set in many infants. It is not unexpected therefore, that infant and young child feeding has been the focus of attention of scientists and planners since long and Global and National Guidelines have been developed for complementary feeding, besides breastfeeding.

8.4 Initiating complementary feeding

Complementary feeding should be timely, i.e. all infants should start receiving foods in addition to breast milk from 6 months onwards (Box 8.1). It should be adequate, or the nutritional value of complementary foods should meet the nutrition gaps required to be filled in with reduction of breast milk. Foods should be prepared and given in a safe manner, implying that steps are taken to minimize the risk of contamination with pathogens. The food should be given in a way that is *appropriate*, which involves ensuring that foods are of appropriate texture, given in sufficient quantity and frequency.

Box 8.1 Timely introduction of complementary foods

Complementary foods should be introduced in infants' diet when the need for energy and nutrients exceeds what can be provided through exclusive and frequent breastfeeding. WHO (2001) recommends the introduction of semi-solid/soft or solid foods in addition to breastfeeding at completion of 6 months of age, i.e. 180 days.

The concept of introducing complementary foods around 6 months of age has been practiced traditionally since ages by the name of "Annaprashan Vidhi" in Hindu community. This ritual marks an infant's intake of food other than milk. This ceremony is commonly referred to in English as "First Rice".

The adequacy of complementary feeding depends not only on the availability of a variety of foods in the household, but also on the feeding practices of caregivers. Feeding young infants require active care and stimulation, where the caregiver is responsive to the child cues for hunger and also encourages the child to eat. This is also referred to as *active or responsive feeding* [1].

8.5 Adequacy and frequency of complementary feeding

Access to adequate complementary foods is a necessary condition for improving infant and young child feeding. Complementary foods are needed to fill the gap between the total nutritional needs of the growing child and nutrients provided by breast milk. An energy gap which starts at 6 months and increases as the child grows (Table 8.1) can be minimized by gradually increasing the energy density of complementary foods with the age of child. Besides energy, gaps exist for other nutrients also, especially iron, zinc, vitamins A and C [18]. To meet the increased nutritional demands, WHO [19] recommends that infants start receiving complementary foods at 6 months of age in addition to breast milk/milk substitute, initially 2–3 times a day between 6 and 8 months, increasing to 3–4 times daily between 9 and 11 months, and 12–24 months with additional nutritious snacks offered 1–2 times per day, as desired.

Table 8.1 Energy needs from complementary foods in infants and young children [19]

Age (months)	Total energy needs (kcal/day)	Energy from breast milk (kcal/day)	Energy from complementary food (kcal/day)
6–8	615	413	202
9–11	686	379	307
12–23	894	346	548

The amount of milk consumed by exclusively breast fed infants at 6 months ranges between 760 and 775 ml/day, with an energy density ranging from 74 to 67 kcal per 100 ml breast milk [20]. Based on the requirements of energy and other nutrients by infants and young children, the amount of these provided by breast milk, the energy and other nutrients that complementary foods need to provide can be estimated.

Due to increased growth velocity during this period leading to age related increased energy and nutrient requirements of the infants and young children, age-specific recommendations for energy and nutrient from complementary foods are presented in Table 8.1 [21].

8.6 Energy and other nutrient intake from complementary foods

8.6.1 Energy intake

The recommended levels of energy intake from complementary foods for infants with average breast milk intake in developing countries are about

200 kcal/d for infants 6–8 months of age, 300_kcal/d for infants 9–11 months of age, and 550 kcal/d for children 12–23 months of age [22]. The amount of energy required from complementary foods has been estimated by subtracting the amount of energy from breast milk from the age-specific total energy needs of infants and children (Table 8.1). These recommendations have been derived for developing countries on the basis of assuming good maternal nutritional status and adequate breast milk volume and composition. In industrialized countries, these estimates differ somewhat (130, 310 and 580 kcal/d at 6–8, 9–11 and 12–23 months, respectively) because of differences in average breast milk intake.

The Indian Recommended Dietary Allowances (RDA) for infants aged 6–12 months give the net energy requirements as 98 kcal/kg body weight of the age group, but does not specify the amount of energy required from complementary foods for this age group [23]. Hence, for practical purpose, the WHO [19] energy requirements are used.

To develop general feeding guidelines for children, information on children with low energy intake from breast milk was used, as these provide the most conservative assumptions regarding the minimum desirable number of meals or energy density of complementary foods needed to ensure adequate total energy intake. Based on these estimates, revised recommendations have been formulated. For an average healthy breastfed infant and young child with average energy density from complementary foods of at least 0.8 kcal/g, it is recommended that complementary foods be fed 2–3 times per day at 6–8 months of age, 3–4 times per day at 9–11 months of age, and 3–4times per day at 12–23 months of age [19].

Recommendations also state that older infants and young children should be provided additional nutritious snacks (such as a piece of fruit or bread or chapatti) offered 1–2 times per day, as desired. Snacks are defined as foods eaten between meals, usually self-fed, convenient, and easy to prepare. The calorific value of these snacks could be increased with addition of oil or fat to these. If energy density or amount of food per meal is low, or the child is no longer breastfed, more frequent meals may be required.

The previous recommendations [21] for children 12–23 months of age were to feed complementary foods 4–5 times per day. It is currently believed, however, that high meal frequency may lead to excessive displacement of breast milk. For this reason, the revised recommendation limits the number of feedings to a maximum of four, even among children in their second year of life. It is thus important to confirm that energy density of the complementary food is 0.8 kcal/g or higher in this age group, to ensure that young children receive sufficient energy from complementary foods (Table 8.2).

Table 8.2 Minimum number of complementary feeds/day to provide energy and nutrient needs of young children [19–22]

Energy density (kcal/g complementary food)	No. of meals		
	6–8 months	9–11 months	12–23 months
0.6	3–4	4	5
0.8	3	3	3–4
1.0	2–3	2–3	3

These guidelines are based on theoretical estimates of the number of feedings required, calculated from the energy needs from complementary foods and assuming a gastric capacity of 30g/kg body weight per density and a minimum energy density of complementary foods of 0.8 kcal/g. Infants with low intakes of breast milk would require higher meal frequencies. Also, as indicated in Table 8.2 when energy density of the usual complementary foods is less than 0.8 kcal/g or infants typically consume amounts that are less than the assumed gastric capacity at each meal, meal frequency would again need to be higher than the values shown.

8.6.2 Other macro and micro-nutrient requirements

It is equally important to ensure that infants and young children in addition to their energy requirements meet their protein and other micronutrient requirements from a combination of complementary foods and breast milk. As indicated above, nutrient requirements from complementary foods have been estimated as the difference between infants and young children's estimated total nutrient needs and the amounts transferred in breast milk to children of different age groups.

With regards to fat content of complementary foods, WHO [19] recommends the amount of fat that should be present in complementary foods to assure that fats provide 30–45% of the total dietary energy together from both breast milk and other foods.

The recommended protein and other micronutrient intakes from complementary foods were estimated by subtracting the amounts provided by human milk from the recommended nutrient intake for each age group. These have then been further expressed as recommended nutrient densities, which have been calculated by dividing the amount of nutrient required from complementary foods by the amount of energy needed from these foods for each age group [21]. In addition to WHO/UNICEF [21] recommendations on micronutrient densities, a revised vitamin and mineral requirements have been published by WHO/FAO [24]. Table 8.3 gives the recommended protein and micronutrient densities required from complementary foods as given by WHO/UNICEF 1998 report [21] and WHO 2002 report [24] assuming average breast milk intake. As mentioned in case of energy requirements, Indian Recommended Dietary Allowances (RDAs) for infants give the recommended nutrient amounts per kg body weight per day and there are no recommendations available for specific amount required from complementary foods, which again poses a problem in using these RDAs for comparison purpose.

The recommended protein, calcium and vitamin A densities are generally met in infants diet consisting of a mixture of cereals and milk or commercial infant formula along with breastfeeding since in developing countries, human milk, commercial infant milk formula, and cow's milk are good sources of vitamin A. Poor vitamin A status during infancy is generally associated with low intake of milk and vitamin A rich food during infancy and occurrence of infectious diseases. This is the reason why vitamin A supplementation first dose is recommended as per the Government of India Policy to be administered to infants between 6 and 12 months though it is administered at the age of 9 months, along with measles vaccine, for using the contact opportunity of the National Immunization Schedule.

As can be seen in the Tables 8.3 and 8.4, the requirements of iron are very high. Infant's iron needs are acquired from two different sources, prenatal reserves and food sources. Before birth, the fetus accumulates iron in the last trimester of pregnancy. Premature infants have limited reserves that are quickly depleted. Healthy term infants are born with iron stores sufficient for the first 6 months of life. At birth, the total body iron content is approximately 75 mg/kg, twice that of an adult man in relation to weight. During the first 6 months of life, total iron body content increases slightly and exclusive breastfeeding is sufficient to maintain an optimal iron balance. Thereafter, with high growth rate, iron requirement increases substantially (Tables 8.3 and 8.4) The Indian RDA for 6–12 months is 1 mg/kg body weight per day (Table 8.4). After 6 months, an infant

Table 8.3 Recommended nutrient densities of complementary food diets as per WHO/UNICEF 1998 [21] and WHO 2002 [24] values

Nutrient	Recommended nutrient densities					
	6–8 months		9–11 months		12–23 months	
	WHO/UNICEF 1998	WHO 2002	WHO/UNICEF 1998	WHO 2002	WHO/UNICEF 1998	WHO 2002
Protein (g/100 kcal)	0.7	1.0	0.7	1	0.7	0.9
Vitamin A (μg RE/100 kcal))	5	31	9	30	17	5
Vitamin C (mg/100 kcal)	0	1.5	0	1.7	1.1	1.5
Iron (mg/100 kcal)	4.0	4.5	2.4	3	0.8	1
Calcium (mg/100 kcal)	125	105	78	74	26	63
Niacin (mg/100 kcal)	1.1	1.5	0.9	1	0.9	0.9
Riboflavin (mg/100 kcal)	0.07	0.08	0.04	0.06	0.05	0.06
Thiamine (mg/100 kcal)	0.04	0.08	0.04	0.06	0.05	0.07
Folate (μg/100 kcal)	0	11	0	9	0	21
Zinc (mg/100 kcal)	0.8	1.6	0.5	1.1	0.3	0.6
Vitamin B_6 (mg/100 kcal)	0.09	0.12	0.08	0.08	0.98	0.08

becomes critically dependent on dietary source of iron, provided through complementary foods. A low amount and/or bioavailability of dietary iron provided through complementary feeding at the age of 6–12 months is one of the important factors contributing to nutritional iron deficiency in infancy.

Table 8.4 Indian recommended dietary allowances for infants (6–12 months) and young children (13–24 months) [23]

Nutrient	RDA	
	6–12 months	13–24 months
Protein (g/d)	1.65 g/kg body weight per density	22 g/d
Vitamin A (μg RE/d)	350	400
Vitamin C (mg/d)	25	40
Iron (mg/d)	1 mg/kg body wt/d	12
Calcium (mg/d)	500	400
Niacin (mg/d)	650 μg/kg body wt/d	8
Riboflavin (mg/d)	60 μg/kg body wt/d	0.7
Thiamine (mg/d)	50 μg/kg body wt/d	0.6
Folate (μg/d)	25	30
Vitamin B6 (mg/d)	0.4	0.9

Box 8.2 Problem nutrients in complementary feeding diets

As per WHO/UNICEF report 1998 [21], "problem nutrients" are defined as those for which there is greatest discrepancy between their content in complementary foods and the estimated amount required by the infant. They can be identified by comparing the estimates of desirable nutrient densities of complementary foods with actual densities of these nutrients in the diets of breastfed children in various populations. Table 8.6 gives the reported nutrient densities of complementary food diets consumed by infants as per different age groups from 4 developing countries: Bangladesh, Ghana, Guatemala and Peru. On comparing the nutrient densities of complementary foods diets consumed by infants in Table 8.5 with the desirable nutrient densities of complementary foods as recommended by WHO/UNICEF (1998) [21] and WHO (2002) [24] in Table 8.3, iron, zinc, vitamin B6 and vitamin A are problem nutrients in complementary feeding diets of developing countries. The same findings have also been reported by studies in other developing countries [25–27], signifying the urgent need to focus on nutrition programming for addressing the deficiencies of iron, zinc, vitamin A and vitamin B6 in developing countries.

8.7 Causes of faulty complementary feeding practices

Undernutrition in children is not simply the outcome of food insecurity but of inappropriate feeding practices, along with poor care practices, lack of safe drinking water and sanitation, resultant infections and mostly poor access to health care services.

Table 8.5 Nutrient densities of complementary food diets consumed by infants in developing countries

Nutrients	Bangladesh[a]	Ghana[b]	Guatemala[c]	Peru[d]
Age group	6–8 months			
No. of infants	50	207	194	107
Protein (g/100 kcal)	1.9	3.3	2.2	2.6
Calcium (mg/100 kcal)	16	35	27	19
Iron (mg/100 kcal)	0.4	1.2	0.5	0.4
Vitamin C (mg/100 kcal)	0.00	0.02	2.30	2.30
Vitamin A (RE/100 kcal)	0	7	87	35
Zinc (mg/100 kcal)	0.2	0.6	0.4	0.4
Vitamin B_6 (mg/100 kcal)	0.02	0	0.05	0
Age group	9–11 months			
No. of infants	66	171	148	99
Protein (g/100 kcal)	2.5	3.1	2.7	2.6
Calcium (mg/100 kcal)	20	40	37	27
Iron (mg/100 kcal)	0.4	1.3	0.6	0.4
Vitamin C (mg/100 kcal)	0.3	0.9	2.4	1.1
Vitamin A (RE/100 kcal)	1	9	62	29
Zinc (mg/100 kcal)	0.3	0.6	0.4	0.4
Vitamin B_6 (mg/100 kcal)	0.03	0	0.07	0

[a] Kimmons et al 2005 [25]
[b] Lartey et al 1999 [28]
[c] Brown et al 2000 [29]
[d] Creed de Kanashiro et al 1990 [30]

Inappropriate feeding practices are often a greater determinant of inadequate intakes and malnutrition, than the availability of foods in the households. Factors such as lack of awareness and knowledge about feeding amount, frequency and type of food contributes significantly to the poor nutritional status among children, even in families where adults meet their daily requirements [2, 31] . For example, in some cases complementary foods are introduced earlier than is desirable, in other cases their introduction is inappropriately delayed. The frequency and amounts of the foods that are offered may be less than required for normal growth, or their consistency or energy density may by inappropriate in relation to the child's needs. Further, reports on prevalence of specific micronutrient deficiencies in early childhood suggests that the specific micronutrients content of these foods is either inadequate or nutrient absorption is impaired by other components of these foods. Frequent microbial contamination of complementary foods and the associated high rates of diarrhoeal disease indicate a need for introduction of measures for improved food safety. Finally, responsive feeding, maternal encouragement to eat, and other psychosocial aspects of care during feeding which again arise due to time constraints of mother and other caretakers and is important for ensuring adequate food and nutrient intake of the child, are generally not addressed [32]. Box 8.3 discusses the findings of a formative study on assessing complementary feeding practices from India.

Box 8.3 Complementary feeding – a challenge to be addressed in rural Uttar Pradesh, India [34]

In a formative study conducted in 6 villages of District Ghaziabad, Uttar Pradesh, India, it was observed that of the total sample only 6% infants were exclusively breastfed till 6 months of age and similarly only 6% were introduced semisolid foods along with breastfeeding at completion of 180 days of age. The age of introduction of complementary foods varied as per the family belief and mothers' breast milk secretion. With regards to frequency of feeding complementary foods, majority (48%) of the mothers reported feeding 1–2 times/day, with only 16% and 5% infants in the age group of 6–8 and 9–12 months receiving recommended frequency of 2–3 times/day and 3–4 times/day, respectively. The consistency of complementary food fed was either very thin like pulse water, fruit juices etc, or solids like *roti*[1], biscuits etc. Lack of awareness, ignorance and mothers' lack of motivation emerged as prime factors responsible for these faulty feeding practices.

The energy and nutrient intake from complementary food suggested monotony and inadequacy in diets fed to infants between 6 and 12 months of age, with no significant difference observed between the mean nutrient intake of 6–8 and 9–12 months age group. Iron density from complementary food was found to be sub-optimal for all the three age groups, though protein and calcium densities were high when compared to standards [22]. Food group analysis showed that consumption of pulses, green leafy vegetable and other vegetables and fruits though present in adults' diets but didn't find place in infants' diet due to age old beliefs and ignorance.

The prevalence of diarrhoea, fever, cough and acute respiratory tract infection was 48, 42, 39 and 12% respectively. The prevalence of infants underweight, stunted and wasted was found to be 27.1%, 24.5% and 16.5%, respectively.

Thus, lack of exclusive breastfeeding till 6 months of age, delayed initiation of complementary foods and inappropriate complementary feeding with respect to the quality, quantity and consistency were observed to be the major factors contributing to high morbidity and malnutrition amongst infants' up till 12 months of age.

Food restrictions due to cultural beliefs are at times causative factors for poor nutritional status, especially in South East Asia, despite steady improvement in incomes and food availability [21]. Ignorance about the easy availability of complementary foods within economic means from the 'family pot', food fads and beliefs, are also major culprits. Urbanization and industrialization have to an extent compounded the problem, due to socio-cultural changes and breakdown of social support systems, with more urban and rural women working outside home, even before child is 3 months. These factors can have adverse effects on infant and young child feeding as summarized below in Box 8.4.

Box 8.4 Determinants of inadequate food intakes and malnutrition in infants and young children

- Lack of awareness and knowledge about feeding amount, frequency and type of food
- Local perceptions about the acceptability of specific foods for young children
- Cultural beliefs and perceptions on mode of feeding e.g. bottle feeding, feeding with hands
- Ignorance about the easy availability of complementary foods
- Inappropriate age of introduction of complementary foods
- Inappropriate energy density and frequency of feeding complementary foods
- Caregiver's education
- Caretaker's especially mother's time commitments to other activities
- Feeding schedule and style
- Feeding environment of the infants

In India, according to NFHS-3 [8], 57 children per 1000 live births die every year. Inappropriate infant feeding practices which are mainly attributable to lack of nutrition awareness within the community, are primarily responsible for the high morbidity and mortality of infants and young children [33].

8.8 Desirable features of satisfactory complementary feeding

Within the framework of the global and national Infant and Young Child Feeding (IYCF) guidelines, the prime characteristic of satisfactory complementary feeding is that foods given should complement rather than replace breast milk, which should continue till at least 2 years age, to meet the nutrient needs of the young child.

The guiding principles for complementary feeding given by WHO [1] and also by the Food and Nutrition Board of the Ministry of Women and Child Development (MWCD) [11], in their National Guidelines on Infant and Young Child feeding, focus on the following aspects:

Duration of exclusive breastfeeding and age of introduction of complementary foods – Exclusive breastfeeding from birth to 6 months of age, with introduction of complementary foods at completion of 180 days of age, while continuing to breastfeed.

Maintenance of breastfeeding – Continued frequent, on-demand breastfeeding until 2 years of age or beyond.

Quantity of complementary foods – Starting at 6 months of age with small amounts of food, increase the quantity of complementary foods fed to the infants from 2 to 3 katori/day (*katori* is a small bowl of medium size with a volume of 150 cc) at 6–8 months of age to 3–4 katori/day and

4–5 katori/day at 9–11 months and 12–23 months of age, while maintaining frequent breastfeeding.

Food consistency, meal frequency and energy density – Gradual progression of food consistency and variety as the infant gets older, adapting to the infant's requirements and abilities. Infants can eat pureed, mashed and semi-solid foods beginning at six months of age. By 9 months of age infants along with semi-solid foods can also eat "finger foods" or snacks. By 12 months, most infants can eat the same types of foods as consumed by the rest of the family but here nutrient density of the foods should be kept in mind and additional fat may be required. Addition of 0.5–1.0 tsp fat or oil in 1 katori of complementary food is recommended to increase density. Foods that may cause choking or items that have a shape and/or consistency that may cause them to become lodged in the trachea, such as nuts, grapes, and raw pieces of carrots must be avoided.

There has to be an increase in the number of times that the child is fed complementary foods as he/she gets older in order to meet the recommended quantity of feeding. The appropriate number of feedings depends on the energy density of the local foods and the usual amounts consumed at each feeding. If energy density or amount of food per meal is low, or the child is no longer breastfed, more frequent meals may be required.

Nutrient content of complementary foods – A variety of foods should be fed to ensure that the age -specific nutrient needs of the infants and young children are met. Meat, poultry, fish or eggs should be eaten daily, or as often as possible, if affordable and culturally acceptable. With vegetarian diets often it might be difficult to meet nutrient needs of infants and young children unless nutrient supplements or fortified products are used. Vitamin A and vitamin C rich fruits and vegetables and iron rich cereals, nuts and green leafy vegetables are recommended to be eaten frequently. Diets with adequate fat with incorporation of cereal-pulse combination should be provided, while avoiding drinks with low nutrient value, such as tea, coffee and sugary drinks such as aerated beverages, which are unnecessary foods as they are a poor source of nutrients and lead to malnutrition [35].

Several commercial complementary foods fortified with nutrients are available for fulfilling the nutrient requirements of the infants and young children, but these are within the reach of only the affluent class of people. The process of complementary feeding can be made economical, sustainable and practical for the masses, if based on local resources and home available foods. If complementary feeding of young children is to become universal, especially in developing countries, there is need to focus on children in low income settings, with consideration for the economic and environmental constraints, common in these countries [21]. Box 8.5 outlines the food based approaches to improve the iron and vitamin A content of complementary food diets.

It is possible to develop appropriate and nutritious complementary foods using appropriate food combinations, in diverse cultural settings, which less privileged mothers can prepare and their children are able to eat.

Box 8.5 Food-based approaches to improve iron and vitamin A content of complementary foods

Dietary improvement

- Increase the intake of iron and vitamin A rich foods (both carotene and retinol)
- In case of iron there is a need for improving meal pattern to enhance iron absorption with including enhancers of iron absorption like consumption of vitamin C rich foods, fermented and germinated foods and meat, fish and poultry especially after 9 months of age. Efforts have to be made to avoid giving the child milk and iron rich food together, as calcium acts as an inhibitor to absorption of iron from the diet.
- For vitamin A, there is a need to include both carotene (from plant-based diet) and retinol (milk, meat and fish diet) in complementary food

Food fortification

- Consumption of iron and vitamin A fortified complementary foods
- Adding 'home fortificants" such as micronutrient sprinkles to the complementary food

Use of vitamin–mineral supplements or fortified products for infant and mother – There should be need based use of fortified complementary foods or vitamin–mineral supplements for the infant. In some populations, breastfeeding mothers may also need vitamin–mineral supplements or fortified products, both for their own health and to ensure normal concentrations of certain nutrients particularly vitamins in their breast milk. Key micronutrients like iron, zinc, calcium, vitamin A and vitamin B12 are needed to be given if diets are plant-based or in non-breast fed infants.

Safe preparation and storage of complementary foods – Practice good hygiene and proper food handling behaviors. Important behaviours include washing caregiver's and children's hands before food preparation and eating, storing foods by covering and keeping at an elevated place, serving foods immediately after preparation, using clean utensils to prepare and serve food, using clean cups and bowls when feeding children, and avoiding the use of feeding bottles which are difficult to keep clean.

Responsive feeding – Practice responsive feeding applying the principles of psycho-social care. This involves feeding infants directly and assisting young children when they feed themselves; being sensitive to their hunger and satiety cues; feeding slowly and patiently, and encouraging children to eat but not forcing them; if children refuse many foods, experimenting with different food combinations, tastes, textures and methods of encouragement; minimizing distractions during meals if the child loses interest easily; remembering that feeding times are periods of learning and love; talking to children during feeding, with eye-to-eye contact.

Feeding during and after illness – Increase fluid intake during illness, including more frequent breastfeeding, and encouraging the child to eat soft, varied, appetizing and their favorite foods. It is observed that the children are fed less amount of complementary foods or at times not fed complementary foods during illness especially during diarrhea due to the fear of them suffering with more diarrhoea episodes. This practice should be discouraged and the mothers and other caretakers should be encouraged to feed the child foods which he/she likes along with breastfeeding during illness. After illness, food should be given more often than usual and the child is encouraged to eat more.

8.9 Measuring the status of complementary feeding

Till recently, there was a lack of evidence and consensus on simple indicators of appropriate feeding practices in children 6–23 months of age which has hampered the progress in measuring and improving the infant feeding practices. In 2001, WHO recommended indicators on measurement of exclusively breastfeeding and complementary feeding practices, which have now been revised and released as definitions by WHO in 2008 [36]. These indicators focus on selected food related aspects of child feeding, amenable to population-level measurement. Table 8.6 gives the list of population-level indicators on IYCF practices which can be used primarily for assessment, targeting, monitoring and evaluation.

Efforts have also been made to develop and use an Infant and Young Child feeding Index (ICFI) for measuring optimal IYCF practices [37]. The ICFI is a composite index of scores for breastfeeding, avoiding bottle feeding, 24-hour dietary diversity (measured by total number of food groups consumed), frequency of feeding of complementary foods and past 7 days food frequency score. The ICFI has been reported to be useful in identifying faulty feeding practices in a sample as well as for monitoring and evaluation of nutrition interventions [38]. Box 8.6 gives the indicators and the scoring system used in the complementary feeding index (CFI) developed by a study in India [39].

Table 8.6 Core indicators of measuring IYCF practices at population level [36]

1	Early initiation of breastfeeding	Proportion of children born in the last 24 months who were put to the breast within one hour of birth
2	Exclusive breastfeeding under 6 months	Proportion of infants 0–5 months of age who are fed exclusively with breast milk during the previous day
3	Continued breastfeeding at 1 year	Proportion of children 12–15 months of age who are fed breast milk during the previous day
4	Introduction of solid, semi-solid or soft foods	Proportion of infants 6–8 months of age who received solid, semi-solid or soft foods during the previous day
5	Minimum dietary diversity	Proportion of children 6–23 months of age who receive foods from 4 or more food groups during the previous day
6	Minimum meal frequency[(a)]	Proportion of breastfed and non-breastfed children 6–23 months of age who receive solid, semi-solid or soft foods (also including milk feeds for non-breastfed children) the minimum[(a)] number of times or more during the previous day
7	Minimum acceptable diet	Proportion of children 6–23 months of age who receive a minimum acceptable diet (minimum dietary diversity and minimum meal frequency) during the previous day
8	Consumption of iron-rich or iron fortified foods	Proportion of children 6–23months of age who receive an iron rich food or iron-fortified food that is specially designed for infants and young children

Note: [(a)]Minimum is defined as 2 times for breastfed infants 6–8 months, 3 times for breastfed children 9–23 months and 4 times for non-breastfed children 6–23 months.

Box 8.6 Variables and scoring pattern for Complementary Feeding Index (CFI) for infants aged 6–12 months in rural India [39]

Indicator	*Variable*		*Scoring*
1. Continued BF[(a)]	Breastfeeding	No Yes	02
2. Bottle feeding	Uses bottles	No Yes	10
3. Timely Initiation of CF[(b)]	CF were initiated on the completion of 6 months (180 days)	No Yes	02
4. Dietary diversity (past 24 hours)	*For infants (6–8 months)*		
	Sum of cereals (grains/tubers) + pulses + milk (other than breast milk)+ GLVs[(c)] and vitamin A rich fruits + egg + others[(d)]	0 1–2 3+	012
	For infants (9–12 months)		
	Sum of cereals (grains/tubers) + pulses + milk (other than breast milk)+ GLVs and vitamin A rich fruits + egg + others	0 1–3 4+	012
5. Food frequency (past 7 days)	Starchy staples (grains/ tubers)	0 1–3 4+	012
	Pulses	0 1–3 4+	012
	Milk (other than breast milk)	0 1–3 4+	012
	Meat/egg	0 1–3 4+	012
	Vitamin A rich fruits and vegetables	0 1–3 4+	012
	Other fruits/vegetables	0 1–3 4+	012
	Foods made with oil, fat or butter	0 1–3 4+	012
	Food frequency score = sum of scores for starchy staples + pulses + milk + meat/egg + vitamin A rich fruits/vegetables + foods made with fat		
6. Meal frequency (past 24 hours)	For infants (6–8 months)		
	No. of times the child was fed in the past 24 hours	0 1 2+	012
	For infants (9–12 months)		
	No. of times the child was fed in the past 24 hours	0 1–2 3+	012

CFI Score Range: Low: =6; Medium: 7–16; High: 17–23

[(a)] BF = Breastfeeding [(b)] CF=Complementary foods; [(c)] GLVs=green leafy vegetables; [(d)] other category includes fruits, other seasonal vegetables, fat and sugar food groups.

8.10 Complementary feeding status – global and India

The recent report of the State of World's children [40], reports the following rates of appropriate complementary feeding amongst 6–9 months infants: Sub-Saharan Africa – 68%, Eastern and Southern Africa – 71%, West and Central Africa – 65%, Middle East and North Africa – 57%, South Asia – 53% and East Asia – 45%. These figures suggest that South Asian countries lag behind the other developing countries in appropriate complementary feeding practices. An analysis of the rates of complementary feeding in South Asian countries have been presented by State of World's Breastfeeding report of South East Asian countries [35]. The rate of complementary feeding in South Asian Countries varies from 22% to 98% (Figure 8.2). In the report Pakistan has been reported to have lowest (22%) complementary feeding rates followed by Afghanistan (29%) and India (35%), while Sri Lanka with 98% has the excellent status regarding complementary feeding practices.

In the recent World Breastfeeding Trend's Initiative India report [41], India scored 69 out of 150 on IYCF indicators with complementary feeding rate (56.7%) getting a score of 3/10. In India, although breastfeeding is almost universal, poor rates of exclusive breastfeeding of only about 46% have been reported by the recent NFHS-3 [8] survey, with late introduction of complementary foods in a high proportion of infants. Timely introduction of complementary foods has been reported to be low, with only almost half of the infants' population (53%) being given complementary foods in addition to breast milk between 6 and 8 months of age [8]. Trends in initiation of breastfeeding and complementary feeding show very minimal upward change over about the last 15–17 years, as reflected in comparison of the three National Family Health Surveys (NFHS) [5, 6, 8], held in 1992, 1998–1999 and 2005–2006. Box 8.7 discusses the state-wide scenario across India of the complementary feeding rates as reported by the State of World's Breastfeeding, India Report [42].

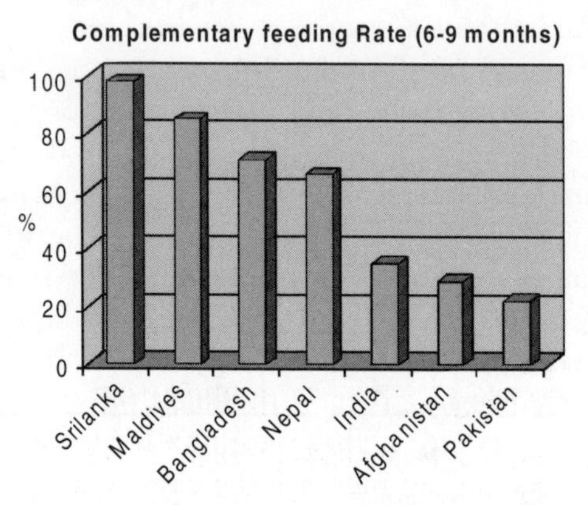

8.2 Complementary feeding rates of infants (6–9 months) in South-Asian countries [35].

Box 8.7 India: State-wide scenario [41]

As presented in the report of the 'State of the World's Breastfeeding India report', India scored 5 or 'poor' amongst 8 South Asian Countries, for timely and appropriate complementary feeding. Differences have been reported across the states with wide variations in under nutrition rates and IYCF practices. Appropriate practices were followed most often in Sikkim and Kerala, where undernutrition figures are relatively lower, but in these states too, a large percentage of infants and young children were not fed appropriately. States which were a little better off were Goa, Manipur, Himachal Pradesh and Delhi. The lowest compliance was observed in states of Andhra Pradesh and Maharashtra. Rural data was even worse than urban. Factors exerting a positive influence on feeding practices were mother's education and income status.

Figure below presents the data emerging on complementary foods started between 6–9 months in two national surveys – NFHS 2 (1998-99) and NFHS 3 (2005-06) as well as the goal stated under the 10th and 11th Five Year Plan (FYP).

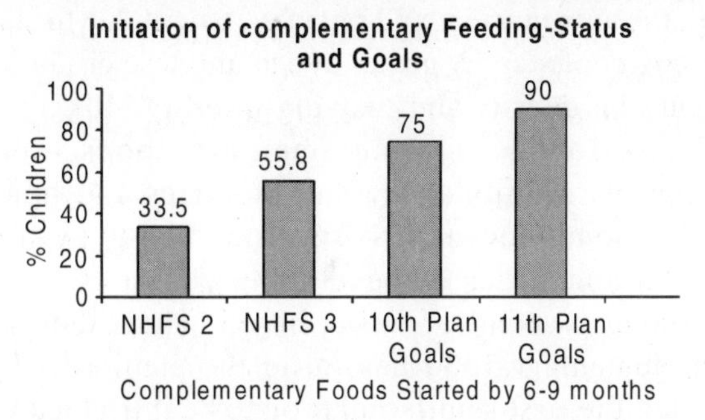

8.3 Target goals for achieving complementary feeding rates as per 10th and 11th five year plan of the government of India [14].

8.11 Low-cost complementary feeding

To provide nutritionally adequate and balanced complementary foods, it is important to have food mixtures or a variety of foods that fulfill all the nutrient and energy needs of the child. The young infant, although developmentally mature to start complementary foods, has a small stomach and can only consume small amounts of food at a time. Thus, energy and nutrient dense meals assume importance. A start made with cereals provides some energy, calcium, iron and zinc besides some other minerals and vitamins. Cereals however have phytates which are inhibitors of iron absorption. They also do not contain vitamins A and C and are not protein dense providing energy and good quality protein. Cereals therefore need to be given with added pulse or animal foods such as milk, meat, eggs etc, if these are unaffordable and culturally acceptable. Oil or nuts help to increase the energy density and further contribute to some of the protective nutrients. Addition of sugar/jaggery also increases nutrient density. In developing countries with cereal based high bulk diet, addition of fat or oil (0.5 to 1 tsp in 1 katori) is recommended with every meal to increase density. Seasonal and locally grown fresh or dehydrated vegetables/fruits are desirable to meet the requirements of micronutrients (especially vitamins A and C, iron and zinc) to ensure nutritional balance. This may sometimes prove a challenge.

Foods prepared could be fresh, modified from the 'family diet', traditional foods or low cost 'Ready to Eat' (RTE) premixes or instant infant foods, requiring only reconstitution. Traditional practices and processes like multimixing, roasting, parching, puffing, fermenting and malting could be used, resulting in beneficial outcomes like improved nutritional balance, reduction in dietary bulk due to dextrinization of starch, reduction in the anti-nutrient and phytate content due to soaking of grains, reduced viscosity of starchy gruels due to amylase production, facilitating increased nutrient density and easy digestibility [40].

Appropriate low cost complementary foods therefore require consideration of traditional feeding practices and home based diets, within the economic means. Diverse food habits exist among various regions and communities of developing countries, although all diets are predominantly cereal or millet based. Thus, the basic component of the complementary food has to be the staple cereal/millet of the region. In fact, the first semi-solid food to be introduced into the child's diet in India and other South Asian countries is usually a cereal based gruel or porridge made with addition of pulse or milk. The cereal use varies region wise. While this may help to initiate the child's eating and swallowing of soft foods, the nutritional balance and quality of foods are important, as mostly small amounts and very thin gruels are given to infants and that also often irregularly. The use of very thin gruel, such as mere cooked cereal starch or watery portion of pulse is low in nutrients and is an in-appropriate practice which should be actively discouraged. Table 8.7 provides an example of a day's sample diet for an infant.

8.12 Different 'home based' complementary foods

8.12.1 Traditional foods

Most of the traditional foods are based on starchy gruels, cereals, cereals with pulse, cereals with milk or a soft seasonal fruit or tuber. Based on the region, there are several traditional foods like *khichri, pongal, dalia, kheer, upma, idli, roti with dal/curd, ragi balls sattu, panjiri,* etc, which are used for infant feeding [41].

However, these are usually not fed in adequate amounts or at the right time. In some countries, like India, 'Annaprashan' ceremony (Box 8.1) is held, when solid food/cereals are first introduced, between 6 months to 1 year of age. However, this is often not followed with continued active feeding of the child with right frequency and consistency.

While some of these foods do provide energy and good quality protein, being based on cereal pulse combination, they lack important protective nutrients. Foods are often only carbohydrate rich and nutritionally unsuitable for the child. It becomes evident therefore, that traditional food and local and regional dietaries need to be identified with their good practices supported. Use of the desirable foods should be encouraged and sustained by focused, universalized nutrition education and awareness programs, emphasizing ways to make these traditional foods nutritionally dense and complete by addition of extra fat/nuts/oilseeds, sugar/jaggery to increase the energy density and fruits/yellow and orange coloured vegetables/green leafy vegetables (GLVs) to provide micronutrients. In vegetarian diet, iron and vitamin A availability of micronutrients is low and therefore use of micronutrient sprinkles has been tried with positive impact [32, 38].

Table 8.7 Sample diet for a day for an infant aged 12 months belonging to low socioeconomic group family in India

Time	Feed	Feed content	Household measures[(a)]
Morning	Sweetened milk with *chapatti* or bread	Milk sugar or jaggery *chapatti* or local bread	3/4th cup 1 tsp 0.5 *chapatti* or 1 slice
Mid-noon	Banana or any other fruit	Banana	1 medium Sized
Noon	Khichri–rice pulse mixture (modified from family pot)	Rice Pulse (Dal) [(b)] DGLV[(b)] Oil	1 bowl (150 cc) 0.5 bowl (75 cc) 0.5 bowl 1 tsp
	Or Chapatti/bread with dal and vegetable (can be mixed in one bowl)	*Chapatti* Dal[(b)] DGLV[(b)] Oil	1.5 *Chapatti* 0.5 bowl 0.5 bowl 1 tsp
Evening	Sweetened milk with *Chapatti* or bread	Milk Sugar or Jaggery *Chapatti* or local bread	3/4th cup 1 tsp 0.5 *chapatti* or 1 slice
	Or Dry take home ration (THR) with milk	Milk THR	3/4th cup 3 tsp
Night	*Chapatti* / bread / rice with *Dal* or vegetable	*Chapatti / rice / bread* *Dal* or Vegetable (GLV or yellow vegetable) Oil	1 *Chapatti or 1 bowl rice* ½ bowl 1 tsp

[(a)] GLV: Green leafy vegetable
[(b)] Cooked

8.12.2 Modified family foods

In the less privileged sections of society, complementary foods are mostly home-made, based on the modified adult diet. However, as indicated by several studies, complementary feeding is delayed and the quantity of solid food given is meager. In fact, modifying the family diet can be the most economical, practical and effective means of ensuring complementary feeding of children, provided a suitable combination of foods is given with incorporation of additional oil or fat and variety gradually increased, to ensure nutritional adequacy and easy adaptation to the home diet. High requirements of iron through dietary source are difficult to meet unless food source is rich in heme iron or fortified food items or "home fortificants" such as sprinkles are incorporated in food (see chapter on child anaemia for details)

Appropriate introduction of semi-solid food can also develop good eating patterns and habits which usually continue till later years. In this respect, the more economical home-based complementary foods have an edge over the high cost commercial foods with little variation in texture, consistency and flavor. Starting with mashed and smooth mixtures at 6 months, the mixtures can progressively be made thicker, with gradual transition to soft chopped and lumpy foods. By 1 year of age, most infants are ready to eat unmodified but 'non-spicy' adult or family diet. Personal hygiene in feeding the child, food safety aspects like well cooked food, fresh food, and food hygiene such as food kept covered are however some important aspects of complementary feeding that also need attention.

One issue of concern that arises is that the underprivileged families often eat only 2 meals per day, while a young child needs to be fed 4–5 times a day or more, due to the limited stomach capacity and high nutrient requirements per unit body weight. Frequent feeding of the family diet, which being predominantly cereal based also tends to be bulky and may be impractical, as the food maybe subject to spoilage. Thus, processes like roasting and malting of cereals are beneficial to reduce dietary bulk. Between meal feedings, use of ready to eat (RTE) infant foods or nutritious snacks that can be stored, facilitate meeting the child's dietary and nutrient needs. Soft seasonal, locally grown and easily available fruit may also be used for between meal feeding.

Thus, awareness creation is needed regarding the ways and means of making the home based infant food as rich in nutrients as possible, within the constraints of time, cost, and other physical facilities. Simple one dish meals with different food groups need to be promoted. A study [45] to assess the amount of GLVs and carrot required to meet the vitamin A requirements of infants and young children, taking into account the contribution of breast milk at different ages between 6 months to 3 years, quantified the amount of GLV needed as 10 g/day (1/4 medium katori raw and 1 tablespoon cooked) for the 6 month infant, 20 g/day at 9 months with reduction in breast milk, and 30 g/d from 1 to 3 years age. From the practical point of view, about 3 times the amount required daily or 1/4 katori cooked GLV could be given twice a week instead of GLV daily [45]. This addition of GLV contributes to the iron and vitamin C content of the complementary food also. Carrot required to provide the same amount of vitamin A is approximately 3 times the quantity of GLV needed at a particular age group.

8.12.3 Ready-to-eat (RTE) infant premixes or instant infant foods

Low cost RTE infant foods, made from grains available in the home, have a major role to play in supporting complementary feeding and its sustainability for the common man, especially in view of the increasing workforce of women outside home and changing social networks affecting the practicality of using only freshly prepared foods. RTE infant foods only require reconstitution with boiled warm water. Other fluids like milk, lassi/buttermilk, coconut milk could also be used, if available and affordable, to increase nutrient density. These RTE premixes, can be easily prepared at home by taking about 3 parts of the staple cereal or millet like *atta, suji, ragi,* rice, *bajra or jowar* and combining with 1 part of a locally available dehusked pulse such as *arhar, chana dal*, *besan* or *moong*, with addition of 0.25 or 0.50 part of some nut or oilseed to increase the energy density. These food items need to be roasted separately, ground finely and mixed well and stored in a clean airtight container for good shelf life. At the time of feeding, 2–4 tablespoons of the mixture can be mixed with boiled water or any other liquid, and sugar/jaggery and a teaspoon of oil added, and fed to the infant. Powdered millets may need sifting initially to reduce the husk content. Seasonal dehydrated GLV or carrot (1–2 g) may also be added to this premix to provide important micronutrients. The consistency of the reconstituted premix can vary depending on the age of the child and if available, some soft seasonal fruit could be chopped or mashed and added. In fact, such a premix could also be used to prepare the already mentioned mid meal snacks for the older child.

Although roasted starchy grains swell less in water as compared to unroasted, the viscosity of the premix gruel or a starchy gruel could be further reduced by using a small amount of amylase rich flour (ARF), which then enables the child to have a higher intake. The efficacy of such foods has been amply shown by the early studies from Gujarat [46] to several more recent field and research studies (Chapter on ARF presents details).

It must also be kept in mind that mothers from the low income group may sometimes find it difficult to prepare even a simple RTE food due to physical and monetary constraints. Therefore community based enterprise to produce RTE foods with an element of income generation, especially for women, assumes significance. For community-based production at low cost, involvement of '*panchayats*', (local governance) women's groups and adolescent girls with NGO's and Government linkages, for training in safe preparation, packaging and marketing to local shops or young child feeding programs, can go a long way in improving complementary feeding of infants and young children. Small scale production units could be attached to rural health centers, fulfilling the need of complementary foods and income generation for the women. Several such successful models are reported. However, an important prerequisite of any such venture is again widespread generation of nutrition awareness resulting in a realization for the need and demand for such foods.

8.13 Promoting improved complementary feeding practices – programs, strategies and challenge ahead

It is evident that appropriate complementary feeding requires a combination of strategies. Establishing appropriate universal and timely introduction of complementary foods has emerged as one major strategy to combat this 'avoidable' undernutrition in young children and could be one of the most economic means of reducing childhood malnutrition. Often, it is not the food insecurity with respect to the child's diet but lack of awareness which results in inadequate intake and undernutrition. What is required is focused and aggressive awareness generation on issues related to complementary feeding such as time of introduction, the foods, texture, frequency and amount, and method of feeding complementary foods including active feeding and feeding during illness. Food fads found interfering with intake of nutritious foods need to be dispelled.

From the point of view of custom, practice, feasibility and cost also, it has been recognized since long that it would be most convenient for mothers to feed their infants and toddlers, an easily modifiable family or home cooked food or traditional foods. Expensive commercial foods as well as biscuits, snacks are not essential and mostly, special foods may not be required to be produced for very young child in situations where family uses appropriate principles of complementary feeding [43].

Ensuring sustainability of improved complementary feeding in addition requires adequate advocacy and awareness among all stakeholders, community participation, encouragement to families and women's self help groups to make low cost infant foods as well as public private partnership for production of the RTE. Production of RTE at community and large scale level from a variety of raw materials available in the household needs to be encouraged along with appropriate marketing strategies of reasonably priced convenient sized packs of complementary foods [47]. Fortification with micronutrients is another strategy which may need to be considered to improve nutrient balance of low cost infant foods, prepared on a large scale. Mixing of micronutrient sprinkles[1] or nutrient-rich pastes has been successfully promoted in some settings, and requires further research.

A review of the working group on breastfeeding and complementary feeding of Standing Committee for Nutrition (SCN) [45] of various intervention strategies to improve IYCF, such as nutrition education on energy rich complementary foods, food with education, fortification of complementary foods and increased energy density and/or nutrient bioavailability of complementary foods via simple technologies, concluded that educational approaches can be effective, but in many situations a greater impact may be seen when they are combined with home-fortification or provision of fortified foods. The biggest challenge for complementary feeding interventions is going to scale with a combination of the most cost-effective components, while assuring adequate delivery and sustainability.

Targeted interventions are thus the need of the hour and interventions maybe at following different levels:

- Interventions at the household level (with a focus on domestically produced foods).
- Interventions at the village or community level (focusing on low volume, community production units and local distribution).
- Interventions at the intermediate level (focusing on intermediate-volume production units and regional distribution).
- Interventions at the central, industrial level (focusing on large volume, industrial production units and widespread distribution).

There is need to identify local feeding practices, common problems associated with feeding appropriate complementary foods and adapt to the feeding recommendations based on guidelines given by WHO [10].

---

1. Sprinkles is a dry, tasteless, single-serving packet to be 'sprinkled' onto food. It includes a mix of iron, vitamins C, D and A, and zinc. Contrary to many other supplements it doesn't change the taste or appearance when mixed into children's food, making it more acceptable to use.

Improvement of complementary feeding has received insufficient attention as a public health intervention and poor feeding practices continue as a major threat to social and economic development in our country. Development of successful interventions to improve child feeding practices, in particular are necessary to begin to overcome earlier insults to child's nutrition status and to mitigate the effects of poverty. Some of the successful models, used across the country, by Government, NGOs, research groups, public nutritionists, for improving infant feeding practices have been based on community participation, active feeding counseling, mobilization of community based voluntary workers, positive deviance approach[2] or advocating what works, nutrition education and counseling of mothers, and frontline workers, involvement of grandmothers and mobilization of self-help groups.

It must be borne in mind that approaches to improving the availability of adequate complementary foods include simple technologies that can be applied in the home or community, and larger-scale industrial production of fortified processed foods that can involve both the public and the private sector. In conclusion, 10 messages for successful complementary feeding are

1. Age of introduction of complementary foods
2. Safe preparation and storage of complementary foods
3. Foods of appropriate consistency for age and development stage
4. Fat and carbohydrate content of complementary foods
5. Energy density of food-addition of fat or oil.
6. Amount of complementary foods needed
7. Appropriate meal frequency
8. Protein and micronutrient content of complementary food
9. Use of supplements or fortified products
10. Continuation of breastfeeding
11. Responsive feeding

The global strategy on IYCF gives due weightage not only to infancy and young child feeding but mother and child dyad and advocates that improved IYCF begins with ensuring the health and nutritional status of women, in their own right, throughout all stages of life [10]. Thus, focusing on improving the complementary feeding is an intervention requiring urgent attention as improved feeding practices during the first 2 years of life is an important key to bridge the gap in the health and nutrition continuum of care.

---

2. Positive Deviance is a process of inquiry and action that looks for children who are well-nourished in spite of the forces working against their nutritional status, and examines the behaviors, beliefs, and practices which enable that child to cope and thrive.

References

1. WHO (2001). 'Complementary Feeding', Report of the Global Consultation and Summary of Guiding Principles for Complementary Feeding of Breastfed Infants. WHO, Geneva.
2. MURRAY CJ, LOPEZ AD (1997). 'Mortality by cause for 8 regions of the world: Global Burden of Disease Study', *Lancet*, **349**, pp. 1269–1276.
3. BLACK RE, ALLEN LH, BHUTTA ZA, CAUFIELD LE, DE ONIS M, EZZATI M, MATHERS C, RIVERA J (2008). Maternal and child undernutrition: global and regional exposures and health consequences. Lancet **371**, pp. 243–260.
4. BRAUN VJ, RUEL M, GULATI A (2008). Accelerating progress towards reducing Child Malnutrition in India: A Concept for Action, IFPRI.
5. NFHS 1 (1991–1992). National Family Health Survey, IIPS, Mumbai, India (1993).
6. NFHS 2 (1998–1999). National family Health Survey, India, International Institute for Population Sciences. Mumbai, India (2000).
7. DLHS (2002). District Level Household Survey: Phase 1 Round II, 2002. Department of Family Welfare, GOI, January 2004.
8. NFHS-3 (2005–2006), National Family Health Survey. Volume I. IIPS, Mumbai, India: 2007.
9. VICTORA CG, ADAIR L, HALLAL PC, MARTORELL R, RITCHER L, SACHDEV HS (2008). Maternal and child undernutrition: consequences for adult health and human capital. *Lancet*, **371**, pp. 340–57.
10. WHO (2003). Infant and Young Child feeding. A Tool for Assessing National Practice, Policies and Program. Geneva.
11. Ministry of Women and Child (MWCD) (2006). National Guidelines on Infant and Young Child Feeding. Food and Nutrition Board, MWCD, GOI 2006.
12. JONES G, STEKETEE RW, BLACK RE, BHUTTA ZA, MORRIS SS and the Bellagio Child Survival Study group (2003). How many child deaths can we prevent this year? *Lancet*, **362**, pp. 65–71.
13. BHUTTA ZA, AHMED T, BLACK RE, COUSENS S, DEWEY K, GLUGLIANI E, et al (2008). What works? Interventions for maternal and child undernutrition and survival. *Lancet*, **371**, pp. 417–440.
14. MWCD (2006). Report of the Working Group on Integrating Nutrition with Health- 11th 5 Year Plan: 2007–2012. MWCD, GOI Nov 2006.
15. LANIGAN JA, BISHOP JA, KIMBER AC, MORGAN J (2001). Systematic review concerning the age of introduction of complementary foods to the healthy full term infant. *Eur J Clin Nutr*, **55**, pp. 309–20.
16. BUTTE N, COBB K, DWYER J, GRANEY L, HEIRD W, RICKARD K (2004). The healthy feeding guidelines for infants and toddlers. *Journal of the American Dietetic Association*, **104**, no. 3, pp. 42–54.
17. BROWN KH, BLACK RE, LOPEZ DE ROMANA G, CREED DE KANASHIRO H (1989). Infant feeding practices and their relationship with diarrhoeal and other diseases. *Pediatrics*, **83**, pp. 31–40.
18. WHO (2002). 'Global Consultation on Complementary Feeding. Report of WHO Expert Consultation. WHO.
19. PAHO/WHO (2003). Guiding principles for Complementary Feeding of Breastfed Child. Washington D, Pan American Health Organisation, WHO.
20. RAMJI S (2006). 'Appropriate Feeding: 6–24 months. Nutrition in Late Infancy and Early Childhood (6–24 months), Nutrition Foundation of India, New Delhi, pp. 32–34.

21. WHO (1998). Complementary Feeding of Young Children in Developing Countries: A Review of Current Scientific Knowledge, Geneva.
22. DEWEY KG and BROWN KH (2003). Update on Technical Issues Concerning Complementary Feeding of Young Children in Developing Countries and Implications for Intervention Programs, Food and Nutrition Bulletin, 24, pp. 5–28.
23. Indian Council of Medical Research (ICMR) (1990). Nutritive Value of Indian Foods. NIN, Hyderabad.
24. WHO (2002). Joint FAO/WHO Expert Consultation. Vitamin and mineral requirements in human nutrition. World Health Organization, Geneva.
25. KIMMONS JE, DEWEY KG, HAQUE E, CHAKRABORTY J, OSENDARP SJM and BROWN KH (2004). Behaviour-change trials to assess the feasibility of improving complementary feeding practices and micronutrient intake of infants in rural Bangladesh. Food and Nutrition Bulletin, **25**, no. 3, pp. 228–237.
26. HOTZ C and GIBSON RS (2001). Complementary feeding practices and dietary intakes from complementary foods amongst weanlings in rural Malawi. *Eur J Clin Nutr*, **55**, pp. 841–849.
27. HUFFMAN SL, GREEN CP, CAUFIELD LE and PIWOZ EG (2000). Improving infant feeding practices: Programs can be effective! *Mal J Nutr*, **6**, no. 2, pp. 139–146.
28. LARTEY A, MANU A, BROWN KH, PEERSON JM, DEWEY KG (1999). A randomised, community-based trial of the effects of improved, centrally processed complementary foods on growth and micronutrient status of Ghanaian infants from 6–12 months of age. *Am J Clin Nutr*, **70**, pp. 391–404.
29. BROWN KH, SANTIZO MC, BEGIN F, TORUN B (2000). University of California, Davis and Instituto Nutricional de Centro America y Panama, unpublished data.
30. CREED DE KANASHIRO H, BROWN KH, LOPEZ DE ROMANA G, LOPEZ T, BLACK RE (1990). Consumption of food and nutrients by infants in Huascar (Lima), Peru. *Am J Clin Nutr,* **52**, pp. 995–1004.
31. GHOSH S (2007). Viewpoint: National family Health Survey 3, 2007. *Indian Pediatrics* **44**, p. 619.
32. RUEL MT, BROWN KH and CAULFIELD LE (2003). Moving Forward with Complementary Feeding, IFPRI, FCND. Discussion Paper No. 146.
33. DEWEY KG (2001). The challenges of promoting optimal infant growth. *J Nutr*, **131**, pp. 1879–1880.
34. Complementary Feeding practices – a challenge to be addressed in rural India (2009). *Pak J Nutr* **8**, no. 4, pp. 505–506.
35. IBFAN Asia (2007). The State of World Breastfeeding South Asia Report.
36. WHO (2008). Indicator for assessing infant and young child feeding practices, Part 1. Definitions. WHO 2008.
37. ARIMOND M and RUEL MT (2002). 'Progress in developing an infant and child feeding index: an example using the Ethiopia Demographic and Health Survey 2000. Food Consumption and Nutrition Division Discussion Paper 143, International Food Policy Research Institute, Washington, DC.
38. ARIMOND M and RUEL MT (2004). 'Dietary Diversity is associated with child nutritional status, 'Evidence from 11 Demographic and Health Surveys, *J Nutr.*, **134**, pp. 2579–85.
39. UNICEF, The State of World's Children (2009). Maternal and Newborn health, New York.
40. BPNI/IBFAN Asia (2008). 'World Breastfeeding Trend's Initiative', India Report. BPNI/IBFAN–Asia.
41. BPNI/IBFAN Asia Pacific (2005). State of Implementation of the Global Strategy for Infant and Young Child Feeding 2005.

42. WHO (2000). 'Department of Child and Adolescent Health and Development. Complementary Feeding Family Foods for Breast Fed Children', *WHO/NDH*, Geneva.
43. SETH V (2006). 'Appropriate Feeding: 6-24 months. Nutrition in Late Infancy and Early Childhood (6–24 months), *Nutrition Foundation of India*, New Delhi, pp. 35–43.
44. SHARMA S and SETH V (1994). 'Quantification of Food Needs of Infants, Preschoolers and Pregnant Mothers, towards meeting their Energy and Vitamin A Requirements', Project Report: Department of Food and Nutrition, Lady Irwin College, New Delhi India (Sponsored by UNICEF).
45. GOPALDAS T (1983). 'Complementary and supplementary foods for young child feeding at household, community, programme and industrial levels', Workshop on Weaning Foods: A Report, College of Home Science. Andhra Pradesh Agricultural University. Hyderabad, India. Pub: UNICEF. July, 1983.
46. GHOSH S (1995). 'Preventing malnutrition: The critical period is 6 months -2 years', *Indian Pediatrics,* **32**, pp. 1057–1058.
47. SCN (2007). 'The Working Group on Breastfeeding and Complementary Feeding', 34th Session of SCN, February 2007, Rome.

9

Options and strategies to reach under-two children through complementary feeding with ARF in the South Asian countries

Tara Gopaldas

Tara Gopaldas is Director at Tara Consultancy Services, Bangalore. She was dean and senior professor at Faculty of Family & Community Sciences at M S University, Baroda (1978–1993); Honorary Director of the WHO Collaborating Centre (1989–1993); Senior Adviser, Planning Commission (1976–1978); Nutrition Adviser & Project Director, CARE-India (1970–1976); Research Executive, Hindustan Levers (1960–1965). Dr. Gopaldas holds a PhD Degree from University of Illinois, Ch-Urbana, USA (1958), MSc in Biochemistry from Indian Institute of Science, Bangalore and BSc in Home Science from Madras University. She is a member of Nutrition Mission of India since 2003 and was President of Indian Dietetic Association of India (1982–1986) and was a UGC National Lecturer (1984–1985).

9.1 Introduction

Most of the 'malnutrition drama' is already over by the time a South Asian child is of two years of age [1]. More than half the world's underweight children live in South Asia [2, 3, 4]. India has about 45 million infants/toddlers (6–24 months) per annum. As against India's 45 million under two; Bangladesh would have about 6 million; Nepal about 1 million; and Sri Lanka about 1 million. The target population for complementary foods in just these four South Asian countries is a staggering 53 million per annum.

This chapter consists of the following sections:

- Section 9.2: Nutritional needs, deficiencies and the role of complementary foods in the age group of under two
- Section 9.3: Options for providing nutrition to overcome deficiencies

- Section 9.4: Technology for development of premixes/complementary foods
- Section 9.5: Delivery channels and mechanisms to improve outreach

9.2 Nutritional needs, deficiencies and the role of complementary foods in the age group of under twos

Section 9.2 focuses on the following three components: nutritional status of children under two in South Asia; nutritional requirements for the under two in South Asia; and role of complementary foods for the under two.

9.2.1 Nutritional status of children under two in South Asia

It is now well recognized that most of the children in Asia under-2 years of age, especially children 6–18 months old are extremely undernourished, underweight and stunted. Generally, data on nutritional status is available for the 'Under Fives' and "Under Threes" and not for the 'Under Twos'. From Table 9.1, it can be noticed that underweight, stunting and wasting is very high in India, Bangladesh and Nepal. The picture is slightly better in Sri Lanka. In South Asia there are several factors operating synergistically to hasten the 'Below Twos' rapid decline into undernutrition, especially so, from his/her sixth month of life.

These are as follows:

- the child may have been low birth weight (LBW), i.e. below 2500 g at birth;
- lack of and/or total unsuitability of complementary foods;
- repeated episodes of diarrhoeal and respiratory infections;
- unhygienic personal, maternal and environmental status;
- unsafe drinking water and poor sanitation;
- limited, distant, slow and non-affordable access to preventive and curative health services;
- poor income levels, illiterate, and working parents;
- ignorance of simple and doable caring practices and large families with narrow or no birth spacing.

Table 9.1 Selected indicators of the nutritional profile of the "under fives" in India, Bangladesh, Nepal and Sri Lanka in 1990 [7]

Indicator	India (%)	Bangladesh (%)	Nepal (%)	Sri Lanka (%)
Children underweight	50	56	49	31
Children stunted	63	51	51	16
Children wasted	17	15	9	NA
LBW babies (<2500 g)	30	50	33	18
Prevalence of vitamin A deficiency	0.70 Night blindness	0.78 Night blindness	0.33 Bitot's Spots	0.6 Bitot's Spots
Prevalence of iron deficiency – Anemia	56	73	78 School children	45 School children
Prevalence of iodine deficiency disorder	23–65	50	40 School children	14 School children
Exclusively breast fed up to 3rd month	51	54	36	24
Breast fed with complementary food (6–9 month)	31	30	80	60
Breast feeding until 20–23rd month	87	67	NA	66

India – India's National Family Health Survey (1992–93) found the prevalence of undernutrition to be very high in the Under Twos. The Survey found more than half (53%) of all children under the age of four to be underweight and a similar proportion (63%) to be stunted. 21–29% of children were severely undernourished according to weight-for-age and height-for-age measures. One in every six children was found to be excessively thin (wasted). It further documented that undernutrition varied substantially by the age of the child, being highest after first six months. Undernutrition was particularly high in Bihar and Uttar Pradesh, while the problem of wasting was most evident in Bihar and Orissa, which also have among the highest infant mortality rates in the country [5]. Recent NFHS-3 data on under-3 children also reveals 40.4% underweight, 44.9% stunted and 22.9% wasted [5a]. A study by Gopalan and coworkers nearly three decades ago, clearly showed that the greatest increase in height in a preschool child (1–5 years) was between the age of 1 and 2 years. It was much less thereafter [6].

Bangladesh [7] – Improper weaning practices were observed and labeled as a cause of early childhood malnutrition in Bangladesh. Too early commencement of complementary feeding (within a month of the child's birth) was also a problem. Semi-solid and solid food (mostly boiled rice) was given to all children by the time they were a year old – but in tiny amounts. The urban and rural poor were similar as regards prolonged breast feeding. But the urban poor gave more snacks, earlier supplements such as rice, extra milk, fish, egg and vegetables to the infant. More complementary food and a better level of hygiene improved their growth even under impoverished conditions. Apparently IEC alone did reduce malnutrition to some extent [8].

Nepal [7] – A Nepal nutrition survey clearly showed that the most critical age in the Nepali child's life was 12–23 months, when 80% were undernourished (weight for age), and 48% had a less than normal height for age [2]. Another study indicated that the prevalence of undernutrition in the under 2 was very high [9].

Sri Lanka [7] – In Sri Lanka about 25% of mothers in urban areas begin giving semisolid food after the fourth month as compared to 6% in rural areas. Solids such as "rusks" and "biscuits" are offered in significant amounts only after the child is six months old [10].

Malnutrition prevalence in children is lower in Sri Lanka than in other South Asian countries. Rural children have a better exclusive breastfeeding pattern compared to their urban counterparts. The "Thriposha" project which promotes a high protein fortified food began in 1972, in collaboration with CARE. Wheat from the PL480 programme was diverted to prepare a weaning food. "Thriposha" is a cereal-based weaning food for the undernourished preschool children, undernourished children in primary grades, anaemic, pregnant and lactating women and ward patients. "Thriposha" contains wheat-based products such as flour and wheat protein concentrate, defatted soy flour, refined soy oil, vitamins and minerals, a percentage of pre-cooked local cereal-based flour. The promotion and intensive coverage of the supplement could be a major task for health planners of Sri Lanka.

It can be seen from Table 9.2 that the child 1–3 years of age is most deficient in vitamin A, vitamin C, riboflavin, calcium, niacin, thiamine, energy protein of high biological value, and iron. Since the nutrients are available to the child from the staple cereal, much of the iron would not be available to the child [11]. Recent studies indicate that most South Asian children are deficient in zinc. The requirement is 5 mg/day [12].

Table 9.2 Average nutrient intake in Indian under-3 in India versus their RDA [6]

Age (years)	Energy (kcal)	Prot (g)	Ca (mg)	Fe (mg)	Vitamin A (μg)	Thaimin (mg)	B2 (mg)	Niacin (mg)	Vitamin C (mg)
1–3	908	23.7	256	10.2	117	0.52	0.37	5.55	14
RDA 1–3	1242	22.0	400	12.0	400	0.60	0.70	8.00	40
% of RDA 1–3	73%	108%	64%	85%	29%	87%	53%	69%	35%

In sum the child needs all the micronutrients (both micro and macro) to be provided in his complementary food.

9.2.2 Nutritional requirements for the under twos in South Asia

Recommended daily allowances (RDA) for the Indian child is viewed to be the most applicable for South Asia. The nutrient requirements for the infant (6–12 months) and children (1–3 years) as recommended by the Indian Council of Medical Research (ICMR), 1992 [13] is set out in Table 9.3.

The Dietary Guidelines for the infant (6–12 months) and the 1–3 year age group as per the National Institute of Nutrition (NIN), 1998, is reproduced in Table 9.4 [14]. It is evident from Table 9.4 that most of our rural, tribal and urban children aged 6–24 months are in no way fortunate enough to receive the balanced diet recommended by the National Institute of Nutrition (NIN). In North and West India the children under two receive miniscule amounts of *dal–roti* (pulse and wheat bread), while in South and East India they receive *rice–sambhar* or *dal* (pulse). The child, fortunately, is on breastmilk right into his third year. The National Family Health Survey found breastfeeding to be universal in India, with 95% of all children born in the 4 years preceding the survey having been breast fed. However, among children aged 6–9 months, less than one-third were receiving solid or mushy food (amount not specified) in addition to breast milk.

Table 9.3 Recommended daily allowances for the infant (6–12 months) and the child (1–3 years) [14]

Group	Infants	Children
Particulars	6–12 (months)	1–3 (years)
Body weight (kg)	8.6	12.2
Net energy (kcal/d)	843	1240
Protein (g/d)	14	22
Fat (g/d)	25	25
Calcium (mg/d)	500	400
Iron (mg/d)	12	12
Zinc (mg/d)	5	5
Vitamin A (μg/d)	350	400
β-Carotene (μg/d)	1200	1600
Thiamine (mg/d)	0.6	0.6
Riboflavin (mg/d)	0.7	0.7
Nicotinic acid (mg/d)	8.0	8.0
Pyridoxine (mg/d)	0.4	0.9
Ascorbic acid (mg/d)	25	40
Folic acid (μg/d)	25	30
Vitamin B12 (μg/d)	0.2	0.2–1.0

Table 9.4 Balanced diet for infants and children [14]

Food groups	Infants (6–12 months) Amount per day (g)	Children (1–3 years) Amount per day (g)
Cereals and millets	45	120
Pulses	15	30
Milk (ml)	500	500
Roots and tubers	50	50
Green leafy vegetables	25	50
Other vegetables	25	50
Fruits	100	100
Sugar	25	25
Fats/Oils (visible)	10	20

Note: Top milk of 200 ml has to be given even in case of breastfed infants.

Items listed in the National Institute of Nutrition (NIN), balanced diet for infants and young children such as top milk, roots and tubers, green leafy vegetables, fruits, fats and oils and sugar are luxuries beyond the means or comprehension of any typical rural or urban, poor Indian household. These expensive items of fruits, vegetables, milk and pluses are the dietary avenue to supply vitamins and minerals to the young child which almost all the low income group (LIG), or even middle-income group (MIG), urban or rural households cannot afford.

9.2.3 Role of complementary foods for the under 2

(i) *Importance of complementary feeding for the under 2* – Complementary nutrition is a nutritional intervention, which aims to make up for the deficit in the child's diet. The supplement provides the child with energy, proteins and micronutrients. Various nutritional programs have demonstrated the importance of complementary nutrition and the difference it has made to the nutritional status of the vulnerable age group.

Data from CARE-India's Project Poshak [15] revealed that

- The experimental group (6–11 months, 12–23 months, and 24–36 months), which received instant corn–soya–milk fully fortified with vitamins and minerals, significantly improved their nutrient intake status versus a matched control group.
- However, one could see glaring deficits in the control group relating to calories, vitamin C, calcium and iron in the infant (6–11 months). The deficit got accentuated with respect to calories, vitamin A and C, calcium and iron in the 12–23 month old child. This is because the volume of breast milk drops and the amount of complementary home diet is very meagre. Data show that the 2–3 year old child is able to fend for himself/herself better than the younger age groups as he/she is practically on the home diet. Great deficiencies in vitamin A and C persist [15]. Consequently most infants have to depend on fortified supplementary food to obtain their RDA of vitamins and minerals, at least partially. Every attempt should be made therefore to see that the complementary or supplementary food
- is fortified with 80–100% of the child's RDA, especially that of vitamin A, B–complex, vitamin C, iron, zinc;
- is low-bulk (soupy) yet high in nutrient density, so that the child can consume all or at least almost all of his/her ration in one sitting. Portion size is very important, especially for the intake of the micronutrients.

- and that the ration gets to the home of most children under two, through delivery channels such as take-home rations (THR) or take home delivery systems (THDS).
  (a) These three important conditions need to converge if children are to benefit from complementary food.
  (b) It is of utmost importance that policy makers, implementers and the public health and nutrition community recognize these facts.
  (c) It is unfortunate that not even nutritionists and dieticians have sufficiently realized that the consistency, nutrient-density and the amounts and infant can consume at a sitting vary enormously for a 6–9 months old; a 9–12 months old; a 12–15 months old infant till the child reaches his/her second birthday. *More operational research and field-testing need to be done in this area.*

(ii) *Timely complementary feeding rates in India* – The Indian National Family Health Survey (1992–93) revealed a wide range among the Indian states as to when food (liquid, semi solid or solid) was first introduced into the diet of an infant, 6–9 months of age. It ranged from a mere 9% in Rajasthan to relatively high 69% in Kerala. Recent NFHS-3 data also shows similar pattern with 31% 6–9 months introduced to semi-solids (Table 9.5). However, no nation-wide survey has been able to quantify the amount of complementary food given to the infant. Such a survey is urgently required to be conducted. (The results of the above survey are shown in Table 9.5).

Table 9.5 Timely complementary feeding rates (%) in Indian states [4]

State	Rate (%)
Rajasthan	9
Assam	39
Bihar	18
Orissa	30
West Bengal	54
Andhra Pradesh	48
Karnataka	38
Kerala	69
Tamil Nadu	57
Gujarat	23
Maharashtra	25
Uttar Pradesh	19
Madhya Pradesh	28
All India	31

Note: Amount of complementary food given is not stated.

9.3 Options for providing nutrition to overcome deficiencies

To restate from Section 9.2, it is seen that a complementary food for the under 2 has to be fully fortified; liquefied or drinkable in consistency; and readily available and affordable.

This section will address the importance of consistency of the complementary food under the following headings:

(1) Problem of feeding the under-2
(2) Concept of amylase-rich-food (ARF)
(3) Advantages of a fully micronutrient-fortified ready-to-eat (RTE) complementary food with ARF

9.3.1 Feeding the under-2

The vast majority of older infants (7–12 months) and young toddlers (13–24 months) in the developing world are chronically undernourished. Most of the undernutrition is associated with growth faltering that occurs in the so-called weaning period (6–24 months) [16]. This condition is associated with a high bulk, low energy diet [17], accompanied with bouts of diarrhoea contributed in large measure by the intake of contaminated left over foods [18]. The most common and first complementary foods to breast milk, which is fortunately one of the most energy and nutrient dense foods [19] are small amounts of soft boiled rice or mashed chapatti or bread or most commonly, viscous cereal gruels or preparations made from rice (Asia), sorghum, finger millet, maize, cassava and plantain (Africa); rice, wheat, millets, tapioca, potato (India) or sweet potato (Papua New Guinea) [20]. The problem is that most poor mothers make a 5% gruel (5 g of a staple cereal flour cooked in 100 ml of water), which becomes thick and voluminous on cooking due to gelatinization and water-binding capacity of the long chain carbohydrate component in the cereal flours. Such gruel would contribute a mere 20 cal/100 g gruel or it would have an extremely poor nutrient density whilst having a high dietary bulk [21]. Further, at 6 months, a child has a poor swallowing reflex and can consume only small portions of semi-solid preparations.

Hence, the dilemma is how to feed enough of the traditional gruel with a high energy density? How can one modify the form and texture of a solid or semisolid complementary preparation to a pour batter consistency? In fact, how can one literally ‘thin’ an extremely thick preparation and make it swallowable yet energy rich for the weaning child?

Table 9.6 Reduction in viscosity of 20% hot paste slurries with the addition of 0.8 g wheat ARF [24]

Hot paste slurries prepared with	Viscosity in centipoise units	
	Control gruel	Experimental gruel
Soya-fortified bulger wheat	22400	1210
Low-fat Marie biscuits	8100	2460
Medium-fat glucose biscuits	15200	5000
High-fat biscuits (salty)	3800	2520
Bread	9200	2360
Khichdi	18000	10700
Chapatti	14800	3600

Note: In all cases 20 g of the powdered material was cooked to boiling in 100 ml water. When ARF was added it was at the expense of the substrate powder.

9.3.2 Concept of amylase-rich-food (ARF)

The concept of amylase-rich-food or ARF [22] directly addresses the twin problems of dietary bulk and poor energy density of most weaning gruels of the poor. ARF is nothing but germinated cereal flours which are extremely rich in the enzyme alpha-amylase. Just tiny or catalytic amounts of any germinated cereal flour can instantly liquefy or reduce the dietary bulk of any viscous multimix gruel in which cereal flour is the main ingredient. The alpha-amylase cleaves the long carbohydrate chains in the cereal flour into shorter dextrins. However, for enzymatic action three conditions are required in the gruel or porridge, namely, it must be homogenous, it must be moist, and it must be hot (at least 70°C). Just half a flat teaspoon of any ARF can reduce even a very high solid concentration of 45 g made up of 25 g flour, 15 g sugar and 5 g oil cooked in 100 ml of water to soupy consistency. This remarkable property makes it possible to offer the child being introduced to semi solid food, a low viscosity yet high energy dense preparation from habitual ingredients that are used for young child feeding even in poor homes. ARF will act equally well on any gruel prepared from homogenized khichidi, or from chapatti, biscuit or bread powder, or soya-fortified bulgar–wheat powder. The single and unique contribution of ARF is that it can permit the mother to mix in much more flour into the gruel and consequently makes it high in energy density, yet low in viscosity and dietary bulk.

Germination of pulses and cereals are part and parcel of the culinary culture of Asia and Africa. ARF preparation is relatively simple as it is broadly based on germination. A small amount of any whole cereal grain (100 g or so) is steeped overnight in 2–3 times its volume of water, the excess water drained, and the moist swollen seeds germinated in a moist dark environment for 24–48 hours till the sprouts are evident. The further steps are sun-drying for 5–8 hours and lightly toasting the grains on a flat skillet to remove any surface moisture. The sprouts and the grains are milled or powdered. This is stored in an air-tight bottle or plastic container. This small amount of ARF for a cost of about 20–40 US cents, will suffice for one child's gruel for one month. It needs to be made also only once a month [23–27]. Summing up the advantages of ARF preparations are

- cheap cost;
- widely known and practiced household technology;
- small amounts to be made only intermittently, and;
- adaptability of making at the household, the community or even at the scaled-up commercial level.

In fact a barley malt, which sells from Rs. 30–40 per kg at current rates, can be directly purchased from beer breweries, and be milled and packaged into 5 g packets with or without the micronutrients, which the mother can buy [28–33]. However, individual packaging will increase costs. Germinated sorghum flour has been used for the same purpose in Tanzania.

9.3.3 Advantages of a fully micronutrient-fortified ready-to-eat (RTE) complementary food with ARF

As explained above, the transformation from a thick or pasty complementary food to a 'drinkable consistency' is the miracle of ARF. An infant/toddler (6–24 months) can easily consume 3–5 times of an isocaloric yet nutrient dense complementary food with ARF versus one without ARF (34–37). It stands to reason that unless the child consumes his/her entire ration of the complementary food, the vitamin and mineral fortificants will also go waste. The liquefied yet nutrient-dense complementary food, therefore becomes the conduit or channel to deliver the entire RDA of micronutrients to the infant and toddler.

9.4 Technology for development of premixes and complementary foods

The following four sub-sections address the issue of technology.

1. India's experience with making complementary foods in the seventies
2. India's expertise in the commercialization of these technologies at the present time
3. Major findings of the Baroda group (1980–1993) on the ARF technology
4. Baroda group's findings can be applied to move forward to the commercial production of appropriate RTE complementary foods and/or sprinklers/sachets that include micronutrients and ARF.

9.4.1 India's experience with making complementary foods in the seventies

In India the technology for preparing simple roasted mixtures from cereals, pulses, oilseeds and jaggery (brown sugar) or sugar has been formulated by many research groups for decades. Almost all have been field tested and were found to promote growth in the child. Many have found their way into community level or state level programmes (Table 9.7). However, the great lacunae in these early attempts at formulating these RTEs for infants, toddlers and preschool children were—

- The concept of ARF the 'liquefier' was not known.
- The mixes were solid. Hence, the most vulnerable under-1 could consume very little of his/her ration.
- None of them were fortified with vitamin–mineral premixes.

Table 9.7 Protein-enriched RTEs for infants, toddlers and preschool children at the community and industrial level [15]

Reference		Product	Ingredients
No.	Community level		
1	Pasricha et al (1973)	Ready-to-mix powder	60 g cereal (wheat, bajri or ragi) 15 g pulse (roasted Bengal gram), an oilseed and 40 g sugar/jaggery.
2	Devadas et al (1974)	Weaning mix	Cereal (cholam, ragi or maize), pulse (roasted green gram or Bengal gram dal), oil seed (roasted groundnut) and jaggery.
3	Gopaldas et al (1975)	Poshak (a)	Cereal (wheat, maize, rice or jowar), pulse (chana dal or mung dal), an oil seed (groundnut) and jaggery in the proportion of 4:2::1:2
		Poshak (b)	Same ingredients as Poshak (a) but in the proportion of 60:17:14:9 as per linear programming.
4	Chandrashekhara et al (1975)	Kerala indigenous food (KIF)	Tapioca rava, soya fortified bulgar wheat (SFBW) rava and groundnut flour.
5	ICMR (1975)	Ready-to-consume mixture	Roasted cereal (cholam, maize, ragi or bajra). Pulse (roasted or sprouted Bengal gram, green gram or fox gram), oil seed (groundnut, groundnut / sesame cake flour).

9.4.2 India's expertise in the commercialization of these technologies at the present time

In the last 10 years, India and other countries have advanced tremendously. Linear programming is used routinely for evolving nutritious low-cost complementary foods. It has the state-of-the art plants or factories in both the private and public sector with large capacities for making complementary or weaning foods. There are technologies such as extrusion; roller/drum drying; spray drying; addition of the entire or a large proportion of the RDA of vitamins–minerals requirements; and the ARF technology (Table 9.8). In additional, the technique of linear programming to obtain least cost multi-mixes to deliver a stated amount of energy and protein is also possible.

Table 9.8 Weaning food formulations developed in various countries [42]

Product	Country	Primary ingredients
Balanced malt food	India (CFTRI)	Cereal, malt, pulses, and skim milk powder
Bal-ahar (dry-blend)	India (FCI formulated by CFTRI)	Wheat flour, groundnut flour, Bengal gram flour and skim milk powder
Flakes (Macaroni process)	India (CFTRI)	Edible groundnut cake flour, Bengal gram flour, green gram flour, wheat flour
Precooked weaning food of different formulae (Roller dried)	India (CFTRI)	Cereal flours, pulses and oilseed cakes
Bal-Amul and Bal-Amul cereal with milk (Roller dried)	India (NDDB formulated by CFTRI)	Cereal flours, pulses, soya flour, skim milk powder
Nestum	India	Soyabean flour, milk powder
Farex	India (Glaxo)	Cereals and milk powder
Lactogen	India (Nestle)	Wheat flour, milk
Incaparina	Columbia	Maize flour, cottonseed flour, soyabean flour, vitamin A, calcium cabonate
Pronutro	S. Africa	Maize flour, soya, groundnut wheat germ, skim milk powder, fish flour
Corn soya milk	USA	Precooked maize, defatted soya flour, skim milk powder, $CaCO_3$, Vitamins
Caplapro	USA	De-germinated maize flour, wheat flour, soya flour, skim milk powder, $CaCO_3$, vitamins
Superasmine	Algeria and Turkey	Hard wheat flour, chick-pea lentil flour, skim milk powder, vitamins
Faffa	Ethiopia	Wheat flour, field pea flour, skim milk powder, chick-pea lentil
Duryea	Colombia	Defatted soya flour, high lysine corn flour, corn starch, milk powder, vitamins, minerals
Peruvita	Peru	Cottonseed flour, Quinoa flour, skim milk powder, sugar, spices, vitamins
Laubina	Beirut	Wheat, chick-pea, and skim milk powder

9.4.3 Major findings of the Baroda University group (1980–1993) on the ARF technology

Between 1980 and 1993, Baroda University established the following:

- Toddlers consumed significantly greater amounts of fully malted mixes of wheat flour, chickpea flour and powdered groundnut flour than equivalent amount of roasted mixes. However, the task of germinating, drying and powdering large quantities of cereal and pulses was cumbersome and laborious [31].

- Catalytic amounts of any germinated cereal grain (malt) powder, such as wheat, millet and barley, can liquefy virtually any cereal based viscous gruel. This is because of their high content of alpha-amylase, which has the power to break down starches into smaller units almost instantly at boiling temperatures. These malt powders were named Amylase-Rich-Food (ARF).
- By virtue of the drinkable consistency, a child could consume three to five times more of the treated food per sitting. Hence, the child received more food energy/nutrients [38, 22]. Traditional gruels were made more energy dense by cooking 40 g of staple flour +5 g of ARF +200 ml water. Toddlers were easily able to consume this amount, so obtaining 180 calories from a typical traditional gruel. Addition of oil and sugar raised the calorie intake to 200–250 Kcal / 200 ml [34].
- The addition of ARF to donated foods such as soya-fortified bulger–wheat powder significantly increased calorie density and intake in infants/toddlers 6–24 months old [26].
- Mothers in urban slums in the eighties were taught to make wheat ARF. They found the germination process laborious. However, they were more than willing to buy 5 g of ready-made ARF as an additive, even at Rs. 2/- per packet or Rs. 60/- per month. Nevertheless, they preferred to buy ARF – treated "fullfeed" packets of 50 g or 100 g for Rs. 3/- or Rs. 5/- each, respectively [39]. The cost would have doubled or tripled by 2009–10.
- ARF was found to liquefy khichadi (a boiled rice/lentil food), chapatti pieces soaked in water, corn–soya mix and soya-fortified bulger–wheat powders [40].
- In a controlled six month trial of infants and toddlers fed a high-energy, low-bulk gruel (with ARF) or an isocaloric high energy, high-bulk gruel (without ARF) in addition to their habitual home diet, intakes of the low-bulk gruel were significantly higher (91 ± 28 ml or 148 ± 46 kcal per ad-lib feed) than intakes of the high bulk gruel (26 ± 11 ml or 42 ± 18 kcal) [35]. Children on the low-bulk gruels also grew faster [36] (Figures 9.1 and 9.2).
- The ARF technology was very successful in nutritional rehabilitation [41]. A major breakthrough was achieved when commercial barley malt (CBM) powder was shown to have the most powerful ARF activity [42].

9.4.4 Application of Baroda University group's findings to commercial production of appropriate RTE complementary foods and/or sprinklers/sachets that include micronutrients and ARF

Liquefaction of complementary foods with ARF promises to be a valuable technology to reduce the burden of malnutrition in infants and toddlers in developing countries. In India, for example, parents from an enormous pool of increasingly mobile, low to middle income families are looking for moderately priced foods that they can buy on a regular and sustained basis. They currently buy expensive brands but feed them in very small quantities. There is a strong habit among most Indians to buy food commodities such as milk and condiments in small amounts for the day. Preliminary participatory research assessments in 2003 have shown that even low-income couples are earnings total incomes of Rs. 4000–5000 per month. They are more than prepared to pay Rs. 3–5 for a single feed of 50 g right through a child's weaning period (6–24 months). The concept of "sachets or sprinklers of CBM + the entire RDA of micronutrients" also appealed to them very much.

CBM can be sourced like any of the other ingredients in complementary foods in the open market or from the local liquor or malt food industry. In India, a good grade CBM costs about Rs. 30 per kg in 2003. In fact the fuel costs of extrusion can be greatly reduced if ARF is added to the slurry prior to extrusion as shown by Buffa in 1971 [43]. CBM sells at only 20 US cents per kg in USA; so USAID, CARE and WFP should seriously consider sourcing this food commodity in addition to soya oil, CSB and SFBW. The government-run ICDS weaning food plants would only require 2000 tonnes of CBM for the 100,000 tonnes of complementary food they produce per annum. The ARF can be blended or mixed into the complementary food with the vitamin–mineral mix at the last stage of processing.

The question might be posed as to why more research with commercial barley malt ARF is needed? There are cogent reasons for large multi-country operational research studies in South Asia as under:

- Commercial barley malt is by far the most powerful ARF that has been tested. Just 5% CBM can liquefy a ready-to-eat ration (50 g in 100 ml boiling water) which wheat ARF cannot do. Hence, a 50 g complementary food in 100 ml of water can delivery an extra 200 kcal + 6 g protein.
- An infant or toddler can easily consume about 100 ml of ARF – treated complementary feed at one sitting.
- A low-bulk or "drinkable" feed fortified with the child's entire RDA of micronutrients (Table 9.9) would also improve the child's micronutrient and nutritional status.
- The concept of a measurable and adequate amount of complementary feed could be introduced through the concept of a daily 50 g packet per day. The concept of "protein size" and hygiene could be introduced through the "daily packed ration". Since the entire amount can be consumed at one sitting, much of the problem of microbial contamination will not arise.
- Extrusion and individual packing are recommended to ensure a shelf

life of more than a year. Simple roasted mixes have a shelf-life of only 3–4 months.

- Rice and green gram are accepted all over South Asia as being the most digestible cereals for the infant.
- The economic position of the low-income group is much better now. Their expectations are higher. They are prepared to pay for their child's nutrition and health, provided such complementary food packets or sachets are affordable and easily available.

The concept could be extended to any population or condition requiring a high-energy, low-bulk food (e.g. geriatrics, tubal feeding, refugee, burn cases, HIV/AIDS, feedings, pregnancy, etc). What is now needed is an organization or company that is ready to take this initiative and bring the technology to a level that will allow this complementary food to be produced commercially.

9.5 Mechanisms to improve acceptability, palatability, utilization and outreach of the donated complementary food in the public sector

Corn–Soya–Blend (CSB) is a food that is widely donated in all the four countries under review to the public sector. Based on a review by CARE – India [45], the following issues are addressed.

(1) Improving acceptability of CSB which is fully fortified with the micronutrients;
(2) Improving palatability of cooked CSB rations;
(3) Improving utilization of CSB;
(4) and Improving outreach of donated foods.

9.5.1 Improving acceptability of CSB

CARE – India in the past supplies corn–soya–blend (CSB) and soya oil (SO) to India's Integrated Child Development Services (ICDS) programme. Table 9.9 depicts the percentage contribution of a single ration of 65 g CSB + 8 g soya oil to the RDA of a child under-2 years of age.

Assuming the child 6–24 months consumes his/her entire ration, this would satisfy the Government of India's (GoI) requirements of delivering 300 kcal and 12 g protein per child per feeding day and address the nutrient gap of calories in their usual diet. However, the nutritional gap in vitamins and minerals remains.

1. CSB + soya oil are excellent complementary foods. The only problem with the CSB is that it is gritty or grainy in texture. When cooked –

Table 9.9 Nutrient value of CSB and oil [45]

65 g ration of CSB + 8 g of oil	Nutrient value	Percentage RDA
Food energy	319 kcal	26
Protein	11.7 g	53
Vitamin A	1105 IU	69
Riboflavin	0.33 mg	47
Folic acid	13.00 mg	43
Vitamin C	26.00 mg	65
Calcium	520.00 mg	130
Iron	11.70 mg	98
Zinc	1.95 mg	39
Iodine	32.50 ppm	108

it becomes pasty and non-homogenous to the touch and taste. It is not appropriate for the early infant or even the late infant. Due to its bulk and pastiness, the 'Below 2' cannot eat his full ration. Further, children upto one year of age, and evens upto two, have a poor swallowing reflex and are slow feeders. Hence, feeds that are nutrient dense but 'liquidy' go down faster, without spillage or waste. There are many options to enhance its acceptability.

- Fine grind it.
- Extrude CSB rather than roast it. Extrusion will powder the product and will thoroughly cook it.
- Blend in Soya oil, extra vitamins, minerals and 5% CBM. This should be done at the final stage.

All these processing actions can be done at the manufacturing end and the specially processed food can be separately bagged and demarcated for children under-2.

2. If this not possible, the composition of the RTE complementary food, which is usually sweetened with sugar (25%), can be slightly modified as under. Five percent of the sugar can be replaced by 5% of CBM. The entire micronutrient RDA of a 1-year-old Indian child [13] or 80% of it should also be incorporated into the RTE.
3. Project Poshak [15] noted that most Indians like a fried/roasted/caramelized smell and flavour. If within manufacturing and/or processing costs, the addition of a synthetic smell/flavour could be considered.
4. Another study reports that about half the mothers in Uttar Pradesh, India felt that the CSB-RTE was not suitable for the 'Below Two'. The RTE had to be made semi-solid with milk or water. They felt the dry RTE choked the young child. However, the CSB – RTE in a semi solid gruel, halwa or dalia form was suitable [44].
5. The concept of 'hot' and 'cold' foods are firmly entrenched in most rural and tribal populations. For instance, especially in Madhya Pradesh and Uttar Pradesh home diets made out of wheat, ghee, milk, jaggery and pulses, all considered 'hot' would be appropriate for the

cold and rainy seasons. Whereas rice, curd, lassi, groundnuts and sugar (cold foods) could be fed to the child in summer. CSB/oil recipes and ingredients likewise could be adapted to the seasons [45].

9.5.2 Improving the palatability of the cooked CSB rations

1. The Regional Profile for 'Malnutrition in South Asia', UNICEF, 1997 strongly recommends the use of the ARF technology as a manageable, practical and traditional technology to increase the energy intake of traditional low energy-gruels [7]. We would go a step further and strongly endorse the adoption of the 'ARF Technology' for the immediate improvement of the CSB–THR ration [46]. CSB–THR rations without ARF are extremely bulky and pasty. Hence, the THR with ARF becomes smooth and semi liquid while retaining all its good nutrition.
2. For the 'Below Twos', especially the 'Below Ones', it is the consistency and texture of the complementary food that are of paramount importance. Most Indian mothers like a caramelized or roasted taste and flavouring. Both the mothers and the babies like it sweet. Intakes by children definitely are better with a sweet tasting preparation.
3. Sweet tasting or 'liquidy' dalia, rabadi or kheer recipes would be most suitable for the early-infant in Madhya Pradesh and Uttar Pradesh. It would be the payasam (milky sweet porridge) counterpart in Andhra Pradesh.
4. The older child (1–2 years) may like laddu (solid sweet made from gram flour ghee, sugar and special spices) which the mother can make by roasting the grainy CSB in the Soya-oil, add some jaggery and fashioning into laddus, halwa, sattu or prashad. Salty preparations would be chappati, paratha, dosai or uppumav. Our interactions with the mothers in Uttar Pradesh (particularly in Uttar Pradesh), Madhya Pradesh & Andhra Pradesh showed that most of the mothers generally wanted to cook only twice (morning and evening) perhaps due to fuel and time constraints. They usually chose to make the same dish that was most convenient for them to make, for instance, chapatti (unleavened bread) in Uttar Pradesh and Madhya Pradesh and uppumav (snack made from broken rice) in Andhra Pradesh. Even sweetening the CSM with jaggery or sugar was a special treat. In short, the mothers were not enterprising about varying the CBM–oil recipes for the 'Below Twos'.

9.5.3 Improving the palatability of cooked CSB rations

Although there is clear evidence that the THR has reached the homes of the 'Below Twos', it is still a question mark as to how much of the THR gets into the stomachs of the 'Below Two'. This is the current problem. There is a lack of sufficient appreciation among all concerned, namely, the policy makers, the bureaucrats, the community and the mothers, that unless a major portion of the THR s fed to the intended 'Below Two', he/she will not improve in weight or health. At the moment, about a fourth to a third of the ration may be consumed by the 'Below Two', while the rest is consumed by other siblings and the family.

Possible solutions are

1. The concept of a full THR for the 'Below Two' has to be actively promoted by the implementing staff, health staff, panchayat, village health practitioners, village school teachers, change agents and adolescent girls and boys.
2. Change Agents, and adolescent girls/boys can advice and ensure that the THR is given to the 'Below Two', when the 'Above Two' is at the aanganwadi. This will greatly minimize sharing.
3. On the nutrition health days, repeated cooking demonstration or 'demos' of the cooked up THR may be done. A single demonstration 'baby' of 6, 9, 12 months can be fed in front of the mother group. They will then learn two important facts:
   (a) The amount that can be consumed by the infant;
   (b) The amount consumed per sitting will increase with age. Even a few months difference in age would make a big difference in consumption. Probably by 18 months, the entire THR ration would be consumed by the child at a sitting.
4. Mothers can be requested to bring their own small bowls or tumblers. These can be calibrated for CSB and oil single rations.

9.5.4 Improve the outreach of supplementary foods for under twos

The Planning Evaluation Organization (PEO), 1976, [47] and the Integrated Child Development Services (ICDS) National Evaluation in 1992 [48], pointed out that children under three could not reach the ICDS or aganwadi centre (AWC). Project Poshak in MP, 1975 [15], also showed that the children below three could not be transported every day to a feeding center for spot feeding. The problem is even more accentuated for the 'Under Two' especially in scattered tribal hamlets, hilly areas or even within a village. CARE – India's baseline survey, 1997 reported that 40% children under-2 years of age were brought to the AWC in the past one week for spot feeding, a figure often grossly over-reported by the AWC workers [49].

Possible solutions are

1. The product should be 'THR' especially for the 'Below Twos'. THR has to be appropriate and demarcated for the 'Below Twos'.

2. THR product should be made attractive and meaningful to the mothers in order that they come regularly to collect the THR for the 'Below Twos'.
3. CARE – India has shown the way by organizing Integrated Nutrition Health Programme (INHP) Days, where both the functionaries of the ICDS (AWW and Supervisors) and Health (ANM) are present. The 'Below Twos' are weighed and the THRs distributed. Mothers willingly help and participate. This is an excellent mechanism and strategy that can be taken up by the entire National ICDS.
4. Possible areas that can be strengthened are counseling on the child's weight 6–9 m, 9–12 m, 12–15 m and so on. The Nutrition and Health staff as well as the mothers will realize how much a cooked portion of a single ration will be and how much of this an infant of a specific age group can consume over a reasonable period of time (say 20 minutes). This is the kind of practical and visual education that will immediately communicate to both ICDS staff and mothers.
5. It would be useful if the NH days are held every 15 days rather than every month. One of the NH days should be exclusively for the 'Below Twos' and one exclusively for her mothers (P & L). The village elders and members of the village panchayat should be encouraged to participate and get actively involved.
6. The strategy of change agents to ensure that the services of ICDS are understood by all; and to roundup all the 'Below Twos', and their mothers is an excellent strategy for outreach. It could be universalized in the ICDS.
7. The setting up of 'seasonal crèches' and enhancing the THR may be considered for both mothers and child beneficiaries. Since, mothers will have to stay back on NH day(s), some monetary compensation for doing so may be considered by the village panchayat.

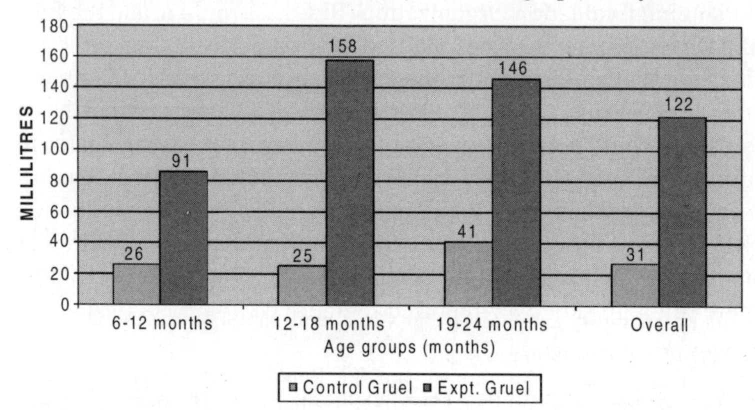

9.1 Mean intake of control and experimental gruels by different age groups for a feeding trial period of 180 days [35].

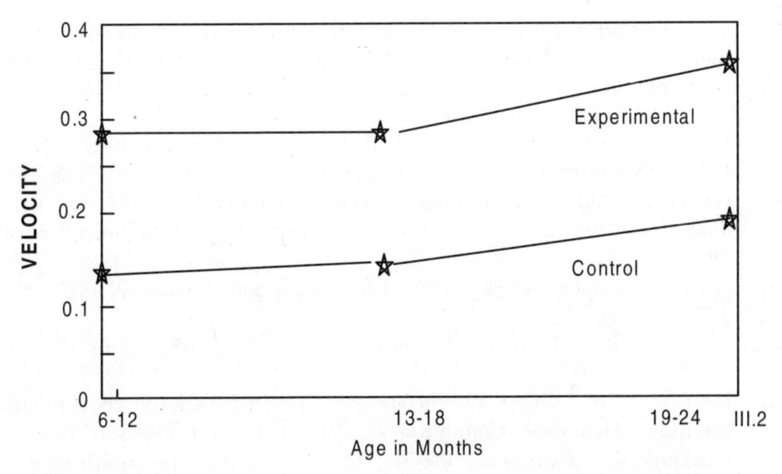

9.2 Growth velocity of children on control and experimental gruels by different age groups for a feeding trial period of 180 days [36].

References

1. Nutrition and Poverty: Papers from the ACC/SCN, 24th Session symposium, Kathmandu, Nepal, March 1997.
2. Nutrition in South East Asia: World Health Organization Regional Office for South-East Asia, New Delhi, 1999.
3. Malnutrition in South Asia: A Regional Profile. UNICEF Regional Office for South Asia, 1997.
4. Complementary Feeding of Young Children in Developing Countries: a review of current scientific knowledge WHO, Geneva, 1998.
5. The National Family Health Survey (MCH and Family Planning), India: Report of the International Institute for Population Science, Bombay, India, 1992–93.
6. GOPALAN C, SWAMINATHAN MC, KRISHNA KUMARI VK, HANUMANTARAO D., VIJAYARAGHAVAN K (1973). Effect of calorie supplementation on growth of undernourished children. *Am J Clin Nutr* vol. 26, pp. 563–566.
7. ROY SK (1997). Complementary feeding in South Asia, in malnutrition in South Asia: A regional profile, pp. 51–73.
8. BROWN LV et al (1992). Evaluation of the impact of weaning food messages on infants feeding practices and child growth in rural Bangladesh. *Am J Clin Nutr* vol. 56, pp. 994–1003.
9. MORTORELL R, LESLIE J, MOOK PR (1984). Characteristics and determinants of child nutritional status in Nepal. *Am J Clin Nutr* vol. 39, pp. 74–86.
10. SOYSA P and SENNAYEKE M (1985). The Introduction of a low-cost weaning food, its acceptability and effectiveness in a well-baby clinic. Ceylon J (ed). *Child Health* vol. 14, pp. 21–26.
11. National Nutrition Monitoring Bureau: Report on the Repeat Survey (1988–90). National Institute of Nutrition, Indian Council of Medical Research, Hyderabad, 1991.

12. SAZAWAL S. et al (1998). Zinc supplementation in young children with acute diorrehea in India. *New England Journal of Medicine* vol. 333, pp. 839–844.
13. Nutrient requirements and recommended dietary allowances for Indians (1992). *The Indian Council of Medical Research*, New Delhi.
14. Dietary Guidelines for Indians – A Manual: The National Institute of Nutrition, Indian Council of Medical Research, 1998.
15. GOPALDAS T, SRINIVASAN N, VARADARAJAN I, SHINGWEKAR AG, SETH R, MATHUR RS, BHARGAVA V: *Project Poshak*, pp. 73, vol. 1, printed by CARE-India, New Delhi, 1975.
16. WATERLOW J and PAYNE PR (1985). The protein gap. *Nature* vol. 258, pp. 113–117.
17. NICOL BM (1971). Protein and calorie concentration. *Nutr Rev* vol. 129, pp. 83–88.
18. ROWLAND MGM, BARRELL R, WHITEHEAD RG (1978). Bacterial contamination in traditional Gambian weaning foods. *Lancet* vol. 1, pp. 136–138.
19. CAMERON M, HOFVANDER Y (1971). Manual on feeding infants and young children. New York: United Nations, p. 73.
20. ALNWICK D, MOSES S, SCHMIDT OG (1987). Improving young child feeding in Eastern and Southern Africa. Canada International Development Research Center, pp. 1–380.
21. MELLANDER O, SWANBERG U (1984). Compact calories, malting and young child feeding. In: Advances in International, Maternal and Child Health. Jelliffe DB, Jelliffe EEP (eds). Oxford: Clarendan Press, pp. 84–85.
22. GOPALDAS T, MEHTA P, PATIL A, GANDHI H (1986). Studies on reduction in viscosity of thick rice gruels with small quantities of an amylase rich cereal malt. *UNU Food Nutr Bull* vol. 8, pp. 42–47.
23. GOPALDAS T, MEHTA P, JOHN C (1987). Bulk reduction of traditional gruels in: Improving Young Child Feeding in Eastern and Southern Africa. Alnwick D, Moses S, Schmidt OG (eds). Canada: International Development Research Centre, vol. 1987, pp. 330–339.
24. GOPALDAS T (1988). Simple traditional methods for reducing the dietary bulk of cereal based diets in rural homes. Proceedings of the 20th Annual Meeting of the Nutrition Society of India, pp. 73–84.
25. GOPALDAS T, DESHPANDE S, JOHN C (1988). Studies on a wheat amylase-rich-food (ARF), *UNU Food Nutr Bull* vol. 10, pp. 50–54.
26. JOHN C, GOPALDAS T (1988). Studies on reduction in dietary bulk of soya fortified bulger wheat gruels with amylase rich food. *UNU Food Nutr Bull* vol. 10, pp. 1–7.
27. DESHPANDE S, NISAR SR, GOPALDAS T (1990). A technology to improve the viscosity, texture and energy density of commercial weaning foods. Abstracts 27th National Conference of Indian Academy of Pediatrics, 1990.
28. MOSHA AC and SVANBERG U (1983). Preparation of weaning foods with high nutrient density using flour of germinated cereals. *UNU Foods Nutr Bull* vol. 5, pp. 10–14.
29. DESIKACHAR HSR (1980). Development of weaning foods with high calorie density and low hot paste viscosity using traditional technologies. *UNU Foods Nutr Bull* vol. 2, pp. 21–23.
30. BRANDTZAEG B, MALLESHI NG, SVANBERG U, DESIKACHAR HSR, MELLANDER O (1981). Dietary bulk as a limiting factor for nutrient intake in pre-school children. III

Studies of malted flour from ragi, sorghum and green gram. *J Trop Pediatr* vol. 27, pp. 184–189.

31. GOPALDAS T, INAMDAR F, PATEL JB (1982). Malted versus roasted young child mixes: viscosity, storage and acceptability trials. *Indian J Nutr Dietet* vol. 19, pp. 327–336.
32. GOPALDAS T (1990). The ARF story. A compendium of research of amylase-rich-food. National/International Workshop on ARF Technology, Baroda, p. 12.
33. GOPALDAS T (1998). Fighting Infant Malnutrition with amylase complementary foods. *Nutriview Issue* vol. 2, pp. 2–4.
34. GOPALDAS T (1991). Technologies to improve weaning food in developing countries. Editorial, *Indian Paediatrics* vol. 28, p. 217.
35. GOPALDAS T and JOHN C (1993). Evaluation of a controlled six months feeding trial on intake by infants and toddlers fed a high-energy, low bulk gruel. *J Trop Paediatr* vol. 38, pp. 278–283.
36. JOHN C and GOPALDAS T (1993). Evaluation of the impact on growth of a controlled six months feeding trial on children (6–24 months) fed a complementary food of a high energy, low bulk gruel in addition to their habitual home diet. *J Trop Paediatr* vol. 39, pp. 16–22.
37. GOPALDAS T (1992). Amylase reactive foods in the Improvement of Young Child. *Diets Proc Nutr Soc*, India.
38. GOPALDAS T (1984). Malted versus roasted weaning mixes. Development, storage, acceptability and growth trials. In: Interfaces between Agriculture, Nutrition and Food Science. KT Acharya (ed). *UNU Food Nutr Bull* Suppl vol. 9, pp. 293–307.
39. GOPALDAS T, DESHPANDE S, VAISHNAV U et al (1991). The transfer of a simple dietary bulk reduction technology of weaning gruels by amylase-rich foods (ARFs) from laboratory to urban slum. *UNU Food Nutr Bull* vol. 13, pp. 318–321.
40. GOPALDAS T (1988). Simple traditional methods for reducing dietary bulk of cereal based diets in rural homes. *Proc Nutr Soc India* vol. 34, pp. 73–84.
41. TAJJUDDIN KM (1990). Studies on nutritional rehabilitation with ARF. Unpublished PhD results.
42. MUJOO R (1993). Studies on commercial barley malt. Unpublished PhD results, 1993.
43. BUFFA A (1971). Food Technology and Development, Part I. Processing low-cost nutritious foods for the world's hungry children. Factors, formulas, processes. *Food Engineering*, pp. 79–106.
44. Consultancy Report by IESSCO Pvt. Ltd., on Uttar Pradesh, India's RTE, Cited as an Appendix in Reference; Pillai G, CARE – India's Integrated Nutrition and Health Programme, 1995–2000.
45. GOPALDAS T and SUNDER G (1998). Addressing Nutritional gaps in Children Under Two in Rural India. Working Paper for CARE – India, 1998.
46. PILLAI G. CARE – India's Integrated Nutrition and Health Programme 1995–2000.
47. Planning Commission Evaluation Report on the ICDSA 1976–78: New Delhi, Planning Evaluation Organization, New Delhi, 1982.
48. National Evaluation of the ICDS: National Institute of Public Cooperation and Child Development, New Delhi, 1992.
49. JOHRI N (1998). CARE – India's INHP Results Reports. Achievements versus plans (FY 1997 Vs FY 1996).

10 Diarrhea and undernutrition

Shariqua Yunus

Shariqua Yunus, MBBS, MD, is currently working as Program Officer (Health and Nutrition) at the United Nation World Food Program (WFP). Prior to this, Dr. Yunus was working with WHO as their focal point for nutrition in India (2006–2009). Her areas of interest include role of nutrition in HIV and AIDS, nutrition in emergencies, community-based management of malnutrition and nutrition in relation to non-communicable disease.

10.1 Introduction

Diarrheal diseases and malnutrition are common in children of developing countries and an interaction between diarrhea and undernutrition has been well established. Undernutrition is the underlying cause of thirty-five percent of global childhood deaths [1]. Diarrhea is one of the primary cause of poor nutrition in the under five children. It is estimated that "the total number of deaths caused directly and indirectly by malnutrition induced by safe water, inadequate sanitation and insufficient hygiene is therefore 860,000 deaths per year in children under five years of age" [1]. Globally improving water, sanitation and hygiene could prevent at least 9.1% of the DALYs (disability adjusted life years – a weighted measure of deaths and disability) or disease burden or 6.3% of all deaths. In developing countries the consequences of unsafe water, inadequate sanitation or insufficient hygiene impact on nutritional status of children.

10.2 Definition of diarrhea

Diarrhea is defined as the passage of loose, liquid or watery stools. However, it is the recent change in consistency and character of stools rather than the number of stools that is more important.

Infants, particularly those who are on breast feeds, during the initial 2–3 months of life may pass many "pasty" or semi-formed stools daily; if they are gaining adequate weight, this should not be considered diarrhea. Again, a recent change in character of stools is more important.

Mothers usually know when their children have diarrhea and often have a local word for diarrhea. In developing countries, diarrhea is common during infancy – the period of accelerated growth. For e.g. in India, the highest prevalence of 18.1% is reported in the age group of 6–11 months [2].

10.3 Types of diarrhea

Acute diarrhea – it is an attack of sudden onset, which usually lasts 3–7 days, but may last up to 10–14 days. It is caused by an infection of the bowel. Only 3–12 percent of acute diarrhea episodes last beyond two weeks. For the purposes of this chapter, we will be considering diarrhea as acute diarrhea.

Chronic/persistent – A diarrheal episode which lasts for more than 14 days is a chronic episode. The delineation of persistent diarrhea as a sub group distinct from acute diarrhea is, as such, arbitrary as the duration of acute diarrhea forms a continuum. Though the cut-off of 14 days for defining persistent diarrhea is illogical but is supported by observations of a significantly high case fatality rate when diarrhoea extends for two or more weeks. A proportion of persistent episodes are associated with growth failure. The persistent episodes with inadequate weight gain or loss of weight are termed prolonged 'malnourishing diarrhea'. It is these cases that have the greatest clinical significance and require careful management.

Acute diarrheal episodes may become chronic because of (i) persistent colonization of upper small intestines by microbes; (ii) dietary allergies; (iii) carbohydrate intolerance because of damage to the brush border of intestinal mucosa, resulting in low levels of disaccharidases; (iv) infants and children with decreased host immunity such as after an attack of measles or delayed repair of intestinal damage due to associated protein –energy malnutrition with increase in being prone to retracted diarrhea (younger infants who are weaned very early develop intolerance to food proteins such as cow's milk or even soya milk); (v) poor personal hygiene and environmental or food contamination may lead to recurrent intestinal infections before the infant recovers from a previous episode; (vi) protozoal infections *Giardia lamblia* or *Entamoeba histolytica*; and (vii) inadequate treatment of acute diarrhea is another important cause.

Dysentery – The clinical syndrome of dysentery is characterized by the presence of blood and pus in the stools, abdominal cramps and fever. Gross blood in stools is the most reliable sign; its presence facilitates early recognition by the mother and the health worker and identifies a clinically severe form of the disease.

10.4 Causes of diarrhea

Agent factors – In developing countries, diarrhea is almost universally infectious in origin. A wide assortment of organisms cause acute diarrhea and many of them have been discovered only in recent years (Table 10.1). The rotavirus has emerged as the single most important cause of diarrhea in infants and children. Nearly all children are infected with rotavirus once before the age of 2 years. Viruses are probably responsible for about one-half of all diarrheal diseases in children aged up to 2 years.

Table 10.1 Pathogens frequently identified in children with acute diarrhea in treatment centers in developing countries [3]

Pathogen		% of cases
Viruses	Rotavirus	15–25
Bacteria	Enterotoxigenic	
	• *Escherichia coli*	10–20
	Shigella	5–15
	• *Campylobacter Jejuni*	10–15
	• *Vibrio cholerae*	5–10
	• *Salmonella (non-typhoid)*	1–5
	Enteropathogenic	1–5
	• *Escherichia coli*	
Protozoans	*Crytosporidium*	5–15
No pathogen found		20–30

Environmental factors – Environmental factors is the major contributory cause of the disease (Figure 10.1) and pertains to mainly ingestion of pathogens, especially in unsafe drinking water, in contaminated food or from unclean hands (Figure 10.1). Inadequate sanitation and insufficient hygiene promote the transmission of these pathogens. Unsafe water, inadequate sanitation or insufficient hygiene contributes to 88% of cases of diarrhea worldwide [1, 4]. These cases results in 1.5 million deaths each year, most being deaths of children. In India, 0.4 million deaths and 13.6 million DALYS lost on account of diarrhea are attributable to lack of safe water, sanitation and hygiene [1]. The category 'diarrhea' includes some more diseases, such as cholera, typhoid and dysentery-all of which have related 'faecal-oral' transmission pathways.

10.5 Diarrhea, morbidity, malnutrition and mortality

Diarrhea is a major public health problem and also a leading cause of morbidity, malnutrition and mortality in the developing countries. Diarrheal diseases contribute the highest fraction of the total global burden of disease in DALYs among diseases with the largest water, sanitation and hygiene contribution (Figure 10.2). Contribution of diarrheal diseases is 39 percent to the water sanitation hygiene related disease burden (Figure 10.3).

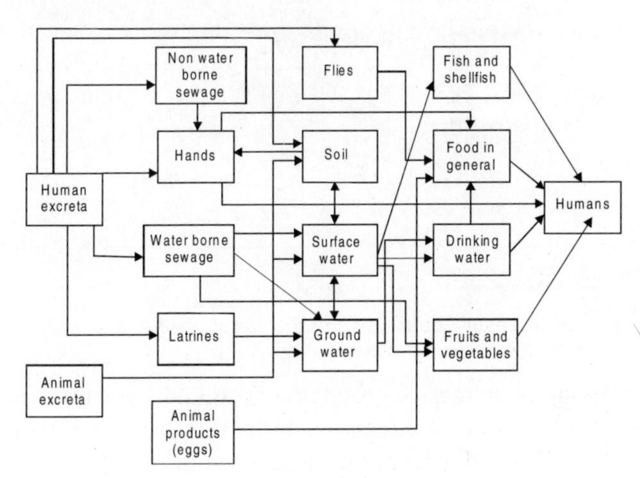

10.1 Faecal–Oral Transmission Pathways [1].

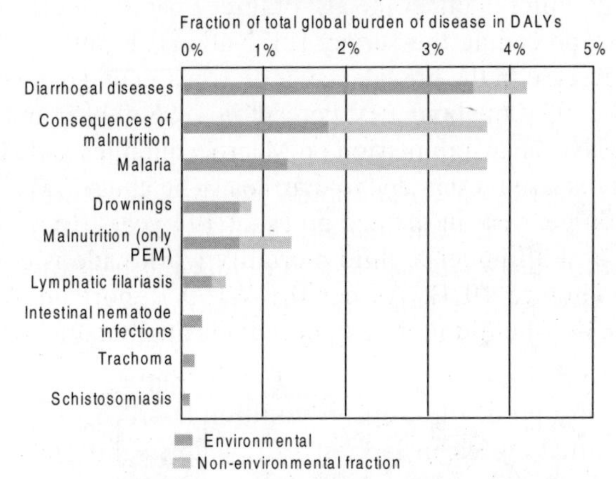

DALY: disability-adjusted life year (which measures the years of life lost to premature mortality and the year lost to disability); PEM: protein-energy malnutrition (which is malnutrition that develops in adults and children whose consumption of protein and energy is insufficient to satisfy the body's nutritional needs).

10.2 Diseases with the largest water, sanitation and hygiene contribution, year 2002 [1].

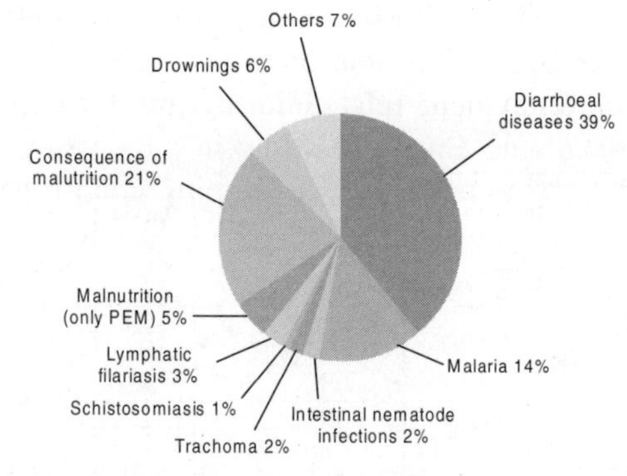

10.3 Diseases contributing to the water, sanitation and hygiene related disease burden [1].

Children belonging to the age group of 0–59 months are most susceptible to diarrhea and other kinds of infections. In India, 9 percent of under-5 year children are found to suffer from diarrhea. A child in India suffers, on an average, 10–15 episodes of diarrhea in the first five years of life. Of these, three to five episodes occur in the first two years of life. Overall, children are ill with diarrhea for 10–20 percent of their first 3 years of life. About 12.1 percent of children under the age of three years suffer from diarrhea in the two weeks preceding the survey [2]. National Health Survey of India indicates a decrease in the prevalence of diarrhea in under-5 years between 1998–99 and 2005–06; about 19.2 percent in 1998–99 [5] and 9 percent in 2005–06 [2]. National Commission on Macroeconomics and Health (2005) estimates the disease burden due to diarrhea to be about 760 cases per 100, 000 population per year in the age group of 1–4 years [6].

About 17% of all under-5 child mortality worldwide is contributed by diarrhea [7] (Figure 10.4). As per the WHO Report on World Health Statistics, 20.3% of child mortality in India is attributable to diarrhea [8].

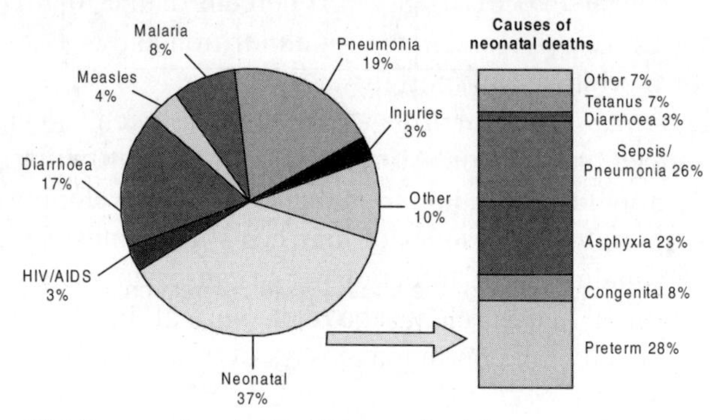

10.4 Causes of under-5 child mortality [7].

A meta-analysis review of child morality due to diarrhea in the developing countries placed global deaths from diarrhea in children under five years of age at 1.87 million; which is 19% of the total child deaths [9]. WHO African and South East Asia regions account for 78% of all diarrhea deaths occurring among children in the developing world; 73% of these are concentrated in just 15 developing countries (Figure 10.5).

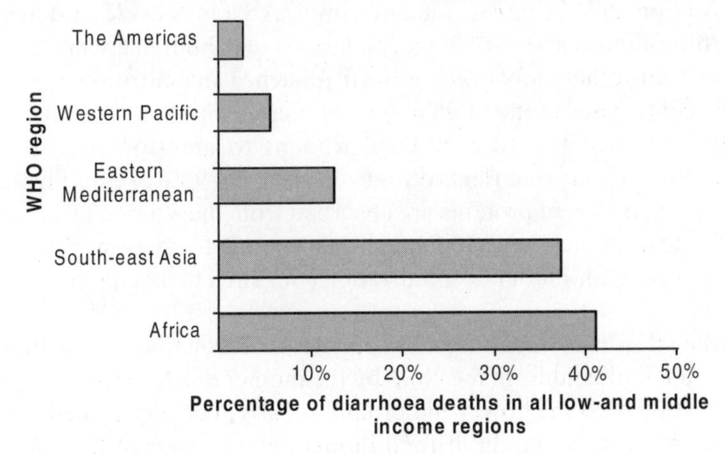

10.5 Distribution of deaths due to diarrhea in five WHO low- and middle-income regions [9].

The two main dangers of diarrhea are malnutrition and death. The more common cause of diarrhea related deaths is dehydration but a substantial proportion of such deaths occur as a result of malnutrition consequent to a series of diarrheal episodes of varying length and severity. Equally important causes of death are dysentery and prolonged malnourishing diarrhea resulting in malnutrition. Diarrhea is rightly referred to as a nutritional disease, because malnutrition is associated with nearly two-thirds of diarrhea-related deaths.

Acute diarrheal diseases contribute to growth retardation in patients. Persistent Diarrhea (PD) exists in 3–20 percent of the total episodes of diarrhea [10]. It leads to worsening of malnutrition and is associated with a high risk of morbidity and mortality.

Role of diarrhea in malnutrition – Diarrhea has been shown to have a significant impact on nutrition. Most field studies identify diarrhea as the major determining factor leading to malnutrition in developing countries.

A child with multiple episodes of diarrhea suffers most severely from protein–energy malnutrition. Infection per se causes excessive catabolism and increases energy requirements above the normal. In addition, diarrhea is further associated with continuous losses of nutrients from the body in the form of stools.

Even a brief episode of diarrhea leads to loss of 1–2 percent of body weight per day. Infants and young children in developing countries are sick for about 10 percent of the time (or nearly 30 days per year) with diarrheal illnesses. Thus, over the time, even the slow and continuous deficit associated with mild illness can accumulate to become a major nutritional deficiency.

Atrophy of the intestinal epithelium in cases of malnutrition causes malabsorption and accentuates malnutrition. A vicious cycle of diarrhea-malnutrition-diarrhea sets in. Since, malnourished children are more prone to suffer from other infections as well; diarrhea malnutrition symptom complex contributes to the large majority of early childhood deaths either directly or indirectly. It would be prudent to mention that despite malabsorption of macronutrients during diarrhea, 80–90% of carbohydrates, 70% of fats and 75% of proteins are absorbed from diets based on common foods. Recent studies have indicated that enteral feeding may result in faster recovery with shorter hospitalization compared to parenteral nutrition [10].

Diarrhea results in impairment of appetite. Additionally, during diarrhea food is often withheld from the child by the mother due to erroneous belief that starvation rests the bowel and promotes early recovery from diarrhea. The practice of withholding of food in fact delays repair of the damaged intestinal lining and return of the ability to produce digestive enzymes. Many a times, the need for continued feeding during diarrhea or on correcting faulty feeding practice prior to illness is not appreciated by medical practitioners and not advised.

10.6 Management of diarrhea

There are three essential elements in the management of diarrhea in children namely, rehydration therapy, zinc supplementation and continued feeding.

10.6.1 Rehydration therapy

During diarrhea, there is an increased loss of water and electrolytes in the liquid stool. Dehydration occurs when these losses are not adequately replaced and a deficit of water and electrolytes develops. The degree of dehydration is graded according to symptoms and signs that reflect the amount of fluid lost.

Oral Rehydration Therapy (ORT) is at the core of management of diarrhea. The term ORT includes complete oral rehydration salts (ORS) solution with composition within the WHO recommended range (Table 10.2), as well as solutions made from sugar and salt, food based solutions and home available fluids (HAF) without insisting on inclusion of both glucose precursor and salt or their presence in specified amounts. It is imperative to stress upon the use of safe and clean water for purposes of preparing the oral rehydration solution.

Table 10.2 Composition of the new ORS formulation [11]

New ORS	grams/litre	Percentage	New ORS	mmol/litre
Sodium chloride	2.6	12.683	Sodium	75
Glucose, anhydrous	13.5	65.854	Chloride	65
Potassium chloride	1.5	7.317	Glucose, anhydrous	75
Trisodium citrate, dehydrate	2.9	14.416	Potassium	20
			Citrate	10
Total	20.5	100.00	Total Osmolarity	245

In India, it is reported that only 26% of children (less than 3 years of age) received ORS supplementation when suffering from diarrhea in contrast of 57% of children who receive neither Oral Rehydration Therapy (ORT) nor fluids in increased amounts when they are sick with diarrhea [1] – see Box 10.1. As presented in Table 10.3, only two infants out of ten in the age group of 6–11 months received ORT or increased fluids and continued feeding despite the fact the diarrhea management policy of Government of India clearly states the various actions to be taken (Box 10.1).

Table 10.3 Percentage of children under age five who had diarrhea in the two weeks preceding the survey, the food offered compared to normal practices and percentage given ORT or increased fluids and continued feeding [1]

Age (in months)	Any diarrhea[(a)]	Amount of food offered (%)			ORT or increased fluids and continued feeding (%)
		More food offered	Much less offered	Same as usual amount of food offered	
<6	10.6	1.7	6.9	23.3	8.9
6–11	18.1	1.9	7.4	30.3	22.3
12–23	13.8	1.7	13.6	39.7	39.6
24–35	8.3	2.3	11.7	43.3	37.1
36–47	5.0	1.9	11.6	45.4	41.0
48–59	3.9	3.2	11.1	41.5	43.2

[(a)]Diarrhea in the two weeks preceding the survey [1]

10.6.2 Zinc supplementation

Zinc is an important micronutrient for a child's overall health and development. Zinc is lost in greater quantity during diarrhea. Replacing the lost zinc is important to help recover and to keep the child healthy in the coming months

A large body of evidence from India and other developing countries shows important therapeutic benefits with zinc administration during and after diarrhea, and some studies also reported reduction in diarrhea morbidity in the subsequent 2–3 months without further supplementation. Apart from reducing the duration and severity of the treated episode of acute diarrhea, zinc treatment in programmatic condition has the potential to decrease hospital admission rates by 15–20%, decrease child mortality by 3–5% and decrease the subsequent episodes of diarrhea and possibly pneumonia over the ensuing 3 months [15]. While ORS remains the mainstay of therapy during acute diarrhea, zinc has an additional benefit in reducing duration and severity of diarrhea. Addition of zinc supplements to ORS for treatment of diarrhea has been shown to substantially reduce use of unwarranted drugs during acute diarrhea [15]. This is likely to reduce emergence of drug resistant entero-bacteria, a major public health problem. The therapeutic benefits of zinc supplementation in acute diarrhea may be attributed to effects of zinc on various components of the immune system and its direct gastrointestinal effects. Government of India Policy on diarrhea Management and zinc supplementation is presented in Box 10.1.

Box 10.1 National programmes for management of diarrhea in India [12, 13]

The Diarrhea Disease Control Programme in India was launched in 1978. The main objective of the programme was to prevent death due to dehydration caused by diarrheal diseases among children less than 5 years of age due to dehydration. Since 1985–86, with the inception of the National Oral Rehydration Therapy Programme, the focus of activities has been on strengthening case management of diarrhea for children under the age of five years and improving maternal knowledge related to use of home available fluids, use of ORS and continued feeding. From 1992–93, the programme became a part of the Child Survival and Safe Motherhood (CSSM) Programme and all activities were integrated with those of the CSSM programme. CSSM was further merged with the Reproductive and Child Health (RCH) program in India following its launch in 1997–98. The second phase of the RCH in 2005 was accompanied by the introduction of the "Integrated Management of Neonatal and Childhood Illnesses (IMNCI)" which was based on the understanding that a child presenting with an illness may require follow up for other related issues as well. The IMNCI guidelines and training package is based on a logical framework of assessment, classification and management of illnesses.

The Government of India has recognized that IMNCI is a superior approach to newborn and child survival and health. IMNCI does not imply that the health workers will not treat individual diseases. Rather, it implies that the workers will broaden their approach to consider and respond to the child and manage the different factors that could be contributing to child's sickness. These guidelines recommend standardized case management procedures based on two age categories: (i) upto 2 months and (ii) 2 months to 5 years. In IMNCI, only a limited number of carefully selected clinical signs are considered, based on their sensitivity and specificity, to detect the disease. A combination of these signs helps in arriving at the child's classification, rather than a diagnosis.

Classification(s) also indicates the severity of the condition. The classifications are color coded: "pink" suggests hospital referral or admission, "yellow" indicates initiation of treatment, and "green" calls for home treatment. A sick young infant up to 2 months of age is assessed for possible bacterial infection, jaundice, and diarrhea. A sick child aged 2 months to 5 years is assessed for general danger signs and major symptoms like cough or difficult breathing, diarrhea, fever, and ear problems. All the children are also routinely assessed for nutritional and immunization status, feeding problems, and other potential problems. The IMNCI strategy provides for home-based care for newborns and young infants. IMNCI strategy promotes the accurate identification of childhood illnesses in outpatient setting and ensures appropriate combined treatment of all major illnesses, strengthens counseling of caretakers, and speeds up the referral of severely ill children. At a referral facility, the strategy aims to improve the quality of care provided to sick children. In the home setting, it promotes appropriate care-seeking behaviors, improved nutrition and preventive care, and the correct implementation of recommended care. The assessment, classification and management of diarrhea remain the same, though the approach proposed under IMNCI reflects a more integrated pattern. For further details, kindly refer to the IMNIC guidelines.

In November, 2006, the Government of India after examining the evidence on the use of zinc in the management of diarrhea among children in the country issued a policy note to the effect. The salient features of the policy note [14] are as:

Zinc (20 mg/day for 14 days) is to be used in the national programme as an adjunct to ORS in the management of diarrhea in children older than 6 months. For children less than six months, zinc in doses of 10 mg/day is dissolved in breast milk to be used for 14 days.

- Zinc is a very safe drug.
- A stable formulation is available.
- It is well accepted by children and mothers.

Apart from reducing duration and severity of the treated episode of acute diarrhea, zinc treatment in the programmatic condition has the potential to decrease hospital admission rates by 15–20 percent, decrease child mortality by 3–5 percent and decrease the incidence of subsequent episodes of diarrhea. To ensure timely intervention and avoid expenditure of parents on unnecessary drugs Government of India has decided to supply zinc along with ORS under Reproductive child Health II/National Rural Health Mission. The critical issue is that zinc tablets must be freely available and accessible round the year in every village. All health personnel including private practitioners and ICDS workers must be included in the network of zinc distribution. In this context, it has been decided that all health personnel including AWW and ASHA will promote use zinc in addition to ORS for diarrhea management and make zinc supplement available at the ICDS centres.

10.6.3 Feeding

Continuation of nutrition feeding is an important element in the management of diarrhea. Feeding of infants and children during diarrhea may be considered under-3 heads:

Breast-fed babies – The infants should continue to be breastfed during an attack of diarrhea. Breastfeeding should be allowed as often as the infant desires it. Stimulation of the receptors of the nipple by continued suckling helps maintain milk production. Breastfeeding reduces severity and complications of acute diarrhea. Withdrawal of breastfeeding during diarrhea, apart from its deleterious effect on nutritional status, is also associated with a higher risk of dehydration compared with continuation of breastfeeding.

Non-breastfed infants – Once the dehydration has been corrected, feeding can be done with full strength milk as there is increasing evidence available on not using diluted milk during any phase of acute diarrhea. Milk cereal mixtures can be used.

Older infants who are receiving both solid and liquid diet including either breast milk or animal milk – The diet should contain adequate amount of calorie dense foods, so that enough nutrients are absorbed from a small quantity of food.

Diet practices – The nutritional management of diarrhea diseases is challenging and should ideally evolve around diets based on low cost, practical and easily available foods acceptable to children of the specific age groups. Milled cereals are preferred to whole cereals. A well-cooked porridge or gruel of rice and lentil is usually well tolerated. Mashed bananas are also good. The diet should be iso-osmolar. These foods should be started 4–6 hours of starting the treatment. Soft drinks and fruit juices with high sugar content should preferably be avoided during diarrhea. Food should be easily digestible and can be given in smaller quantities at shorter intervals.

Culture-specific beliefs influence feeding during diarrhea. The source of ideas is both folklore and existing philosophy of medical community. The medical community needs to upgrade its understanding based on recent carefully done research.

Behavioral studies show that in India, some mothers offer less than usual amount of food to infants during diarrhea and often receive endorsement from physicians to do so. More often food intake is already low, prior to illness, due to use of dilute hypocaloric semi-solid complementary foods and less than required frequency of feeding. Children who need care for diarrhea are usually the children in a community whose feeding behaviour is likely to have been faulty. Diarrhea is therefore a great opportunity to introduce and influence proper complementary feeding practices.

Details of dietary management of acute diarrhea are presented in Box 10.2. The dietary management of persistent diarrhea is not discussed as it is outside the scope of this chapter.

Box 10.2 Recommendations for dietary management of acute diarrhea [15]

- Children should continue to be fed during acute diarrhea because feeding is physiologically sound and prevents or minimizes the deterioration of nutritional status that normally accompanies such illness.
- In acute diarrhea, breastfeeding should be continued uninterrupted even during rehydration with ORS.
- Optimally energy dense foods with the least bulk that are recommended for routine feeding and available in the household should be offered during diarrhea, in small quantities but frequently, at least once every 2–3 hours.
- Staple foods do not provide optimal calories per unit weight and these should be enriched with fats and oils or sugar, e.g. khichri with oil, rice with milk or curd and sugar, mashed banana with milk or curd, mashed potatoes with oil and lentil.
- Foods with high fibre content, e.g. coarse fruits and vegetables should be avoided.
- In non-breast fed infants, cow or buffalo milk can be given undiluted after correction of dehydration together with semisolid foods. Milk should not be diluted with water during any phase of acute diarrhea. Alternatively, milk cereal mixtures, e.g. dalia, sago, milk–rice mixture, can be used.
- Routine lactose-free feeding, e.g. soy formula is not required during acute diarrhea even when reducing substances are detected in the stools. Lactose malabsorption meriting dietary modification is very uncommon in acute diarrhea. It may be required in very few infants in whom diarrhea persists beyond 8–10 days with progressive weight loss and $\geq$1 percent reducing substances in stools.
- During recovery, an intake of at least 125% of the normal diet eaten by the child should be attempted with nutrient dense foods. Such feeding should continue until the child reaches pre-illness weight and ideally until the child achieves normal nutritional status, as measured by expected weight for height or weight for age. This might take several weeks or longer, depending on the degree of deficit. The child must be offered an extra meal after an episode of diarrhea.
- Caution must be exercised to avoid hyper-osmolar foods like heavily sweetened juices, soft drinks and bottled or canned sweet drinks as they are hyper-osmolar and might aggravate diarrhea.

10.7 Prevention of diarrhea

Proper treatment of diarrheal diseases is highly effective in preventing death, but has limited impact on the incidence of diarrhea. Health staff working in treatment facilities is well placed to teach family members and motivate them to adopt preventive measures. Mothers of children being treated for diarrhea are likely to be particularly receptive to such messages. Overloading mothers with information should be avoided, only one or two of the following points most appropriate for the particular mother and child should be selected and need to emphasized. The basic diarrhea prevention strategies are presented in Box 10.3.

Box 10.3 Basic diarrhea prevention strategies

- The babies under 6 months of age should be exclusively breastfed.
- Complementary feeding practices should be improved.
- Clean water for drinking and washing should be used.
- Hand washing should be encouraged.
- Latrines should be used.
- There should be quick and sanitary disposal of babies' stools.
- Children should be given measles immunization.

(i) *Breastfeeding* – During the first 6 months of life, infants should be *exclusively* breastfed. This means that the healthy baby should receive breastmilk and *no other foods or fluids*, such as water, tea, juice, cereal drinks, animal milk or formula. Exclusively breastfed babies are much less likely to get diarrhea or to die from it than are babies who are not breastfed or are partially breastfed. Breastfeeding should continue until at least 2 years of age. The baby should be put to the breast immediately after birth and should not be given any other fluids including water. The advantages of breastfeeding should be explained to mothers using simple language. If breastfeeding is not possible, cow's milk (modified if given to infants younger than 6 months) (see Box 10.4) or milk formula should be given from a cup. This is possible even with very young infants. Feeding bottles and teats should *not* be used because they are very difficult to clean and easily carry the organisms that cause diarrhea. Careful instructions should be given on the correct hygienic preparation of milk formula using water that has been boiled briefly before use.

Box 10.4 The modification required for cow's milk [15]

Dilution is recommended during the first two months of infancy to reduce the solute load on the kidney. The dilution recommended is as below:

	Infant's weight (kg)			
	3	4	5	6
Cow's milk (ml)	70	100	150	180
Sugar (g)	5	10	10	10
Water(ml)	20	20	0	0
Energy	64	103	135	153
Protein	2.1	3.0	4.5	5.4

Instructions

- Place milk, water and sugar in a pan
- Bring to boil and then cool
- Pour into feeding vessel

(ii) *Use of safe water* – To reduce the risk of diarrhea the cleanest available water should be used and it should be protected from contamination. Box 10.5 presents the details.

Box 10.5 Use of safe water

- Water should be collected from the cleanest available source.
- Bathing, washing, or defecation should not be allowed near the source. Latrines should be located more than 10 m away and downhill.
- Animals should be kept away from protected water sources.
- Animals should be kept away from protected water sources.
- Water should be collected and stored in clean containers. The container should be emptied and rinsed every day.
- The storage container should be covered and children or animals should not be allowed to drink from it.
- Water should be collected and stored in clean containers. The container should be emptied and rinsed every day.
- The storage container should be covered and children or animals should not be allowed to drink from it.
- Water should be removed from the storage container with a long handled dipper that is kept especially for the purpose so that hands do not touch the water.

There are numerous things mothers should do to decrease the chances of someone in her family getting sick with diarrhea. Listing these for the mother may not be the best way to get her to remember all of them. Instead, the health care workers should find out how much the mother knows and what she is already doing and then add to her knowledge.

Health care workers should ensure that mothers or care givers know about the basic diarrhea prevention strategies.

If fuel is available, water should be boiled for making food or drinks for young children. Water needs only to be brought to a rolling boil, i.e. when water has just started boiling Vigorous or prolonged boiling is unnecessary and also result in fuel wastage.

The *amount* of water available to families has as much impact on the incidence of diarrheal diseases as the *quality* of water. This is because larger amounts of water facilitate improved hygiene. If two water sources of water are available, the better quality water should be stored separately and used for drinking and preparing food.

(iii) *Hand washing* – All diarrheal disease agents can be spread by hands that have been contaminated by faecal material. The risk of diarrhea is substantially reduced when family members practice regular hand washing. All family members should wash their hands thoroughly after defecation, after cleaning a child who has defecated, after disposing of a child's stool, before preparing food, and before eating/feeding the child. Good hand washing requires the use of soap or a local substitute, such as ashes or soil, and enough water to rinse the hands thoroughly.

(iv) *Food safety* – Food can be contaminated by diarrheal agents at all stages of production and preparation, including: during the growing period (by use of human fertilizers), in public places such as markets, during preparation at home or in restaurants, and when kept without refrigeration after being prepared. Individual food safety practices should also be emphasized. Health education for the general population should stress the following key messages concerning the preparation and consumption of food:
   - Raw food should not be eaten except undamaged fruits and vegetables that are peeled and eaten immediately;
   - Hands should be hashed thoroughly with soap after defecation and before preparing or eating food;
   - Food should be cooked until it is hot throughout;
   - Food should be eaten while it is still hot, or reheated thoroughly before eating;
   - All cooking and serving utensils should be washed and thoroughly dried after use;
   - Cooked food and clean utensils should be kept separately from uncooked food and potentially contaminated utensils;
   - It should be ensured that the food cooked is consumed the same day; and
   - Food should be protected from flies by means of fly screens.

(v) *Use of latrines and safe disposal of stools* – An unsanitary environment contributes to the spread of diarrheal agents. Because the pathogens that cause diarrhea are excreted in the stools of an infected person or animal, proper disposal of faeces can help to interrupt the spread of infection. Faecal matter can contaminate water where children play, where mothers wash clothes, and where they collect water for home use. Every family needs access to a clean, functioning latrine. If one is not available, the family should defecate in a designated place and bury the faeces immediately. Stools of young children are especially likely to contain diarrheal pathogens; they should be collected soon after defecation and disposed of in a latrine or buried.

The launch of "Total Sanitation Campaign" in India and efforts to address to sanitation through the National Rural Health Mission (NRHM) are the concentrated efforts to improve the sanitation situation in India (Box 10.6).

(vi) *Measles immunization* – Measles immunization can substantially reduce the incidence and severity of diarrheal diseases. Every infant should be immunized against measles at the recommended age.

A meta-analysis on impacts of diarrheal disease reduction by intervention/area revealed 25–37% reduction in diarrhea frequency by each of the intervention. Water, sanitation and hygiene interventions interact with one another and impact of each intervention may vary widely according to local circumstances. Based on local conditions, interventions need to be prioritized.

Table 10.4 Impact on diarrheal disease reduction by intervention area [18]

Intervention area	Reduction in diarrhea frequency (%)
Hygiene	37
Sanitation	32
Water supply	25
Water quality	31
Multiple	33

Box 10.6 Initiatives of the Government of India for improving sanitation situation

(a) *Total sanitation campaign* [16] – Individual health and hygiene is largely dependent on adequate availability of drinking water and proper sanitation. There is, therefore, a direct relationship between water, sanitation and health. Consumption of unsafe drinking water, improper disposal of human excreta, improper environmental sanitation and lack of personal and food hygiene have been major causes of many diseases in developing countries. India is no exception to this. Prevailing high infant mortality rate is also largely attributed to poor sanitation. It was in this context that the Central Rural Sanitation Programme (CRSP) was launched in India in 1986 primarily with the objective of improving the quality of life of the rural people and also to provide privacy and dignity to women. Later CRSP strategy was modified with a "Demand driven approach" and the revised approach in the programme was titled as "Total Sanitation Campaign" (TSC). The TSC programme emphasizes more on information, education and communication (IEC), human resource development and capacity development activities to increase awareness amongst the rural people and generation of demand for sanitary facilities. The programme is being implemented with a focus on community led and people centered initiatives. The objectives of TSC are as follows:

- Bring about an improvement in the general quality of life in the rural areas.
- Accelerate sanitation coverage in rural areas.
- Generate felt demand for sanitation facilities through awareness creation and health education.
- Cover schools/anganwadis in rural areas with sanitation facilities and promote hygiene education and sanitary habits among students.
- Encourage cost effective and appropriate technologies in sanitation.
- Eliminate open defecation to minimize risk of contamination of drinking water sources and food.
- Convert dry latrines to pour flush latrines, and eliminate manual scavenging practice, wherever in existence in rural areas.

The strategy is to make the Programme 'community led' and 'people centered'. A "demand driven approach" is being adopted with increased emphasis on awareness creation and demand generation for establishing and usage of sanitary facilities in houses, schools and for cleaner environment. Alternate delivery mechanisms are being adopted to meet the needs.

(b) *Formation of Village Health and Sanitation Committees (VHSC)* [17] – Sanitation is considered as an important determinant of health under NRHM: Under the National Rural Health Mission, for institutionalizing community led action for health "Village Health and Sanitation Committees" are being formed at the village level. Of the various roles assigned to the committee. VHSC is also responsible for *Participatory Rapid Assessment*: to ascertain the major health problems and health related issues in the village. Estimation of the annual expenditure incurred for management of all the morbidities is also being encouraged. Mapping of health resources and the unhealthy influences within village boundaries is being done through participatory methods with involvement of all strata of people. The health mapping exercise aims to provide quantitative and qualitative data to understand the health profile of the village. The database includes information on number of households – caste, religion and income ranking, geographical distribution, access to drinking water sources, status of household and village sanitation, physical approach to village, nearest health facility for primary care, emergency obstetric care, transport system as well as morbidity pattern.

References

1. PRUS-USTUN A, BOS R, GORE F, BARTRAM H (2008). Safe water, better health: costs, benefits and sustainability of interventions to protect and promote health. World Health Organization, Geneva.
2. International Institute for Population Sciences. National India Fact Sheet. National Family Health Survey 3; 2005–06.
3. FRICKER J (1993). Children in the Tropics. No. 204.
4. UNICEF (2006). Progress for Children: A Report Card on Water and Sanitation. No. 5, September 2006.
5. International Institute for Population Sciences. National Family Health Survey 2; 1998–99.
6. Burden of Disease in India (2005). National Commission on Macroeconomics and Health. Ministry of Health and Family Welfare.
7. BRYCE et al (2005). WHO estimates of the causes of death in under five children. Lancet vol. 365, no. 1147–1152.
8. Report of World Health Statistics. World Health Organization, Geneva, 2008.
9. CB PINTO, VELEBIT L, SHIBUYO K (2008). Estimating child mortality due to diarrhea in developing countries: a meta-analysis review. *Bulletin of the World Health Organization* vol. 86, no. 710–717.
10. MEHTA M (1996). Nutritional management of diarrheal diseases. *Indian Pediatrics* vol. 33, pp. 149–157.
11. Oral Rehydration Salts: Production of the new ORS, WHO/FCH/CAH/06.1
12. PARK K (2009). Intestinal Infections. Park's Textbook of Preventive and Social Medicine 20th edition. Jabalpur: M/S Banarsidas Bhanot, p. 200.
13. INGLE GK, MALHOTRA C. Integrated management of neonatal and childhood illnesses: an overview. *Indian Journal of Community Medicine* vol. 32, no. 2 (2007-04-2007-06).
14. Government of India. Ministry of Health and Family Welfare, Department of

Family Welfare, Child Health Division. Use of Zinc as an alternate therapy in the treatment of diarrhea, 2006, no. Z 28020/06/2005-CH.
15. Draft Guidelines for Management of Diarrhea in Children for Medical Officers and Health Workers. India, August 2007.
16. Guidelines on Central Rural Sanitation Programme (2004). Total Sanitation Campaign. Department of drinking water supply, Ministry of Rural Development, Government of India.
17. Framework for implementation of the National Rural Health Mission. Ministry of health and family welfare, Government of India. Nirman Bhavan, New Delhi.
18. FEWTRELL L, KAUFMANN RB, KOY D, ENANARIA W, HALLER L, COLFORD JM JR (2005). Water, sanitation and hygiene interventions to reduce diarrhea in less developed countries: a systematic review and meta-analysis. *The Lancet* vol. 5, no. 1, pp. 45–52.

11

Prevention and management of protein energy malnutrition

Siddarth Ramji

Siddarth Ramji, MD, is professor in the Department of Pediatrics, Maulana Azad Medical College, New Delhi. His research interest include neonatal and child health, particularly nutrition amongst the low birth weight babies. He has been a member of several task forces of government and scientifice bodies.

11.1 Introduction

The most recent estimates of the global burden of malnutrition in under 5 children are that 178 million (one-third of all children) are stunted, 112 million are underweight, 55 million are wasted (19 million having severe acute malnutrition) and 13 million children are born each year with intrauterine growth retardation [1]. Together they account for 21% of all under-5 deaths. Besides increased risk of mortality and morbidity, recent reviews have also provided compelling evidence for links between stunting and reduced cognition and economic productivity, and for trans-generational effects resulting in small babies and increased risk of childhood under-nutrition, when accompanied by rapid weight gain with chronic diseases such as high blood pressure, metabolic and cardiovascular disorders. There is therefore sufficient reason to both prevent and appropriately manage malnutrition in early childhood if both the short- and long-term consequences are to be avoided.

11.2 Clinical syndromes of malnutrition

The classification of protein energy malnutrition (PEM) is primarily clinical (anthropometry and other clinical changes). Traditionally three syndromes have been described amongst severely malnourished children – kwashiorkor, marasmus and marasmic-kwashiorkor.

Kwashiorkor is characterized by a weight for age between 60% and 80% of reference median with edema. These children are usually apathetic, irritable and inactive; usually have hepatomegaly, skin changes (desquamating hyperpigmented patches exposing raw areas of skin, fissures at flexures) and depigmented hair. Anorexia, intermittent diarrhea and vomiting after feeds are frequent complaints. Decreased serum albumin, anemia and signs of vitamin A deficiency are commonly associated in these children.

Marasmic children are grossly emaciated due to wasting of muscles and subcutaneous fat, having weight for age < 60% of reference median and may be stunted and have no edema. These children are often irritable and unlike children with kwashiorkor may have good appetite for food. The skin and hair are usually dry and depigmented, and the hair is usually sparse. When children with features of marasmus have edema they are classified as marasmic-kwashiorkor.

Children are classified as underweight (below –2 z-score from the median for weight-for-age), stunted (below –2 z-score from median for length/height for age), wasted (below –2 z-score from the median for weight-for length/height) and severly stunted (below 3 z-score from the median for length/height for age) based on the WHO standards. Severe malnutrition includes children who are severly wasted or severly stunted.

11.3 Prevention of malnutrition

Malnutrition in childhood is the result of a complex interplay of socio-cultural, economic, health and biological factors, the details of which are presented elsewhere in this book. Eliminating and preventing malnutrition requires a change in economic and socio-cultural environment. However, these are beyond the realms of interventions that public health specialists or nutritionists can do. We therefore need to identify interventions that can be applied at scale without adding to the economic burden of nations.

11.3.1 Evidence-based interventions to improve child nutrition

Critical evaluation of evidence-based literature would help in identifying such interventions that could be applied to scale for improving childhood nutritional status. This section provides an overview of strategies that could potentially prevent malnutrition. Table 11.1 summarizes the interventions that have evidence for affecting child undernutrition.

11.3.2 Low birth weight and fetal-growth restriction

The NFHS-3 survey for India reports a low birth weight incidence of about 21.5%. Though exact data is not available, it is estimated that about half of them are expected to have experienced fetal-growth retardation. Is there any evidence to suggest that they could contribute to the stunting or underweight amongst under-five children, especially in the developing nations? In a prospective study from the slums of Dhaka [3], about 1600 newborns were followed till 12 months. The prevalence of

Table 11.1 Interventions that could affect child undernutrition

Sufficient evidence for universal implementation	*Intervention with insufficient or variable effectiveness evidence*	*Implementation in specific contextual situations*	*Interventions with little or no effect*
Breastfeeding promotion (Individual & group counseling)	Baby friendly hospital initiatives	Delayed cord clamping at birth	Mass media promotion of breastfeeding
Behavioral change communication for improved complimentary feeding	Dietary diversification strategies, home gardening	Conditional cash transfer programs (with nutritional education)	Growth monitoring
Vitamin A supplementation/ fortification	Cooking in iron pots	Iron fortification and supplementation programs	Vitamin D supplements
Zinc supplementation including in diarrhea	Iodine supplements	Deworming	Preschool feeding programs
Universal salt iodisation		Insecticide treated bednets	
Hand washing/hygiene interventions			
Treatment of severe acute malnutrition			

low birth weight in that population was about 46%, and 70% of LBW babies were growth retarded (<–2SD weight for age of NCHS reference standards). The follow-up revealed little or no catch-up in growth in weight with the mean Z-score being at –2.38 at birth and at –2.34 at 12 months. The mean length for age Z-scores also revealed no catch up and was lower at 12 months than at birth. Sayers et al [4] have reported the growth outcomes at 11 years of an aboriginal cohort of term growth retarded infants from Australia. The IUGR children were lighter by 4 kg and shorter by 2 cm than the non-IUGR children. Data from developed parts of the world suggest that a larger proportion of IUGR infants show catch up, compared to those from developing countries, yet about 44% are below the 5 percentile weight for age at 18 months and almost 13% are stunted at 12 months [5, 6]. Thus, the evidence suggests that a large proportion of IUGR remain underweight during early childhood and a smaller proportion remain stunted. The magnitude of persistent postnatal growth restriction amongst IUGR infants is probably larger amongst poorer communities, and could possibly contribute to the burden of underweight and stunted children being reported from these regions of the world. It appears logical to assume that the burden of malnutrition could potentially be reduced by reducing the burden of LBW, improving postnatal nutrition of LBW or both. LBW or fetal growth retardation causality has a complexity similar to that of postnatal malnutrition and there exists very little evidence supporting strategies that significantly contribute to its reduction. Some of the potential interventions include improving adolescent and maternal nutrition besides other socio-economic and medical interventions. The intrauterine re-programming induced by fetal growth restriction doesn't seem amenable to post-natal interventions for growth promotion. In fact, attempts to feed these children to improve their growth centiles are more likely to result in adult cardiovascular and metabolic disease without much increase in obesity amongst these children [7]. *There is at present no evidence to support that improved nutrition of IUGR infants promotes significant growth and thus reduces post-natal growth failure amongst these sub-set of children.*

Breastfeeding promotion

Breastfeeding has always been touted as an important strategy for child health and survival. Several publications also have underscored the unique nutritive values of breast milk and its potential long-term impact. What has not been very clear is its impact on nutritional status of children during the first 2 years of their life. A recent systematic review has observed that while breastfeeding promotion has an impact on reduction of child mortality, it has no significant impact on child nutrition especially stunting [8]. The exclusively breastfed children in the WHO Growth reference study were about 360 g and 100 g heavier at 4 and 6 months respectively, compared to the children in the NCHS reference growth curves derived from predominantly non-breastfed children [9]. After 6 months non-breastfed children gain more weight than breastfed children, although their median lengths are similar. *Though breastfeeding doesn't impact on undernutrition, it is an important strategy that must be promoted because of its large benefit on child survival.*

Complimentary feeding

The transition from breastfeeding to family foods is a critical period for preventing child malnutrition. Complimentary feeding interventions are usually targeted in children of 6–24 months which is the peak age for growth faltering, micronutrient deficiencies and illness in most developing countries. After 2 years it is much more difficult to reverse the effects of malnutrition, especially stunting and some of these effects may be permanent.

It is very difficult to assess the impact of complimentary feeding alone on growth since most trials have used fortified foods as the intervention. Improving the energy density of foods may have a benefit on growth in societies where traditional foods are low in energy density, and children are unable to compensate by increasing the quantum/volume of food intake. In most trials and programs, educational inputs are important co-interventions. The most common educational messages in most studies included continued breastfeeding during complimentary feeding, use of thick porridges for feeding, using animal food source, dietary diversity, responsive feeding and personal hygiene [8]. It has been observed that in food secure populations, educational intervention for complimentary feeding without provision of additional food resulted in a modest reduction in stunting (height for age Z-score (HAZ) was 0.25 (95% CI, 0.01–0.49) scores higher in the educational intervention group). On the other hand, in food insecure population, educational interventions alone had little impact on stunting; provision of complimentary foods reduced stunting (with or without education); the fed group had HAZ scores higher by 0.41 (95% CI 0.05–0.76) [10]. Thus, in situations with fragile food security, educational interventions alone have little impact on nutritional status, specially stunting. In such situations access to food must accompany educational interventions for any impact on nutritional status.

Nutritional education

Interventions composed of primarily nutritional education appear to have lesser impact on the nutritional behaviours of families and nutritional status of children, than interventions that incorporated child care, health and feeding components into it.

A community-based cluster randomized trial in Bangladesh [11], demonstrated that nutritional educational interventions targeted to mothers of infants of 6–9-month old could prevent malnutrition amongst young children (Box 11.1). The study also suggested that the cost of preventing malnutrition in one child using the UNICEF's "food-health-care" nutritional triangle model ranged from USD 21 to 37.

It is also important to note that the targeted nutritional interventions are more effective in reduction of malnutrition when implemented early before onset of malnutrition, than after they become undernourished. In a cluster randomized trial in Haiti [12], the study compared two programs – a preventive model consisting of behavioral changes and communication component, which targeted all children of 6–23 months, and a recuperative model which provided, in addition, food assistance to all underweight children (WAZ score <–2) of 6–60 months. At follow-up, stunting, underweight and wasting were all 4–6 percentage points lower in the preventive arm. The weight for age, height for age and weight for height Z-scores were all higher in the preventive group compared to the recuperative group. The effect was more in children exposed to the full span of the intervention of 6–24 months than in those exposed for shorter duration. The effect on nutrition status was observed independent of the quality of the delivered intervention or the population's utilization of health-care services.

A key to the success of any health-care intervention is when communities participate in identifying their problems and its solutions, and participate in the implementation of the intervention. A good success story is the 'Dular' project in India, an initiative of the UNICEF to strengthen

Box 11.1 Preventing malnutrition through nutrition and health education in rural Bangladesh

Mothers of infants aged 6–9 months were provided messages on feeding, care of the child and health seeking. Focus group discussions with the mothers at baseline formed the basis for developing culturally appropriate messages used in the study. Along with these messages they were demonstrated the preparation of energy and protein rich local complimentary foods such as *khichari* (see Table 11.2). Both the quantitative and qualitative aspects of complimentary foods were explained to caregivers and separate feeding pots were identified in the household to provide estimates of the food intake of the infants. These interventions were provided by community health workers/counselors to small groups of women (6–8 per group). Nutrition education sessions were provided once a week for 3 months and then once every 2 weeks for another 3 months. The comparison group received standard nutritional counselling twice weekly under its integrated nutrition program.

Table 11.2 Ingredients and preparation of *Khichri* [11]

Khichri – ingredients and preparation		
Ingredients	*Quantity*	
Rice	2 fistful (65 g)	Required amount of rice, lentil, oil boiled in water. After 10 min potato, vegetables and egg/meat/fish added. If green leafy vegetables are used, they are added 5 min after boiling of rice. After that cooking pot is covered and allowed to cook for 25 minutes. After cooking the expected weight of *khichri* was about 650 g. Mothers instructed to cook in the morning and serve the amount in 5–6 servings to the child within 12 h.
Lentil	1 fistful (25 g)	
Oil	5 teaspoonfuls (18.8 g)	
Potato	1 medium size (50 g)	
Onion	1 medium size (17.6 g)	
Pumpkin/ Vegetables	1 piece (26 g)	
Garlic/ginger	½ tespoonful (4 g)	
Salt	¾ teaspoonful (3 g)	
Egg/meat/fish*	1 piece (55 g)	
Water	4 glasses	

At the end of 1 year more mothers in the intervention group were giving 3 more times/day of complimentary feed (88.5%), khichari as the main complimentary food (15.4%), adding extra oil in food (61.3%) and using a separate pot for the child (91.8%) compared to the control group (24.5%, 4.4%, 21.5% and 76.8% respectively). At the end of the observation period, the children in the intervention arm had a higher weight gain (1.89 versus 1.31 kg, $p<0.001$). The proportion of normal and mildly malnourished children were higher in the intervention arm (88.9% versus 61.5%, $p>0.001$). The length for age Z-scores were also significantly higher in the intervention group compared to the control arm.

community participation and the ICDS. Community mobilization by local resource persons, inter-sectoral participation and networking resulted in improved maternal and child care. It was noted that in Dular project areas children received complimentary feeds earlier and there was a 45% lower prevalence of severe malnutrition [13].

Educational interventions for improving complimentary feeding are effective in populations which have sufficient means to procure appropriate foods. In populations with food insecurity, educational interventions would benefit only when provided along with food supplements.

Food fortification including multiple micronutrient supplementations (MMN)

Food fortification has been considered a complimentary strategy for improving the growth of children less than 2 years. A systematic review evaluated [10] six efficacy trials on the effect of fortification of complimentary foods on growth. Three trials involved home fortification of complimentary foods with micronutrient supplements (as sprinkles or crushed tablets). The other studies used cereal/legume mixes or a milk formulation. In all studies, the control group received unfortified foods. The only study that showed an effect on growth was a study from India which used a milk formulation. The children in the intervention group gained significantly more weight (0.21 kg, 95% CI 0.12, 0.31 kg) and had greater mean length (8.6 ± 1.14 versus 8.1 ± 1.37 cm).

Review of 13 trials and 2 systematic reviews using multiple micronutrient supplementation on growth [8], noted that it increased the weight for age Z-score (WAZ) by 0.12 (95% CI 0.01, 0.23) compared to iron supplementation. Trials with three or more micronutrient supplementations resulted in 9.24 g/dl increase in haemoglobin (95% CI 5.13, 13.35) compared to trials using either placebo, one or two micronutrients. It thus appears that while food fortification improves weight gain, it appears to have inconsistent effect on linear growth and does not appear to impact on the prevalence of stunting.

Using ready-to-use nutritional "multimix" supplements appears an attractive preposition for combating nutritional problems in pre-school children. In a randomized controlled trial amongst pre-school children in Brazil, the intervention arm received 10 g/day of a multimix (composed of rice bran, wheat flour, cassava, safflower seeds) added to the routine school meals each day for 6 months [14]. At the end of the observation period there was no significant difference in weight, height or haemoglobin levels between the two groups. It appears that these strategies do not improve nutritional status of pre-school children.

There appears to be little benefit of micronutrient supplementation or fortification, except for iodine, on micronutrient status of young children.

Micronutrient supplementation

Amongst the several micro-nutrient deficiencies, iron, zinc and vitamin

A appear most important in most developing countries. Review of randomized controlled trials (RCT) and systematic reviews on iron supplementation [8] indicate that iron-supplemented children had an average of 7.4 g/dl higher haemoglobin concentration compared to un-supplemented group (95% CI 6.1–8.7). Based on these observations, it has been estimated that reduction in the prevalence of anemia could range from 38% to 62% in non-malarial areas, while in malaria hyper-endemic regions it could range from 6% to 32%. Fortification with iron alone in school children reduced prevalence of anemia by 70% (RR 0.30, 95% CI 0.17–0.51). Similarly, studies on use of sprinkles for home fortification in targeted children resulted in increase of haemoglobin (weighted mean difference 5.7 g/dl, 95% CI 1.78–9.57) and reduction in iron deficiency, anemia (RR 0.54, 95% CI 0.42–0.70) compared to placebo [8]. With regard to zinc it was observed while zinc reduced diarrheal morbidity and also child mortality, it had a significant beneficial impact on child nutrition. The average effect size for change in weight was 0.31 (95% CI 0.18–0.44). Similarly the mean effect size for change in height was 0.35 (95% CI 0.19–0.55) [8]. Vitamin A supplementation in the neonatal period has been used for mortality reduction and its effects have been equivocal. Its impact on undernutrition has not been demonstrated.

Evidence suggests that untargeted iron supplementation should not be used in children as it may be detrimental in children. Zinc supplementation appears to have a positive effect on nutritional status of children, besides its benefit in reducing diarrheal episodes.

Conditional cash transfers (CCT)

Conditional cash transfers are becoming an increasingly popular program for poverty alleviation. The idea behind CCT is simple: to receive cash transfer, the families must undertake certain activities (such as regular health exams or regular attendance of children at school). In food insecure households in Central and South America, interventions of conditional cash transfer resulted in decline in prevalence of underweight from 15% to 10% and a 10% reduction in stunting from about 40% [8].

Deworming children

An important issue is whether routine deworming as an adjunct intervention contributes to improved nutritional state in children. Review of published studies indicates that deworming children resulted in non-significantly higher haemoglobin compared to placebo. Single dose of a deworming agent resulted in a significant increase in weight by 0.24 kg (95% CI 0.15–0.32 kg), while multiple dosing resulted in a weight increase of 0.10 Kg (95% CI 0.04–0.17). Mebendazole for deworming significantly reduced the risk of wasting by almost 47%. Deworming also improved increase in height. A single-dose strategy increased height by 0.14 cm (95% CI 0.04–0.23), while multiple dose by 0.07 cm (95% CI 0.01–0.15) [8]. *Routine deworming has no benefit on the nutritional status of children. In areas with heavy worm infestation, it could possibly impact by reducing anemia prevalence.*

Growth monitoring

The need for growth monitoring of children to assess their nutritional and health status is undisputed. However, what is currently being debated is its impact in bringing about a change in childhood malnutrition status and utilization of health services. Studies (including projects from India such as the Tamil Nadu integrated nutrition project) have shown that children whose growth has been monitored, and whose mothers receive good nutritional counselling have better nutritional status. However, results from large scale programs have been equivocal. While interventions from Brazil have shown a benefit; those from the India (ICDS program) and Bangladesh (BINP) have not shown any benefit [15]. The reasons for this disparity in observations may lie in the effectiveness of nutritional counselling by the workers. For growth monitoring activities to be effective, counselling must be done well, but most often they are done badly. In spite of the equivocal evidence on its benefits, it provides several contact points for families to access health services. There is a need to strengthen growth promotional activities beyond just charting children's weight on a monthly basis. In resource limited setting, growth charting may be limited to contacts at birth and during the immunization visits (6, 10, 14 weeks and 9 months) and sick child visits. Routine weight charting may be discontinued beyond 12 months in those children who show good growth; follow-up monitoring is required only in children showing growth faltering or those whose weight for age < –2SD. The capacity of health workers must be improved in terms of their knowledge and counselling skills so that effective nutritional education can be imparted to mothers. Growth monitoring should not be an end in itself, it should be the means of improving child health. *Current evidence does not support growth monitoring as a strategy to reduce undernutrition in children.*

11.4 Managing malnutrition

Traditionally while mild-moderate forms of malnutrition have been treated on an outpatient basis and at home, severe acute malnutrition has been treated on an inpatient basis. This has historically been the textbook teaching, because most of the cases of severe acute malnutrition came late with physiological derangements and multiple complications. However, inpatient treatment is associated with huge opportunity and economic costs both to the families and health-care providers. These costs are often unaffordable and inpatient-treatment programs are associated with low coverage, low recovery, high mortality and high default rates. Review of global experience suggests that both delivery systems, namely inpatient (hospital or nutrition rehabilitation units) and outpatient (community) therapeutic care can be equally effective in treating children with malnutrition. It has become increasingly evident that children with severe acute malnutrition without complications can be treated as effectively as outpatients compared to the inpatient program at lower costs and default rates [16].

11.4.1 Inpatient (hospital) care

Convention has been to admit all children with severe malnutrition – weight for height <70% of reference median or below 3 standard deviations of mean or those with symmetrical edema. However, admission criteria that use clinical signs along with mid-upper arm circumference measurement that can be used even by primary-care providers, especially in under-resourced scenario, are depicted in Table 11.3. The treatment during the first week consists of managing complications such as hypoglycaemia, hypothermia, dehydration, sepsis and other problems. Feeding the child as early as possible is an important component of initial treatment. Since these children are usually unable to tolerate large amounts of protein, they need a diet low in protein and high in carbohydrate. During initial treatment a formula F-75 (75 kcal per 100 ml) is used to feed the child (Table 11.4). The goal is to provide the child 130 ml/kg of this formula. If the child's appetite is poor then the child is fed via a nasogastric tube. Once appetite improves, the child enters the rehabilitation phase which involves increase in feeding to achieve catch up growth, stimulate emotional and sensorial development. Catch up growth is facilitated by providing an F-100 (100 kacl/100 ml) (Table 11.4) dietary formula. This formula should be continued till the child reaches 90% of median weight for height. Once the child is eating well, becomes interested in its surroundings, has no edema, is free of illness, and is gaining at least 5 g/kg/day for 3 successive days, treatment can be shifted to non-residential care in a nutritional rehabilitation centre or clinic.

Table 11.3 Criteria for selecting children with severe acute malnutrition (age 6–59 months or 65–110 cm height as proxy for age) outpatient and inpatient care

Outpatient therapeutic care (No complications)	Inpatient care (With complications)
MUAC < 115 mm	Bilateral pitting edema grade 3[(a)]
OR	OR
Bilateral pitting pedal edema grade 1 or 2* with MUAC $\geq$ 115 mm	MUAC < 115 mm and bilateral pitting edema grade 1 or 2
AND	
all of the following: • Good appetite • Clinically well • Alert	OR MUAC < 115 mm OR bilateral pitting edema grade 1 or 2 AND one of the following: • Anorexia • Lower respiratory tract infections • Severe palmar pallor • High fever • Severe dehydration • Not alert

[(a)] *Grade 1 – mild edema on both feet and ankles; Grade 2 – moderate edema on both feet and legs, hands or lower arms; Grade 3 – severe generalized edema, including both feet, legs, hands, arms and face*

Table 11.4 Composition of F-75 and F-100 dietary formula

Ingredient	Amount	
	F-75	F-100
Fresh milk or equivalent	30 ml	75 ml
Sugar	6 g	2.5 g
Cereal flour (or powdered puffed rice)		
Vegetable oil	2.5 g	7 g
Water to make	2.5 g	2.0 g
	100 ml	100 ml

Milk cereal diets do need cooking. Mix the flour, milk or milk powder, sugar, oil in a measuring jug. Slowly add cooled, boiled water up to 100 ml. Transfer to cooking pot and whisk the mixture vigorously. Boil gently for 4 minutes, stirring continuously. Some water will evaporate, so transfer the mixture to measuring jug and add enough water to make 100 ml. Cooking can be avoided if you use puffed rice powder or commercial pre-cooked rice preparation as cereal flour. Give additional vitamins and minerals. Multi-vitamin supplement at twice RDA (should contain vitamin A, C, D, E and B_{12} and not just vitamin B-complex), folic acid; 5 mg on day 1, then 1 mg/day, zinc; 2 mg/kg/day, copper; 0.3 mg/kg/day and iron 3 mg /kg/day.

11.4.2 Community management of severe acute malnutrition

Community-based therapeutic care (CTC) is a community-based therapeutic intervention based on the principles of access, coverage and cost-effectiveness. The three basic premises of this model are that if malnourished subjects gain early access to a nutritional program before their condition deteriorates and stay in the program till recovery, the success rates are high. Second, to be sustainable and effective, community-based programs must involve the target populations. Third, for these programs to remain sustainable, investment must be made in social mobilization so that the key stakeholders can benefit from the positive feedback from individual success stories. CTC can be provided through day care nutrition centres, health clinics or domiciliary care. A recent review has analyzed the efficacy and effectiveness of these therapeutic models [17].

11.4.3 Health clinics

Inpatient care of severely malnourished children has socio-economic dimensions that limit its acceptability. Ashraf et al [18] developed and prospectively evaluated a day-care clinic approach in Bangladesh. All children received protocolized management with antibiotics, micronutrients and milk-based diet from 8:00 am to 5:00 pm each day, while mothers were educated on continuation of care at home. They were transitioned to the day-care nutrition rehabilitation unit following resolution of acute illness. About 264 children were enrolled; 78%, 21% and 1% had marasmus, marasmus–kwashiorkor and kwashiorkor, respectively. One-third had pneumonia, 35% had diarrhea, and 17% had both pneumonia and diarrhea. Successful management was possible in 82% children, 12% discontinued treatment and 6% referred to hospitals.

11.4.4 Day-care nutritional centres

These were envisaged as a simple building where upto 30 malnourished children could attend 6–8 hours for 5–6 days in a week, and receive three meals a day for about 3–4 months. Mothers would help to cook and clean, and learn good feeding and child care practices. Most studies did not document a benefit as default rates were high, sustainability difficult, and their popularity appears to have waned. However, only the program in Bangladesh appears to have been effective [18] (Box 11.2).

Box 11.2 Managing malnutrition through Day care nutritional centres: Bangladesh experience

The nutritional centres were set up in the poorest areas of Dhaka and facilities donated and were maintained by the local nutritional councils. The centres were open for 8 hours a day and manned by volunteers from the Urban Health Extension Program (UHEP). UHEP provided trained the volunteers, food and technical support. Each centre had 5 volunteers and 25 children, and the centres were supervised by weekly visits by physicians. At enrollment each child was given high dose of vitamin A and immunization and antibiotics if signs of infection were present. The children were provided 3 meals and 2 snacks/day. Locally available, low-cost and energy densed food, such as stuffed paranthas, lentils, halwa, khichuri, potato and high energy milk (1 kcal/ml). Mothers actively participated in meal preparation. Mothers were providing education on prevention of malnutrition, diarrhea, family planning, child care and hygiene.

Children who completed the treatment had a weight gain of approximately 5 g/day over 4 weeks. No children died. The reasons for non-attendance included disruption of care of other children at home, loss of wages and girl child. Maintenance of these facilities without aid is a problem and therefore the sustainability of this model is questionable.

11.4.5 Domiciliary care

The first step is identifying cases of severe acute malnutrition who qualify for community based or domiciliary care. Traditionally, the existing therapeutic programs have used either weight for age or weight for height of median reference (or Z scores), for identifying children needing inpatient care. Recognizing the difficulties of recording height by front line community health workers, the Integrated Management of Childhood Illness (IMCI) guidelines used weight for age and/or presence of severe visible wasting, severe pallor or bilateral pedal edema' as criteria for screening children for inpatient care. However, often recording weights or objectifying severe pallor are problems in the community. The present recommendations using mid-upper arm circumference (MUAC), edema and complications for identifying children in need of outpatient therapeutic care or inpatient care are depicted in Table 11.3. It is important that all children are assessed by a trained health worker who can assess MUAC, respiratory rate, edema, pallor, temperature, hydration status, alertness and appetite. A vital step in the decision-making process is the child's appetite. Appetite is assessed by giving the child some therapeutic diet or ready to use therapeutic food (RUTF) and see if the child eats it freely. It is vital that the child is provided sufficient time and a calm environment to eat the food.

11.4.6 Nutritional treatment

Energy dense therapeutic diets with low bulk are essential in the initial phase of management. However, these should be economical, available, and acceptable. These diets could be (i) home based (prepared/modified from the family pot); or (ii) ready-to-use therapeutic food (RUTF). Table 11.5 provides the typical ingredients of an RUTF. The first commercial RUTF was Plumpy'nut, which is a mixture of peanut butter, milk powder, oil, sugar, mineral/vitamin and protein mix (each packet of 92 g provides 500 kcal). This compares with the F-100 formula used in dietary rehabilitation of severe malnourished children in hospitals. Commercially available international RUTF may not be suitable, acceptable, cost-effective and sustainable in most resource poor settings [19]. Local production of RUTF is however possible [20] (see Box 11.3). Each child needs about 200 kcal/kg/day of therapeutic diet. Feeding should be frequent (6 to 8 times per 24 hours), active, and hygienic. The mother must be counselled that the child consumes the therapeutic food before consuming other foods. If the mother is still breastfeeding, then she is asked to give the therapeutic diet after the breastfeed. The child is followed weekly at the centre (this could be a health centre, an anganwadi centre or even the clinic of a registered medical practitioner (RMP)). The child should receive mineral and multiple micronutrient supplements as per standard WHO protocol for inpatient management of such children.

Box 11.3 Local production of RUTF

For producing a few hundred kilos of RUTF needed each week, small scale production is possible. It requires a small room dedicated to food production and free of rodents and other pests, and a 40-L planetary bakery mixer. Such mixer can mix 25 kg of RUTF per batch. Oil and peanut butter should be directly added to the mixing bowl and combined at a mixing speed of 105 rpm till homogenous. A Z-shaped kneader blade rather than wire whisk device should be used to minimize the amount of air incorporated into the mixture. The sugar, milk powder and vitamin and mineral mixture are hand mixed as dry powder in a separate dedicated plastic container and then added into the electric mixing bowl. The RUTF are then mixed at 105 rpm for 6 minutes, 210 rpm for 6 minutes, and 323 rpm for 6 minutes. The RUTF can then be poured or hand packed into plastic bottles containing 250g; a typical daily dose for a malnourished child.

Table 11.5 Recipe for typical RUTF

Ingredients	% weight
Full fat milk	30
Sugar	28
Vegetable oil	15
Peanut butter	25
Mineral–vitamin mixture	1.6

11.4.7 Medical treatment

At admission into the therapeutic program, each child should receive a single dose of vitamin A (it is not given if child has received it during the last 1 month or if edema is present). In children with edema it should be given before they leave the program, Amoxicillin (thrice a day) for 7 days, and in malarial areas appropriate anti-malarial medication. On the first follow-up visit, a single dose of Folic acid (5 mg) should be given, and Mebendazole/albendazole (in children ≥ 12 months) as single dose on the second follow-up visit. The child must be immunized as per the prevalent national guidelines.

11.4.8 Follow-up visits

A recommended schedule for follow-up visits is weekly for 8–12 weeks at facility or at home. If home visits are possible, 2 contacts/week for the first 2 weeks is recommended. After 8–12 weeks the child should be followed once a month till 6 months. But experience in Africa suggests that children who have stayed in the program for 8–12 weeks and have recovered, remain nutritionally well for about 12 months even without follow-up visits.

11.4.9 Recovery and discharge from home-based program

A child could be considered recovered if he/she has been on follow-up for a minimum of 2/3 months, has an MUAC>115mm, is edema free for at least 2 weeks, shows sustained weight gain (weight gain each week for at least 3 weeks), is clinically well and infection free. The guidelines for community management of severe malnutrition are summarized in Table 11.6 [21].

Table 11.6 Guidelines for community management of acute severe malnutrition

- Children between 6 and 59 months only should be considered for community management of severe malnutrition
- Children eligible for enrollment are those with MUAC < 115 mm (or weight for height <70% of WHO reference median or < 3 SD of reference mean) with complications (*see* Table 11.3 for details)
- RUTF or locally available nutrient dense food can be used for rehabilitation.
- If RUTF is used, the children should receive 150–220 kcal/kg/day
- Children should receive appropriate mineral and vitamin supplements
- Medications could include antibiotics and/or anti-malarials at entry into program and deworming
- Criteria for effectiveness of treatment is a weight gain of at least 5 g/kg/day
- Discharge from the therapeutic program can be considered when MUAC >115mm and the child is edema free.

The success story with RUTF in domiciliary management of malnourished children is depicted in Box 11.4.

Box 11.4 Home-based therapy of malnutrition with RUTF-Malawi experience [22]

Children of 10–60 months were randomly allocated to receive either standard therapy (F-100 formula during inpatient stay and at discharge a supplemented maize-soy blended flour) or RUTF (a locally produced RUTF which provided 175 kcal/kg/day and 5.3 g/kg/day). The children were followed up 2 weekly at clinic for assessment and receipt of food supplements. Children who received RUTF were more likely to achieve a weight for height Z-score >–2 compared to those on standard therapy (79% versus 46%); less likely to relapse or die (8.7% versus 16.7%). The home RUTF group also had fewer episodes of cough, fever or diarrhea on follow-up.

11.5 Guidelines for management of mild-moderate malnutrition

Non-severe forms of malnutrition are managed at home by counselling and educating care providers on feeding and care of the child. The IMCI feeding guidelines provide a good backbone for implementing nutrition management of children with milder forms of malnutrition (Table 11.7).

Table 11.7 IMNCI feeding guidelines (6–59 months)

6–12 months	12 months up to 2 years	2 years or older
• Breast feed as often as possible • Give atleast 1 cup of complimentary foods per serving • Give the child 3 servings/day if breast fed; if not atleast 5 servings/day • Keep the child on your lap and feed with your own hands • Wash your and child's hands with soap and water before each feed	• Breast feed as often as possible • Give atleast 1.5 cup of complimentary foods per serving • Give the child 5 servings/day • Sit by the child's side and help finish the food • Wash your child's hands with soap and water before each feed	• Give family foods in 3 meals each day • Give the child also 2 snacks of nutritious food each day • Ensure the child finishes the serving • Teach the child to wash hands before each meal

11.6 Conclusion

Malnutrition in childhood is the result of multiple causes with a complex web of interactions. Its prevention requires a change in economic and socio-cultural environment. Amongst the most effective interventions are those of nutritional and educational counselling of care providers. Sustainability of these impacts requires community mobilization and empowerment.

Evidence suggests that uncomplicated severe acute malnutrition can be managed at home, and duration of stay of those needing hospital admissions can also be curtailed and dovetailed with the community management program, to reduce costs to families and the health system.

References

1. BLACK RE, ALLEN LH, BHUTTA ZA, CAULFIELD LE, DEONIS M, EZZATI M, MATHERS C, RIVERA J (2008). Maternal and child undernutrition: global and regional exposures and health consequences. *The Lancet* **371**, no. 9608, pp. 243–260.
2. WHO (2006). WHO Multicentric Growth Reference Study Group. WHO Child Growth Standards: Length/height for age, weight for age, weight-for-length, weight-for-height and body mass index-for age: Methods and Development Geneva: World Health Organisation, 2006.
3. ARIFEEN SE, BLACK RE, CAULFIELD LE, ANTELMAN G, BAQUI AH, NAHAR Q, ALAMGIR S, MAHMUD H (2000). Infant growth patterns in the slums of Dhaka in relation to birth weight, intrauterine growth retardation and prematurity. *Am J Clin Nutr* **72**, no. 4, pp 1010–1017.
4. SAYERS S, MACKERRAS D, HALPIN S, SINGH G (2007). Growth outcomes for Australian Aboriginal children aged 11 years who were born with intrauterine growth retardation at term gestation. *Paediatr Perinat Epidemiol* **21**, no. 5, pp 411–417.
5. Fitzhardinge PM and Inwood S (1989). Long-term growth in small-for-date children. *Acta Paediatr Scand Suppl* **349**, pp 27–33, discussion 34.
6. KARLBERG J and ALBERTSSON-WIKLAND K (1996). Growth in full-term small-for-gestational-age infants: from birth to final height. *Pediatr Res* **38**, no. 5, pp 733–739. Erratum in: *Pediatr Res* (January 1996), **39**, no. 1, pp 175.
7. BHARGAVA SK, SACHDEV HPS, FALL CHD, OSMOND C, LAKSHMY R, BARKER DJP, BISWAS SKD, RAMJI S, PRABHAKARAN D, REDDY KS (2004). Relationship of serial changes in childhood body-mass index to impaired glucose tolerance in young adulthood. *N Engl J Med* **350**, no. 9, pp 865–875.
8. BHUTTA ZA, AHMED T, BLACK RE, COUSENS S, DEWEY K, GIUGLIANI E, HAIDER BA, KIRKWOOD B, MORRIS SS, SACHDEV HP, SHEKAR M; Maternal and child undernutrition study group (2008). What works? Interventions for maternal and child undernutrition and survival. *Lancet* **371**, no. 9610, pp 417–440.
9. DEONIS M, ONYANGO AW, BORGHI E, GARZA C, YANG H; WHO Multicentre Growth Reference Study Group (2006). Comparison of the World Health Organization (WHO) Child Growth Standards and the National Center for Health Statistics/ WHO international growth reference: implications for child health programmes. *Public Health Nutrition* **9**, pp 942–947.
10. DEWEY KG AND ADU-AFARWUAH S (2008). Systematic review of the efficacy and effectiveness of complimentary feeding interventions in developing countries. *Matern Child Nutr* **4**, no. 1, pp 24–85.
11. ROY SK, JOLLY SP, SHAFIQUE S, FUCHS GJ, MAHMUD Z, CHAKRABORTY B, ROY S (2007). Prevention of malnutrition among young children in rural Bangladesh by a food-health-care educational intervention: A randomized, controlled trial. *Food Nutr Bull* **28**, no. 4, pp. 375–383.
12. RUEL MT, MENON P, HABICHT JP, LOECHL C, BERGERON G, PELTO G, ARIMOND M, MALUCCIO J, MICHAUD L, HANKEBO B (2008). Age-based preventive targeting of food assistance

and behaviour change and communication for reduction of childhood undernutrition in Haiti: a cluster randomised trial. *Lancet*, **371**, no. 9612, pp 588–595.

13. DUBOWITZ T, LEVINSON D, PETERMAN JN, VERMA G, JACOB S, SCHULTINK W (2007). Intensifying efforts to reduce child malnutrition in India: an evaluation of the Dular program in Jharkhand, India. *Food Nutr Bull* **28**, no. 3, pp 266–273.
14. GIGANTE FP, BUCHWEITZ M, HELBIG R, ALMEIDA AS, AROUJO CL, NEUMANN NA, VICTORA C (2007). Randomized clinical trial of the impact of a nutritional supplement "multimixture" on the nutritional status of children enrolled at preschools. *J Pediatr (Rio J)* **83**, no. 4, pp 363–369.
15. ASHWORTH A, SHRIMPTON R, JAMIL K (2008). Growth monitoring and promotion: review of evidence of impact. *Matern Child Nutr* **4**, pp 86–117.
16. COLLINS S, SADLER K, DENT N, KHARA T, GUERRERO S, MYATT M, SABOYA M, WALSH A (2006). Key issues in the success of community-based management of severe malnutrition. *Food Nutr Bull* **27**, no. 3, pp. S49–S82.
17. ASHWORTH, A (2006). Efficacy and effectiveness of community-based treatment of severe malnutrition. *Food Nutr Bull* **27**, no. 3, pp. S24–S48.
18. ASHRAF H, AHMED T, HOSSAIN MI, ALAM NH, MAHMUD R, KAMAL SM, SALAM MA, FUCHS GJ (2007). Day-care Management of Children with Severe Malnutrition in an Urban Health Clinic in Dhaka, Bangladesh. *J Trop Pediatr* **53**, no. 3, pp 171–178.
19. National workshop on Development of guidelines for effective home based care and treatment of children suffering from acute severe malnutrition (2006). *Indian Pediatr* **43**, no. 2, pp 131–139.
20. MANARY MJ (2006). Local production and provision of ready-to-use-therapeutic food (RUTF) spread for the treatment of severe childhood malnutrition. *Food Nutr Bull* **27**, no. 3, pp S83–S89.
21. WHO, UNICEF and SCN informal consultation on Community-Based Management of Severe Malnutrition in Children (2006). SCN Nutrition Policy Paper No. 21. *Food Nutr Bull* **27**, no. 3.
22. CILIBERTO MA, SANDIGE H, NDHEKA MJ, ASHORN P, BRIEND A, CILIBERTO HM, MANARY MJ (2005). Comparison of home based therapy with ready-to-use therapeutic food (RUTP) with standard therapy in the treatment of malnourished Malawian children: a controlled, clinical effectiveness trial. *Am J Clin Nutr* **81**, no. 6, pp. 864–870.

12

Severe acute malnutrition in children

Kamal Raj

Kamal Raj, a public-health physician, graduated from Osmania University Hyderabad, India. He is post graduate in Community Nutrition in Low-Income Countries from the University of Sweden. Currently, Raj is Nutrition Specialist with UNICEF (India country office). Raj has a vast experience of working in treating war victims and displaced and refugee children in a number of countries. Raj's specific interest is in the subject of management of severe acute malnutrition (SAM) and infant young child feeding (IYCF) practices of children who are infected and affected with HIV/AIDS.

12.1 An overview

Severe acute malnutrition (SAM) is defined by a very low weight for height (below -3 Z-scores of the median WHO growth standards), by visible severe wasting, or by the presence of nutritional edema (Table 12.1). Acute malnutrition is classified into severe acute malnutrition (SAM) and moderate acute malnutrition (MAM) according to the degree of wasting and the presence of edema. It is severe acute malnutrition if the wasting is severe with mid-upper-arm circumference (MUAC) <115 mm or W/H -3 SD WHO growth standards or there is edema. Acute malnutrition is defined as moderate acute malnutrition if the wasting is less severe (MUAC between 115–125 mm, W/H -2SD WHO growth standards); edematous cases are always classified as severe [1].

Table 12.1 Diagnostic criteria for SAM in children aged 6–60 months [2]

Indicator	Measure	Cut-off
Severe wasting[(b)]	Weight for height[(a)]	–3 SD
Severe stunting[(b)]	MUAC	< 115 mm[(d)]
Bilateral edema[(c)]	Clinical sign	

[(a)] Based on WHO standards
[(b, c)] Independent indicators of SAM that require urgent action
[(d)] Cut-off increased from 110 to 115 mm to define SAM [2]

12.2 Clinical features

A path-physiological change that takes place in children with severe acute malnutrition (SAM) is very complex. Studies have shown that even experienced paediatricians have difficulties in understanding and diagnosing case of SAM correctly. Nutritional deficiencies are common in children with severe acute malnutrition. Angular stomatitis resulting from B vitamin deficiency is frequently observed. A smooth tongue in a SAM child can be due to B_{12} or chronic foliate deficiency. Oral Candida is very common and affects the mouth, esophagus, stomach and colon. Disseminated Candida is a common infection that does not respond to routine antibiotics – most children need nystatin or ketoconazole. Gentian violet is not sufficient. Many children with SAM develop very thin skin with tissue fluid seeping through.

Anemia is common among these children. Another common condition is photophobia, which is seen in more than half of the children, and in such cases eye ball can get injured during examination. All patients have gross osteoporosis, but fractures are rare. Affected hair becomes straight and discoloured; most malnourished children go bald. The ease with which the hair is pulled out is a measure of the reduction in protein synthesis and it is a useful sign in diagnosis of SAM. Blond hair has no prognostic significance. Scorbutic rosary is due to chronic Vitamin C or copper deficiency.

Multiple small green mucoid stools are a common feature of malnutrition. Counting the stools can give a false impression of diarrhea. It is due to changes in the colonic metabolism and is not related to infections such as Entaemoeba. An orange stool when exposed to atmosphere turns green in malnourished children.

Severely malnourished children have abnormal kidney and liver function; metabolizing and excreting drugs become difficult due to changed levels of the enzymes [3].

12.3 Severe acute malnutrition and mortality

Severe acute malnutrition (SAM) remains a major killer of children under five years of age. SAM contributes to one million child deaths every year [1]. Globally, it is estimated that there are nearly 26 million children who are severely acutely malnourished [1–4]. Most of these SAM children live in South Asia and in Sub-Saharan Africa (Box 12.1). In India currently 8.1 million children are severely wasted (severe acute malnutrition). India has 31.2% of the world's severely wasted children and the largest pool of severely wasted children worldwide [5]. Details on SAM prevalence are presented below:

Box 12.1 Wasting and stunting in children in Africa and India

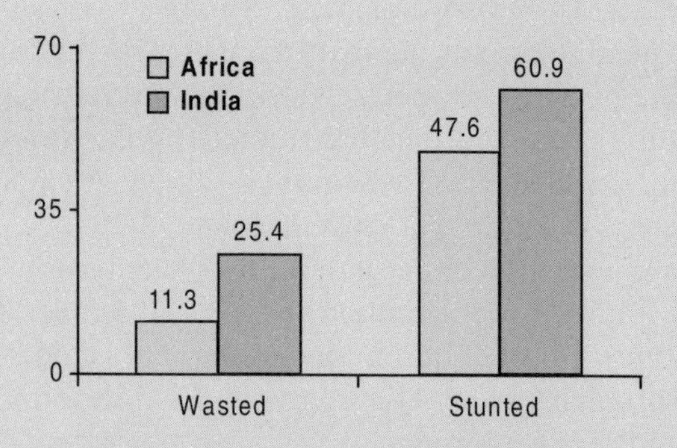

12.1 Percentage prevalence of wasting and stunting in Africa and India.

In India, the rates of wasting and stunting is 25% and 61%, while severe form of wasting and stunting is reported to be 6.4 and 23.7 respectively [6]. The percentage prevalence is much higher than the sub-Saharan African countries (Figure 12.1), even though the latter is one of the most food insecure regions in the world. One of the most important contributing factors for the situation in Africa is that the prevention and out-reach programmes are very well-designed. In Africa, severe malnutrition is addressed through effective implementation of well-designed strategies constituting community- and facility-care components with clear guidelines, treatment protocols in place with regular trainings, and capacity building of health workers and community workers. In India, no such guidelines are in place for care of SAM children [5].

Severe acute malnutrition (SAM) can be a direct cause of child death, or it can act as an indirect cause by dramatically increasing the case fatality rate in children suffering from such common childhood illnesses such as diarrhea and pneumonia.

The risk of death is 5–20 times higher in severely malnourished children compared to well-nourished children. On an average, mortality rate in SAM children is estimated to be 9 times higher than those in well-nourished children [5]. Using existing studies of case fatality rates in several countries, WHO has extrapolated mortality rates of children suffering from severe acute malnutrition (Table 12.2).

Table 12.2 Mortality rate in children with severe acute malnutrition [1]

Country	Mortality rate
Congo, Democratic Republic of the	21%
Bangladesh	20%
Senegal	20%
Uganda	12%
Yemen	10%

12.4 Management of severe acute malnutrition (SAM)

Along with efforts to prevent undernutrition, therapeutic programs are needed as "safety nets" in parallel with prevention programs (Box 12.2). Management of SAM calls for a specialized care considering the vulnerable health situation of children due to altered physiological state which involves multiple organ systems of the body. Until recently, the gold standard for management of SAM, as per the WHO recommendation, is to admit severely malnourished children to hospitals as inpatients for a period of at least a month. This requires many trained staff and substantial inpatient bed capacity. In places where such facilities are available, sufficient attention can be paid to the quality of care and there is adequate evidence that this approach can substantially decrease case fatality rates in both stable environment and emergency situations. However, the limitations of a hospital-based approach for addressing a large number of children, particularly when hospital capacity is poor, have been recognized for more than 30 years. Moreover hospital stays of several weeks for a child and mother are disruptive for families, especially when the mother has other children at home or when her labour is essential for the economic survival of the household. As a result, hospital-based management of severe malnutrition has been perceived as efficacious, but not effective, on a large scale, either as part of routine health services or in emergencies. Moreover, institution-based care reduces family or community involvement.

Box 12.2 Prevention and management of SAM – a parallel effort

Malnutrition, severe or otherwise, is estimated to be a contributing factor in over 50% of child deaths. Moderate malnutrition contributes more to the overall disease burden than severe malnutrition, since it affects many more children, even if the risk of death is lower. Preventing all forms of malnutrition therefore need to be accorded a high priority in developing countries. Reduction in child malnutrition depends on interventions during fetal development and early childhood. Preventive nutrition interventions need to focus on high priority population groups–women during pregnancy and lactation and young children. Children under 24 months of age require special attention since this is the period when the children are growing most rapidly and are most vulnerable to irreversible deficits in growth and development .However, existing prevention programs are inadequate, especially in the poorest countries or in countries undergoing an emergency crisis. Many children therefore go on to become severely malnourished, even when prevention programs are in place, and these children will require treatment. Therapeutic programs are required to be implemented in parallel with prevention programs [7].

In view of the above and also considering the fact that in many poor countries, majority of children who have severe acute malnutrition are never brought to health facilities; it has been felt that only an approach with a strong-community component can provide them with the appropriate care. In recent years, there has been a significant development in the treatment of SAM at community level.

WHO and UNICEF recommend two major approaches for the treatment of SAM: facility- /hospital-based approach for clinical management (using the WHO protocol) and home- or community-based approach, an integrated response to acute malnutrition without medical complications. Facility-based management refers to treatment in a hospital or centre that provides skilled medical and nursing care on an inpatient basis. The term community-based management refers to treatments that are implemented with some external input, such as that provided by health worker for diagnosing the condition, instituting treatment, and monitoring the condition of child at home [7].

Severe malnutrition is both a medical and a social disorder. Addressing SAM therefore requires an integrated approach that combines facility and community-based quality feeding and care. Every child with SAM requires therapeutic food and care in a timely manner, for life saving and rapid weight gain and recovery. Care for children with SAM requires early case detection (before the development of medical complications), optimal therapeutic feeding and care protocols, and access to therapeutic foods. Successful management of the severely malnourished patients requires that both medical and social problems be recognized and corrected. If the illness is viewed as being only a medical disorder, the patient is likely to relapse when he/she returns home.

The first step is to identify SAM children through a nutritional survey and the second step is to provide therapeutic feeding and other required treatment until the child regains its normal weight.

12.4.1 Identification of SAM Children

Identification of SAM may be based on: (i) clinical criteria (presence of *visible severe wasting* or *bipedal edema*); or (ii) mid-upper-arm circumference (MUAC) of 11.5 cm in children 6–59 months of age. The cut-off recommended for screening using MUAC is as follows:

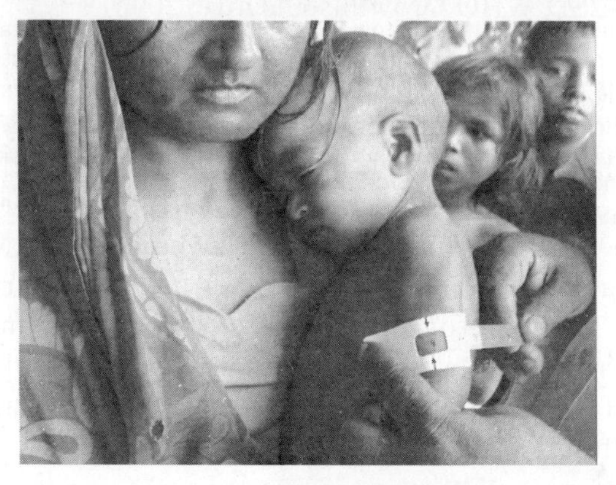

(a) MUAC criteria

Screening – Mid-upper-arm circumference (MUAC)

- Severe acute malnutrition (SAM): MUAC < 115 mm;
- Moderate acute malnutrition (MAM): MUAC = ≥115 and <125 mm; and
- Normal: MUAC ≥125 mm

(b) Clinical criteria

Bilateral pitting edema

- 0 = Absent
- + = Mild: both feet/ankles (Grade 1)
- ++ = Moderate: both feet, plus lower legs, hands, or lower arms (Grade II)
- +++ = Severe: generalized oedema including both feet, legs, hands, arms and face (Grade III)

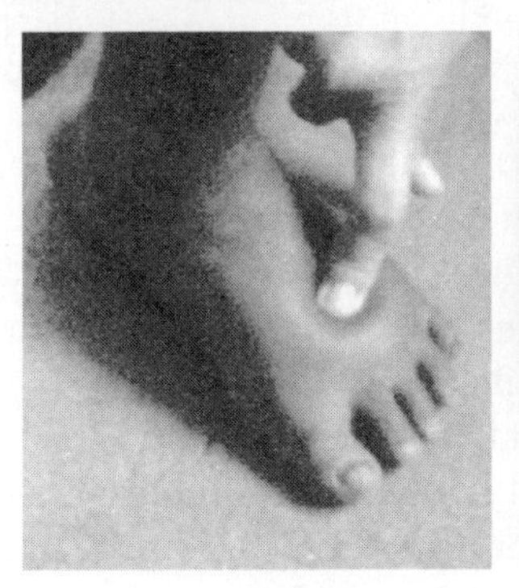

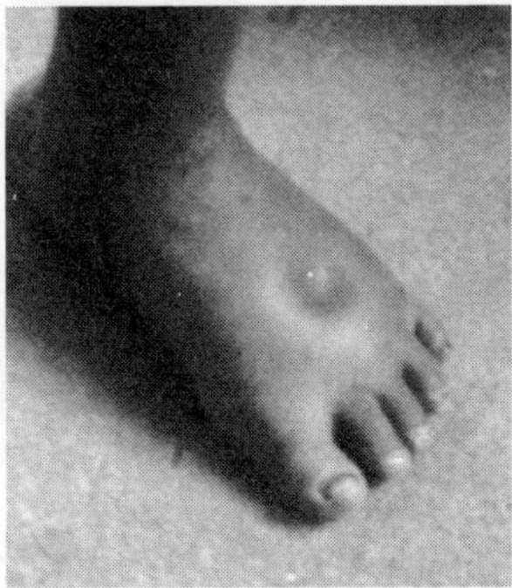

(c) Weight for height criteria (using WHO 2006 standards—see Box 12.3)

- SAM: –3SD WHO Growth Standards (2006)
- MAM: –2SD WHO Growth standards (2006)

MUAC tape is the most appropriate screening tool and has an advantage over all other methods, considering its simplicity, acceptability, precision, cost, accuracy, and the predictive value. In Bangladesh, Uganda and Malawi, MUAC has been successfully used for accelerating identification and for achieving a high coverage of SAM children for treatment in a short period [5]. The other anthropometric criterion of "weight for height" for diagnosis of SAM is complicated and operationally not feasible, as it requires use of many tools and complex calculation. This criterion may create confusion amongst the health workers or other grass-root workers.

Box 12.3 Programmatic implications of using WHO child growth standards

In 2006, the World Health Organization released new child growth standards. The introduction of the WHO new standards, with the Z-score criterion (weight-for-height –3 Z-score), for identifying children for admission into SAM-treatment programs has some important programmatic implications. Using < -3 Z-score implies the inclusion of children who are younger but have relatively higher weight-for-height on admission compared with the National Centre for Health Statistics (NCHS) reference that uses weight-for-height <70% of the median criterion for SAM case detection. Using the WHO standards in developing country situations results in 2–4 times increase in the number of infants and children falling below -3 SD compared to using the former NCHS reference. The introduction of the WHO child growth standards (and MUAC <115 mm) to identify SAM children will increase the caseload for therapeutic feeding programmes; however, at the same time, more children will be detected earlier and in a less-severe state; thereby resulting in faster recovery and lower case-fatality rates. Increasing number of children with SAM identified using the new WHO cut-offs has cost and human resource implications, especially in resource-poor settings [9].

Efforts to identify severely malnourished children need to be undertaken at community as well as at the outpatient department (OPD) and emergency ward within the hospital. In fact, every available opportunity for identification of SAM must be utilized so that maximum children are covered. All possible contact opportunities with children need to be exploited including home visits, immunization outreach sessions, community health centre, primary health centre (PHC) network and clinics.

It is important that most peripheral child health workers or community workers are encouraged to identify severely malnourished children. Verification of identified SAM cases, if required and feasible, be undertaken by higher level of functionaries. Role of family members, including mothers, traditional birth attendants, link workers in the community (community volunteers, village adolescents, etc.), in identification of SAM children is therefore considered essential. In India, formal linkages between registered medical practitioners (RMPs) and government functionaries can be developed for identification and referral of SAM children in the community.

12.4.2 Therapeutic feeding programs – admission and discharge criteria

Therapeutic feeding

Details of therapeutic feeding such as F-75, F-100 are presented in Box 12.4 and on RUTF in Box 12.6.

Box 12.4 Details of therapeutic feeding [10]

Therapeutic milk F-100

F-100 should be used in accordance with the recommendations of doctors and nutritionists. This product contains all the nutrients necessary in the treatment of severe malnutrition; therefore it is recommended not to add anything else.
Recommended use – Do not distribute to families. Use only in therapeutic feeding centres.
Composition – Skimmed milk powder, vegetable fat, whey powder, malto-dextrin, sugar, mineral and vitamin complex.
Preparation – Each sachet contains the quantity necessary to be added to 2 litres of boiled water in order to obtain 2.4 litres of therapeutic milk.

Therapeutic milk F-75

F-75 therapeutic milk is to be used during the first phase of the dietetic treatment of severe malnutrition.
F-75 therapeutic milk must be used in accordance with the recommendations of doctors and nutritionists. It is advisable to use this milk during phase 1 of the dietetic treatment of severe malnutrition (rehydration phase, treatment of medical complications and beginning of the nutritional rehabilitation). As this milk is not intended to gain weight to the child, its use should be restricted to phase 1 of the treatment.
During the second phase, the standard therapeutic milk formula F-100 is used.
F-75 therapeutic milk contains all the nutrients necessary for the treatment, therefore it is recommended not to add anything else.
Recommended use –
To be administered at the rate of 135 ml/kg/day in 8–12 meals per day. As the energy density is 75 kcal for 100 ml, this is equivalent to 100 kcal/bodyweight/day.
Composition –
Skimmed milk powder, vegetable fat, sugar, malto-dextrin, vitamin and mineral complex.

Admission criteria

All children of 6–59 months who fulfil any of the following three criteria have SAM and should be treated and offered therapeutic feeding in one of the available settings:

- (Weight/height or length) W/H or W/L < –3 Z-score (2006 WHO standards) or
- MUAC < 115 mm or
- Presence of bilateral oedema (+ and ++ admission to out-patient; +++ admission to in-patient care) [as explained above]

Admission and discharge from feeding programmes are based on MUAC or weight-for-height Z-score, using the WHO standards for children of 6–59 months. Separate reference charts for boys and girls be used for admission and discharge until further evidence supports using a combined reference chart [6].

MUAC continues to be used as an independent criterion for admission to therapeutic feeding program. The recommended current revised cut-off for identification of severe acute malnutrition of MUAC is <115 mm.

Discharge criteria

The recommended discharge criteria for therapeutic feeding programs are as follows:

- *Percentage weight gain of 15%.* This criterion can be used for all children admitted to therapeutic feeding programs, either on weight-for-height or on MUAC.
- *Weight-for-height > -1 Z-score WHO standards.* This criterion can be used when children are admitted according to weight-for-height.
  - For children with edema, the same discharge criteria should be applied using the weight-after-edema has disappeared as the baseline. For children who have a weight-for-height above -3 SD or an MUAC above 115 mm after edema has disappeared, discharging after two weeks is usually sufficient to prevent relapse.

12.4.3 Community-based and facility-based care

The care of SAM is presented under the following two sections:

(a) Community-based care
(b) Facility-based care

Community-based management of SAM is based on early detection and assessment of children with SAM who have no medical complications. Those with complications, evidenced by loss of appetite assessed by conducting an appetite test (Box 12.5), require facility-based treatment. Evidence suggests that about 80% of children with SAM who have been identified through active case findings, or through sensitization and mobilizing communities to access decentralized services themselves can be treated at home [1]. The community-based component of the treatment of severe malnutrition is recommended to be closely linked with the facility-based component so that children who are ill or who are not responding to treatment can be referred to the facility-based treatment. On the other hand, children admitted to facility-based care, which have regained their appetite, can be transferred for continued care in the community. Figure 12.2 presents a matrix of SAM management.

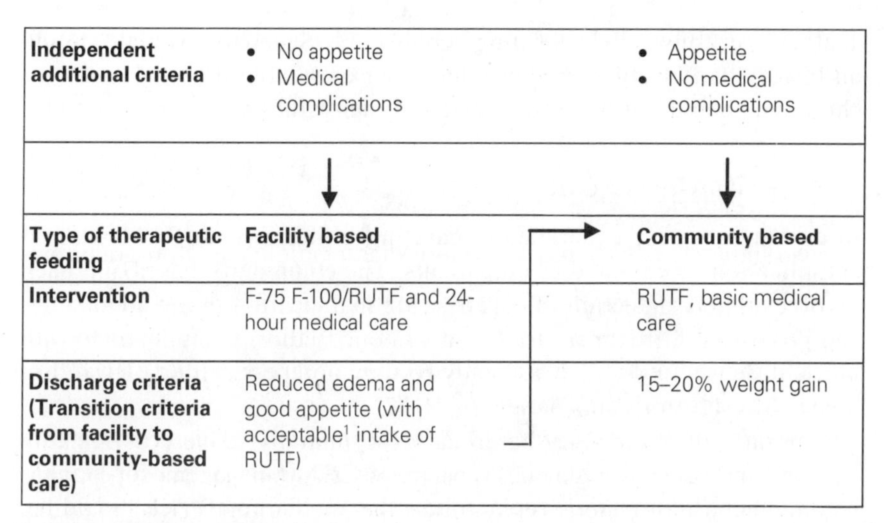

Independent additional criteria	• No appetite • Medical complications	• Appetite • No medical complications
	↓	↓
Type of therapeutic feeding	**Facility based**	**Community based**
Intervention	F-75 F-100/RUTF and 24-hour medical care	RUTF, basic medical care
Discharge criteria (Transition criteria from facility to community-based care)	Reduced edema and good appetite (with acceptable[1] intake of RUTF)	15–20% weight gain

12.2 SAM management [2].

[1]Child eats atleast 75% of their calculated RUTF ration for the day.

Box 12.5 Appetite test

Poor appetite occurs with significant metabolic disturbance, intoxication, infection, and liver disease. Poor appetite is often the only sign of severe metabolic malnutrition and physiological de-compensation. Even a slight reduction of appetite can lead to malnutrition.

Appetite test is recommended to be conducted in a separate quiet area. The first step is to explain to the mother how the test will be done. This is followed by the mother washing her hands and sitting comfortably with the child in her lap. A mother is then advised to offer calorie-dense food to the child. The ingredients of the recommended food comply closely with that of ready-to-use therapeutic food (RUTF) together with micronutrient and vitamin mix. The test usually takes a short time but may take up to one hour. The child must not be forced to consume the food and must be offered plenty of water to drink from a cup as he/she is taking the calorie-dense food.

A child who finishes eating the minimum recommended amount of food is considered as having "passed" the test and is advised to be managed at the community-based care. On the other hand, if a child is able to continue the minimum recommended amount of food than this child is considered to have not passed the test and is referred for an in-patient/facility-based care.

When a child fails the appetite test than such a child directly gets admitted into the facility for further management. A child with a failed appetite test should not be treated at the community level. Children who pass the appetite test are examined by the community nurse or health worker or doctor for complications. Based on the assessment, it is determined whether a child is to be treated as an out-patient (community-based care) or in-patient. A child with serious medical complication is advised to be referred for in-patient treatment; these complications include the following: severe vomiting, hypothermia, pneumonia, extensive infection, very weak, apathetic, unconscious and fitting/convulsions. Severe dehydration based on history and changes in appearances are unreliable in a malnourished child and should not be used to diagnose dehydration.

(a) Community-based Care

In community-based therapeutic care, all children with SAM without complications are treated as outpatients. The community-based approach involves timely detection of severe acute malnutrition in the community and provision of treatment for those without medical complications with nutrient-dense foods such as ready-to-use therapeutic food (RUTF) at home. Box 12.6 presents details on RUTF.

Programs of community-based care substantially reduce case-fatality rates and increase coverage rates substantially. SAM management programs recommend use of generic ready-to-use therapeutic foods (RUTF) with a defined composition and are designed to increase access to services, reduce opportunity costs, encourage early presentation and compliance, and thereby increase coverage and recovery rates. This approach promises to be a successful and cost-effective treatment strategy. However, community-based management of severe wasting will only be effective if the affected children have timely and un-interrupted access to safe, palatable, and nutrient-rich ready-to-use therapeutic foods. Therefore, successful management of severe malnutrition does not require sophisticated facilities and equipment neither highly qualified personnel. It does, however require that each child be treated with appropriate feeding along with proper care and affection.

Successful management of severe acute malnutrition in community settings, however, depends on three crucial factors. First, a provision for horizontal integration of programs for community management of acute malnutrition with existing health-system interventions, so that moderately and severely malnourished children with any complications are promptly recognized and referred for receiving essential lifesaving interventions in addition to food. There is little to gain from supply of therapeutic feeding such as RUTF alone if effective and timely treatment for malaria, pneumonia and diarrhea is not available. Second, in HIV-endemic populations, ensuring rapid and continued access to antiretroviral and ancillary support strategies for children with severe acute malnutrition is critical and the key to ensuring that children survive and benefit from nutrition interventions. Third, and perhaps the most important, is community mobilization and ensuring creation of demand and early detection which is extremely critical for community management of acute malnutrition, especially, large-scale programs that manage severe acute malnutrition.

Success of community-based care of SAM children

Experience in Ethiopia showed that in community-based therapeutic care, families became key participants in the rehabilitation of their children. Recovery rates were noted to be comparable with international standards, and coverage far exceeded that of traditional centre-based care. The success of community-based therapeutic care programs is evident from experiences of 21 implemented programs in Malawi, Ethiopia, and North and South Sudan between 2000 and 2005. A total of 23,511 cases of SAM were treated, and out of these coverage rate was 73% and recovery rate was 79.4%, and mortality rate was reported to be 4.1%. Of the SAM children, 76% were treated solely as out-patients [8]. A study in Malawi compared therapeutic feeding program coverage of severely malnourished children achieved by a community-based therapeutic care (CTC) program and a therapeutic feeding centre (TFC) program operating in neighbouring districts. Results revealed that CTC gave substantially higher program coverage than a TFC program [9]. Findings of a study from Niger suggest that satisfactory results for the treatment of severe malnutrition can be achieved using a combination of home- and hospital-based strategies [5].

Community-based management of severe acute malnutrition could prevent the deaths of millions of children if properly combined with a facility-based approach for those malnourished children with medical complications and implemented on a large scale. Details regarding feeding, medicine and counselling are presented below.

(i) Feeding

Children identified for home-based management are treated at community level with the use of nutrient-dense foods such as ready-to-use therapeutic foods (Plumpy Nut, BP100, or locally made RUTF) or other nutrient-dense foods at home. Children are required to eat a definite amount of RUTF as supplement (Box 12.6), along with breastfeeding or other home foods, until the discharge criteria from such special feeding are met. In some settings, production of locally appropriate therapeutic diet using locally available nutrient-dense foods with added micronutrients supplements may be possible but care needs to be taken to produce therapeutic food with adequate macro as well as micronutrient. Adequacy of nutrients is critical and appropriate feeding is essential not only for adequate weight gain but also for recovery to normality, i.e. children should return to physiological, immunological and anthropometric normality. In fact the rate of weight gain by itself is an inadequate measure of recovery of normality [3].

Box 12.6 Ready-to-use therapeutic food (RUTF)

RUTF are high-energy-fortified foods. WHO recommends RUTF for children 6–59 months for home-based management of SAM children [1].

RUTF has a similar nutrient composition as F-100, which is the therapeutic diet used in hospital settings. But unlike F-100, RUTF are not water-based, meaning that bacteria cannot grow in them. RUTF contains iron while F-100 does not. RUTF has been remarkably useful in treatment of SAM and MAM, even normal children at times of hardship.

RUTF should be given to children only after 6 months of age.

WHO recommendation: exclusive breast feeding to children below 6 months.

RUTF spread is an edible lipid-based paste that is energy dense, resists bacterial contamination, and requires no addition of water or cooking. RUTF are soft and can be consumed easily by children from the age of 6 months onwards. The primary production principles include grinding all ingredients to particle size <200 microns, producing the food without the introduction of water, and embedding the protein and carbohydrate components of the food into the lipid matrix. The most widely used RUTF spread is a mixture of milk powder, sugar, vegetable oil, peanut butter, vitamins and minerals.

RUTF foods can be used safely at home without refrigeration and even where hygiene conditions are not optimal.

Nutritional value

100 grams of RUTF (Nutriset's Plumpy net) – Kcalories (545), of which 10% protein calories (at least half of the proteins contained in the foods should come from milk products) and 59 % lipidic calories.

Vitamins – Vitamin A (910 μg), Vitamin D (16 μg), Vitamin E (20 mg), Vitamin C (53 mg), Vitamin B1 (0,6 mg), Vitamin B2 (1,8 mg), Vitamin B6 (0,6 mg), Vitamin 12 (0,53 μg), Vitamin K (21 μg), biotin (65 μg), folic acid (210 μg), pantothenic acid (3,1 mg), niacin (5,3 mg).

Minerals – Calcium (320 mg), phosphorus (394 mg), potassium (1111 mg), magnesium (92 mg), zinc (14 mg), copper (1,78 mg), iron (11,53 mg), iodine (110 μg), sodium (189 mg), selenium (30 μg).

RUTF spread can be produced in quantities sufficient to treat several hundred children using a plenary mixer in a clinic. RUTF cost about US$ 3 per kilogram when locally produced. A child with SAM will need 10–15 kg RUTF given over a period of 6–8 weeks. Production of larger quantities of RUTF spread can be achieved in partnership with local food companies. Production sufficient to meet the needs of several thousand children can be achieved with a dedicated production facility using technology appropriate for use in the developing world. Care must be taken to avoid aflatoxin contamination, and quality control testing of the product is essential.

The development of RUTF has allowed much of the management of SAM out of hospitals. RUTF is a paste-form spread which requires no adding of water. It can be safely and easily produced in small or large quantities in most settings worldwide. Several countries in Africa such as Niger, Congo, Malawi and Ethiopia are manufacturing RUTF following appropriate technology transfer.

The development of RUTF has allowed much of the management of SAM out of the earlier traditional facility care. In Malawi, a large scale home-based therapy with RUTF-yielded acceptable results with respect to recovery and case fatality of 6–60-month old children without requiring formally medically trained personnel. In addition 1–5-year-old children with malnutrition and good appetite were successfully treated with home-based therapy with RUTF [10].

A controlled, comparative, clinical effectiveness trial in Southern Malawi compared the recovery rates (defined as reaching a weight-for-height Z-score > –2) among 10–60-month-old children with moderate and severe wasting, kwashiorkor or both receiving either home-based therapy with RUTF or standard in-patient therapy. It was found that home-based therapy with RUTF was associated with better outcomes for childhood malnutrition than standard therapy when compared for recovery rates, relapse, case fatality and prevalence of fever, cough and diarrhea [11].

During periods of food insecurity in developing nations, a recurrent challenge is to reach out to the affected populations in rural areas where malnutrition is widespread but distance or geographic location makes health services inaccessible. These areas may also be without trained health personnel or a health-care structure to treat malnutrition. In such situations, home-based therapy with RUTF is effective in treating malnutrition. For example in rural Malawi, home-based therapy and RUTF were used to successfully treat children with severe malnutrition by village-health aides with nearly 94% of the children recovering from SAM. The results demonstrate that home-based therapy with RUTF administered by trained village-health aids is an effective approach to treating malnutrition in areas lacking health services.

In Malawi, home-based treatment of 1–5-year olds with RUTF, both locally produced and imported RUTF, were similar in efficacy in treatment of severe childhood malnutrition. Results of a study from Senegal indicate that home-based rehabilitation of severely malnourished children with locally produced RUTF was successful in promoting catch-up growth. The locally produced RUTF was as well accepted as the imported version and led to similar weight gain [12].

The efficacy of RUTF and F-100 in promoting weight gain in malnourished children was compared in 70 severely malnourished Senegalese children (6–36 months) who were randomly allocated to receive 3 meals of either F-100 (n=35) or RUTF (n=35) in addition to the local diet. It was found that the energy intake and the rate of weight gain were significantly greater in those receiving RUTF than in those receiving F-100, whereas time to recovery was significantly shorter in the RUTF group. In India the acceptability and energy intake of imported RUTF was compared with cereal-legume-based *khichri* among malnourished children 6–36 months. RUTF and *khichri* were both well-accepted. However, the energy intake from RUTF was higher due to its better energy density [13].

Lessons learnt [14] from experiences in Africa indicate the following:

1. A community-based approach using RUTF makes effective SAM management possible in settings where in patient treatment is just not possible.
2. Large numbers of children can be treated with community-based approach.
3. Outcome of community-based management of SAM with RUTF is atleast as good as inpatient management in terms of survival.
4. Outcome of management with RUTF is superior to management with blended flours in terms of weight and height gain and presumably of survival.

(ii) Routine medicine

Children with SAM suffer from infections; they need appropriate medicines to treat any existing infections, along with essential micronutrient deficiencies.

The following chart presents the medicines and nutrients recommended to be given to children admitted directly to the out-patient or for community-based care (Table 12.3).

12.3 Routine medicines for systemic treatment of SAM children – community-based care [3]

Vitamin A	1 dose at admission (recommended dose as presented below age wise) For children with bilateral pitting oedema (additional one single dose on discharge) 6 months to 1 year: 100,000 IU 1–5 years: 200,000 IU
Folic acid	1 dose at admission
Amoxicillin	1 dose at admission + 7-day treatment at home
Malaria	According to national protocol
Measles vaccine	1 dose on the 4th week (4th visit)
Iron	No (RUTF contains required amounts of Iron)
Albendazole	1 dose on the 2nd week (2nd visit) only for children ≥12 months 1–2 years: 200 mg; 2–5 years: 400 mg

(iii) Nutrition and health counseling

Nutrition health counseling is an important component in the community-based care of SAM and is a critical factor contributing to success of SAM management. Community worker should be assigned the task of providing nutritional counseling to mother of a SAM child. Health workers therefore need to be well-trained in technical issues as well as in counseling skills. Field-level functionaries play an extremely crucial role in ensuring regular home visits are made and mothers counseled in order to ensure compliance to the treatment advised as well as for ensuring long-term sustainability of the nutritional status of children. Conducive environment needs to be fostered for counseling. Besides the primary care giver, counseling of other decision-makers in the family is important. Uniformity and accuracy in the messages is essential. Content of the message needs to be simple, appealing, logical, short, technically correct, culturally acceptable, and practical. These messages need to be backed up by appropriate services. Capacity building of counselors is essential.

(iv) Surveillance

Following the enrolment in the community-care component, each child is assessed weekly on the following criteria:

- MUAC
- Edema
- Weight
- Body temperature
- Appetite
- Standard clinical signs (stool, vomiting, etc.)

Anthropometry (MUAC and weight) are recommended to be used only by the health workers or trained child care frontline workers. Recommended frequency of follow-up visits by the health worker is as follows: (i) first 2 weeks: 2 contacts/week separated by at least 48 hours; (ii) 3rd to 8th week: once a week; (iii) from the 8th week onwards till 6 months: every 4 weeks (shift back to weekly follow up if any danger signs occur again); and (iv) end point: 6 months or MUAC of 115 mm and more, whichever is later.

The recommended anthropometric norms for satisfactory improvement are as follows:

- No further weight loss from the baseline in a non-edematous child: at first follow-up visit; and weight gain of at least 5g/day/kg body weight, irrespective of age, at any weekly follow-up visit. These are as per the Sphere minimum standards. (Minimum standards: Reference values have been developed by the Sphere project, which are applicable to both normal as well as emergency situations. These standards give an indication of what might be considered "acceptable" and "bad" functioning under average conditions where the other programs are also functioning).

- Based on findings of the surveillance, following assessment, analysis, classification and actions are recommended:
  (a) *Recovered.* The child on a follow-up for a minimum period of 12 weeks is free of edema for at least 2 weeks, achieves mid-upper-arm circumference of 115 mm or more, is gaining weight regularly, is free of infection, and immunized for age.
  (b) *Non-responder (within first 4 weeks).* Child does not lose edema in 4 weeks or does not start gaining weight in 2 weeks. If the child develops a danger sign at any time during first 4 weeks, the child should be referred to a hospital. If no danger sign develops, it is advisable to discuss with local health provider and decide on future management;
  (c) *Relapse (after 4 weeks).* Edema reappears or there is no weight gain in two consecutive visits or the child develops danger signs. The child should be referred to hospital;
  A child being treated at home that deteriorates (non-responders or relapse cases described above) or develops a complication should be transferred to in-patient care for a few days before continuing their treatment at home. It is only appropriate to refer SAM patients to facilities where the proper training in the care of the severely malnourished has been accomplished; in particular, the staff in emergency wards need to understand that the standard treatment of complications given to children can lead to the death of a child if the child is severely malnourished. For e.g., the management of a severely malnourished child if it includes IV infusions and multi-drug regimens can lead to fluid overload and can die from heart failure and other organ failures. Children with severe acute malnutrition is not an easy condition to diagnose correctly, it is commonly misdiagnosed as it is viewed very clinically and not with a public health point of view. The two arms of the program should be integrated so that there is smooth transfer of SAM children from one to the other mode of treatment.
  (d) *Defaulter.* These are children who are not traceable for at least two recommended visits. It is important to track such cases.

(b) In-patient facility-based care

The treatment of SAM occupies a unique position between clinical medicine and public health. Hospitals treating SAM are commonly challenged with extremely ill patients who need intensive medical and nursing care. Most of these medical-care facilities are in the poorest parts of developing countries with severe capacity constraints, in particular, very few skilled staff. Additionally, the caregivers of children come from economically disadvantaged families whose existence depends on daily labour. Admitting their children into a medical-care facility puts great demands on their time. Such constraints need to be taken into account to achieve an impact at a population level.

It is well-documented that high case fatality rates in children with SAM can be substantially reduced by methodically following standardized treatment protocols such as the WHO protocol for in-patient management [15].

Experiences of over the past decade indicate that the survival of malnourished children improves substantially if the WHO guidelines are followed systematically. A halving of deaths, from 40% to 20% has been regularly reported when the guidelines are followed to a large extent including special feeds, antibiotics, electrolytes avoiding intravenous fluids except in shock and not giving diuretics for edema are followed [16]. A meticulous follow-up of guidelines has been reported to reduce the mortality to below 10%. This involves appropriate training, supervision and monitoring of treatment and attentiveness to danger signs, and a high level of diligence in performing all tasks. Successful implementation of WHO protocol in hospital settings has been reported from Bangladesh and South Africa [17, 18]. In India and Bangladesh, WHO-modified guidelines for the treatment of SAM have been used for a small number of children [19, 20]. In such modified protocols, nutrient adequacy, as attained in milk-based therapeutic diets such as F-75 and F-100, is observed to be difficult to achieve with low-cost local foods combined with micronutrient supplements.

(i) Phases of management

Phase I – Patients without an adequate appetite and/or an acute major medical complication are initially admitted to an in-patient facility (in hospitals or at health centres) for Phase-1 treatment. The children are given milk-based formula like F-75 (refer to Box 12.4) to promote recovery of normal metabolic function and nutrition–electrolytic balance. This is a period of stabilization of SAM children.

Transition phase – Once the child in Phase 1 stabilizes and is ready to continue further in the out-patient, a transition phase is introduced because a sudden change to large amounts of diet, before physiological function is restored, can be dangerous and lead to electrolyte disequilibrium. During this phase the patients start to gain weight with the milk-based formula F-100 (see Box 12.4) and increased energy is introduced.

Criteria to progress from Phase 1 to transition phase:

- Return of appetite
- Beginning of loss of edema

Phase II – For all in-patients, as soon as they regain their appetites and are ready for Phase II, they should be treated as out-patients, and an out-patient program should be in place to take care of these patients who have come out of the transition phase (Figure 12.2).

(ii) Surveillance

Following the enrolment in the facility-care component, each child is recommended to be assessed daily on the following criteria:

- Weight
- Degree of edema (0 to +++)
- Body temperature (twice)
- Standard clinical signs (stool, vomiting, dehydration, cough, respiration and liver size)
- A record is taken (on the intake chart) if the patient is absent, vomits or refuses a feed, and whether the patient is fed by naso-gastric tube or is given IV infusion or transfusion.

It is important that the MUAC is checked weekly, and height once in three weeks.

It needs to be appreciated that many children have psycho-social deprivation and in emergency situations, many have seen parents or relatives suffer or die. Such children require a caring environment and love. There is no place for strict staff, oppressive rules, or blame of the parents. The mother is the primary carer and her wishes need to be always considered.

(iii) Diagnosis and treatment of complications

When a patient develops a complication, always transfer him/her to Phase 1 for treatment (in-patients are transferred back to Phase 1 and out-patients to facility-based treatment).

WHO-management protocol recommends the following 10 steps to be followed in 2 phases – stabilization and rehabilitation [15].

1. Treat/prevent hypoglycemia
2. Treat/prevent hypothermia

3. Treat/prevent dehydration
4. Correct electrolyte balance
5. Treat/prevent infection
6. Correct micronutrient deficiency
7. Start cautious feeding with F-75
8. Achieve catch up growth by feeding F-100 after appetite returns
9. Provide sensory stimulation and emotional support
10. Prepare for follow-up after recovery

Details of hospital-based care, presented in WHO-management protocol, are essential to be followed. Details with reference to item 3 on rehydration is presented below as an example of the complex details of management that need to be taken into consideration.

(a) Treat/prevent dehydration

Since SAM children are *sensitive* to excess sodium intake. Treating a malnourished child who is not really dehydrated with IV fluids is very dangerous. Misdiagnosis of dehydration and giving inappropriate treatment is the commonest cause of death in severe malnutrition. The treatment of dehydration is *different* in the severely malnourished child from the normally nourished child. *Infusions are almost never used and are particularly dangerous.* ReSoMal (ORS with low sodium content) must not be freely available in the unit – but only taken when prescribed. The management is based mainly on accurately monitoring changes in weight of the child. Severely wasted patients cannot *excrete excess* sodium and retain it in their body. This leads to volume overload and compromise of the cardiovascular system. The resulting heart failure can be very acute *(sudden death)* or be misdiagnosed as pneumonia.

(i) Diagnosis

- History of recent change in appearance of eyes
- History of recent fluid loss. No oedema – Oedematous patients are over-hydrated and not dehydrated (although they are often hypovolaemic from septic shock)
- Check the eyes lids to see if there is lid-retraction – a sign of sympathetic over-activity
- Check if the patient is unconscious or not
- Oedema comes from salt and water excess – over hydration.

A conscious oedematous patient must *never* be given intravenous fluids.

(ii) Monitoring rehydration

Fluid balance is measured at intervals by *weighing* the child – the change in weight gives a very accurate estimate of fluid balance. It is recommended not to attempt to measure the volume of fluid lost since this is much less accurate and very time-consuming – it is quick and accurate to weigh the child. It is recommended to monitor the following every hour: the respiration and pulse rate, the heart sounds, in order to monitor the size of the liver, it is recommended to mark the liver edge on the skin with a pen before any rehydration treatment starts.

It is advised to *only* rehydrate until the weight deficit (measured or estimated) is corrected and then *Stop* – *Do* not give extra fluid to "prevent recurrence".

If child is conscious, give ReSoMal and if un-conscious give IV fluids – Darrow's solution or half saline and 5% glucose or Ringer lactate and 5% dextrose at 15 ml/kg in the first hour and reassess the patient. If the patient is improving, give 15 ml/kg in every 2nd hour and if not improving strongly suspect that the patient has developed Septic shock and treat accordingly.

(iii) Reassess status of hydration

Formally reassess in one hour, if there is no weight gain, and then increase the rate of administration of ReSoMal by 5 ml/kg/h. Later reassessing every hour becomes important if there is clinical improvement but there are still signs of dehydration; continue with the treatment until the appropriate weight gain has been achieved.

If there is no weight gain and there is deterioration in a child's condition with the re-hydration therapy, then the diagnosis of dehydration was definitely wrong. Stop and start the child on F-75 or equivalent diet.

For diagnosis and treatment of other dehydration, heart failure, anemia, hypoglycaemia and fever, it is essential to follow the WHO protocol. Box 12.7 presents the WHO "Emergency Treatment Wall Chart".

Box 12.7 WHO emergency treatment wall chart [21]

Emergency treatment of severely malnourished children

Severely malnourished children are different from other children. So they need different treatment.

Condition	Immediate action
Treat shock Shock is if the child is lethargic or unconscious and cold hands **Plus either:** Slow capillary refill (longer than 3 seconds) or Weak fast pulse	**If child is in shock,** 1. Give oxygen 2. Give sterile 10% glucose (5 ml/kg) by IV 3. Give IV fluid at 15 ml/kg over 1 hour, using one of the following solutions in order of preference: • half-strength Darrow's solution with 5% glucose (or dextrose) • Ringers' lactate with 5% glucose* or • half-normal saline with 5% glucose* or **if either of these is used, add sterile potassium chloride (20 mmol/l) if possible.*
Monitor closely: use the Critical Care Pathway Initial Management Chart	4. Keep the child warm. 5. Measure and record pulse and respirations every 10 minutes. If there are signs of improvement (pulse and respiration rates fall), repeat IV 15ml/kg for one more hour If there are no signs of improvement after the 1st hour of IV fluid, assume child has septic shock. In this case: 1. Give maintenance fluids (4 ml/kg/h) while waiting for blood. 2. Order 10 ml/kg fresh whole blood and when blood is available, stop oral intake and IV fluids. 3. Give a diuretic 4. Transfuse whole fresh blood (10 ml/kg slowly over 3 hours). If signs of heart failure, give packed cells instead of whole blood.
Treat severe dehydration Assume severe dehydration if there is history of watery diarrhea, thirst, hypothermia, sunken eyes, weakness or absent radial pulse, cold hands and feet, reduced urine output.	**Do not give IV (intravenous) fluids except in shock** 1. Give ReSoMal 5 ml/kg in every 30 min for 2 hours (orally or by NG). Do not give standard ORS to severely malnourished children. 2. Measure and record pulse and respirations every 30 minutes. 3. Give ReSoMal 5–10 ml/kg/hour for next 4–10 hours in alternate hours with F-75. **STOP** rehydration if 3 or more signs of rehydration or any signs of over hydration (increased respiratory rate and pulse rate, increase oedema and puffy eyelids). Only give ReSoMal for up to 10 hours. **Monitor during rehydration for signs of over-hydration:** • increasing pulse and respiratory rate • increasing oedema and puffy eyelids Check for signs at least hourly. Stop if pulse increases by 25 beats/minute and respiratory rate by 5 breaths/minute.

Treat very severe anemia Very severe anemia is Hb less than 4 g/dl	**If very severe anemia (**or Hb 4–6 g/dl and respiratory distress): 1. Stop all oral intake and IV fluids during the transfusion. 2. Look for signs of congestive failure. 3. Give furosemide 1 ml/kg IV at the start of the transfusion. 4. If no signs of congestive failure, give whole fresh blood 10 ml/kg body weight slowly over 3 hours. If signs of heart failure, give 5–7 ml/kg packed cells rather than whole blood.
Treat hypoglycaemia Hypoglycaemia is a blood glucose <3 mmol/L Assume hypoglycaemia if no dextrostix available	Perform Dextrostix test on admission, before giving glucose or feeding. **If hypoglycaemia is suspected and no dextrostix are available or if it is not possible to get enough blood for test, assume that the child has hypogly caemia and give treatment immediately without laboratory confirmation.** **If conscious:** 1. Give a bolus of 10% glucose (50 ml) or sugar solution (1 rounded teaspoon sugar in 3 tablespoons of water). Bolus of 10% glucose is best, but give sugar solution or F-75 formula rather than wait for glucose. 2. Start feeding straightaway: feed after every 2 hours (12 feeds in 24 hours). Use feed chart to find amount to give and feed every 2–3 hours day and night. If unconscious, give glucose IV (5 ml/kg of sterile 10% glucose), followed by 50 ml of 10% glucose or sucrose by NG tube.
Treat hypothermia Hypothermia is a rectal temperature <35.5°C (95.9°F) or an underarm temperature <35°C (95°F).	**If hypothermia** For all children: 1. Feed straightaway and then every 2–3 hours, day and night. 2. Keep warm. 3. Use the kangaroo technique, cover with a blanket. Let mother sleep with child to keep child warm. 3. Keep room warm, no draughts. 4. Keep bedding/clothes dry. Dry carefully after bathing (do not bathe if very ill). 5. Avoid exposure during examinations, bathing. 6. Use a heater or incandescent lamp with caution, do not use hot bottle water or fluorescent lamp.
Emergency eye care Corneal ulceration	**If corneal ulceration,** 1. Give Vitamin A immediately (<6 months 50,000 IU, 6–12 months 100,000 IU, >12 months 200,000 IU) 2. Instill one drop atropine (1%) into affected eye to relax the eye and prevent the lens from pushing out.

Condition	Immediate action
Treat hypothermia Hypothermia is a rectal temperature <35.5°C (95.9°F) or an underarm temperature <35°C (95°F).	**If hypothermia** For all children: 1. Feed straightaway and then every 2–3 hours, day and night. 2. Keep warm. 3. Use the kangaroo technique, cover with a blanket. Let mother sleep with child to keep child warm. 3. Keep room warm, no draughts. 4. Keep bedding/clothes dry. Dry carefully after bathing (do not bathe if very ill). 5. Avoid exposure during examinations, bathing. 6. Use a heater or incandescent lamp with caution, do not use hot bottle water or fluorescent lamp.
Emergency eye care Corneal ulceration	**If corneal ulceration,** 1. Give Vitamin A immediately (<6 months 50,000 IU, 6–12 months 100,000 IU, >12 months 200,000 IU) 2. Instill one drop atropine (1%) into affected eye to relax the eye and prevent the lens from pushing out.

In case a child does not respond to treatment, steps to be followed are presented in Figure 12.3.

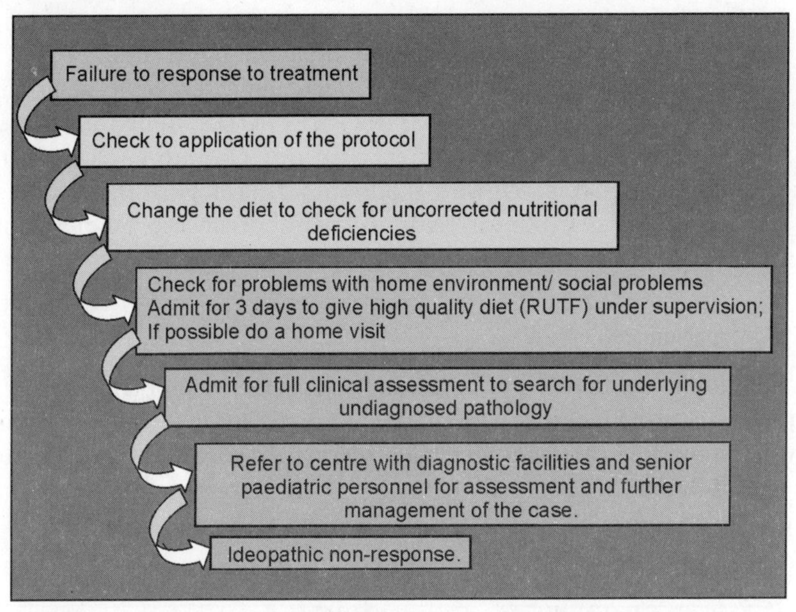

12.3 Steps to follow when children fail to respond to treatment [22].

(b) Special problems observed with individual children – in-patients and out-patients

Apart from problems encountered with children who have failed responding to the treatment, there are other following issues, observed in both in-patients as well as out-patients, which need to be taken care of:

(i) In-patients

- Insufficient food provided. Reasons could be food taken by siblings or caretaker, sharing of caretaker's food, vitamin or mineral deficiency, mal-absorption, psychological trauma (particularly in refugee situations and families living with HIV/AIDS).
- Rumination may occur. Rumination is a condition which occurs in up to 10% of severely malnourished, emotionally impaired children. This condition is suspected when a child eats well, but fails to gain weight. Children with this condition regurgitate food from the stomach into the mouth, and then vomit part of it and swallow the rest. This usually happens when they are ignored. It is important that children are observed for such signs by the care taker. Such children are usually thought to have vomiting without diarrhea because they often smell of vomit, and may have vomit-stained clothes or bedding. They are often unusually alert and suspicious, may make stereotyped chewing movements, and do not appear distressed by vomiting. Rumination is best treated by staff members who have experience with this problem and give special attention to the child.
- Infections like diarrhea, dysentery, pneumonia, tuberculosis, urinary infection/ Otitis media, malaria, HIV/AIDS, schistosomiasis/ leishmaniasis, hepatitis/cirrhosis are common. Congenital abnormalities (e.g., Down's syndrome), neurological damage (e.g., cerebral palsy), inborn errors of metabolism are other serious underlying diseases.

(ii) Out-patients

In addition to the details presented under (i), specific problems observed with SAM out-patient cases are sharing of foods within the family, sibling rivalry, unwilling caretaker, caretaker overwhelmed with other work and responsibilities.

(c) Innovative models for care of severely malnourished

(i) Nutrition Rehabilitation Centre (NRC) is an approach tried in many countries, including a few states in India. The approach is new and requires in-depth review before it is considered to be scaled up to other parts of the country. In NRCs, children receive treatment for the complications associated with severe wasting and are fed formula F-75 or F-100 in quantities adapted to their metabolic needs. Children and their mothers stay in the NRC for 2–4 weeks, with the associated opportunity cost to the child's mother and siblings. The NRC treatment has two phases – stabilization phase and rehabilitation phase. The stabilization phase at NRCs usually lasts for 2–5 days. During this period, metabolism of children gets stabilized, infections are under control, and appetite returns. The following 21–30 days is the rehabilitation phase that aims at rebuilding the child's wasted tissues.

The limitation of NRC is evident from the efforts undertaken in large state of India, Bihar. There are eight NRCs that provide care to about 120 children per month. For effective management of SAM, the state government would need to establish over 5,500 NRCs and recruit over 8,300 staff to provide care for estimated 1,000,000 children annually with severe wasting. The NRC model is costly. Moreover, it is estimated that, 80–90% of children who are admitted to NRCs do not have medical complications and can therefore be considered for community therapeutic care program described under A.

(ii) Community Therapeutic Care (CTC) model

The CTC delivery model was conceived, developed, and implemented in complex emergency contexts. CTC model is a community-based model and seeks to provide fast, effective and cost-efficient assistance in a manner that empowers the affected communities. CTC equips communities to deal more effectively with future periods of vulnerability and therefore is a model which creates a platform for long-term solutions to the problems of food security and public health. Experience of implementing CTC in transitional and developmental contexts is currently being acquired in Bangladesh, Ethiopia, Malawi and Zambia.

CTC is complementary to traditional Therapeutic Feeding Centres (TFCs) and Supplementary Feeding Programs (SFP), integrating them into a broader framework that better takes into accounts the social, economic and political realities of food insecurity and malnutrition. Through decentralizing distributions, engagement with communities, working with local health care providers and outreach, CTC improves access to services, case finding and follow up. An international humanitarian nongovernmental organization "Concern Worldwide" has piloted this model and is now implementing and researching CTC approaches to manage acute malnutrition [23].

12.5 Monitoring and evaluation of SAM management program

Effectiveness of each intervention must be reviewed at regular intervals. International standards put forward by Sphere have provided benchmarks to monitor and evaluate emergency nutrition programming (Sphere represents a unique voluntary initiative comprising a broad array of humanitarian actors with aim to improve the quality of assistance to people affected by disasters.) [24]. Reference values have been developed by the Sphere project, which are applicable to both normal as well as emergency situations. They give an indication of what might be considered "acceptable" and "bad" functioning under average conditions where the other programs are also functioning. These standards are as follows:

Recovery rate = No. of patients discharged for recovery / Total no. of exits

Death rate = No. of patients died in the programme / Total no. of exits

Defaulter is a patient who is absent from the programme for 2 consecutive weighing.

Defaulter rate = No. of true defaulters / Total no. of exits

Length of stay – This indicator should be calculated only for the recovered patients[1] for each category.

Mean length of stay = sum of (No. of days for each recovered patient) / No. of recovered patients

Rate of weight gain – The average weight gain is calculated for all recovered patients for each patient category. The rate of weight gain for an individual is calculated as the discharge weight minus the minimum weight multiplied by 1000 to convert the weight gain to grams. This is then divided by the minimum weight. Lastly, this total weight gain is divided by the number of days from the day of minimum weight to the day of discharge, to give g/kg/d.

Average weight gain (g/kg/day) = Total individual weight gains/Total no. of individuals

Box 12.8 Management of SAM in India

The development of the community-based approach for the management of severe acute malnutrition provides a new impetus for putting the preventive measure into practice and re-visit guidelines of management of SAM in developing countries. It is urgent that SAM management, along with preventive action, is added to the list of cost-effective interventions to reduce child mortality. A consultation meeting was held in India in 2009 to review the global lessons learned and reach a consensus on medical nutrition therapy (MNT).

Consensus Statement of the National Consensus Workshop on Management of SAM Children through Medical Nutrition Therapy held on 26th and 27th November

2009 [25] is as follows: "In India 8.1 million children are estimated to suffer from severe acute malnutrition (SAM). In a nation marching ahead on the economic front, the magnitude and serious consequences of SAM among children makes it unethical not to urgently initiate measures to prevent and treat SAM. Protecting lives and promoting optimum development of SAM children is also a human rights issue. Up to 15% under-5 children with SAM require in-patient management because of medical complications. The remaining 85% (without medical complications) can be managed through a community- and/or home-based care approach. There is an urgent need to update both facility- and home-based care recommendations for the management of SAM among children in India, on the basis of latest evidence. Medical Nutrition Therapy (MNT) is only a component of the entire process of managing SAM children and being a time-limited therapeutic intervention it should not be viewed as being in conflict with the objective and accepted process of attaining food and nutrition security or promoting appropriate Infant and Young Child Feeding (IYCF) practices for children with or without SAM. However, adequate caution should be exercised to ensure that MNT for SAM does not interfere with measures for the holistic prevention of childhood undernutrition. Ready-to-use therapeutic food (RUTF) as per WHO and UNICEF specifications is a medical nutrition therapy based on sound scientific principles with a balanced composition of type I and type II nutrients. Apart from anthropometric recovery, RUTF results in physiological and functional (including immunological) recovery. It has a specific composition which has been tested and proved effective in functional recovery of SAM children. RUTF should not be confused with ready-to-use food (RTUF) or any other products or preparations. Global evidence, primarily from Africa, indicates that RUTF-based nutrition therapy is effective for facility- and home-based management of SAM children who do not have medical complications, and can be scaled up for community or home-based management for children over six months of age. Pilot experience from India (Bihar and Madhya Pradesh) suggests that RUTF is effective for nutritional therapy of SAM children and can also be scaled up. Similar experience from Maharashtra has been reported with other locally formulated products. Other models from West Bengal and Gujarat, on a smaller scale, have also showed similar weight gains with locally formulated products. There is a suggestion from observational data in Madhya Pradesh that RUTF may be superior to standard treatment with F-100 and IAP formulations. However, there is no head-to-head comparison of effectiveness of RUTF with locally formulated products. Further, all of these experiences from India relate to weight gain and not to height gain or physiological or functional recovery. A qualitative study undertaken in mid 2009 from six states of India suggests that against the backdrop of fragile food security and faulty feeding practices, mothers who are time-constrained tend to reach out to market foods to feed their children, which may be of sub-optimal nutrition quality. Further, the families do not recognize the signs of undernutrition until children develop severe malnutrition and medical complications.

Considerable sensitivities exist regarding the possibility of commercial exploitation of undernutrition through aggressive marketing and supply of international product-based nutrition therapy and erosion of (i) exclusive breastfeeding during the first six months of life; and (ii) continued breastfeeding between 6 and 24 months of life. Further, any action has to be in consonance with the Infant Milk Substitutes Feeding Bottles, and Infant Foods (Regulation of Production, Supply and Distribution) Act 1992 as amended in 2003 (IMS Act) *(http://www.bpni.org/docments/IMS-act.pdf)* and the Supreme Court orders on the Right to Food Act *(http://www.righttofoodindia.org and http://www.sccommissioners.org).* Indian manufacture of RUTF is feasible, can be scaled up and even industrial production for export has been started by at least a couple of units. The fear of commercialization can be obviated by following principles of (i) non-proprietary product; (ii) partially decentralized manufacture with public-sector involvement; (iii) public health system being the sole procurement agency with a specific strategy that ensures purchase from multiple producers; and (iv) prescribed product, which is not freely available. Product-based nutrition therapy including RUTF can be introduced on a pilot basis at scale (district or state level) utilizing existing systems for sustainability. The pilot project should be introduced when a delivery design and plan of action is developed and is in place as a part of the larger system to deal with childhood undernutrition. RUTF should be used only:

- As therapeutic and not supplementary feeding
- Above six months of age
- For a limited time period (4–8 weeks) until the child recovers from SAM, which should be defined in explicit treatment protocols

MNT could be operationalised by the health ministry through the Integrated Management of Newborn and Childhood Illnesses (IMNCI) module, which also has a component for the management of SAM. The Integrated Child Development Services (ICDS) system could converge for the identification and referral of children with SAM and the follow-up of these children after their discharge from therapeutic feeding. To aid the evaluation process in an observational manner, outcome measures should be recorded after some time of operationalisation of intervention program and include follow-up of rehabilitated children. Regulatory issues would need to be resolved between the two nodal authorities (Drug Controller General of India and Food Safety and Standards Authority of India) before MNT can be operationalised. The feasibility of manufacturing, regulation and registration as a food, and use and distribution as a drug should be explored. Food and nutrition security and preventive aspects should be ensured during treatment for and after recovery from SAM to prevent relapses. Urgent research issues include:

- Comparison of RUTF with home-based and locally formulated products
- Physiological recovery and longer benefits of the above treatments
- Effect of introduction of RUTF on breast feeding
- Operationalisation and economic analysis in different settings

References

1. WHO/WFP/UNSCN/UNICEF (2007). Community-based management of severe acute malnutrition. A joint statement.
2. WHO / UNICEF. WHO child growth standards and the identification of severe acute malnutrition in infants and children (2009). A joint statement by WHO and UNICEF.
3. GOLDEN M AND GRELLETY I. State of the Art Training on Integrated Management of Severe Acute Malnutrition, hosted by NRHM, ICDS, Maharashtra State Nutrition Mission, Organised by UNICEF Delhi, 24–27th November, 2008, Pune.
4. LINKAGES PROJECT. Complementary feeding. http://www.linkagesproject. org/technical/compfeeding.php (accessed on May 2010).
5. AIIMS (2009). National Consensus Workshop on Management of SAM Children through Medical Nutrition Therapy. Compendium of Scientific Publications, A Summary, 26–27th November, 2009.
6. NATIONAL FAMILY HEALTH SURVEY (NFHS–III), 2005–2006. International Institute for Population Sciences, Mumbai, and ORC Macro, Calverton; September 2007, 274–284.

7. PRUDHON C, PRINZO ZW, BRIEND A, BERNADETTE MEG, MASON JB (2006). Proceedings of the WHO, UNICEF and SCN information consultation on community-based management of severe malnutrition in children, *Food and Nutrition Bulletin* **27**, no. 3, pp S99–S104.
8. THE LANCET EDITORIAL (2007). Ready-to-use therapeutic foods for malnutrition. *The Lancet* **369**, no. 9557, p 164; and COLLINS, S, DENT, N, BINNS, P, BAHWERE, P, SADLER, K, HALLMAN, A (2006). Management of severe acute malnutrition in children. *Lancet* **369**, no. 9563, pp 1992–2000.
9. SANDIGE H, NDEKHA MJ, BRIEND A, ASHORN P and MANARY M (2004). Home-based treatment of malnourished Malawian children with locally produced or imported ready-to-use food. *J Pediatr Gastroenterology and Nutrition* **39**, no. 2, pp 141–146.
10. LINNEMAN Z, MLTILSKY D, NDEKHA M, MANARY MJ, MALETA K, MANARY MJ (2007). A large-scale operational study of home-based therapy with ready-to-use therapeutic food in childhood malnutrition on Malawi. *Matern Child Nutr* **3**, no. 3, pp 206–215.
11. CILIBERTO MA, SANDIGE H, NDEKHA MJ, ASHORN P, BRIEND A, CILIBERTO HM, MANARAY MJ (2005). Comparison of home-based therapy with ready-to-use therapeutic food with standard therapy in the treatment of malnourished children: a controlled clinical effectiveness trial. *Am J Clin Nutr* **81**, no. 4, pp 864–870.
12. SADLER K, MYATT M, FELEKE T, COLLINS S (2007). A comparison of the program coverage of two therapeutic feeding interventions implemented in neighbouring districts of Malawi. *Public Health Nutr* vol 10, no. 9, pp 907–913.
13. DUBE B, RONGSEN T, MAZUMDAR S, TANEJJA S, RAFIQUI F, BHANDARI N, BHAN MK (2009). Comparison of ready-to-use therapeutic food with cereal legume-based Khichri among malnourished children. *Indian Pediatr* vol 46, no. 5, pp 383–388.
14. BRIEND A. Therapeutic nutrition for SAM children: Summary of African experience. National Consensus Workshop on Management of SAM children through Medical Nutrition Therapy, AIIMS Delhi, November 26–27, 2009.
15. WHO (1999). Management of Severe Malnutrition: A manual for Physicians and other senior health workers WHO, Geneva 1999. http://whqlibdoc.who.int/hq/1999/a57361.pdf (accessed in January 2007).
16. ASHWORTH A, JACKSON A UAUY R (2007). Focusing on malnutrition management to improve child survival in India. *Indian Pediatr* **44**, no. 6, pp 413–416.
17. HOSSAIN MI, DODD NS, AHMED T, MIAH GM, JAMIL KM, NAHAR B, MAHMOOD CB (2009). Experience in managing severe malnutrition in a government tertiary treatment facility in Bangladesh. *J Health Popul Nutr* **27,** no. 91, pp 72–80.
18. ASHWORTH A, CHOPRA M, MCCOY D, SANDERS D, JACKSON D, KARAOLIS N, SOGAULA N, SCHOFIELD C (2004). WHO guidelines for management of severe malnutrition in rural South African hospitals: effect on case fatality and the influence of operational factors. *Lancet* **363**, no. 9415, pp 1110–1115.
19. PARAKH A, DUBEY AP, GAHLOT N, RAJESHWARI K (2008). Efficacy of modified WHO feeding protocol for management of severe malnutrition in children: a pilot study from a teaching hospital in New Delhi, India. *Asia Pac J Clin Nutr* **17**, no. 4, pp. 608–611.
20. HOSSAIN MM, HASSAN MQ, RAHMAN MH, KABIR A, HANNAN AH, RAHMAN AKMF (2009). Hospital management of severely malnourished children: comparison of locally adapted protocol with WHO protocol. *Ind Pediatr* **46**, no. 3, pp 213–218.
21. WHO (2003). Guidelines for inpatient treatment of severely malnourished children. WHO, Geneva.

22. State of the art training on integrated management of SAM by Professor Michael Golden and Dr. Yvonne Grellety, Pune, India 2008.
23. The sustainability of community-based therapeutic care (CTC) in non-emergency contexts. http://www.fantaproject.org/downloads/.../CTC_a_Manual_v1_Oct06.pdf.
24. Humanitarian charter and minimum standards in disasters. http://www.sphereproject.org/.
25. SACHDEV HPS, KAPIL U and VIR S (2010). Consensus Statement: National Consensus Workshop on Management of SAM children through Medical Nutrition Therapy. Indian Paediatrics, **47** (August 17), p. 661.

13

Prevention and management of overweight and obesity in children

Anura Kurpad and *Sumathi Swaminathan*

Anura Kurpad, MD, PhD, FAMS, a physiologist and nutritionist, is the Dean of St John's Research Institute, and Head of the Nutrition Division. His primary interests are in energy and protein metabolism and requirements, body composition, adaptation to undernutrition, and in fetal development.

Sumathi Swaminathan, PhD, is a nutritionist. She is an honorary lecturer at St John's Research Institute, with interest in childhood obesity. Dr Swaminathan is currently conducting epidemiological studies in overweight and obesity in urban and rural regions.

13.1 Introduction

Over the past decade, there is an increased focus on childhood overweight and obesity that has developed into a world-wide phenomenon both in the developed and the developing nations. The World Health Organization [1] reports that world-wide 22 million children under the age of 5 are obese. Obesity is defined as a condition in which excess body fat has accumulated to an extent that health may be adversely affected. It is debatable whether obesity is merely a condition or a disease [2]. It seems reasonable to call it a disease, and to make a public policy for the prevention of obesity more definitive in terms of disease prevention and management. In 2004, Bray [3] suggested that obesity meets the criteria needed to call it a disease. It has an etiology – an imbalance between energy intake and expenditure. It has a pathogenesis in the feedback systems involving neurochemicals in the brain, and the neural and endocrine messages that respond to the intake of food. The pathology of obesity lies in its enlarged fat cells, including cytokines, procoagulants, inflammatory peptides, and angiotensinogen. These secretory products of fat cells and the increased mass of fat are responsible for the associated metabolic diseases, such as diabetes, hypertension, heart disease, sleep apnea, and some sorts of cancer. Treatment consists of techniques to alter the balance between energy intake and energy expenditure. Obesity and overweight are major risk factors for many diseases.

Since overweight and obesity result from an imbalance between energy intake and expenditure, it makes sense that preventive strategies are also dependent on modulating these variables successfully. In normal healthy children, a homeostatic regulation ensures a balance between energy intake and expenditure, and energy storage for growth (approximately 84 kJ/day), thereby resulting in the maintenance of body weight and body stores [4, 5].

13.2 Maintenance of energy balance

Energy intake, energy expenditure and energy storage in the body result in the energy balance in children. This homeostatic regulation is governed by the first law of thermodynamics, that is, energy cannot be created or destroyed. Energy intake is defined as the caloric or energy content of food as provided by the major sources of dietary energy: carbohydrate (16.8 kJ/g), protein (16.8 kJ/g), fat (37.8 kJ/g) and alcohol (29.4 kJ/g). Most of the energy expended is for the basal metabolic rate (BMR) which is for the maintenance of basic physiologic functions for sustenance of life such as heart beat and respiration. Since under most measurement situations, the resting metabolic rate or resting energy expenditure (REE) is more practical with the rate being approximately 3% more, BMR and REE are used interchangeably. The REE in an average child is roughly 2.94 kJ/ minute. The other components of energy expenditure are the thermic effect of a meal (TEM), which is the energy expended to digest, metabolize and store ingested macro-nutrients, and physical activity or activity energy expenditure (AEE). TEM comprises about 10% of the caloric content of a meal while AEE is the most variable component of energy expenditure dependent on an individual (Figure 13.1). Apart from these, children require additional energy for growth. However energy cost of growth relative to total energy needs is small, except in the first few months of life.

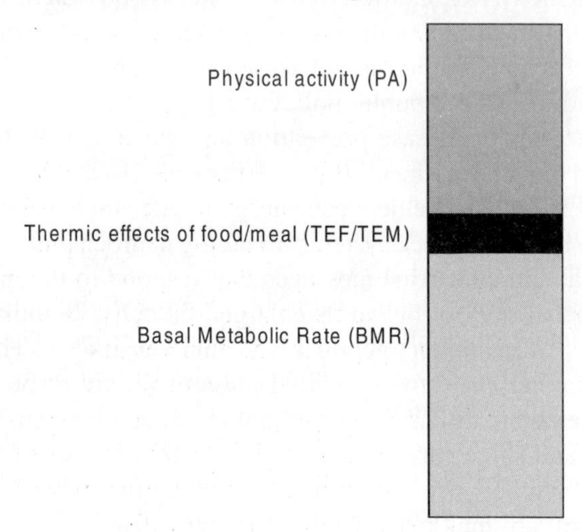

13.1 Components of energy expenditure.

When energy intake exceeds energy expenditure, a state of positive energy balance occurs. Normally, ingested carbohydrate is used up immediately for energy, and through adaptive processes any excess is stored as glycogen for urgent needs (e.g. exercise). However no such adaptive mechanism exists for fat and therefore fat with low metabolic costs for storage, is the preferred energy store in the body [4].

Regulation of energy intake occurs through short-term signals that control hunger, food intake and satiety, and through long-term signals that relate to the conservation of energy stores, lean tissue or both. In the short term regulation, gastro-intestinal signals provide important inputs to the brain and the hormones released from the stomach and intestines are inhibitory. For example, the YY_{3-36}, the major circulating form of peptide YY (PYY), a gut hormone produced by the L cells of the small intestine produced in this manner, when infused into lean or obese subjects led to a decrease in food intake by approximately 30%. However, ghrelin, a peptide produced by the stomach and proximal small intestine, stimulates food intake, and has been observed to decline after a meal and to rise before the next meal. In Prader-Willi syndrome, ghrelin levels are elevated and marked by hyperphagia. In long-term regulation, the adipose tissue is involved in the feedback regulation of energy balance by production of a number of peptide hormones. Leptin and adiponectin are two of the most important ones. The absence of leptin produces massive obesity, and treatment of leptin-deficient individuals reduces food intake and body weight. However, in obese people leptin has little or no effect on both food intake and body weight, as they are leptin resistant leading to already high levels of leptin in the circulation [6, 7, 8].

13.3 The epidemic of obesity in children

The current epidemic which is largely a result of rapid urbanization with consequent rapid changes in demographic, nutritional and socio-economic transition has resulted in increased energy intake due to modern food processing and marketing techniques, coupled with the decline in energy expenditure because of automation, mechanized transport and increases in sedentary occupation and leisure pursuits, for example, use of computers and television [9, 10, 11, 12].

Overweight and obesity in children are most common in the North America, United Kingdom and South-Western Europe [1]. In the latest report by Centers for Disease Control, in the United States, 13% were obese, (more males than females), while 15.8% were overweight, with linear increases from 25.1% in 1999 to 28.8% of overweight/obese children from high schools [13]. In the United Kingdom, prevalence of overweight in children aged 2–10 years increased from 23% to 28% from 1995 to 2003 [1]. Overweight data from 79 out of 147 developing countries on pre-school children, using the criteria of weight-for-height above 2 standard deviations (SD) from the National Center for Health Statistics/World Health Organization international reference (1978), indicated that 3.3% children below 5 years of age were overweight in 1995, with the percentage highest in Latin America and Caribbean (4.4%), followed by Africa (3.9%) and then Asia (2.9%). However, in absolute numbers Asia had the highest numbers of overweight children [14].

In the most recent analysis of prevalence in 60 out of 191 regions of the World Health Organization, the most dramatic increase is in the industrialized countries. From the 1970s to the 1990s, prevalence doubled or tripled in large countries of Canada and United States in North America, Brazil and Chile in South America, Australia and Japan in the Western Pacific, Finland, Germany, Greece, Spain and United Kingdom in Europe, with prevalence ranging from 20% to 30%. Estimated figures of overweight and obesity for school-aged children in the year 2010, is 1 in 5 in urban China (which was 1 in 8 in 1997), 46% in the Americas, 41% in the Eastern Mediterranean region, 38 % in the European region, 27% in Western Pacific region and 22% in South East Asia [15]. An increasing gradient in immigrant populations from the first generation of immigrants to the third has been demonstrated, in Hispanic and Asian-American adolescents, indicating an important role of acculturation or assimilation into lifestyles in industrialized countries being a risk factor for obesity [16].

A matter of concern, especially in the lower and middle income countries, is the transition from undernutrition to overnutrition problems, causing a double burden of both under- and overnutrition. For example, in Brazil between 1975 and 1997, prevalence of overweight in children between 6 and 18 years of age increased from 4.1% to 13.9%, while prevalence of underweight decreased from 14.8% to 8.6% [15, 17]. Prevalence rates of overweight and obesity in school children in India reported from studies from various regions vary from 4% to 30% [18–24].

Box 13.1 Trends of childhood obesity in India

In urban school children in Delhi [24], prevalence increased from 16 % in 2002 to 24 % in 2006–2007.
In Ernakulam district in Kerala, prevalence increased from 4.94% in 2003 to 6.57% in 2005.

Probable causes of childhood obesity in India

1. Rapid urbanization and globalization with marked changes in food availability and consumption, as well as changes in physical activity patterns.
2. High prevalence of low birth weight.
3. High prevalence of stunting. Nutritional stunting causes changes such as lower energy expenditure, higher susceptibility to the effects of a high fat diet, lower fat oxidation and impairment in regulation of food intake which could result in later obesity [25, 26, 27].

13.4 Developmental aspects of growth, weight gain and later obesity (Figure 13.2)

Adipose tissue is found in the fetus after the 14th week of gestation. At birth, about 13% of the body mass consists of adipose tissue doubling to about 28% at the end of the first year for a normal weight infant. The percentage of fat in the body mass of children again increases during puberty. During the first year of life, fat accumulation is characterized by increase in the volume of adipocytes. However, during the pubertal period fat accumulates largely through an increase in the number of adipocytes, without further change in the fat cell volume. Two mechanisms play a role in this process; one regulates the breakdown or storage of fat within the cell through lipolytic and lipogenic mechanisms, and another which regulates the number of cells through proliferation from pre-adipocytes or removal through apoptosis or merger of fat cells. Age-dependent differences are seen in the formation of adipose cells from pre-adipocytes, with maximum proliferation and capacity for differentiation during the first year of life and just before puberty. Unlike adults, adipose tissue in children has a higher proportion of smaller fat cells, indicating a higher rate of formation of new cells in childhood.

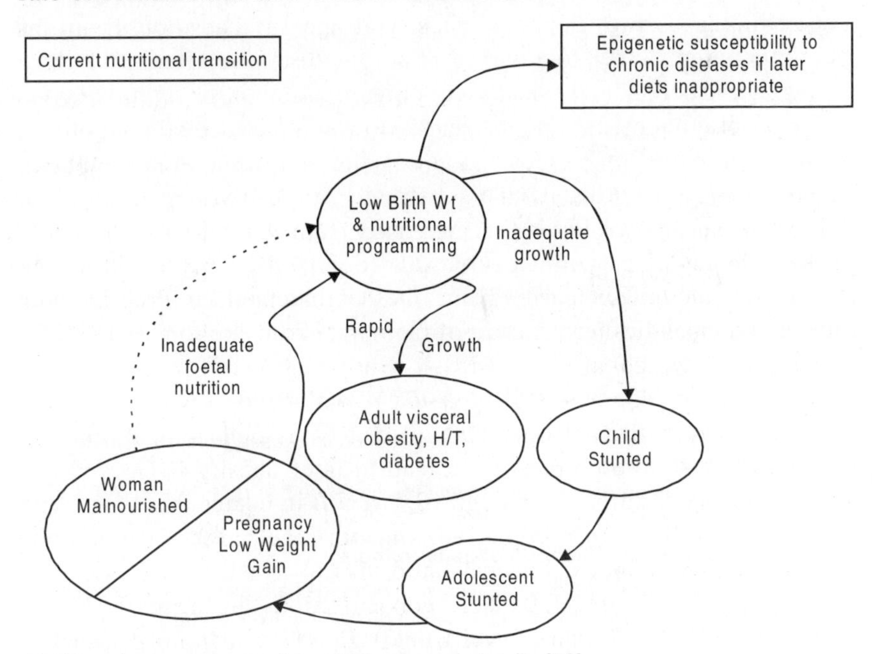

13.2 Developmental aspects weight gain and obesity [12].

The pubertal growth spurt is associated with significant changes in body composition, with girls tending to accumulate more fat than boys.

Fat gain occurs in both boys and girls in early adolescence, but then ceases and even reverses temporarily in boys, but continues through adolescence in girls. Body Mass Index (BMI) as a measure of body fatness in adolescents is influenced by maturation status, race and distribution of body fat [28].

A number of factors are related to obesity during childhood as well as in adolescence and adulthood.

13.4.1 Intra-uterine period and birth weight

The earliest evidence pertaining to undernutrition of the mother during the period of pregnancy and later obesity came from the Dutch famine study [29]. This report in 1976 consisted of several natural cohorts based on their intra-uterine exposure to the Dutch famine. During World War II, the Germans restricted food for the population of Northern Holland and consequently food intake declined from approximately 1500 kcal to approximately 1000 kcal for about a 6-month period. The cohort, exposed to famine in the last trimester, was found to have a reduced prevalence of obesity at the age of 18 years. However, individuals exposed to famine in the first 2 trimesters of pregnancy had an increased prevalence of obesity at age 18. These observations were attributed firstly, to a period of adipocyte replication in the third trimester and secondly, to the nascent organization of the hypothalamus in earlier pregnancy. Hence, the responsiveness to caloric intake might be set by the responsiveness of the hypothalamus and sympathetic nervous system to intra-uterine substrate availability.

Evidence is also available linking higher birth weights (>3500 g) with overweight and obesity in late adolescence [30]. However, this has been attributed to increase in lean body mass rather than fat mass. Programming of lean body mass rather than that of fat mass, could explain associations between birth weight and later BMI. The association of low birth weight with a smaller proportion of lean mass, and hence lower metabolic activity, could with environmental influences associated with energy-dense diets have the propensity to lead to later obesity [31]. A recent study of obese children (mean age 10.4 years) indicates that those with high birth weights had a higher adiponectin level, higher whole-body insulin sensitivity index, lower hepatic insulin resistance index, lower plasma insulin and free fatty acid concentrations during oral glucose tolerance test (OGTT), and lower trunk fat percent than normal or low birth weight children [32]. There is a great deal of recent literature on this issue, which is out of the scope of this chapter; interested readers are referred to recent reviews on the subject [28, 33].

13.4.2 Weight gain in infancy, childhood and adolescence

Rapid weight gain, especially during infancy, has been shown to be associated with obesity in later life. A rapid weight gain pattern from birth to 4 months [34] and during the period of infancy [35] has been associated with obesity in childhood and young adulthood. A recent study [32] has shown that increased fetal growth and infant weight gain between 0 and 2 years were associated with relative protection from the development of central obesity and insulin resistance among obese children and adolescents, possibly an indicator of healthy obesity. However, rapid weight gain after 4 years led to insulin resistance.

Body mass index increases through infancy and then drops from the second to the fifth year. There is then, a gradual rise from the sixth year of life through adolescence. This sudden increase around 5–7 years of age is termed "adiposity rebound". Early adiposity rebound is probably a reflection of rapid weight gain during infancy and possibly early maturation [29]. An early adiposity rebound is associated with increased risk of adult obesity. The likelihood of children with very early adiposity rebound (by 43 months) being obese at the age of 7 years was found to be high (OR 15.00, 95 % CI: 5.32 to 42.30) in the Avon Longitudinal Study of Parents and Children (ALSPAC). Early adiposity rebound (44–61 months) too, showed an association (OR 2.01, 95 % CI: 0.81 to 5.2) [35]. A study of 1400 adults in Delhi [36], India, indicated that children with early adiposity rebound of 5 years or younger had the highest body mass index in later childhood, and this persisted into adulthood. These children had the lowest ponderal index (body weight in kg^3/height (cm) × 100) at birth, the lowest body mass index from birth to 2 years of age.

Catch-up growth is a property in human growth wherein children return to their genetic trajectory after a period of growth arrest or delay, for example because of illness. This is most commonly observed in the first 2 years of life, especially after severe intra-uterine growth restraint. These children have been shown to have greater BMI, percentage body fat and total fat mass and central fat distribution [35, 37]. Concentrations of cord blood leptin are positively related to ponderal index at birth but inversely related to weight gain in infancy, and thus low concentrations of this hormone at birth may provide a signal for catch-up growth through reduced inhibition of satiety [37]. Cord leptin concentrations (a surrogate measure of fat mass) of newborn children in the Pune Maternal Nutrition Study, were similar to that of newborns from a white Caucasian population recruited in the study although mean birth weights were lower, suggesting higher adiposity in Indian babies [38].

During adolescence the location of body fat changes and is a period of increased risk of development of obesity, especially in girls. In men, ~10 % of adult obesity begins in early adolescence, while in women this proportion is ~ 30% [29]. A link between early age of onset of menarche to obesity has been observed. However, findings in the Bogalusa Heart Study [39] and the study conducted at National Institute of Child Health and Human Development Study of Early Child Care and Youth Development [40] indicate that much of the apparent influence of menarcheal age on adult obesity, is inversely, due to the influence of childhood obesity on both menarcheal age and adult obesity.

13.4.3 Stunting

Stunted children (height-for-age below 2 SD of standard growth reference charts) constitute one-third of the children globally, mainly in the developing countries [28]. Although stunting indicates the level of long-term undernutrition in the population, it has also been linked to the overweight observed in Russia, Brazil, Republic of South Africa and China due to the nutrition transition [41]. Childhood nutritional stunting was associated with impaired fat oxidation, a factor predicting obesity since dietary fat that is not oxidized has to be stored [42]. This is a matter of concern as it adds to the burden of obesity in developing economies.

13.5 Assessment of overweight and obesity in children

There are several commonly used tools to assess overweight and obesity in children. The most common is the body mass index, followed by the waist circumference, skinfolds and bio-electrical impedance analysis.

13.5.1 Body mass index (BMI)

As the primary purpose for assessing overweight and obesity is to estimate the risk to health at the individual level and to compare populations and to facilitate monitoring of obesity, these assessments are primarily based on anthropometry, with body mass index being most widely used both clinically and epidemiologically followed by waist circumference. BMI is used as it is closely correlated with body fatness. The adult BMI cut-offs are not appropriate for children as they are still growing [28, 43, 44]. Age and sex specific BMI cut-offs are needed for proper classification of overweight and obesity in children for the primary reason that BMI increases with normal growth and maturation after the period of adiposity rebound. At present, the World Health Organization's sex-specific body mass index (the weight in kilograms divided by the square of the height in meters) for age charts is used extensively to assess overweight and obesity in children from birth to 19 years of age [45, 46]. The present standards for age and sex specific BMI charts, have evolved from the Multi-centre growth reference study of the World Health Organization for children from birth to the age of 5 years from Brazil, Ghana, India, Norway, Oman and the USA. Recently, the WHO 2007 charts for the 5–19 year age group has been released by reconstructing the 1977 NCHS/WHO growth reference from 5 to 19 years, using the original sample (a non-obese sample with expected heights), supplemented with data from the WHO Child Growth Standards (to facilitate a smooth transition at 5 years) [46]. The 2007 BMI values for both sexes at +1 SD (25.4 kg/m^2 for boys and 25.0 kg/m^2 for girls) are equivalent to the overweight cut-off used for adults (>25.0 kg/m^2), while the +2 SD value (29.7 kg/m^2 for both sexes) compares closely with the cut-off for obesity (>30.0 kg/m^2). These growth charts are given in the Appendix.

Prior to this, different measures and definitions were used to identify overweight and obese children. Therefore, comparisons across populations from different countries and within regions were a major problem, as different criteria were used. Table 13.1 indicates the criteria used for the past few decades to define overweight and obesity. Apart from these, several countries had developed reference charts using local data (for example France, UK, Singapore).

Table 13.1 Criteria used to evaluate overweight and obesity in children prior to 2006 and 2007 growth charts [99]

Classification	Overweight	Obesity	Data and reference population	Source
WHO Reference	Child (6–9 years): WHZ> 2[(a)] Adolescent (10–18 years): BMI 85th percentile (called as "at risk" overweight)	Child (6–9 years): no reference Adoles-cent (10–18 years): BMI ≥ 85th perce-ntile and subsca-pular and triceps skinfolds ≥ 90th percentile	US NHANES 1 data (1971–74)	[93]
IOTF reference	≥ BMI-for-age cut-offs derived from BMI-age curves passed BMI of 25 at age 18	≥ BMI-for-age cut-offs derived from BMI-age curves passed BMI of 30 at age 18	Data from USA, Brazil, Britain, Hong Kong, the Netherlands and Singapore	[94]
"Old" US BMI percentiles	≥ BMI 85th perce-ntile (called as "at risk" overweight)	≥ BMI 95th percentile (called as "overweight")	US NHANES 1 data (1971–74)	[95]
"New" US BMI percentiles (2000 CDC Growth Chart)	≥ BMI 85th percentile (called as "at risk" overweight)	≥ BMI 95th perce-ntile (called as "overweight")	US NHANES data (1971–1994)	[96]
European – French BMI reference	≥ BMI 90th percentile	≥ BMI 97th percentile	Data from the French population	[97, 98]

WHO – World Health Organization; WHZ – weight-for-height z score; NHANES – National Health and Nutrition Examination Survey; IOTF – International Obesity Task Force; BMI – Body Mass Index; CDC – Centers for Disease Control and Prevention.

(a) A z-score of 2 corresponds to the 97.7th percentile.

13.5.2 Waist circumference

The waist circumference is a good indicator of fatness and health risks in children. However, although waist circumference is a very useful measure of fat distribution in children, appropriate cut-off points for high or low health risks have not yet been developed [28, 47, 48]. Abdominal visceral fat as measured by the DEXA instrument correlates highly with waist circumference [47]. Evidence exists linking accumulated visceral adipose tissue to increased health risks and metabolic disorders in children. In research studies, childhood waist circumference is more efficient than BMI in predicting insulin resistance, blood pressure, serum cholesterol and triglyceride levels [48].

13.5.3 Skin-fold thickness

Skin-folds are predictive of total body fat. The skin-folds at the triceps, biceps, supra-iliac and sub- scapular regions are normally taken using skin-fold calipers. However, there is little evidence to indicate that it performs better than BMI as an indicator of body fat. Hence it is not recommended for routine clinical use to assess overweight in children, although it is used extensively for research. Moreover, there is a lack of reference data in children [48].

13.5.4 Bio-electrical Impedance analysis (BIA)

McCarthy et al [49] have developed centile curves from 1985 children aged 5–18 years using the total fat body fat results from a bio-impedance segmental body composition analyzer. The shape of the fat curves obtained matched the changes in fat patterning with human growth especially during puberty when there is an increase in lean mass in boys, while there is an increase in fat mass in girls. These changes are not reflected in BMI curves. These curves have been proposed as an alternative or as an addition to using the body mass index curves.

13.6 Risk factors for overweight and obesity

13.6.1 Genetic and gene–environment interactions

Studies on twins, siblings, and family, both nuclear and extended, have indicated that an individual's chances of being obese are increased when relatives are obese. The results of a study based on Danish Adoption Register indicate that there is a strong influence of genetic factors in obesity. Twin studies on heritability show that for body mass, body mass index and fat mass, quantitative sex differences were observed and genetic variance of 84%, 85% and 81% of total variation in men and 74%, 75% and 70% in women for each of these respective three parameters were observed. [50] Other studies also indicate a heritability factor of 40–70%. The Human Obesity Genome Map results [51] up to the year 2005 have identified 253 quantitative trait locis (QTL) from 61 genome-wide scans.

One may erroneously conclude that since genes account for so much of variation in BMI, environment may have no impact. However genes are expressed in appropriate environments. The present rapid increase in overweight and obesity is an indication that environmental conditions for obesity expression are being created [28]. The study of how phenotype affects gene expression is called epigenetics. It has been shown that fetal programming occurs during the intra-uterine period wherein the fetus adapts to reduced nutrients and these physiological adaptations lead to life-long changes in structure and function of the body [52]. Parental obesity could mediate obesity in children through both genetic and shared environmental factors leading to familial clustering. Among low income children, maternal obesity in early pregnancy doubled the risk of obesity between 2 and 4 years of age [53]. Large babies tend to become overweight when there is a parental history of overweight. The risk of becoming overweight adolescents was approximately 5 to 7 times higher when the mother was overweight [54]. Offspring of women who had diabetes during pregnancy are more likely to become obese later in childhood and to have a higher prevalence of impaired glucose tolerance than the off-spring of women who are non-diabetic [28]. In a multi-ethnic sample in the U.S., it was found that increasing hyperglycemic values lead to an increased risk of offspring obesity at 5 to 7 years of age [55]. The odds ratio of adolescent overweight was 1.4 (CI: 1.1–2.0) among children born to mothers with gestational diabetes mellitus (GDM) [56].

Ethnicity also plays a role, although one may take ethnicity to really represent a gene-environment interaction. Insulin resistance has been observed in British South Asians. The same trend was also observed in British Asian children compared to British children, reflecting an increased sensitivity to adiposity [57]. In the US, non-white teens (Hispanic, African Americans) were also shown to be more likely to have metabolic syndrome compared to white children [58].

13.6.2 Environmental factors

A drastic change has occurred in the environment both at home and in the community. This environment has had an effect on the way children eat. Socio-economic status seems to have an effect on overweight in children in the developed countries. The odds of developing overweight were higher in children from the lower socio-economic status in the European Youth Heart Study [59]. Low socio-economic status was related to high BMI in children 6–18 years of age which was mediated by the poor quality of breakfast [60]. In India, prevalence of overweight and obesity in children seems to be higher in the higher socio-economic groups [18, 24].

With the advent of globalization and its focus on freer movement of capital, technology, goods and services, major changes in lifestyles linked to diet, physical activity have occurred leading to the problem of overweight and obesity [10]. In the past decade, major developments in food manufacturing, processing and retail sectors have occurred. The agricultural policies and the multifarious industries contributing to all aspects of the food chain are responsible for the progressive cheapening of meat, butter, oils, fats and sugars, whilst the relative price of fruits and vegetables increased [12].

The changing nature of food supply globally, with fresh food sales and marketing decreasing and supermarkets, hypermarkets emerging with increased consumer demand for processed foods, food marketing and promotion through mass media, food advertising and food prices, have contributed in various ways to the "obesigenic" environment. Liberalization of direct foreign investment and trade liberalization has also resulted in increased availability of processed foods of greater variety. Global agricultural policies also have a bearing on the types of foods being marketed. Both food intake and physical activity have been affected through these changes [10, 61]. Tobacco usage has also had an impact, with maternal smoking being associated with subsequent adiposity in children [35, 62].

13.6.3 Dietary factors

Breast-feeding

In a study by Von Kries [62] on over 9357 German children, aged 5–6 years, breastfeeding was reported to be a significant protector against overweight and obesity – with 35 % reduction in adulthood if children are breast fed up till 3–5 months. This association was however not observed with obesity at the age of 5 years [63]. Breastfeeding could have a programming effect in preventing obesity as it is found that breastfed children have higher insulin levels.

Energy-dense foods

Energy Density (ED) refers to the amount of energy per gram of food and depends on the content of fat, carbohydrate, protein and water. Water has the greatest impact on energy density, as it contributes to weight without energy. Fibre also decreases the energy density of foods. The high energy of fat influences energy density. Energy dense foods have been implicated in the increase in overweight and obesity in children. These foods can reduce satiety and increase appetite, leading to over-eating in adolescents [48]. Data from the ALSPAC study revealed that a higher dietary pattern consisting of a high dietary energy density, low fiber intake and a high fat intake at ages 5 to 7 years was associated with higher odds of excess adiposity at 9 years of age [64]. Preference for energy-dense foods (e.g. sweet, fatty) is likely to be an evolutionary trait conferring survival advantage in periods of scarcity [11].

The World Health Organization (2003) [65] has cautioned the use of sugar-sweetened beverages by children as evidence that each glass of sugar-sweetened beverage consumed increases the risk of obesity in children by 60%. Energy dense foods are also micro-nutrient poor. Dietary carbohydrates are not directly responsible for weight gain, but indirectly they may play a role by inducing a reduction in fat oxidation, especially in children who drink large quantities of soft drinks with high sugar content [66].

Frequency of eating away from home

Worldwide eating foods away from home have been implicated as a cause for increased energy intakes [61, 67–69]. Outside the home the type of foods consumed as snacks are often high in fat, sugar and/or starch. Portion sizes, especially in fast food joints have increased to promote their food products. Large portion sizes also have the propensity to increase energy intake even from the pre-school period [70, 71]. Research has indicated that very young children have an innate control of appetite and are able to match intake to energy needs. But this biological mechanism can be overridden by environmental and social factors in older children [28].

13.6.4 Physical inactivity

Globally, more people are driven by technology based, comfort oriented lifestyles, resulting in changes in the activity patterns of children towards more sedentary living. Physical activity is an important determinant of body weight and physical activity and physical fitness are important modifiers of morbidity and mortality in adults. Children who regularly participate in at least 3 hours per week of sports activities are protected against total and regional fat accumulation, with increase in lean and bone mass and physical fitness compared to children who do not participate in sports activities [72]. Television viewing, video games and computer games have been associated with childhood obesity in a few studies. Time spent viewing television is considered to be a major contributor to obesity [73, 74]. Studies on obese and non-obese children have also shown that decreased physical activity could either be a cause or a consequence of obesity. A study conducted on obese and non-obese children in Hong Kong [75] showed a significant difference between the 2 groups in the amount of time spent on sedentary activities, with the obese group spending 51% more time than non-obese children. The ratio of active-to-sedentary waking time was 0.6 for obese children and 1.9 for non-obese children. In a school study of 4700 school children aged between 13 to 18 years the percentage of children overweight was higher in those with lower physical activity [18]. This behavior could then track to adulthood and these children will continue to be obese adults as well as be prone to other non-communicable diseases.

Evidence regarding the dietary and physical activity factors which promote or protect against overweight and obesity are presented in Table 13.2.

Table 13.2 Evidence table for factors that might promote or protect against overweight and weight gain [100]

Convincing	Regular physical activity High dietary NSP/fibre intake		Sedentary lifestyles High intake of energy dense foods[a]
Probable	Home and school environments that support healthy food choices for children Breastfeeding		Heavy marketing of energy dense foods[a] and fast food outlets Adverse social and economic conditions (developed countries especially for women) High sugar drinks
Possible	Low glycemic index foods	Protein content of the diet	Large portion sizes High proportion of food prepared outside the home (western countries) "Rigid restraint/periodic disinhibition" eating patterns
Insufficient	Increased eating frequency		Alcohol

[a] Energy dense foods are high in fat and/or sugar; energy dilute foods are high in NSP/fibre and water such as fruit, legumes, vegetables and whole grain cereals.

13.6.5 Other plausible factors

A few plausible causes for which evidence exists and which are relevant to children are sleep debt, endocrine disruptors, reduction in variability in ambient temperature, pharmaceutical preparations, increasing gravida age of the mother and intergenerational effects [76].

Several cross-sectional studies have indicated that the number of hours of sleep in children is inversely related to BMI [74, 77]. Although sleep and weight gain could be related through hormonal factors causing decreased levels of leptin and increased levels of ghrelin, it could also be associated with an increased sympatho-adrenal secretion of cortisol and catecholamines. Additionally, too little sleep and impaired quality of sleep may affect the chronobiology and adipocyte function adversely [78].

Environmental endocrine disruptors are lipophilic, environmentally stable, industrially produced substances that can affect endocrine function and include dichlorodiphenyltrichloroethane, some polychlorinated biphenols, alkyl phenols, organophosphates, phthalates, carbamates, heavy metals, solvents, etc [76, 79]. These industrial chemical toxins could cause weight gain by interfering with weight homeostasis possibly by causing alterations in weight controlling hormones, altered sensitivity to neuro-transmittors, or altered activity of the sympathetic nervous system. Chemicals with estrogenic activity like diethylstilbesterol, a synthetic estrogen also causes weight gain [79].

Being in the thermo-neutral zone (TNZ), that is, the range of ambient temperature in which energy expenditure is not required for homeothermy increases energy stores. With increase in air-conditions, the time spent in TNZ has increased. Some pharmaceutical preparations induce weight gain. Some examples are medications like anti-depressants, anticonvulsants, anti-diabetics, steroid hormones, antihistamines and protease inhibitors. The usage of most of these pharmaceuticals has increased in the past three decades [76].

Increase in gravida age has also been implicated in some studies for increasing odds (~7%) of obesity in the offspring. Intergenerational effects could also lead to obesity, and this influence could date to two generations back when oocytes form in the grandmother and this could occur partly through epigenetic (e.g. methylation) events. Maternal obesity and resulting diabetes during gestation and lactation could possibly promote the same conditions in subsequent generations [76].

13.7 Consequences of overweight or obesity

Pediatric overweight and obesity has resulted in several co-morbidities which were considered rare in children earlier. There is a rising prevalence of, for instance, Type 2 diabetes, which was unheard of even about a decade ago. Obesity driven insulin resistance, impaired glucose metabolism and cardio-vascular risk factors are also evident in overweight and obese children.

13.7.1 Long-term consequences in adulthood

Whether childhood obesity tracks into adulthood is an important question that has to be answered so that measures to prevent obesity in childhood are of more relevance. Meta-analysis of several studies indicates that the more extreme the obesity of the child, the more the risk of obesity in adulthood. About 26–41% of obese pre-school children and about 42–63% of obese school-age children were obese as adults. The risk of adult obesity was at least twice as high for obese compared to non-obese children [80].Other health consequences of overweight and obesity have been listed in Table 13.3.

13.8 Children at special risk of obesity

At an individual level, children with physical disabilities like cerebral palsy, those treated for epilepsy, adolescents with Type 1 diabetes, children on centrally acting drugs like anti-depressants, those treated with glucocorticoids, and those with psychological problems are prone to obesity. Likewise children with specific genetic disorders such as Downs's syndrome,

Table 13.3 Health consequences of childhood overweight and obesity [25, 44, 78]

Metabolic/Endocrine
Type 2 diabetes mellitus
Insulin resistance/impaired glucose tolerance
Metabolic syndrome
Menstrual abnormalities in girls
Hypercorticism
Polycystic ovary syndrome
Cardio-vascular
Atherosclerosis
High blood pressure
Dyslipidemia
Abnormalities in left ventricular mass
Abnormalities in endothelial function
Raised triglycerides
Pulmonary
Asthma
Obstructive sleep apnea
Gastroenterological
Non alcoholic fatty liver disease
Non-alcoholic steatohepatitis
Cholelithiasis
Gastro-esophageal reflux
Renal
Proteinuria
Orthopaedic
Increased risk of fracture
Flat feet
Blounts disease
Slipped capital femoral epiphysis
Ankle sprains
Neurological
Idiopathic intra-cranial hypertension
Psychological
Low self-esteem
Depression
Other
Raised C reactive protein/ systemic inflammation
Long-term consequences
Tracking of obesity to adulthood
Cardiovascular risk factors in adulthood
Impact on adult morbidity and pre-mature mortality

Prader-Willi Syndrome, Duchenne muscular dystrophy (DMD), Albright hereditary osteodystrophy (AHO), Fragile X syndrome, Bardet-Biedl syndrome and some single gene disorders are prone to obesity. Some endocrine disorders, for e.g. Cushing's syndrome, hypothyroidism, hyperadrenocorticism also cause obesity [28, 47, 81].

13.9 Prevention

With the massive increases in the epidemic of overweight and obesity, and with treatment being a more difficult option, the major strategy will be to focus on prevention of overweight and obesity which target environmental factors. The main aim of prevention is to decrease the prevalence of obesity during the period of childhood as well as to prevent modifiable risk behaviors tracking into adulthood. Prevention strategies include encouragement of an active lifestyle as well as healthy eating. At the population level, the World Health Organization [2, 43] recommends 3 modes of preventive measures: universal prevention, selective prevention and targeted prevention.

1. *Universal prevention* – Targeted at the population as a whole. The aim of this is to stabilize the level of obesity and eventually lower the incidence and hence prevalence of obesity. This is achieved through lifestyle modifications of improvement in diet and increase in physical activity levels and reduction in smoking and alcohol consumption.
2. *Selective prevention* – Educate sub-groups of populations with a high risk of obesity so that they can deal effectively with risk factors which may be genetic and which pre-dispose them to obesity.
3. *Targeted prevention* – Aims to prevent weight gain and reduce the number of people with weight related disorders in those individuals who are already overweight or in those who are not yet obese but with biological markers associated with excess adiposity.
   WHO 2003 [65] recommends some preventive strategies in infants, children and adolescents:

Infants and young children

- The promotion of exclusive breast-feeding during the first 6 months.
- Avoiding the use of added sugars and starches when feeding formula.
- Instructing mothers to accept their child's ability to regulate energy intake rather than to force-feed them.
- Assuring the appropriate micro-nutrient intake needed to promote linear growth.

Children and adolescents

- Promote an active lifestyle
- Limit television viewing

- Promote intake of fruits and vegetables
- Restrict intake of energy-dense and micro-nutrient-poor foods (e.g. packaged snacks)
- Restrict intake of sugar-sweetened soft drinks

Additional measures include modifying the environment to enhance physical activity in schools and communities, creating more family interactions (e.g. family meals), limiting exposure of young children to heavy marketing practices of energy-dense, micro-nutrient poor foods and providing necessary information and skills to make healthy food choices. Promotion of age appropriate serving sizes, consuming adequate amounts of dietary fiber, fruits and vegetables, avoiding use of sugar-sweetened drinks and limiting the intake of salt is required [82].

Recent dietary reference intakes recommend [83] a fat intake of 30–40 percent of energy in children 1–3 years old and 25–35% in children 4–18 years old, a carbohydrate intake of 45–65% of energy in all children and protein intakes of 5–20% energy in children 1–3 years old and 10–30% of energy in children 4–18 years old.

Monitoring the growth of children, is important such that there is an improvement of linear growth in the first 2 years of life (the period when length recovery takes place) while rapid excessive weight gain is prevented relative to height thereafter. Weight should be monitored to prevent a rapid weight gain of ≥1 SD in weight-for age z score during the first year of infancy, the period of adiposity rebound as well as during the pre-pubertal phase. In fact, preventive steps should begin before conception, starting a healthy weight before pregnancy and avoiding either excessive or low weight gain during pregnancy. Since a link between maternal and child malnutrition and later chronic disease exists, concerted effort to achieve a marked reduction in LBW is a priority. If young girls and women have sufficient intakes of animal protein, folic acid and vitamin B12, prevalence of LBW can decrease [84, 85, 86, 87].

In developing countries, avoidance of overfeeding to stunted population groups should be ensured. Nutrition programs designed to control or prevent undernutrition need to assess stature in combination with weight to prevent providing excess energy to children of low weight-for-age but normal weight-for height [66]. It is important to monitor obesity prevention programmes so that they do not lead to the development of clinical eating disorders or risky behavior such as smoking to control weight [16].

With evidence pointing towards the increase in overweight and non-communicable diseases, probably tracking through to adulthood all over the world, promotion of physical activity during the childhood years should be a public health priority.

The WHO (2003) [65] recommends

- At least 30 minutes of cumulative moderate physical activity everyday (walking/ brisk walking as well as other appropriate, healthy and enjoyable physical activities and sport for all actions), with children of all ages requiring an additional 20 minutes of vigorous physical activity three times a week. Moderate intensity exercise of a non-structured nature facilitates most of the disease prevention goals and health promoting benefits.
- Restrict TV viewing, video games and use of computers to a total of ≤2 hours per day.

At the present date, the WHO website [88] indicates that 60 minutes of moderate- to vigorous-intensity physical activity each day that is developmentally appropriate and involves a variety of activities is the minimum required for children between 5 and 18 years of age, although the official recommendations are not yet released.

Further recommendations [89] to promote physical activity especially in Indian children are as following:

At the parent–child level – This includes encouragement of parents to promote physical activity from the period of infancy, by stimulating and encouraging the child to walk and play once he/she learns to do so, support for children's participation in appropriate, enjoyable physical activities, familial participation in games and sports activities and household chores (for example, walking, swimming and other recreational activities), restricting TV viewing to less than 2 hours a day.

At the school–student level – Physical education must be compulsorily integrated into the school and college curriculum. Emphasis on competition should not be the sole objective. Emphasis should be placed on play and activities rather than "exercise". In sporting events, participation should be stressed and competition deemphasized. Lack of space in the school for play activities should be compensated for by obtaining permission to use public playgrounds for the children so that all students in the school avail of the physical education classes. Suitable games should be conceived for children with mild and major disabilities and this should be incorporated in the physical education program. Elementary school students should develop basic motor skills that allow participation in a variety of physical activities, and older students should become competent in a select number of lifetime physical activities they enjoy and succeed in. Discourage the use or withholding of physical activity as punishment.

At a government–community level – Playground facilities and safe play areas for children should be increased and adequate infrastructure provided, especially in urban areas. Safe and level pedestrian paths for the public to walk should be provided. Mass media should be used to promote physical activity.

13.9.1 Effectiveness of intervention programmes to prevent obesity in children

The goal of intervention programmes is to promote healthy eating, active living and positive self-esteem rather than to achieve ideal body weight. An effective intervention programme should use a multi-strategic approach involving multi-levels of the society which is aimed at both population and the individual [16]. Modifications in diet include increasing the intake of fruits and vegetables, reducing the use of snacks and soft drinks and fats, while modifications in physical activity are targeted at reducing sedentary behavior, by watching less television or playing video games and increasing activity to moderate intensity.

Systematic reviews of these programmes have shown that most of these programs have been conducted as randomized control trials in school-based settings or in clinics. Intervention effects were stronger in adolescent age group than pre-adolescents, females than males, in programmes with parental involvement, those in which focused short and simple messages were relayed over a short period of time than long term periods. Very few long-term follow-ups have been done and hence sustainability of prevention programmes, which is most important, is not known [16, 90, 91]. The "Trim and Fit" (TAF) programme initiated by the Singapore government in 1992 [92] as a concerted effort to prevent childhood obesity by initiating changes in school catering, nutrition education, and increased physical activity, was effective in reducing obesity rates, although it was highly criticized for focusing on children with weight or fitness problems leading to stigmatization and eating disorders. TAF was also seen to be a reverse acronym for FAT. This programme was scrapped due to these problems, and the Ministry of Education initiated another programme targeting all school children called the Holistic Health Framework (HHF).

In India, a comprehensive programme for prevention of childhood obesity [24] called MARG has been initiated. This programme aims to promote nutrition and physical activity by education through lectures and leaflets, and through staging drama, skits and debates. The aim is to target 5 lakh children in 15 cities of North India.

13.10 Management and treatment

The basis of management of overweight and obesity in children differs from that of adults, in that prevention of weight gain is more important rather than weight loss as lean body mass increases as children get older and growth cannot be curbed. This eventually ensures that fat mass stays constant and leads to normal body weight. Essentially both the family and child are involved in the process of management and an increase in daily activity and healthy eating habits is recommended. Higher energy expenditure can be achieved more effectively through increased general activity in schools and play rather than through competitive and structured sports. Encouragement is given to curb TV viewing, videogames and computer which is a source of major physical inactivity. In diets of obese children, only small reductions in energy intake should be made so that sufficient energy and nutrients are available to ensure normal growth and development [16, 43]. Care must be taken to provide adequate nutrition as it has been observed that energy restriction in obese children on well-controlled weight reduction diets have led to reduction in height velocity [16].

Pharmacotherapy is used only in extreme cases.

The guiding principles [6] for treatment of overweight should be:

- Establish individual treatment goals and approaches based on the child's age, degree of overweight, and presence of co-morbidities.
- Involve the family or major caregivers in the treatment.
- Provide assessment and monitoring frequently.
- Consider behavioral, psychological and social correlates of weight gain in the treatment plan.
- Provide recommendations for dietary changes and increases in physical activity that can be implemented within the family environment and that foster optimal health, growth and development.

Box 13.2 International Obesity Task Force (IOTF)

The IOTF is part of the International Association for the Study of Obesity (IASO) The task force is a "global network of expertise, a research led think tank and advocacy arm of International Society for the Study of Obesity".
IOTF works in collaboration with the World Health Organization, other NGOs and stakeholders to address the challenge of alerting the world to the growing health crisis of obesity and to persuade governments to act immediately on this rising problem
It has key experts looking at obesity in relation to:
Prevention
Childhood obesity
Management
Economic costs

(*Source:* http://www.iotf.org/)

Overweight and obesity in childhood is a major public health problem in the present world and unless preventive action is taken using all collaborative resources of the community and governments, the problem will escalate to such proportions that lead to major economic losses.

References

1. World Health Organization (WHO). Preventing chronic diseases: A vital investment, WHO Global Report, Geneva (2005): http://www.who.int/chp/chronic_disease_report/en/
2. World Health Organisation (WHO). Obesity: preventing and managing the global epidemic. Report of a WHO Consultation, World Health Organisation Tech Rep Ser 894. Geneva (2000), pp.1–253.
3. BRAY GA (2004). Obesity is a chronic, relapsing neurochemical disease. *Int J Obes Relat Metab Disord* **28**, pp. 34–38.
4. GORAN MI and TREUTH MS (2001). Energy expenditure, physical activity and obesity in children. *Pediatr Clin North Am* **48**, pp. 931–953.
5. GORAN MI (2001). Metabolic precursors and effects of obesity in children: a decade of progress, 1990–1999. *Am J Clin Nutr* **73**, no. 2, pp. 158–171.
6. DANIELS SR, ARNETT DK, ECKEL RH, GIDDING SS, HAYMAN LL, KUMANYIKA S, ROBINSON TN, SCOTT BJ, ST JEOR S, WILLIAMS CL (2005). Overweight in children and adolescents: pathophysiology, consequences, prevention and treatment', *Circulation* **111**, pp.1999–2012.
7. KLOK MD, JACOBSDOTTIR S, DRENT ML (2007). 'The role of leptin and ghrelin in the regulation of food intake and body weight in humans: a review', *Obes Rev* **8**, pp. 21–34.
8. CHAUDHRI OB, WYNNE K, BLOOM SR (2008). Can gut hormones control appetite and prevent obesity? *Diabetes Care*, **31**, pp. S284–S289.
9. UUSITALO U, PIETINEN P, PUSKA P (2002). 'Dietary transition in developing countries: Challenges for chronic disease prevention. *In* Globalization; diets and non-communicable diseases', Geneva, World Health Organization, pp. 1–25.
10. POPKIN BM (2006). Global nutrition dynamics: the world is shifting rapidly toward a diet linked with non-communicable diseases', *Am J Clin Nutr,* **84**, pp. 289–298.
11. MAZIAK W, WARD KD, STOCKTON MB (2008). Childhood obesity: Are we missing the big picture?' *Obes Rev* **9**, pp. 35–42.
12. JAMES WPT (2008). The epidemiology of obesity: the size of the problem, *J Intern Med* **263**, pp. 336–352.
13. Centers for Disease Control and Prevention (CDC) (2008). Youth Risk Behavior Surveillance – United States 2007, *MMWR Morb Mortal Wkly Rep* **57** (SS 4). URL: www.cdc.gov/mmwr.
14. DE ONIS M, BLÖSSNER M (2000). Prevalence and trends of overweight among preschool children in developing countries. *Am J Clin Nutr* **72**, pp. 1032–1039.
15. WANG Y, LOBSTEIN T (2006). Worldwide trends in childhood overweight and obesity. *Int J Pediatr Obes* **1**, pp. 11–25.
16. FLYNN MAT, MCNEIL DA, MALOFF B, MUTASINGWA D, WU M, FORD C, TOUGH SC (2006). Reducing obesity and related chronic disease risk in children and youth: a synthesis of evidence with 'best practice' recommendations. *Obes Rev* **7**, pp. 7–66.
17. WANG Y MONTEIRO C, POPKIN BM (2002). Trends of obesity and underweight in older children and adolescents in the United States, Brazil, China, and Russia. *Am J Clin Nutr*, **75**, pp. 971–977.
18. RAMACHANDRAN A, SNEHALATHA C, VINITHA R, THAYYIL M, KUMAR CK, SHEEBA L, JOSEPH S, VIJAY V (2002). Prevalence of overweight in urban Indian adolescent school children. *Diabetes Res Clin Prac* **57**, pp. 185–190.

19. SHARMA A, SHARMA K, MATHUR KP (2007). Growth pattern and prevalence of obesity in affluent school children of Delhi. *Public Health Nutr* **10**, pp. 485–491.
20. RAJ M, SUNDARAM KR, PAUL M, DEEPA AS, KUMAR R (2007). Obesity in Indian children: Time trends and relationship with hypertension. *Natl Med J India* **20**, pp. 288–293.
21. LAXMAIAH A, NAQALLAH B, VIJAYARAGHAVAN K, NAIR M (2007). Factors affecting prevalence of overweight among 12 to 17 year old urban adolescents in Hyderabad, India. *Obesity (Silver Spring)* **15**, pp. 1384–1390.
22. SRIHARI G, EILANDER A, MUTHAYYA S, KURPAD AV, SESHADRI S (2007). Nutritional status of affluent Indian school children: what and how much do we know? *Indian Pediatr* **44**, pp. 204–213.
23. SWAMINATHAN S, THOMAS T, KURPAD AV, VAZ M (2007). Dietary patterns in urban school children in South India. *Indian Pediatr* **44**, pp. 593–596.
24. BHARDWAJ S, MISRA A, KHURANA L, GULATI S, SHAH P, VIKRAM NK (2008). Childhood obesity in Asian Indians: A burgeoning cause of insulin resistance, diabetes and sub-clinical inflammation. *Asia Pac J Clin Nutr* **17**, pp. 172–175.
25. SAWAYA AL and ROBERTS S (2003). Stunting and future risk of obesity: Principal physiological mechanisms. *Cad Saude Publica* **19**, pp. S21–S28.
26. SAWAYA AL, GRILLO LP, VERRESCHI I, DA SILVA AC, ROBERTS SB (1998). Mild stunting is associated with higher susceptibility to the effects of high fat diets: Studies in a shantytown population in São Paulo, Brazil, *J Nutr* **128**, pp. 415S–420S.
27. HOFFMAN DJ, ROBERTS SB, VERRESCHI I, MARTINS PA, DE NASCIMENTO C, TUCKER KL, SAWAYA AL (2000). Regulation of Energy intake may be impaired in nutritionally stunted children from the shanty towns of São Paulo, Brazil. *J Nutr* **130**, pp. 2265–2270.
28. LOBSTEIN T, BAUR L, UAUY R (2004). IASO International Obesity Task Force. Obesity in children and young people: a crisis in public health. *Obes Rev* vol 5, pp. 4–85.
29. DIETZ WH (1997). Periods of risk in childhood for the development of adult obesity-what do we need to learn? *J Nutr* **127**, pp. 1884S–1886S.
30. SEIDMAN DS, LAOR A, GALE R, STEVENSON DK, DANON YL (1991). A longitudinal study of birth weight and being overweight in late adolescence. *Am J Dis Child* **145**, pp. 782–785.
31. SINGHAL A, WELLS J, COLE TJ, FEWTRELL M, LUCAS A (2003). Programming of lean body mass: a link between birth weight, obesity, and cardiovascular disease. *Am J Clin Nutr* **77**, pp. 726–730.
32. BOUHOURS-NOUET N, DUFRESNE S, DE CASSON FB, MATHIEU E, DOUAY O, GATELAIS F, ROULEAU S, COUTANT R (2008). High birth weight and early postnatal weight gain protect obese children and adolescents from truncal adiposity and insulin resistance: metabolically healthy but obese subjects? *Diabetes Care* **31**, pp. 1031–1036.
33. ROGERS I (2003). EURO-BLCS Study Group. The influence of birth weight and intra-uterine environment on adiposity and fat distribution in later life. *Int J Obes Relat Metab Disord* **27**, pp. 755–777.
34. STETTLER N, KUMANYIKA AK, KATZ SH, ZEMEL BS, STALLINGS VA (2003). Rapid weight gain during infancy and obesity in young adulthood in a cohort of African Americans. *Am J Clin Nutr* **77**, pp. 1374–1378.
35. REILLY JJ, ARMSTRONG J, DOROSTY AR, EMMETT PM, NESS A, ROGERS I et al (2005). Avon Longitudinal Study of Parents and Children Study team. Early life risk factors for obesity in childhood cohort study. *BMJ* **330**, pp. 1357–1363.

36. BHARGAVA SK, SACHDEV HS, FALL CHD, OSMOND C, LAKSHMY R, BARKER DJP, DEY BISWAS SK, RAMJI S, PRABHAKARAN D (2004). Relation of serial changes in childhood body mass index to impaired glucose tolerance in young adulthood. *N Engl J Med* **350**, pp. 865–875.
37. ONG KKL, AHMED ML, EMMETT PM, MICHAEL A, PREECE MA, DUNGER DB (2000). Association between postnatal catch-up growth and obesity in childhood: prospective cohort study. *BMJ* **320**, pp. 967–971.
38. YAJNIK CS (2004). Early life origins of insulin resistance and Type 2 diabetes in India and other Asian countries *J Nutr* **134**, pp. 205–210.
39. FREEDMAN DS, KHAN LK, SERDULA MK, DIETZ WH, SRINIVASAN SR, BERENSON GS (2003). Bogalusa Heart Study. The relation of menarcheal age to obesity in childhood and adulthood: the Bogalusa heart study. *BMC Pediatr* **30**, no. 3, p. 3.
40. LEE JM, APPUGLIESE D, KACIROTI N, CORWYN RF, BRADLEY RH, LUMENG JC (2007). Weight status in young girls and the onset of puberty *Pediatrics* 119, pp. e624–e630.
41. POPKIN BM, RICHARDS MK and MONTEIRO CA (1996). Stunting is associated with overweight in children of four nations that are undergoing the nutrition transition. *J Nutr* **126**, pp. 3009–3016.
42. HOFFMAN DJ, SAWAYA AL, VERRESCHI I, TUCKER KL, ROBERTS SB (2000). Why are nutritionally stunted children at increased risk of obesity? Studies of metabolic rate and fat oxidation in shantytown children from Sao Paulo, Brazil. *Am J Clin Nutr* **72**, pp. 702–707.
43. World Health Organisation, International Association for the Study of Obesity, International Obesity Taskforce. The Asia-Pacific Perspective: Redefining obesity and its treatment. Sydney: Health Communications, 2000.
44. NEOVIUS M, LINNÉ Y, BARKELING B, RÖSSNER S (2004). Discrepancies between classification systems of childhood obesity. *Obes Rev* **5**, pp. 105–114.
45. SEIDELL JC, DOAK CM, DE MUNTER JSL, KUIJPER LDJ, ZONNEVELD C (2006). Cross-sectional growth references and implications for the development of an international growth standard for school-aged children and adolescents. *Food Nutr Bull* **27**, no. 4, pp. S189–S198.
46. DE ONIS M, ONYANGO AW, BORGHI E, SIYAM A, NISHIDA C, SIEKMANN J (2007). Development of a WHO growth reference for school-aged children and adolescents. *Bull World Health Organ* **85**, pp. 660–667.
47. DANIELS SR, KHOURY PR, MORRISON JA (2007). Utility of different measures of body fat distribution in children and adolescents. *Am J Epidemiol* **152**, pp. 1179–1184.
48. KREBS NF, HIMES JH, JACOBSEN D, NICKLAS TA, GUILDAY P, STYNE D (2007). Assessment of child and adolescent overweight and obesity. *Pediatrics* **120**, pp. S193–S228.
49. MCCARTHY HD, COLE TJ, FRY T, JEBB SA, PRENTICE AM (2006). Body fat reference curves for children. *Int J Obes*, **30**, pp. 598–602.
50. SOUREN NY, PAULUSSEN AD, LOOS RJ, GIELEN M, BEUNEN G, FAGARD R, DEROM C, VLIETINCK R, ZEEGERS MP (2007). Anthropometry, carbohydrate and lipid metabolism in the East Flanders Prospective Twin Survey: heritabilities. *Diabetologia* **50**, pp. 2107–2116.
51. RANKINEN T, ZUBERI A, CHAGNON YC, WEISNAGEL SJ, ARGYROPOULOS G, WALTS B, PÉRUSSE L, BOUCHARD C (2006). The Human Obesity Gene Map: The 2005 Update. *Obesity* 14, pp. 529–644.

52. LOKE KY, LIN JBY, MABEL DY. 3rd College of Pediatrics and Child Health Lecture (2008). The past, the present and the shape of things to come. *Ann Acad Med Singapore* **37**, pp. 429–434.
53. WHITAKER RC (2004). Predicting preschooler obesity at birth: The role of maternal obesity in early pregnancy. *Pediatrics* **114**, pp. e29–36.
54. FRISANCHO AR (2000). Prenatal compared with parental origins of adolescent fatness. *Am J Clin Nutr* **72**, pp. 1186–1190.
55. HILLIER TA, PEDULA KL, SCHMIDT MM, MULLEN JA, CHARLES M-A, PETTITT DJ (2007). Childhood obesity and metabolic imprinting. *Diabetes Care* **30**, pp. 2287–2292.
56. GILLMAN MW, RIFAS-SHIMAN S, BERKEY CS, FIELD AE, COLDITZ GA (2003). Maternal gestational diabetes, birth weight, and adolescent obesity. *Pediatrics* **111**, pp. e221–226.
57. WHINCUP PH, GILG JA, PAPACOSTA O, SEYMOUR C, MILLER GJ, ALBERT KGM, COOK DG (2002). Early evidence of ethnic differences in cardiovascular risk: cross sectional comparison of British South Asian and white children. *BMJ* **324**, pp. 635–639.
58. GOODMAN E, DANIELS SR, MORRISON JA, HUANG B, DOLAN LM (2004). Contrasting prevalence of and demographic disparities in the World Health Organization and National Cholesterol Education Program Adult Treatment Panel III definitions of metabolic syndrome among adolescents. *J Pediatr* **145**, pp. 445–451.
59. KRISTENSEN PL, WEDDERKOPP N, MØLLER NC, ANDERSEN LB, BAI CN, FROBERG K (2006). Tracking and prevalence of cardiovascular disease risk factors across socio-economic classes: A longitudinal substudy of the European Youth Heart Study. *BMC Public Health* **6**, p. 20.
60. O'DEA JA, WILSON R (2006). Socio-cognitive and nutritional factors associated with body mass index in children and adolescents: possibilities for childhood obesity prevention. *Health Educ Res.*, **21**, pp. 796–805.
61. ST-ONGE M-P, KELLER KL, HEYMSFIELD SB (2003). Changes in childhood food consumption patterns: a cause for concern in light of increasing body weights, *Am J Clin Nutr*, **78**, pp. 1068–1073.
62. VON KRIES R, KOLETZKO B, SAUERWALD T, VON MUTIUS E, BARNERT D, GRUNERT V, VON VOSS H (1999). Breast feeding and obesity: cross sectional study. *BMJ*, **319**, pp. 147–150.
63. BURDETTE HL, WHITAKER RC, HALL WC, DANIELS SR (2006). 'Breastfeeding, introduction of complementary foods, and adiposity at 5 y of age'. *Am J Clin Nutr.*, 83, pp. 550–558.
64. JOHNSON L, MANDER AP, JONES LR, EMMETT PM, JEBB SA (2008). 'Energy-dense, low-fiber, high-fat dietary pattern is associated with increased fatness in childhood'. *Am J Clin Nutr*, **87**, pp. 846–854.
65. WORLD HEALTH ORGANIZATION (2003). Annual global move for health initiative: A concept paper, Geneva.
66. JÉQUIER E (2001). Is fat intake a risk factor for fat gain in children? *J Clin Endocrinol Metab*, **86**, pp. 980–983.
67. ADAIR LS, POPKIN BM (2005). Are child eating patterns being transformed globally? *Obes Res*, **13**, pp. 1281–1299.
68. FRENCH SA, STORY M, NEUMARK-SZTAINER D, FULKERSON JA, HANNAN P (2001). Fast food restaurant use among adolescents: associations with nutrient intake, food

choices and behavioral and psycho-social variables, *Int J Obes Relat Metab Disord.* 25, pp. 1823–1833.

69. NICKLAS TA, DEMORY-LUCE D, YANG S-J, BARANOWSKI T, ZAKERI I, BERENSON G (2004). Children's food consumption patterns have changed over two decades (1973–1994): The Bogalusa Heart Study. *J Am Diet Assoc.*, **104**, pp. 1127–1140.
70. FISHER JO, ROLLS BJ, BIRCH LL (2003). Children's bite size and intake of an entrée are greater with large portions than with age-appropriate or self-selected portions, *Am J Clin Nutr.*, **77**, pp. 1164–1170.
71. COLAPINTO CK, FITZGERALD A, TAPER LJ, VEUGELERS PJ (2007). Children's preference for large portions: Prevalence, determinants, and consequences, *J Am Diet Assoc.*, **107**, pp. 1183–1190.
72. ARA I, VICENTE-RODRIGUEZ G, PEREZ-GOMEZ J, JIMENEZ-RAMIREZ J, SERRANO-SANCHEZ JA, DORADO C, CALBET JAL (2006). Influence of extra-currricular sport activities on body composition and physical fitness in boys: a 3 year longitudinal study, *Int J Obes* (London), **30**, pp. 1062–1071.
73. HANCOX RJ, POULTON R (2006). Watching television is associated with childhood obesity: but is it clinically important? *Int J Obes* (London), **30**, pp. 171–175.
74. KURIYAN R, BHAT S, THOMAS T, VAZ M, KURPAD AV (2007). Television viewing and sleep are associated with overweight among urban and semi-urban South Indian children, *Nutr J*, **6**, pp. 25–28.
75. YU CW, SUNG YT, SO R, LAM K, NELSON EA, LI AM ET AL (2002). Energy expenditure and physical activity of obese children: cross-sectional study, *Hong Kong Med J.*, **8**, pp. 313–317.
76. KEITH SW, REDDEN DT, KATZMARZYK PT, BOGGIANO MM, HANLON EC, BENCA RM et al. (2006). Putative contributors to the secular increase in obesity: exploring the roads less traveled, *Int J Obes* (London), **30**, pp. 1585–1594.
77. YU Y, LU BS, WANG B, WANG H, YANG J, LI Z, LIULIU WANG, GENFU TANG, HOUXUN XING XIPING XU, ZEE PHYLLIS C, XIAOBIN WANG (2007). Short sleep duration and adiposity in Chinese adolescents'. *Sleep*, **30**, pp. 1688–1697.
78. ASTRUP A. (2006). 'Have we been barking up the wrong tree: can a good night's sleep make us slimmer?' *Int J Obes* (London), **30**, pp. 1025–1026.
79. NEWBOLD RR, PADILLA-BANKS E, SNYDER RJ, PHILLIPS TM, JEFFERSON WN (2007). 'Developmental exposure to endocrine disruptors and the obesity epidemic'. *Reprod Toxicol,* **23**, pp. 290–296.
80. SERDULA MK, IVERY D, COATES RJ, FREEDMAN DS, WILLIAMSON DF, BYERS T (1993). 'Do obese children become obese adults? A review of literature. *Prev Med,* **22**, pp. 167–177.
81. REILLY JJ, METHVEN E, MCDOWELL ZC, HACKING B, ALEXANDER D, STEWART I, KELNAR CJH (2003). 'Health consequences of obesity'. *Arch Dis Child*, **88**, pp. 748–752.
82. KREBS NF, JACOBSEN MS (2003). 'American Academy of Pediatrics Committee on Nutrition. Prevention of pediatric overweight and obesity', *Pediatrics.*, **112**, pp. 424–430.
83. Panel on Macronutrients. Subcommittees on Upper Reference Levels of nutrients and Interpretation and Uses of Dietary Reference Intakes, and the Standing committee on the Scientific Evaluation of Dietary Reference Intakes. (2002). Dietary Reference Intakes for Energy, Carbohydrate, Fiber, Fat, Fatty acids, Cholesterol, Protein and Amino-acids (Macro-nutrients). Washington DC. *National Academies Press.*

84. UAUY R, KAIN J, MERICQ V, ROJAS J, CORVALÁN C (2008). 'Nutrition, child growth and chronic disease prevention'. *Ann Med.*, 40, pp. 11–20.
85. RODE L, HEGAARD HK, KJAERGAARD H, MØLLER LF, TABOR A, OTTESEN B (2007). 'Association between maternal weight gain and birth weight'. *Obstet Gynecol.*, **109**, pp. 1309–1315.
86. JAMES WP (2005). 'The policy challenge of coexisting undernutrition and nutrition-related chronic diseases'. *Matern Child Nutr.*, **1**, pp. 197–203.
87. STETTLER N (2007). 'Nature and strength of epidemiological evidence for origins of childhood and adult obesity in the first year of life'. *Int J Obes.*, 31, pp. 1035–1043.
88. World Health Organization website (Accessed 9th November 2009). http://www.who.int/dietphysicalactivity/factsheet_recommendations/en/
89. KURPAD AV, SWAMINATHAN S, BHAT S (2003). 'IAP National Task Force for Childhood Prevention of Adult Diseases: The effect of childhood physical activity on prevention of adult diseases'. *Indian Pediatr,* 41, pp. 37–62.
90. STICE E, SHAW H, MARTI CN (2006). 'A meta-analytic review of obesity prevention programs for children and adolescents: the skinny on interventions that work'. *Psychol Bull.*, Vol.13, pp. 667–691.
91. SUMMERBELL CD, WATERS E, EDMUNDS LD, KELLY S, BROWN T, CAMPBELL KJ (2005). 'Interventions for preventing obesity in children'. *Cochrane Database Syst Rev*, Issue 3. Art No: CD001871. DOI: 10.1002/14651858.CD001871.pub2.
92. GILL TP (1997). 'Key issues in the prevention of obesity', *Br Med Bull.*, **53**, pp. 359–88.
93. World Health Organisation (WHO), Physical status: the use and interpretation of anthropometry. Report of a WHO Expert Committee, World Health Organ Tech Rep Ser 854, Geneva (1995), pp. 1–452.
94. COLE TJ, BELLIZZI MC, FLEGAL KM, DIETZ WH (2000). 'Establishing a standard definition for child overweight and obesity worldwide: international survey'. *BMJ* **320**, pp. 1240–1243.
95. MUST A, DALLAL GE, DIETZ WH (1991). ' Reference data for obesity: 85th and 95th percentiles of body mass index (wt/ht^2) and triceps skinfold thickness'. *Am J Clin Nutr.,* **53**, pp. 839–846.
96. KUCZMARSKI RJ, OGDEN CL, GRUMMER-STRAWN LM, FLEGAL KM, GUO SS, WEI R, MEI Z, CURTIN LR, ROCHE AF, JOHNSON CL (2000). 'CDC growth charts: United States', *Adv Data.* **314**, pp. 1–27.
97. POSKITT EM (1995). 'Defining childhood obesity: the relative body mass index (BMI)'. European Childhood Obesity Group, *Acta Pediatr.*, **8**, pp. 961–963.
98. ROLLAND-CACHERA MF, COLE TJ, SEMPE M, TICHET J, ROSSIGNOL C, CHARRAUD A (1991). 'Body mass index variations: centiles from birth to 87 years'. *Eur J Clin Nutr* **45**, pp. 13–21.
99. WANG Y, MORENO LA, CABALLERO B, COLE TJ (2006). ' Limitations of the current World Health Organization growth references for children and adolescent'. *Food Nutr Bull.,* **27**, pp. S175–S188.
100. SWINBURN BA, CATERSON I, SEIDELL JC, JAMES WPT (2004). Diet, nutrition and the prevention of excess weight gain and obesity. *Public Health Nutrition* **7**, pp. 123–146.

APPENDIX [Source: WHO website]

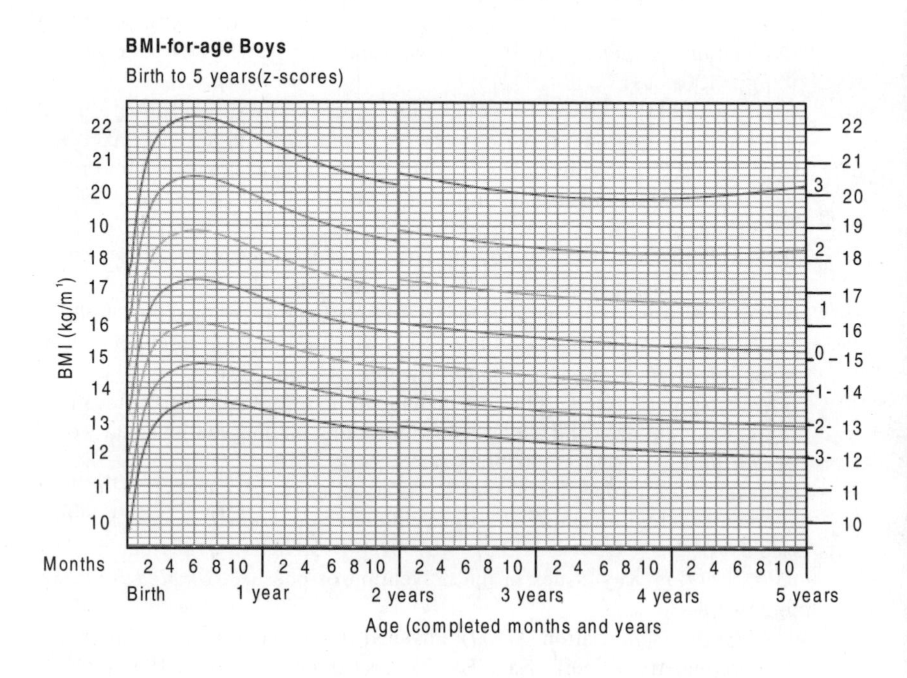

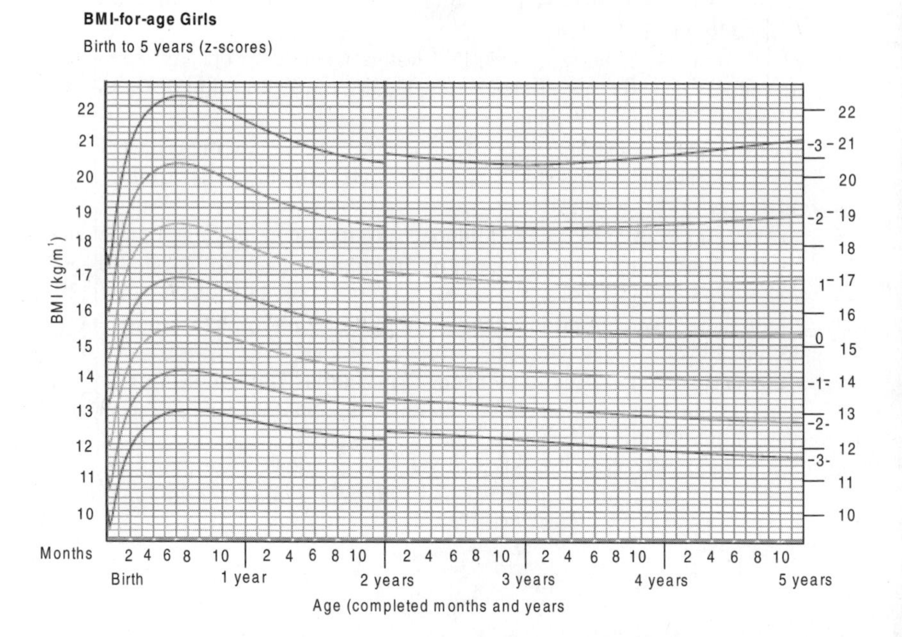

BMI-for-age Boys

Birth to 5 years (percentiles)

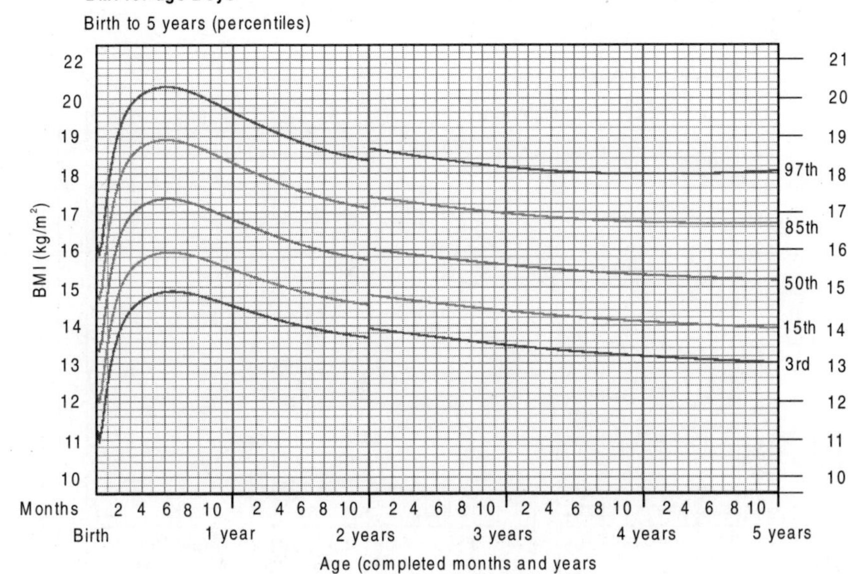

BMI-for-age Girls

Birth to 5 years (percentiles)

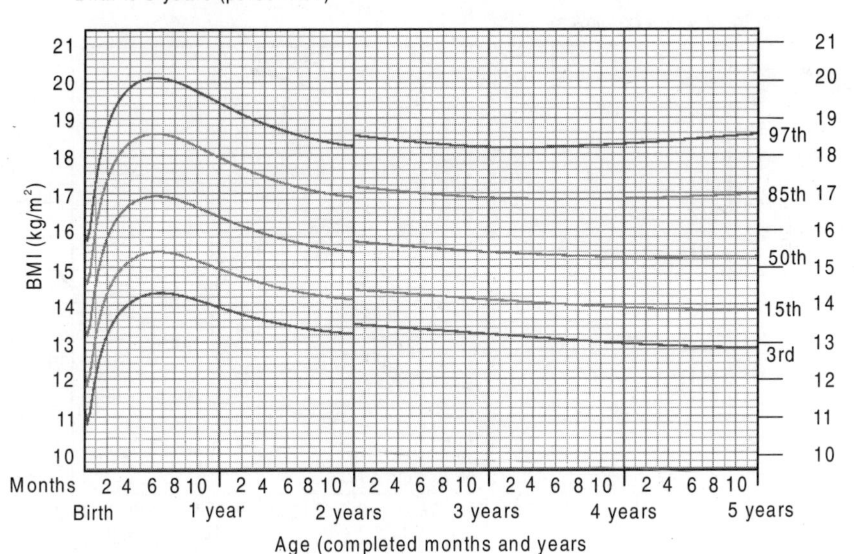

BMI-for-age Boys

5 to 19 years (z-scores)

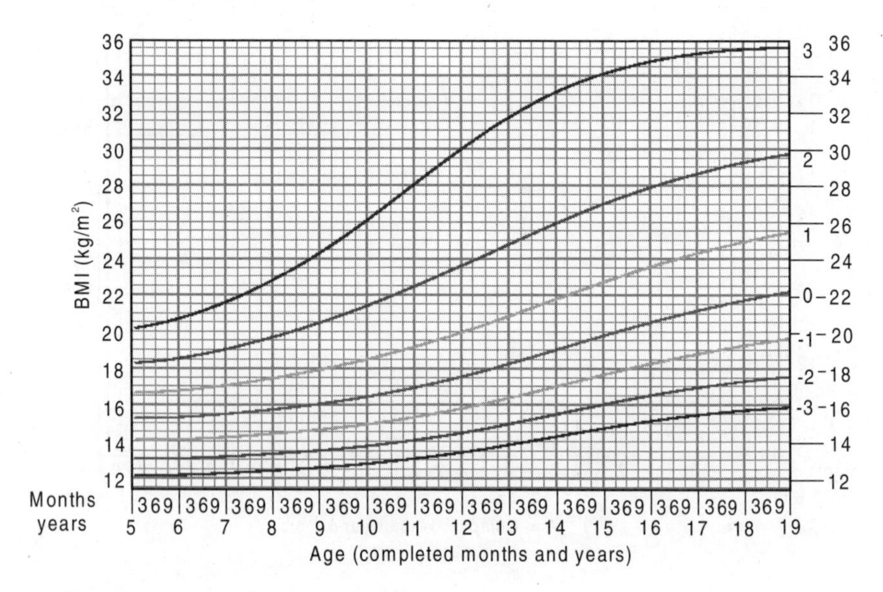

BMI-for-age Girls

5 to 19 years (z-scores)

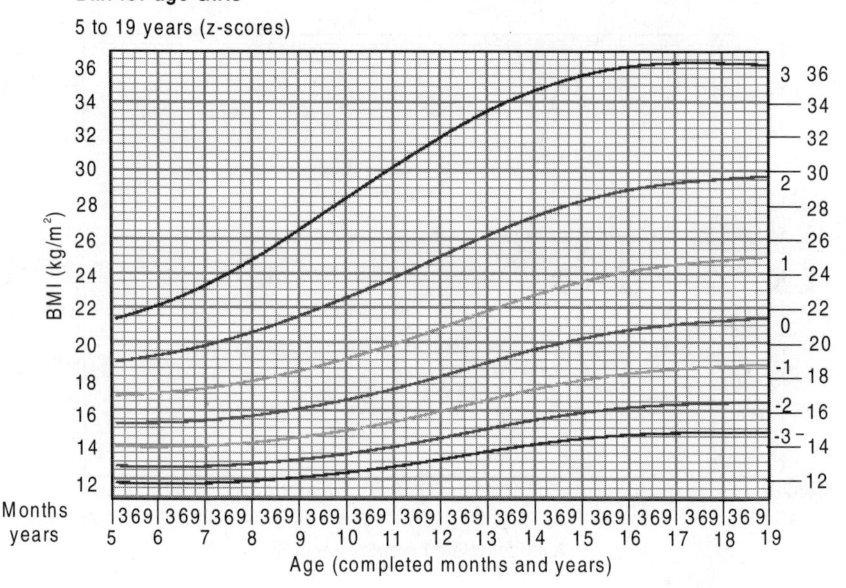

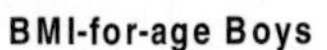

BMI-for-age Boys

5 to 19 years (percentiles)

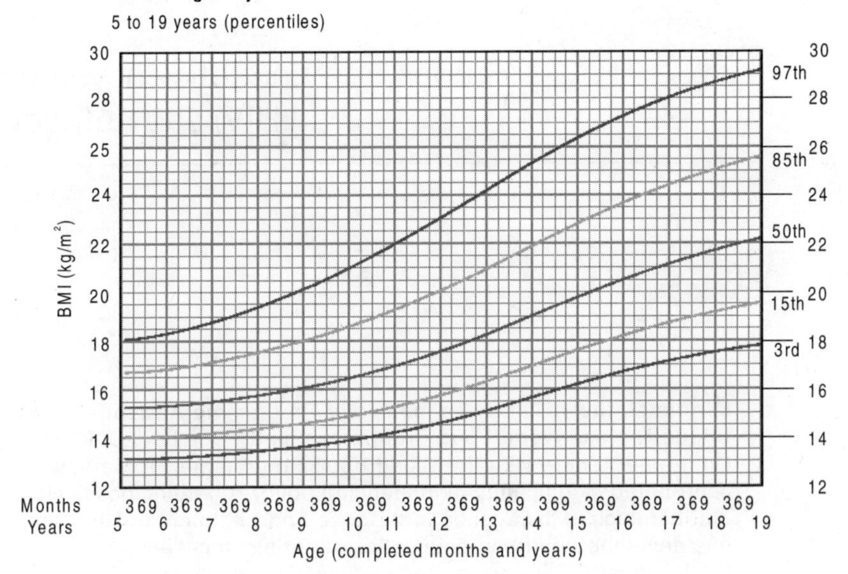

BMI-for-age Girls

5 to 19 years (percentiles)

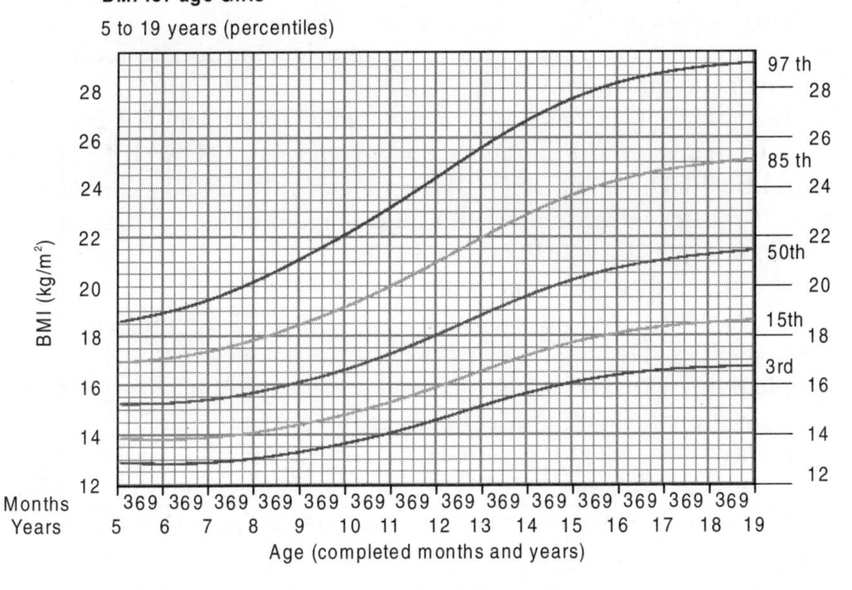

14

Human immunodeficiency virus (HIV) and nutrition

Minnie Mathew

Minnie Mathew, PhD, was the senior Programme Adviser with the United Nations World Food Programme till 31 October 2009. During her tenure with the World Food Programme, Dr Mathew contributed significantly in influencing policy regarding positioning nutrition high in the agenda in the care and treatment of HIV. She has developed nutrition-counseling materials in collaboration with the National AIDS Control Society (NACO), which are being used all over the country.

14.1 Introduction

Human immunodeficiency virus (HIV) is a retrovirus that can lead to acquired immunodeficiency syndrome (AIDS), a condition in humans in which the immune system begins to fail, leading to life-threatening opportunistic infections.

HIV infection in humans is a pandemic. As of January 2006, the Joint United Nations Programme on HIV and AIDS (UNAIDS) and the World Health Organization (WHO) estimated that AIDS has killed more than 25 million people since 1981, making it one of the most destructive pandemics in history. In 2007, 33.3 million (30.6–36.1 million) people were estimated to be living with HIV, 2.5 million (1.8–4.1 million) people became newly infected and 2.1 million (1.9–2.4 million) people died of AIDS [1]. India is a low-prevalence country with 2.47 million people living with HIV with a national prevalence of 0.36% as reported by the National Aids Control Organisation (NACO) in 2006 [2]. It may be pointed out that this (National Family Health Survey (NFHS-3)) data is based on a household survey among the general population, and excludes high-risk groups such as sex workers, men having sex with men (MSM), injecting drug users (IDUs), truckers and so on. NFHS-3 [3] suggests a prevalence figure of 0.28 %. If the high-risk groups are also taken into account – as they have been by NACO – then the prevalence estimate rises.

Infection with HIV occurs by the transfer of blood, semen, vaginal fluid, or breast milk. Within these bodily fluids, HIV is present as both free-virus particles and virus within infected immune cells. The four major routes of transmission are unprotected sexual intercourse, contaminated needles, and transmission from an infected mother to her baby at birth, or through breast milk. Transmission through blood transfusions or infected blood products can be eliminated by appropriate screening of blood products for HIV. Of significance to nutritionists is the mother-to-child transmission since it entails feeding options for the infant.

The transmission of the virus from the mother to the child can occur in utero during the last weeks of pregnancy and at childbirth. A number of studies suggest that about 50–80% vertical transmission of HIV takes place at around the time of birth. In the year 2003 upto 30th November, out of 57,781 AIDS cases reported to NACO, 1,551 (2.68%) cases are due to mother-to-child transmission (MTCT) [4]. In the absence of treatment, the transmission rate between the mother and child is 25%. However, with drug treatment, this can be reduced to 1%. Breastfeeding also presents a risk of infection for the baby and therefore guidelines on infant feeding for infants born to mothers with HIV have been developed (described later in the chapter).

HIV primarily infects vital cells in the human immune system such as helper T cells (specifically CD4+ T cells), macrophages and dendric cells. HIV infection leads to low levels of CD4+ T cells through three main mechanisms: firstly, direct viral killing of infected cells; secondly, increased rates of infected cells; and thirdly, killing of infected CD4+ T cells by CD8 Cytotoxic lymphocytes that recognize infected cells. When CD4+ T cell numbers decline below a critical level, cell-mediated immunity is lost, and the body becomes progressively more susceptible to opportunistic infections. If untreated, eventually most HIV-infected individuals develop AIDS (Acquired Immuno Deficiency Syndrome) and die. About one in ten remains healthy for many years, with no noticeable symptoms. A strong immune defense reduces the number of viral particles in the blood stream, marking the start of the infection's clinical latency stage. Clinical latency can vary between 2 weeks and 20 years.

Good nutrition is a key for living longer with HIV. This chapter focuses on the key principles of good nutrition which is important for people living with HIV. While good nutrition can help in building the immune system, it does not over time preclude treatment.

14.2 The clinical course of infection, immune system and infection

Infection with HIV is associated with a progressive decrease of the CD4+ T cell count and an increase in viral load. The stage of infection can be determined by measuring the patient's CD4+ T cell count, and the level of HIV in the blood.

The initial infection with HIV generally occurs after transfer of body fluids from an infected person to an uninfected one. The first stage of infection, the primary, or acute infection, is a period of rapid viral replication that immediately follows the individual's exposure to HIV leading to an abundance of virus in the peripheral blood with levels of HIV commonly approaching several million viruses per millilitre. This response is accompanied by a marked drop in the numbers of circulating CD4+ T cells (T cells belong to a group of white blood cells known as Lymphocytes, and play a central role in cell mediated immunity). This acute viremia is associated virtually in all patients with the activation of CD8+ T cells [5], which kill HIV-infected cells, and subsequently with antibody production, or seroconversion. The CD8+ T cell response is thought to be important in controlling virus levels, which peak and then decline, as the CD4+ T cell counts rebound to around 800 cells per ml (the normal value is 1200 cells per ml). A good CD8+ T cell response has been linked to slower disease progression and a better prognosis, though it does not eliminate the virus. During this period (usually 2–4 weeks post-exposure) most individuals (80–90%) develop an influenza or mononucleosis-like illness called acute HIV infection, the most common symptoms of which may include fever, pharyngitis, rash, mouth and esophagal sores, and may also include, but less commonly, headache, nausea and vomiting, enlarged liver/spleen, weight loss, thrush, and neurological symptoms. Infected individuals may experience all, some, or none of these symptoms. Symptoms have an average duration of 28 days and usually last at least a week although duration of symptoms may vary. Because of the non-specific nature of these illnesses, it is often not recognized as a sign of HIV infection. Even if patients go to their doctors or a hospital, they will often be misdiagnosed as having one of the more common infectious diseases with the same symptoms. Consequently, these primary symptoms are not used to diagnose HIV infection as they do not develop in all cases and because many are caused by other more common diseases. However, recognizing the syndrome is important because the patient is much more infectious during this period.

HIV directly attacks and destroys the cells of the immune system. Nutritional deficiencies affect the functioning of the immune system that may influence viral expression and replication, further affecting HIV-disease progression and mortality.

People with HIV and AIDS, whose immune systems are compromised, have difficulty in resisting a variety of serious infections and conditions. Infections affect the nutritional status by reducing the dietary intake and nutrient absorption, and by increasing the utilization and excretion of protein and micronutrients as the body mounts its 'acute phase response' to invading pathogens. This leads to increased utilization of antioxidant vitamins (e.g. vitamins E and C, and beta-carotene) as well as several minerals (e.g. iron, zinc, selenium, manganese and copper), which are used to form antioxidant enzymes. 'Oxidative stress' occurs when there is an imbalance between the pro-oxidants and antioxidants, causing further damage to cells, proteins and enzymes. Our immune system is an efficient, complex defence system which protects us against bacteria, viruses, and other disease-causing organisms.

Immune-system maintenance requires a steady intake of all the necessary vitamins and minerals. This can be accomplished by eating a well-balanced diet including plenty of fruits and vegetables and yoghurt products on a regular basis. Regular consumption of fermented dairy products such as yoghurt may enhance the immune defences in the gut.

Energy intake has an important influence on immune activity. Undernourished people are at greater risk from infections. Weight-reduction schemes using diets with less than 1200 kcal per day can also reduce immune function. Excessive energy intake may also compromise the immune system's ability to fight infection. Obesity is linked to an increased rate of infectious disease. Diets that are high in fat seem to depress the immune response and thus increase the risk of infections. Reducing fat content in the diet can increase immune activity. This might not just affect infections but could also strengthen the type of immune cells, which can fight tumour cells. It is important to include oily fish, nuts, soy or linseed oil in the diet since a right balance of different fatty acids is important. Multivitamin and mineral fortification and supplements can boost immunity.

14.3 Treatment for HIV infection

There is currently no vaccine or cure for HIV or AIDS. The only known method of prevention is avoiding exposure to the virus. There is an antiretroviral treatment, known as post-exposure prophylaxis which is believed to reduce the risk of infection if begun directly after exposure.

Current treatment for HIV infection consists of antiretroviral therapy/ART. Box 14.1 presents details on ART.

Box 14.1 Antiretroviral therapy (ART)

Antiretroviral (ARV) drugs inhibit the replication of HIV. When ARV drugs are given in combination, HIV replication and immune deterioration can be delayed, and survival and quality of life improved.

WHO recommends that in resource-limited settings, a single first-line regimen should be identified for the treatment of the majority of new patients. This regimen consists of 2 nucleoside analogs and either a non-nucleoside or abacavir, or a protease inhibitor. Zidovudine (ZDV)/3TC is the initial recommendation for a dual nucleoside analog with d4T/3TC, ZDV/ddl and ddl/3TC as possible alternatives. Efavirenz and nevirapine are recommended non-nucleosides, while recommended protease inhibitors include ritonavir-boosted PIs (indinavir, lopinavir, saquinavir) or nelfinavir. A second line regimen needs to be chosen to substitute first line regimens when needed (for toxicity or treatment failure).

Effective HIV and AIDS care requires antiretroviral therapy (ART) as a treatment option. Without access to ART, people living with HIV and AIDS cannot attain the fullest possible physical and mental health and cannot play their fullest role as actors in the fight against the epidemic, because their life expectancy will be too short.

ART has been highly beneficial to many HIV-infected individuals. ART allows the stabilisation of the patient's symptoms and viremia, but it neither cures the patient, nor alleviates the symptoms and high levels of HIV, often ART resistant, return once treatment is stopped. Moreover, it would take more than a lifetime for HIV infection to be cleared using ART. Despite this, many HIV-infected individuals have experienced remarkable improvements in their general health and quality of life, which has led to a large reduction in HIV-associated symptoms. Non-adherence and non-persistence with ART is the major reason for most individuals failing to benefit from it. The reasons for non-adherence and non-persistence with ART may include poor access to medical care, fear of side effects, stigma in the absence of inadequate social support and drug abuse.

The timing for starting HIV treatment is still debated. There is no question that treatment should be started before the patient's CD4 count falls below 200, and most national guidelines say to start treatment once the CD4 count falls below 350; but there is some evidence from cohort studies that treatment should be started before the CD4 count falls below 350. Delaying treatment in patients with CD4 counts >200 does not appear to increase risk of progression. Viral load, while highly predictive of progression in untreated HIV disease, does not predict clinical response to antiretroviral therapy. Patients started on antiretroviral therapy with CD4 counts >350 are likely to experience considerable toxicity as well as emergence of drug-resistant virus in the absence of a compelling clinical benefit. Initiation of therapy should be based on CD4 count and the patient's ability to comply with complex and potentially toxic regimens [6].

Many ARV drugs are inconvenient to take and are associated with unpleasant effects including nausea, diarrhea, headache, and central nervous system toxicity. They may also cause occasional life-threatening adverse effects such as hypersensitivity reactions, acute hepatitis, lactic acidosis, and pancreatitis. Furthermore, long-term use of ARV has been linked with increased risk of myocardial infarction. If therapy can safely be delayed most patients would prefer to wait. Secondly, the absolute risk of AIDS-related diseases has been felt to be sufficiently low at CD4 counts above 250 that delay can be considered, given the disadvantages of treatment [7].

In India the National AIDS Control Organization (NACO) [8] recommends ART when the CD4 count is below 200 if the patient is asymptomatic or has mild symptoms. With advanced symptoms, it suggests treatment if CD4 is <350 and initiating ART before CD4 drops below 200. For People Living with HIV (PLHIV) with severe and advanced symptoms, treatment is recommended irrespective of CD4 count. In India, free ART is provided through ART centres managed by the State AIDS Control Societies (SACS).

ART is not without side effects. Some of these related to nutritional intake and nutritional status include nausea and vomiting, abdominal pain, diarrhea, vomiting, lack of appetite, dry mouth and anaemia. These will be considerably reduced over a period of time and therefore should not influence adherence to ART.

Metabolic alterations occur resulting in fat-redistribution syndrome, with central obesity and loss of subcutaneous fat.

Development of hyperglycemia and lipid abnormalities may increase the risk of diabetes, heart disease, and stroke. Insulin resistance, a common side-effect of medications used to treat HIV, increases the risk of diabetes, especially in patients who are older or have a family history of the disease.

Food and drug interactions are an important issue for effectiveness and tolerability of ART regimens. All these conditions warrant dietary modifications.

14.4 HIV and implications on nutrition status

Nutrition is a life-sustaining treatment and the role of nutrition in the treatment of HIV is critical. HIV affects each person differently. Anorexia and oral/gastrointestinal symptoms such as pain, nausea, vomiting, malabsorption and diarrhea may arise from HIV infection, secondary infections, encephalopathy or drug therapies. Inability to eat food, which is associated with complicated medical regimens or fatigue adds to the nutritional risk. Opportunistic infections are associated with increased resting energy expenditure, and ART may be associated with increased or decreased resting energy expenditure. Clinically, these symptoms may prevent adequate nutritional intake resulting in continued weight and lean tissue loss, vitamin or mineral deficiencies and poor nutritional status. Chemical dependency and socioeconomic factors can limit access to proper food and nutrition.

The malnutrition that results can itself contribute to an increased immuno-compromised state.

Poor nutritional status may result from multiple causes: depressed appetite, poor nutrient intake and limited food availability; chronic infection, malabsorption, metabolic disturbances, and muscle and tissue catabolism; fever, nausea, vomiting and diarrhea; depression; and the side effects of drugs used to treat HIV-related infections.

HIV-infected patients may be at nutritional risk at any point in their illness. Severe malnutrition and weight loss, particularly loss of lean tissue, and delayed weight gain and height velocity in children, can affect morbidity and mortality.

14.4.1 Weight loss and wasting in HIV and AIDS

The wasting syndrome typically found in adult AIDS patients is a severe nutritional manifestation of the disease. Wasting is usually preceded by a change in appetite, repeated infections, weight fluctuations, and subtler changes in body composition such as changes in the lean body mass (LBM) and body cell mass, which are more difficult to measure than changes in weight alone [9]. Due to illness, appetite is usually lost while there is an increase in nutritional requirements. In such situations, weight loss can be dangerous with a reduction in body's ability to fight off infections and recover.

Weight loss in PLHIV typically follows two patterns: slow and progressive weight loss from anorexia and gastrointestinal disturbances; and rapid, episodic weight loss from secondary infections. Even relatively small losses in weight (5%) have been associated with decreased survival in PLHIV and are therefore important to monitor [10]. Weight loss and wasting in PLHIV develop as a result of three overlapping processes: (i) reduction in food intake, (ii) metabolic alterations, (iii) nutrient malabsorption and effect of drugs.

(1) Reduction in food intake may be due to painful sores in the mouth, pharynx, and/or oesophagus. Fatigue, depression, changes in mental state and other psychological factors may affect the appetite and interest in food. Economic factors affect food availability and the nutritional quality of the diet. Drugs or opportunistic illnesses may cause symptoms that make eating unappealing. Some drugs also alter your sense of taste or smell, and this may, in turn, affect your diet.

(2) Side effects from medications, including nausea, vomiting, metallic taste in the mouth, diarrhea, abdominal cramps and anorexia also result in lower dietary intake that can cause the weight loss associated with HIV and AIDS. Reduction in food intake is believed to be the most important cause of the slow and progressive weight loss experienced by PLHIV.

(3) Metabolic alterations due to the impact of infection on protein, fat and carbohydrate metabolism result in increased energy and protein requirements as well as in inefficient utilization and loss of nutrients. Changes in metabolism occur during HIV infection due to severe reduction in food intake as well as from the immune system's response to the infection. When the intake of food is restricted, the body responds by altering the production of insulin and glucagon, which regulate the flow of sugar and other nutrients in the intestine, blood, liver and other body tissues. Over a period of time, the body uses up its carbohydrate stores from muscle and liver tissue and begins to break down body protein to produce glucose. This process causes protein loss and muscle wasting.

(4) Nutrient malabsorption accompanies frequent bouts of diarrhea due to a compromised immune system. Some HIV-infected individuals have increased permeability and other intestinal defects even when asymptomatic [11]. It is possible that HIV infection itself, particularly of the intestinal cells, may cause epithelial damage and nutrient malabsorption [12]. Malabsorption of fats and carbohydrates is common at all stages of HIV infection in both adults and children [13]. Fat malabsorption, in turn, affects the absorption and utilization of fat-soluble vitamins (vitamins A and E), further compromising the nutritional and immune status.

Weight normally fluctuates by a few kilograms but a loss of 3–5 % of normal body weight is not normal and it is important to understand the cause of the weight loss, and what might be done to prevent it. Equally important are the signs of muscle wasting – thinning in the arms, legs, buttocks, and face. This implies examining the diet to ensure adequate intake of calories to prevent the body from using its stored resources. It may mean increasing the amount of calories or protein in the diet and exercise.

Although weight loss is a common symptom of HIV, there are actions that can be taken to prevent it. Because HIV-related weight loss has many causes, different solutions may be appropriate at different times. It is important to identify the underlying problems. There could be intestinal infections, which prevent proper food absorption. Drugs taken for opportunistic infections can cause nausea. Or there could be a loss of appetite. It is easier to address the problem by identifying the underlying cause.

Omega-3 fatty acids have been proposed for the treatment of HIV-related problems in more than one ways. Box 14.2 presents details on omega-3 fatty acids and mechanism reported in small trails. Large scale trials have not been studied.

Box 14.2 Omega-3 fatty acids – role in HIV

Fish oil contains omega-3 fatty acids, "good fats" that have many potential health-promoting properties. HIV-induced weight loss involves inflammation and responds to treatment with anti-inflammatory drugs. Fish oil also has anti-inflammatory effects. HIV lipodystrophy (HIVL) is associated with increased in vitro release of pro-inflammatory cytokines from subcutaneous adipose tissue, implying a heightened systemic inflammatory state, independent from ART. Omega-3 fatty acids, being anti-inflammatory, play a vital role in HIV.

Studies suggest that poor absorption of fats and carbohydrates occurs at all stages of HIV infection in both adults and children and results in excess nutrient loss. Poor absorption of fat, specifically, reduces the absorption and use of fat-soluble vitamins (such as vitamins A and E). This can further compromise nutrition and immune status.

Fish oil ingestion can boost the activity of enzymes related to metabolism. Specifically, enzymes related to fatty acid beta-oxidation, omega-oxidation, and malic were 1.2-, 1.6-, and 1.7-fold higher in the fish oil-supplemented diet, compared to those only receiving the high fat diet.

Oxidative stress occurs when there is an imbalance between the pro-oxidants and antioxidants – in other words, when there are not enough antioxidants to meet the demands of the pro-oxidant cytokines. This stress is believed to increase HIV replication and transcription, leading to higher viral loads and disease progression. For this reason, many studies have examined the impact of antioxidant vitamin supplementation on HIV transmission and disease progression. Omega-3 fatty acids can serve as an antioxidant and relieve the 'Oxidative stress'.

14.4.2 Metabolic changes in HIV

One of the earliest, often undetected, signs of HIV infection is deterioration of the small intestine where absorption of nutrients occurs. Moreover, it appears that there is an increase in requirements for certain nutrients. These are the two primary reasons. For many HIV cases, there is a decrease in many of the body's vitamins and minerals.

A number of metabolic disorders have been reported among patients on ART, such as high serum lipids and elevated liver enzymes. However, results are still limited and controversial [14].

Persons on ART can develop lipodystrophy. Typical symptoms of the syndrome may include a loss of subcutaneous fat in the face, arms, and legs; increased fat deposits in the abdomen and upper back; changes in cholesterol and other blood lipids; and insulin resistance. The metabolic complications of this condition become more significant as patients spend more time on ART. Persons on this therapy may develop type-2 diabetes, which is four times the usual risk; and concerns are also increasing about the related risk of heart disease.

Preliminary results from a study conducted by Bernasconi et al. [15] point to protease inhibitors as a cause of elevated uric acid, triglyceride and total cholesterol values. Metabolic and body composition changes associated with ART have been well documented in HIV-infected adults, but there have been few reports in children. A study conducted by Meneilly et al. [16] showed that a significant number (62%) of children on ART develop changes in metabolic parameters or body composition, although the relationship to use and duration of ART is unclear. The long-term clinical implications of these changes have yet to be determined. Puberty seems to be the time when HIV-infected children taking potent ARV are more likely to develop lipodystrophy and metabolic complications, especially in children with a severe underlying HIV infection. Once developed, lipodystrophy and metabolic changes seem to be extremely stable with time [17].

Puberty seems to be the time when HIV-infected children taking potent ARV are more likely to develop lipodystrophy and metabolic complications, especially in children with a severe underlying HIV infection.

14.4.3 Nutrition in common HIV-related conditions

(a) *Diarrhea* is common amongst people with HIV. It can be caused by HIV itself, or by infections in the intestine. Intestinal infections are often caused by the same bacteria and parasites that cause food poisoning. They can be serious for people with HIV and need to be treated.

Diarrhea has been reported as a side effect of some antibiotics. With some drugs, diarrhea goes away after the first few weeks of treatment – but some people find that it becomes a permanent feature of living with the drug. The severity of diarrhea can also differ between people. Diarrhea can cause loss of valuable nutrients.

Diet needs to be modified or changed if there is diarrhea. Fatty food can worsen diarrhea. Dairy products in the diet may also contribute to diarrhea because of lactose intolerance. Eating bananas, chicken and fish can help restore levels of potassium, which are commonly depleted in people with bad diarrhea.

Coffee, carbonated beverages, raw vegetables and spicy food should be avoided as these can make diarrhea worse. High-fibre foods such as brown rice and whole grain bread contain lots of nutrients, but they can also contribute to diarrhea. These may be replaced with white bread and rice during bouts of diarrhea. Some fruits and vegetables are also high in fibre (like corn for example) and may contribute to diarrhea. Other fruits and vegetables are easily tolerated and some may even help stop diarrhea. Since there is a loss of water and minerals in diarrhea, drinking extra water can help in rehydration.

(b) *Nausea* has many causes and is a common side effect of many HIV drugs. It is important to determine what is making you nauseous. Nausea can be a sign of gastrointestinal infections or other intestinal problems.
Changes in the diet will help. In extreme conditions, it may not be possible to eat anything. Small frequent sips of ginger drinks or soup will help. Even if not eating, body fluids need to be replaced. In addition, it is not advisable to go without solid foods for more than two days. Generally, cold foods without much of an odour are easier to take in conditions of nausea. Several small meals will be easier to take than one large one. Food should be eaten slowly. Lying down immediately after a meal can also cause nausea.

(c) *Oral conditions* may have an impact on food intake. Mouth or throat infections like thrush, dental problems, or mouth ulcers can all be painful barriers to eating. The best way to resolve this problem is to treat the infection or have the necessary dental work. When these problems cannot be quickly resolved, there are strategies to help in consuming appropriate nutrients over the short term. Milk is good if there is no lactose intolerance. This will provide nutrients. Soft moist foods can be consumed. Fats will not only soften foods but are also a good source of energy. Straw can be used for liquids if most of the problems are located in the mouth. Heating food too much can be avoided as hot foods can cause pain, especially for those with dental problems.
Changes in the tissues of the mouth are associated with deficiencies in some vitamins, particular B complex vitamins and vitamin C. Since these deficiencies have been observed in people with HIV, B complex supplement or a vitamin C supplement might help ward off oral problems. The role of B complex vitamins and vitamin C in preventing oral conditions has not been well studied.

(d) *Lack of appetite*. Rather than eating a whole dinner at frequent intervals, small snack-like meals can be eaten. Protein and nutrient intake can be increased with high protein snacks like nuts, seeds, puddings, cheese or peanut butter and crackers. Taking walks before meals or other exercises can stimulate appetite. It is good to keep favourite foods on hand as there is greater likelihood of eating more. Doctor can prescribe drugs, which are appetite stimulants. These drugs can help in eating more.

(e) *Lactose intolerance.* A large percentage of people with HIV seem to become lactose intolerant. One study found that 70% of HIV+ participants were lactose intolerant. This means that dairy products like milk, cheese and ice cream may cause diarrhea, gas, and bloating. Lactose is also added into a lot of processed foods. Lactose is sometimes added to prepare foods/meals, so if one can tolerate only very small amounts of lactose, it's important to check food labels and lists of ingredients. One should look not only for milk and lactose among the contents, but also for such words as 'whey', 'curds', 'milk by-products', 'dry milk solids', and 'non-fat dry milk powder'. These words denote that the food contains lactose. Several products with lactose content are available in India as well as other developing countries. Examples include:

- Bread and other bakery foods
- Candies
- Pancake, biscuit, or cookie mixes
- Breakfast cereals
- Soups
- Non-dairy powdered coffee creamers
- Margarine
- Salad dressings

There are products especially designed for lactose-intolerant people, including lactase capsules that can be taken before eating. Many people find these capsules helpful, particularly if taken on occasional basis, so they don't have to worry when they go out to dinner. There are also lactose-reduced dairy products. For many people, being lactose intolerant may mean avoiding dairy products altogether. Since dairy products are good sources of protein it is important to get additional protein from sources other than dairy products along with calcium and vitamin D supplements to avoid deficiencies of those vitamins. Whey protein, an expensive product, is used by some people to supplement protein intake; whey protein is derived from dairy products. However, whey protein formulas or products are often lactose reduced, it is important to check the lactose content.

14.5 Nutritional requirements for People Living with HIV (PLHIV)

14.5.1 Energy requirements

Studies point to low-energy intake combined with increased energy demand due to HIV and related infections as the major driving forces behind HIV-related weight loss and wasting. Based on the increased resting energy expenditure (REE) observed in studies on HIV-infected adults, it is recommended that energy needs be increased by 10% over accepted levels for otherwise healthy people. The goal is to maintain body weight in asymptomatic HIV-infected adults. Although studies on energy expenditure have not shown an increase in the overall total energy expenditure (TEE), this may have been the result of individuals compensating by reducing activity-related energy expenditure (AEE). Since maintaining physical activity is highly desirable for preserving the quality of life and for maintaining muscle tissue, it is undesirable that energy intake should only match a reduced level of AEE. The estimated energy requirement therefore allows for normal AEE levels in addition to an increased level of REE.

Energy requirements of adults

Increased energy intake of about 20–30% is recommended for adults during periods of symptomatic disease or opportunistic infections (OI) to maintain body weight.

HIV doesn't kill anybody directly. Instead, it weakens the body's ability to fight disease. Infections, which are rarely seen in those with normal immune systems, are deadly to those with HIV. People with HIV can get many infections (OIs). Many of these illnesses are very serious, and they need to be treated. Some can be prevented too.

This takes into account the increase in REE due to HIV-related infections. However, such intakes may not be achievable during periods of acute infection or illness, and it has not been proven that such high intake levels can be safely achieved during such periods. Moreover, it is recognized that physical activity may be reduced during HIV-related infections and the recommended increased intake is based on the energy needed to support weight recovery during and after HIV-related illnesses. Intake should therefore be increased to the extent possible during the recovery phase, aiming for the maximum achievable up to 30% above normal intake during the acute phase.

Energy requirements of children

Few studies exist on the energy expenditure in HIV-infected children. The energy requirements of children can vary according to the type and duration of HIV-related infections, and whether there is weight loss along with acute infection. Although the finding of increased REE in asymptomatic disease has not been replicated in children, similar to asymptomatic HIV-infected adults, an average increase of 10% of energy intake is recommended to maintain growth. Based on clinical experience and existing guidelines to achieve catch-up growth in children irrespective of the HIV status, energy intakes for HIV-infected children experiencing weight loss need to be increased by 50 to 100% over established requirements for otherwise healthy uninfected children. In the absence of specific data to support specific recommendations for managing severe malnutrition in HIV-infected children, existing WHO guidelines [18] are advised to be followed. Research is needed on the specific energy requirements of HIV-infected children. WHO guidelines are the basis of the following requirements for various nutrients.

Energy requirements of pregnant and lactating women

Pregnancy is a particularly vulnerable time for women because their nutritional requirements of energy, vitamins and minerals increase by up to 30%, yet their usual daily intakes are frequently below the recommended dietary allowance (RDA) for healthy pregnant women. Malnutrition during pregnancy, therefore, may further erode the immune status of HIV-infected women and make them more vulnerable to disease progression, although this hypothesis has not yet been proven.

Specific data are absent regarding the impact of HIV and AIDS and related conditions on the energy needs during pregnancy and lactation, over and above those requirements already identified for non-infected women. Thus, for now, the recommended energy intake for HIV-infected adults should also apply to pregnant and lactating HIV-infected women.

14.5.2 Protein requirements

Protein is important to PLHIV because it is the primary component of muscle, and plays a crucial part in many of our metabolic processes. When PLHIV lose weight, they often lose muscle. This is called muscle wasting. It is important to eat enough food to prevent the body from using the energy stored in the body as muscle. Research also suggests that a high-protein diet and regular exercise may help PLHIV to avoid muscle wasting. Eating more protein may also help to regain lost muscle mass. An approximate rule of thumb is 100–150 g/day for HIV-positive men and 80–100 g/day for HIV-positive women. The protein intake should not be greater than 15–20% of the total calories; a diet extremely rich in protein can stress the kidneys.

14.5.3 Fat requirements

PLHIV may experience medication-related high cholesterol and triglyceride levels, requiring caution with regard to cardiovascular disease (CVD). Omega-3 fatty acids, a type of polyunsaturated fat found in fish and other foods such as flaxseeds, beans, peas, are protective against

CVD. The amount of saturated, monosaturated and polyunsaturated fat in the diet should be 7:10:10 percent, respectively of the total caloric intake.

14.5.4 Requirement of micronutrients

The role of micronutrients in HIV and AIDS has special importance in individuals and populations with marginal or low micronutrient intakes. Studies from both industrialized and developing countries report that PLHIV have decreased absorption, excessive urinary losses, and low blood concentrations of vitamins A, B_1, B_2, B_6, B_{10}, C, E, as well as of folate, beta-carotene, selenium, zinc and magnesium [19, 20]. Currently, it is not known whether these deficiencies are independent markers of disease progression resulting from a compromised immune system, or whether they are causally related to the development or exacerbation of the symptoms of HIV and AIDS. This distinction is important to determine whether the nutritional deficiencies can be reversed, and whether nutritional therapy and management can slow or alter the course of the disease.

Antioxidants

The process of breaking down food into energy involves a chemical reaction called oxidation. Food break down is one of many oxidative processes in our bodies. During this process, molecules called free radicals are produced. Although free radicals are a normal part of the oxidation process, they can damage the membranes of the body's cells in much the same way that rust damages the body of a car. To control this process the body produces an antioxidant, called glutathione, in the walls of the cells. External sources of antioxidants present in food are beta-carotene, selenium and vitamins A, C and E.

During HIV infection, many researchers have observed an increase in free radicals. The cause of this increase is not completely understood. A decrease in antioxidants in general and glutathione in particular has also been observed. Having low levels of glutathione in the body is associated with a lower survival time for PLHIV.

Vitamin A requirements of adults

Of all the micronutrients, the role of vitamin A in HIV has received the greatest attention. This is because of its well-known role in affecting child morbidity and mortality, as well as early observations that vitamin A status was associated with increased risk of mother-to-child transmission (MTCT) of HIV; HIV viral load in breast milk, vaginal secretions [21, 22]; progression to AIDS; adult survival; and infant morbidity and mortality. The potential for vitamin A supplementation to positively impact the course of HIV and AIDS was promising to pursue, since vitamin A is beneficial in HIV-negative populations, is inexpensive, and relatively easy to administer with minimal side effects.

Several studies in Africa have measured the impact of vitamin-A supplementation on various HIV-related outcomes in children. In South Africa, supplementation of vitamin A in HIV-infected children reduced morbidity due to diarrhea by about 50% in one study and improved immune status in another study. In Tanzania, vitamin-A supplementation reduced all-cause mortality by 63% among HIV-infected children in the age group of 6 months to 5 years, and was associated with a 68% reduction in AIDS-related deaths and a 92% reduction in diarrhea-related deaths.

Periodic vitamin A supplementation has been shown to reduce all-cause mortality and diarrhea-related morbidity in vitamin-A-deficient children, including HIV-infected children. In keeping with WHO recommendations, 6 to 59 month old children born to HIV-infected mothers living in resource-limited settings should receive periodic (every 4 to 6 months) vitamin A supplements (100,000 IU for infants 6–12 months of age and 200,000 IU for children >12 months of age). Currently, there is insufficient evidence to recommend an increased dose or frequency of vitamin A supplementation in HIV-infected children.

According to published reports, daily antenatal and postnatal vitamin-A supplementation for HIV-infected women in well-designed, randomized controlled trials was not able to reduce the MTCT of HIV; on the contrary, in some settings, it actually increased the risk. Thus, daily intake of vitamin A by HIV-infected women during pregnancy and lactation should not exceed one RDA.

In areas of endemic vitamin A deficiency, WHO recommends that a single high dose of vitamin A (200,000 IU) be given to women as soon as possible after delivery, but no later than six weeks after delivery. Research is under way to assess further the effect of single-dose, postpartum vitamin A supplementation among HIV-infected women.

Micronutrients and anemia

Anaemia is a common problem among PLHIV, affecting asymptomatic HIV-infected adults and children as well as people with AIDS. The causes of anemia associated with HIV and AIDS are not well understood. Anemia may result from cytokine-induced suppression of red blood cell (RBC) production; chronic inflammation; opportunistic infections (OIs) and/or reduction in dietary intake (including iron), absorption and retention.

Anemia may also be caused by certain antiretroviral (ARV) drugs (e.g. zidovudine, which suppresses bone marrow function and synthesis of RBCs), as well as by nutritional deficiencies of iron, folate, riboflavin, and vitamins A and B_{12}.

Studies have found that anaemia is associated with HIV-disease progression and a two-to-four-fold increased risk of death in HIV-infected individuals. The risk increases with the severity of the anaemia. One longitudinal study in Europe found that the risk of death increased by 57% for every 1 g/dl decrease in the haemoglobin level in HIV-infected subjects, after controlling for CD4 cell counts, viral load, and use of ARVs. This risk was greater than the risks observed with a 50% reduction in the CD4 cell count and a 'log' increase in the HIV viral load. On the other hand, studies also suggest that reversing anaemia can slow down the progression of HIV disease and prolong survival [23].

It is worthwhile to mention that although anaemia is common among PLHIV, advanced HIV disease may also be characterized by an increase in iron stores in the bone marrow, muscle, liver and other cells. This accumulation of iron is probably a result of the body's attempts to withhold iron from plasma, although other factors (e.g. use of zidovudine, cigarette smoking and blood transfusions) may also play a role. Increased iron stores can predispose to microbial infection and also cause oxidative stress, with implications for HIV-disease progression. Additional research is required to identify approaches for managing anaemia in PLHIV.

(i) Iron–folate supplementation for pregnant and lactating women

Iron–folate supplementation is a standard component of antenatal care for preventing anaemia in pregnant women and improving foetal iron stores. WHO recommends daily iron–folate supplementation (400 μg of folate and 60 mg of iron) during the first six months of pregnancy to prevent anaemia, and twice-daily supplements to treat severe anaemia.

As with other chronic infections, HIV causes disturbances of iron metabolism and anaemia. In view of iron's potential adverse effects, for example, its pro-oxidant activity, which might accelerate disease progression, research on the safety of iron supplementation in adults and children with HIV infection is recommended. Based on available evidence, however, the approach to caring for HIV-infected women is the same as that for uninfected women.

(ii) Multiple micronutrient supplements

Observational studies indicate that low blood levels and decreased dietary intake of some micronutrients are associated with faster HIV-disease progression and mortality, and increased risk of HIV transmission. However, the methodological limitations of these studies preclude definitive conclusions about the relationship between micronutrient intake and blood levels, and HIV infection.

Studies have shown that even people who eat good food are likely to have vitamin and mineral deficiencies when they have HIV. Zinc, selenium, magnesium, carotenoids and vitamins A, B_2, B_6, B_{12}, and E intakes have all been shown to be often low. This can happen before visible sicknesses occur, and before the stage that we call AIDS. Supplementation has been shown to be associated with significant slowing of disease progression.

Some studies show that supplements of, for example, B-complex vitamins, and vitamins C and E can improve immune status, prevent childhood diarrhea and enhance pregnancy outcomes, including better maternal weight gain during pregnancy, and a reduction in foetal death, preterm birth and low birth weight. The effect of these micronutrients on HIV disease progression and mortality is under study.

Several neurological problems in HIV disease have been attributed to nutritional deficiencies, especially that of vitamin B_{12}. Low intake of B-complex vitamins is associated with faster progression of HIV disease. PLHIV should be able to get enough of most of these vitamins from supplements that are taken as pills.

Vitamin E is necessary for proper functioning of the immune system. It increases humoral and cell-mediated immune responses, including antibody production, phagocytic and lymphocytic responses, and resistance to viral and infectious diseases [24]. Vitamin E is one of the few nutrients (another is vitamin A) for which supplementation at higher than daily recommended levels have been shown to increase immune response and resistance to disease. The oxidative stress created by HIV and related opportunistic infections (OIs) increases the utilization of the antioxidant vitamin E. Deficiency, in turn, further debilitates the immune system because of its role in immune stimulation and functioning, leaving PLHIV more susceptible to OIs.

A study in Zambia among AIDS patients suffering from persistent diarrhea found that oral supplementation with vitamin E and other nutrients did not affect either mortality or diarrhea-related morbidity, possibly because of severe fat malabsorption accompanying late-stage disease.

Selenium deficiency impairs the immune system and has been associated with faster HIV disease progression and reduced survival in adults [25] and children [26]. Selenium is believed to play an important role in metabolizing reactive oxygen species ('free radicals') and reducing oxidative stress because it is an essential cofactor for glutathione perodixase, an antioxidant enzyme.

Findings of a study conducted in France suggest that selenium (and beta-carotene) supplementation may reduce the impact of oxidative stress on HIV disease. Zinc plays a role in HIV infection because HIV requires zinc for gene expression, replication and integration. Thus, persons with HIV infection may have low plasma zinc levels yet higher zinc intakes may be associated with faster HIV replication and disease progression.

Zinc supplementation among AIDS patients, however, has shown substantial benefits. In a study in Italy, daily zinc supplementation (200 mg/day) for one month reduced the incidence of OIs (particularly *Pneumocystis carinii* and *Candida*), stabilized weight, and improved CD4 cell counts among adults with AIDS who were also receiving ART as compared with controls who received ART but no zinc supplementation. These findings suggest that zinc supplementation should be approached cautiously and must take into account dietary intake of the mineral. Zinc supplementation, in short courses and carefully monitored, may be useful for strengthening resistance to OIs in persons with AIDS [27].

Studies have shown that even people who eat well and adequately are likely to have vitamin and mineral deficiencies when they have HIV infection. Normal recommended dietary levels for vitamins and minerals are often not adequate for PLHIV. Food alone is not enough. Supplementation has been shown to be associated with significant slowing of disease progression. Multiple micronutrient supplements may be needed during pregnancy and lactation. Pending additional information, micronutrient intakes at the RDA level are recommended for HIV-infected women during pregnancy and lactation.

The optimal micronutrient supplement composition that will be safe, ensure nutritional adequacy, and potentially produce the greatest benefits in HIV-infected pregnant and lactating women in different settings has not yet been defined. Additional research is required to determine the safety of nutrient supplements such as zinc, iron and vitamin A, and to determine whether different multiple micronutrient supplements are needed for HIV-infected women compared with uninfected women.

HIV-infected adults and children should consume diets that ensure micronutrient intakes at RDA levels. However, this may not be sufficient to correct nutritional deficiencies in HIV-infected individuals. Several studies raise concerns that some micronutrient supplements, e.g. vitamin A, zinc and iron, can produce adverse outcomes in HIV-infected populations. Safe upper limits for daily micronutrient intakes for PLHIV still need to be established. Some efforts being undertaken in this context are presented in Box 14.3.

14.6 HIV and appropriate support

(a) Nutrition guidelines

Appropriate nutrition is important for PLHIV. Many studies have shown that people living with HIV who are malnourished are likely to get sick more often, and have shorter survival times than other HIV+ people. Poor nutrition has also been observed to weaken the immune system.

There is a need to balance the amount of energy consumed as food with the amount of energy the body needs to maintain itself, and to conduct daily activities. The body may also be less capable of taking in nutrients and therefore energy. This is called malabsorption. Malabsorption may be caused by bacterial or parasitic infections in the intestines. It may be caused by changes in the intestines due to HIV. Malabsorption may occur in conditions of diarrhea caused by drugs taken.

PLHIV need to pay attention to their diet to get the best possible nutrient balance. They may also need to supplement certain specific nutrients. If a person with HIV does not take in enough nutrients, their energy intake is decreased and they may begin to lose weight. Following guidelines will help to stay healthy and get the nutrients needed.

- Healthy dietary principles
- Maintenance of lean body mass and normal growth in children and the treatment of wasting
- Management of metabolic complications due to drug therapies
- Management of drug and food or nutrient interactions
- Management of gastrointestinal symptoms that may influence the types and amount of food ingested
- Appropriate use of nutritional supplements
- Role of exercise
- Food safety
- Nutrition during pregnancy
- Access to infant formula and food as an alternative to breastfeeding

(b) Some dietary guidelines for PLHIV

Nutritional management is integral to the care of all patients with HIV. HIV results in complicated nutritional issues for patients, and there is growing evidence that nutritional interventions influence health outcomes in PLHIV.

This means eating well, which is important since the immune system requires protein to fight infection. But in order for the body to properly use the protein, fat and carbohydrate in food, it needs adequate levels of vitamins and minerals.

Because many of the weight-loss problems seen in HIV are related to low food intake, many small meals throughout the day, rather than 2 or 3 large ones, is suggested. Having HIV is unlikely to mean drastic changes to the diet – a good diet will consist of a balance of the following items:

(i) Carbohydrates

Carbohydrates make up most of the Indian's diet. Carbohydrates can be simple sugars. They can also be complex carbohydrates, which are long strings of sugar molecules linked together. Complex carbohydrates are found in breads, cereals, and pastas, as well as in fruits and vegetables. They provide energy as well as vitamins and minerals. They are usually the most desirable sources of carbohydrates. Simple sugars are fine in moderation, especially if they help increase intake of other nutrients by making the meals more appealing.

Carbohydrates are important because they provide the body with quick, easily used energy. Carbohydrates help you maintain the energy balance, so that the body does not have to draw on stored energy sources like fat and muscle. Fruits and vegetables provide vitamins, minerals, fibre and energy. One should eat five portions a day. A portion is equal to a whole piece of fruit, a heaped serving spoon of vegetables, a small glass of fruit juice, or a handful of dried fruit. Meat, poultry, fish, eggs, beans nuts provide protein, minerals and vitamins. One should eat two or three portions per day. A portion is equal to two medium-sized eggs, a 100 g piece of meat, a 150 g piece of fish, or a small can of baked beans. Dairy products such as milk, cheese, and yoghurt provide vitamins, minerals and calcium. Three portions can be eaten per day. A portion is equal to a third of a pint of milk, a small pot of yoghurt, or a matchbox-sized piece of cheese.

(ii) Fats

Fats such as cooking oils, butter, margarine, meat and other protein-based foods provide energy, essential fatty acids and the fat-soluble vitamins A, D, E and K. They also provide calcium and phosphate. It is recommended that about one-third of the daily calorie intake should come from fats. Eating too much fat can lead to weight gain and increased levels of blood fats. This can increase chances of developing cardiovascular disease and some cancers. There is no increased need for fats for PLHIV.

Some PLHIV have difficulty in absorbing fats. It may be due to intestinal damage caused by opportunistic infections, or by HIV itself.

Steatorrhea can cause diarrhea, bloating, or changes in the colour of the stool. If one has steatorrhea, very little of the fat eaten is absorbed. Since it is still important to have some fat in the diet, it is important to drink liquid supplements or other products that contain a type of fat called MCT (medium-chain triglycerides). This type of fat is easy to absorb.

Excessive amounts of saturated fats can raise the body's cholesterol levels. Saturated fats are animal fats like those found in butter, or as part of red meat. High triglyceride and cholesterol levels are associated with a higher risk of heart attacks and stroke. Recently, both high triglyceride and cholesterol levels have been observed in some PLHIV on ART.

In some studies, polyunsaturated fats (found in some vegetable oils such as corn and peanut oil, and in most margarines) been shown to reduce T-cells, and with them the functioning of the immune system. While these studies were not HIV-specific, it may still be wise for PLHIV to avoid eating a lot of polyunsaturated fat. Polyunsaturated fats are much less likely to increase cholesterol than saturated fats.

Monounsaturated fats are also found in vegetable oils like olive oil and canola oil. These are not suspected of being immune suppressive. Monounsaturated fats do not normally increase cholesterol levels like saturated fats, but they are sometimes modified when heated during processing. For this reason, many people look for olive oil that is "cold pressed".

Omega-3 fatty acids are called essential fatty acids because they must be present in the diet. The body can't manufacture them. They are found in the oils of most fish and seafood, as well as in flaxseed and some beans and peas. Eating foods rich in omega-3 fatty acids has been shown to reduce the risk of heart attack, and to have a positive influence on cell-mediated immunity (the part of the immune system most damaged by HIV infection). Studies on PLHIV have shown that by using omega-3 fatty acids reduced triglyceride levels and, if they had no new opportunistic illnesses, it helped them gain weight.

(c) Fluids

Fluid helps replace water lost in sweat and urine. Water also transports nutrients throughout the body and keeps the kidneys functioning in a healthy way. By sweating, and losing lot of fluid in other ways, like vomiting or diarrhea, one can lose important minerals. As in normal condition, PLHIV should drink at least 8 glasses of water a day.

Box 14.3 highlights the positive impact of nutrition supplement and counselling for PLHIV

Box 14.3 People living with HIV (PLHIV) – Impact of Nutrition Supplements and Counselling– A field trial on integrating nutrition support as a part of care and treatment of PLHIV

World Food Programme in collaboration with Tuberculosis Research Institute in a non-randomized interventional study of PLHIV in Tamil Nadu, India found that PLHIV were more malnourished, anaemic and hypoproteinemic than socio economically matched controls. It was noted that in resource poor setting, with a high background level of malnutrition, HIV infection resulted in adverse nutritional status of individuals. Decrease in the body weight, BMI, mid-arm and hip circumferences with a reduction in the FFM (fat free mass that is, total mass minus fat mass) and BCM (body cell mass) (in males) and triceps skinfold thickness and percent body fat (in females) may be the earliest indication of decline in the nutritional status of HIV-infected patients.

The intervention group received nutritional supplement in the form of 3 kg pack of a blended micronutrient fortified food every month to be consumed 100 g/day (100 g of the supplement provides 400 calories, 15% protein, 6% fat fortified with vitamins A, B_1, B_2, B_{12}, C, Niacin and folic acid). The control group did not receive supplement for the first 6 months. Both groups received nutritional counselling, prophylaxis and psychosocial support.

Anthropometric, laboratory and dietary assessments were done at baseline and at 6 months for all patients. Body composition by BIA (bioimpedance analysis) measured in a sub-group of patients, repeated at 6 months. Quality of life using WHO–Quality of life index protocol was assessed every 6 months. Data was entered in Excel/EpiInfo and analyzed using SPSS statistical package. Both the intervention and Control Groups were compared at baseline. Paired t-test used to compare values at 0 and 6 months.

After 6 months of nutritional supplementation there was a significant increase in weight, BMI and mid-arm circumference (MAC). CD4 cell count remained unchanged in the intervention group but decreased significantly in controls without nutritional supplementation. Though all sub-groups showed improvement, weight gain was maximum in the lowest CD4 count strata. Men and women with CD4<200 showed increase in body fat content.

Based on the findings of the above study (Box 14.3), integration of nutritional support (counselling and nutrition supplementation) for PLHIV was recommended to be included into National AIDS Control Programme of India (see Box 14.4).

Box 14.4 National AIDS Control Programme, India

National Aids Control Organization (NACO) was established in 1992, under Ministry of Health and Family Welfare [23]. NACO formulates policy and implements programs for prevention and control of HIV and AIDS in India. NACO coordinates and manages the National AIDS Control programme (NACP). At the state level, the state governments have established State AIDS Control societies for effective management and implementation of National AIDS Control Programme at the state level. First two phases of NACP have been completed and the third Phase of the NACP III (2007–2012) has placed the highest priority on preventive efforts, while at the same time seeking to integrate prevention with care, support and treatment. According to NACP III, there will be investment in community care centres to provide psychosocial support, outreach services, referrals and palliative care to PLHIV.

In March 2007, NACO approved a programme to provide nutritional supplement to children enrolled under their ART programme in the country. Under this programme, fortified powdered supplement made of wheat, gram and soya is being provided free of cost to children receiving ART. This is processed by roasting/extrusion and is fortified with micronutrients and trace elements which help in improving immunity of people living with HIV. Each ration will provide one RDA as specified by WHO. The programme aims at partially meeting the nutritional needs of over 3000 children currently enrolled under the ART programme in the country. The programme has been undertaken in collaboration with technical support from several international agencies including Clinton Foundation and WFP.

In the state of Tamil Nadu, under the Tamil Nadu State Aids Control Society, nutrition interventions of the programme included free nutritional supplements and nutrition counselling to PLHIV with case-specific advice to people such as pregnant women. The programme estimated to benefit over 15,000 PLHIV. As part of its efforts to increase the quality of life and life expectancy of people living with HIV and AIDS, in March 2007, the Tamil Nadu government in partnership with WFP launched the nutritional supplement support programme known as "Nutriplus programme". In this programme, nutritional support was provided to PLHIV registered at all 20 anti-retroviral therapy (ART) centres in Tamil Nadu.

(iii) Eating safely

PLHIV are vulnerable to many infections because their immune system is damaged. This includes food-poisoning infections like Salmonella. Proper preparation and storage of food is a very important part of staying healthy. Proper food handling and storage minimizes the risk of food borne illnesses and is very important for people with weakened immune systems as is the case in HIV.

Following food safety measures are recommended

- Use only pasteurized milk.
- Never use products whose "sell by" or "best used by" labels have passed.
- Wash hands with soap and water frequently.
- Carefully wash all cutting boards after chopping vegetables.
- Store hot leftovers in a shallow, small container. Reheat until hot to touch throughout.
- Don't keep leftovers for more than three days. When in doubt, throw it out.
- Avoid raw eggs.

- Wash all fruits and vegetables. Peeling eliminates some risk of bacteria.

(iv) Infant-feeding guidelines for infants born to mothers with HIV

A woman infected with HIV can transmit the virus to her child during pregnancy, labour or delivery, or through breastfeeding. Mother-to-child transmission (MTCT) is by far the most significant route of transmission of HIV infection in children below the age of 15 years. In 2005 alone, 700,000 children were reported to have acquired HIV infection. HIV can be transmitted during pregnancy, during childbirth, or breastfeeding. Without intervention, the risk of transmission from an infected mother to her child ranges from 15% to 25% in developed countries and from 25% to 45% in developing countries. This difference is largely attributed to breastfeeding practices (Table 14.1).

Table 14.1 Estimated risk and timing of MTCT in the absence of interventions

During pregnancy	5–10%
During labour and delivery	10–15 %
During breastfeeding	5–20%
Overall without breastfeeding	15–25%
Overall with breastfeeding to 6 months	20–35%
Overall with breastfeeding to 18–24 Months	30–45%

It is a public health responsibility to prevent HIV infection in infants and young children, and to support optimal breastfeeding to prevent mortality and illness due to diarrhea and respiratory infections. AIDS has increased the mortality of children less than five years of age in high-prevalence areas, both through direct infection and because of the reduced levels of care that a family living with HIV can provide. Although only part of this increase in mortality is the result of HIV infection through breastfeeding, it is important to have clear guidelines on infant and young child feeding, including the effects of HIV.

Breast feeding is normally the best way to feed an infant. Breast feeding mothers of infants and young children who are known to be HIV-infected should be strongly encouraged to continue breastfeeding [28].

Exclusive breastfeeding is recommended for HIV-infected women for the first six months of life unless replacement feeding is acceptable, feasible, affordable, sustainable and safe (AFASS – Box 14.5) for them and their infants before that time. When replacement feeding is acceptable, feasible, affordable, sustainable and safe (AFASS), avoidance of breastfeeding by HIV-infected women is recommended. At six months, if replacement feeding is still not acceptable, feasible, affordable, sustainable and safe (Box 14.5), continuation of breastfeeding with additional complementary foods is recommended, while the mother and baby continue to be regularly assessed. All breastfeeding should stop once a nutritionally adequate and safe diet without breast milk can be provided [28].

Regarding infant-feeding choices, NACO [29] states: Breast feeding provides the infant with all required nutrients and immunological factors that help to protect against common infections. This protection is reduced when the child is given water or any other substance during exclusive breastfeeding. Mixed feeding, i.e. breast milk and formula feeds combined, is the most hazardous form of infant feeding. Exclusive replacement feeding is the ideal option but it may not be affordable and feasible, where safe drinking water, fuel or clean utensils are scarce. In such scenario HIV-infected women should be counselled during the antenatal period about infant-feeding choices and to make an informed decision.

The mother who has chosen not to breast-feed must be able to prepare feeds hygienically and should be advised to use cup feeding and not bottle feeding. In case replacement feeding is not possible, exclusive breastfeeding for the first six months of life with early cessation is recommended. The risks of HIV transmission especially if combined with ART may be less than 0.5%, if exclusive breastfeeding is done. If family support is not present, exclusive breastfeeding may be difficult and the parent(s) may need consistent psycho-social support. When the child reaches the age of six months or earlier, breastfeeding should be stopped within two weeks while ensuring the comfort level of both mother and infant. At the same time, good quality complementary foods should be introduced, ensuring adequate amounts of energy proteins and micronutrients.

HIV-infected mothers should be counselled about infant-feeding choices during pregnancy (ante-natal period) and to decide before delivery. During the post-natal period, she should be counselled again to support her decision and to note if there is a change of decision on infant-feeding options. As with the PPTCT recommendations, “HIV-positive women are counselled on feeding options in order for them to make an informed decision on how they would like to feed their infants”.

Box 14.5 AFASS

Acceptable

The mother perceives no barrier, cultural or social, to replacement feeding and has no fear of stigma. She will be able to cope with pressure from family and friends to breastfeed.

Feasible

The mother has adequate time, knowledge, skills and other resources to prepare the replacement food and feed the infant up to 12 times in 24 hours.

Affordable

The mother and family can purchase formula, including all ingredients, fuel, clean water, soap and equipment, without compromising the health and nutrition of the family, and also possible increased medical costs.

Sustainable

Availability of a continuous and uninterrupted supply and dependable system of distribution of formula for as long as the infant needs it.

Safe

Replacement foods are correctly and hygienically prepared and stored, and fed in nutritionally adequate quantities, with clean hands and with clean utensils, preferably by cup.

Evidence has shown that early breastfeeding cessation is associated with increased morbidity and mortality in HIV-exposed infants. Improved adherence, longer duration of exclusive breastfeeding can be achieved in HIV-infected and HIV-uninfected mothers given consistent messages on the meaning and significance of exclusive breastfeeding and frequent, high quality counselling. HIV-infected mothers who need ARVs for their own health should have antiretroviral therapy and this is likely to decrease transmission. Mothers with severe HIV but not yet on ARVs may adopt replacement feeding but it is important that the consider AFASS criteria. HIV-positive infants benefit from continued breastfeeding.

There is no doubt that breast milk can transmit HIV or that an infant's chances of survival when living in a poor or rural community are greatly decreased by not practicing breastfeeding. The challenge is how health systems can, at scale, help individual women, whether infected with HIV or not, appreciate the inherent risks and opportunities of their environment and make appropriate decisions about how to feed their infants. For scientists, the challenge is to study and understand the evidence and possible prejudices in this crucial component of child survival.

Based on these principles, a number of countries have developed guidelines for feeding young children. The national guidelines for infant and young child feeding in India [30] refers to the risk factors such as breast pathology like sore nipples or even sub-clinical mastitis during breastfeeding that increase transmission and are preventable problems through good breastfeeding and lactation management support to mothers.

Box 14.6

All HIV-infected mothers should receive counselling, which should include provision of general information about meeting their own nutritional requirements and about the risks and benefits of various feeding options and specific guidelines in selecting the option most likely to be suitable for their situation. The manifold advantages of breastfeeding even with some risk of HIV transmission should be explained to the HIV-positive mothers.

If artificial feeding is NOT affordable, feasible, acceptable, safe and sustainable (AFASS), then only exclusive breastfeeding must be recommended during the first six months of life. These guidelines imply that till one can ensure all these 5 AFASS factors, it would not be safe to select artificial feeding by HIV-positive mothers.

The danger of mixed feeding should be explained to the HIV-infected mothers. Sometimes mothers may choose to artificially feed the baby, but under some social pressures they also breastfeed the child. An artificially fed baby is at less risk than the baby who receives mixed feeding, i.e. both breastfeeding and artificial feeding. All breastfeeding mothers should be supported for exclusive breastfeeding up to six months. If the woman chooses not to breastfeed, she should be provided support for artificial feeding to make it safe.

To achieve appropriate infant-feeding practices in HIV-positive mothers, capacity building of counsellors and health workers including doctors and nursing staff is mandatory to ensure either 'exclusive feeding', or 'exclusive artificial feeding' as chosen by the mother.

In the absence of safe water, hygiene, and community acceptance exclusive breastfeeding should be promoted until the infant is 6-month old rather than just during the first few months of life. The continued risks of serious morbidity and mortality in infants if breastfeeding is stopped early at around six months stresses the need for continued contact and counselling with mothers during the first months of the infant's life. Counselling will also help in guiding her decisions about feeding practices beyond 6 months. Incorrect use of commercial infant formula can result in diarrheal illness and malnutrition.

(v) Exercise and PLHIV

Several studies have shown that aerobic exercise improves quality of life for people with HIV. For example exercise can

- Increase muscle mass
- Boost the immune system
- Reduce cholesterol and triglyceride levels
- Regulate sleep patterns
- Reduce stress

- Enhance self-image
- Regulated bowel function
- Increase appetite and energy levels

In early HIV infection, loss of muscle mass occurs even before any apparent weight loss. Increasing muscle mass may help increase long-term survival with HIV. It is possible to increase muscle mass, which it is metabolically active tissue, as opposed to fat, which is not. Increased muscle mass can boost the total amount of energy the body produces. In turn, elevated energy levels can enhance the immune system even more.

Moderate exercise is beneficial to the immune system, by increasing T4 Helper Cells, T8 Killer Cells, and Natural Killer Cells. Immune enhancement may be due to the reduced stress levels and improved self-image of people who exercise.

Exercise can reduce cholesterol and triglyceride levels. Some HIV medications increase the amount of fat in the blood, but exercise can help protect against the associated risk of heart disease.

Moderate exercise can improve mood and offer an important way of maintaining a healthy self-image.

Exercise can include anaerobic exercise or resistance training includes activities such as weight lifting and working out with rubber bands. These activities are more beneficial for increasing muscle or strength. Aerobic exercise includes activities such as brisk walking, cycling, swimming, running, or vigorous dancing.

A *combination* of both aerobic and anaerobic types of activity is best. Because aerobic activity tends to promote weight loss, individuals who have trouble maintaining their weight may want to primarily focus on anaerobic activity. Participating in lower impact aerobic activities such as walking can provide benefits without burning excess calories.

Besides these popular forms of exercise like swimming, cycling, aerobics, running, and weight training (sometimes called resistance training), there are a number of movement-based exercises, such as yoga, which help maintain muscle tone and suppleness whilst also having meditative or relaxing qualities.

One should be aware of over-exercising. Warning signs include fatigue and increased minor infections. In case a person feels sick (dizzy or nauseated) after a 10–15 minute warm-up period, one should go easy during work-out or stop exercising until one feels better.

Some studies have also suggested exercise has beneficial effects on the immune system such as increasing CD4+ cells. Exercising to the point of exhaustion, however, has been shown to be immune suppressive. The biggest benefit of exercise for PLHIV may be the building and retention of muscle mass. Exercise, including working out with weights, and swimming, has been shown to improve muscle function and to build lean muscle mass in PLHIV. Such exercise reduces serum triglyceride levels and normalizes blood lipids without requiring the addition of drugs. This would be beneficial to patients who are already consuming too many drugs.

(vi) Nutrition Counselling

Nutritional counselling is helpful for PLHIV to make an informed choice of the right type of foods in relation to their nutritional and HIV status, and other disease conditions that they experience. When dietary counselling is combined with oral nutritional supplements, there is additional evidence for its value.

Nutritional counselling has been shown to be effective; it has also been shown to influence health outcomes in HIV infection (Box 14.7).

Efforts to strengthen nutrition counselling, care and support for HIV-infected persons should be balanced with efforts to alleviate the overall burden of malnutrition, regardless of HIV status. Nutrition guidelines should be appropriate to local resources, and programmatic and clinical environment with the treatment and management of the disease.

Box 14.7 Effectiveness of counselling on nutritional care

A study reported by Tabi et al. [31] on the effectiveness of nutritional counselling as an intervention to improve health outcomes for HIV-positive patients in Ghana, West Africa. Using secondary-analytic data of recorded monthly weights of 25 PLHIV, whose ages ranged from 21 to 60 years, with a mean of 39.4 years (sd = 10.13) were obtained and analysed. It was found that PLHIV responded favourably to nutritional counselling about protein dietary intake as an intervention to improve weight gain. Repeated measures showed a statistically significant weight gain ($P = 0.008$). They conclude that in the absence of ART, nutrition counselling can be an effective intervention for PLHIV in developing countries. The health and nutritional status of the patients can be improved through nutritious food, allowing them to lead longer and better quality lives. It was concluded that nutritional care and support should be essential elements of a comprehensive approach to HIV.

Nutrition counselling should be based on nutrition and dietary assessment. The purpose of this assessment is to gather information about the current nutritional status and dietary practices and to identify risk factors for developing future nutritional complications. The nutritional status assessment should include at least the measurement of weight, height and haemoglobin. This will help in the calculation of Body Mass Index or BMI. Measurement of mid-upper arm circumference can help in a crude estimation of muscle wasting.

The dietary assessment should include information on usual eating patterns and intake, appetite and eating problems, and household food security. All medications taken on a daily basis should be noted so that nutrient interactions and/or contraindications can be identified.

Nutrition counselling, care and support begin with an assessment of the specific circumstances, including the nutritional status, diet and the social and other conditions that could prevent the person from achieving adequate dietary intake.

For HIV-infected persons who are asymptomatic, emphasis should be placed on the need to stay healthy by improving eating habits and the nutritional quality of the diet, maintaining weight (or gaining adequate weight), preserving lean body mass, continuing physical activity and ensuring an understanding of food safety.

For individuals who are experiencing HIV-related infections and illnesses and/or weight loss, the main objective is to minimize the nutritional consequences of the infections by obtaining immediate treatment, maintaining the greatest possible food intake during acute infection, increasing food intake during the recovery period, and continuing physical activity as much as possible so as to preserve lean body mass.

For individuals who have advanced disease or persistent HIV-related infections and illnesses, the main objective is to provide comfort and palliative care, with modification of the diet according to the symptoms and with encouragement for eating.

For persons on ART, the focus of nutrition counselling should be on management of drug and food interactions and other side effects of treatment. Advice related to treatment and counselling on nutrition issues related to ARV and OI treatment cover the timing of pill ingestion in relation to meals, the minimizing and management of nutrition-related side-effects of prescribed medications (e.g. nausea and vomiting), and the consequences of long-term ARV treatment for body fat distribution and metabolism. Nutrition advice and counselling should also cover the food and water requirements related to ARV drug regimens. Advice should be given on how to cope with body fat distribution and the metabolic changes underlying or new conditions that require dietary modifications, e.g. diabetes mellitus, should be monitored during follow-up care.

For pregnant and lactating mothers, it is critical that counselling focuses on issues referred in the section on "infant feeding".

WFP in collaboration with NACO have developed nutrition counselling materials adopting the principles described above. These materials have been provided to all ART and ICTC centres in India. Counsellors all over the country have received training on the use of nutrition counselling materials.

References

1. UNAIDS, WHO, AIDS EPIDEMIC UPDATE (2007). Joint United Nations Programme on HIV/AIDS (UNAIDS) and World Health Organization.
2. NATIONAL AIDS CONTROL ORGANIZATION. Ministry of Health and Family Welfare, Government of India. 2006.
3. NATIONAL FAMILY HEALTH SURVEY (NFHS-3), International Institute for Population Sciences, 2005–06.
4. HIV/AIDS SURVEILLANCE IN INDIA (as reported to NACO as on 30th November 2003). http://www.naco.nic.in/indianscene/overv.htm.
5. LICHTERFELD M, KAUFMANN DE, et al. Loss of HIV-1specific CD8+ T cell Proliferation after acute HIV Infection and restoration by vaccine-induced HIV-1 specific CD 4+ T cells. JEM (Journal of experimental medicine), **200**, no. 6701–6712.
6. CHAISSON RE (2002). When to start antiretroviral therapy? *9th Conf Retrovir Oppor Infect Feb 24 28 2002 Wash State Conv Trade Cent Seattle Wash Conf Retrovir Oppor Infect 9th 2002 Seattle Wash.* 2002 Feb 24–28; 9: abstract no. S17.
7. PHILLIPS AN, GAZZARD BG, CLUMECK N, LOSSO MH, LUNDGREN JD (2007). When should antiretroviral therapy for HIV be started? *BMJ* **334**, pp 76–78.
8. NACO, MINISTRY OF HEALTH AND FAMILY WELFARE, GOVERNMENT OF INDIA (2007). Antiretroviral therapy guidelines for HIV-infected adults and adolescents including post-exposure prophylaxis.
9. BABAMETO G, KOTLER DP (1997). Malnutrition in HIV infection. *Gastroenterol Clin North Am* **26**, no. 2, pp 393–415.
10. MACALLAN DC (1999). Wasting in HIV infection and AIDS. *J Nutr* **29**, no. 1, pp 238S–242S.
11. KEATING J, BJARNASON I, SOMASUNDARAM S, MACPHERSON A, FRANCIS N, PRICE AB, SHARPSTONE D, SMITHSON J, MENZIES IS, GAZZARD BG (1995). Intestinal absorptive capacity, intestinal permeability and jejunal histology in HIV and their relation to diarrhea. *Gut* **37**, no. 5, pp 623–629.
12. ULLRICH R, ZEITZ M, HEISE W, L'AGE M, HOFFKEN G, RIECKEN EO (1989). Small intestinal structure and function in patients infected with human immunodeficiency virus (HIV): evidence for HIV-induced enteropathy. *Ann Intern Med* **111**, no. 1, pp 15–21.
13. SEMBA RD, TANG AM (1999). Micronutrients and the pathogenesis of human immunodeficiency virus infection. *Br J Nutr* **81**, pp 181–189.
14. VALADAS E (2004). Metabolic changes in HIV-infected patients on HAART. European Society of Clinical Microbiology and Infectious Diseases. *Fourteenth European Congress of Clinical Microbiology and Infectious Diseases*, Prague/ Czech Republic, May 1–4, 2004.
15. BERNASCONI E, CAROTA A, MAGENTA L, PONS M, RUSSOTTI M, MOCCETTI T (1998). Metabolic changes in HIV-infected patients treated with protease inhibitors. *Int Conf AIDS* **12**, pp 88 (abstract no. 178/12375).
16. MENEILLY G, FORBES J, PEABODY D, REMPLE V, BURDGE D (2001). Metabolic and body composition changes in HIV-infected children on antiretroviral therapy. *Program Abstr 8th Conf Retrovir Oppor Infect Conf Retrovir Oppor Infect 8th 2001 Chic Ill.* 2001 Feb 4–8; **8**, p 239 (abstract no. 650).
17. BEREGSZASZI M, DOLLFUS C, LEVINE M, FAYE A, DEGHMOUN S, BELLAL N, HOUANG M, CHEVENNE D, HANKARD R, BRESSON JL, BLANCHE S, LEVY-MARCHAL C (2005). Longitudinal evaluation and risk factors of lipodystrophy and associated

metabolic changes in HIV-infected children. *Acquir Immune Defic Syndr* **40**, no. 2, pp 161–168.

18. WORLD HEALTH ORGANIZATION (WHO). *Nutrient requirements for people living with AIDS: Report of a technical consultation*, Geneva, 13–15 May, 2003.
19. FRIIS H, MICHAELSEN KF (1998). Micronutrients and HIV infection: a review. *Eur J Clin Nutr* **52**, pp 157–163.
20. TANG AM, SMIT E (1998). Selected vitamins in HIV infection: a review. *AIDS Patient Care STDS* **12**, no. 4, pp 263–273.
21. NDUATI RW, JOHN GC, RICHARDSON BA, OVERBAUGH J, WELCH M, NDINYA-ACHOLA J, MOSES S, HOLMES K, ONYANGO F, KREISS JK (1995). Human immunodeficiency virus type 1-infected cells in breast milk: association with immunosuppression and vitamin A deficiency. *J Infect Dis* **172**, no. 6, pp 1461–1468.
22. JOHN GC, NDUATI RW, MBORI-NGACHA D, OVERBAUGH J, WELCH M, RICHARDSON BA, NDINYA-ACHOLA J, BWAYO J, KRIEGER J, ONYANGO F, KREISS JK (1997). Genital shedding of human immunodeficiency virus type 1 DNA during pregnancy: association with immunosuppression, abnormal cervical or vaginal discharge, and severe vitamin A deficiency. *J Infect Dis* **175**, no. 1, pp 57–62.
23. BAUM MK, SHOR-POSNER G, LU Y, ROSNER B, SAUBERLICH HE, FLETCHER MA, SZAPOCZNIK J, EISDORFER C, BURING JE, HENNEKENS CH (1995). Micronutrients and HIV-1 disease progression. AIDS **9**, no. 9, pp 1051–1056.
24. MEYDANI SN, HAYEK M (1992). Vitamin E and immune response. In: Chandra RK (ed). *Nutrition and Immunology*. St John's, Newfoundland: ARTS Biomedical, pp 105–28.
25. BAUM MK, SHOR-POSNER G, LU Y, ROSNER B, SAUBERLICH HE, FLETCHER MA, SZAPOCZNIK J, EISDORFER C, BURING JE, HENNEKENS CH (1995). Micronutrients and HIV-1 disease progression. AIDS **9**, no. 9, pp 1051–1056.
26. CAMPA A, SHOR-POSNER G, INDACOCHEA F, ZHANG G, LAI H, ASTHANA D, SCOTT GB, BAUM MK (1999).. Mortality risk in selenium-deficient HIV-positive children. *J Acquir Immune Defic Syndr Hum Retrovirol* **15**, pp 508–513.
27. MOCCHEGIANI E, MUZZIOLI M (2000). Therapeutic application of zinc in human immunodeficiency virus against opportunistic infections. *J Nutr* **130**, no. 5S, pp 1424S–1431S.
28. NACO AND IAP (2006). Guidelines for HIV care and treatment on infants and children.
29. WHO / UNICEF / UNAIDS / UNFPA (2006). HIV and infant feeding new evidence and programmatic experience. Report of a technical consultation.
30. GOVERNMENT OF INDIA (2006). Ministry of women and Child Development, National guidelines on infant and young child feeding.
31. TABI M, VOGEL, RL (2006). Nutritional counselling: an intervention for HIV-positive patients. *J Adv Nurs* **54**, no. 6, pp. 676–682.

15
Vitamin A metabolism

Ravinder Chadha

Ravinder Chadha, PhD, is an Associate Professor at the Department of Food & Nutrition, Lady Irwin College, Delhi University. She is engaged in teaching Public Nutrition courses to undergraduate and post graduate students. Her doctoral research work was in the area of vitamin A deficiency among school-age children.

15.1 Introduction

Vitamin A plays a vital role in human metabolism, being involved in a number of regulatory and other physiological processes. Understanding the role of vitamin A in human body and its physiological processing is important for effectively correcting vitamin A deficiency which remains a public health problem throughout much of the world. The present chapter focuses on the processing of dietary vitamin A, its transport in the circulation and assessment of vitamin A status.

15.2 Discovery of vitamin A

Vitamin A was the first vitamin to be discovered. In the year 1913, recognition of the dietary requirement for vitamin A began with the independent observations of McCollum and Davis [1, 2] and Osborne and Mendel [3] that there was a factor in certain fats which was essential for growth of rats. This lipid soluble growth factor which could be found in animal fats and fish oils was called “fat-soluble A”. It was also observed by Osborne and Mendel that the green parts of plants contain relatively high amounts of “fat soluble A” activity. However, it was Steenbock [4] who concluded from a comparative study of the growth-promoting activities of white and yellow maize in 1919 that there was a definite relationship between the fat-soluble A and the yellow plant pigments. This was further substantiated by Moore [5] who demonstrated that the livers of rats given a diet deficient in vitamin A but with massive amounts of carotene (derived from yellow plant pigments) for 1–3 months contained very high amounts of vitamin A. The chemical relationship between β-carotene and retinol was conclusively established by the classical work of Karrer et al [6, 7] as it became obvious that carotene is converted to retinol in the animal body. Though the knowledge of the metabolism of vitamin A and carotenoids has advanced dramatically over the years it continues to be an area of active research.

15.3 Occurrence and sources

All vitamin A present in the body must be derived from the diet as humans as well as other animal species have no capacity for de-novo vitamin A synthesis. Vitamin A is a generic term to designate any compound possessing the biological activity of retinol. The active forms of vitamin A are retinol (alcohol form), retinal (aldehyde form) and retinoic acid (acid form). Nearly 90–95% of total vitamin A reserves are usually in the liver in the form of retinyl esters which is the storage form of vitamin A (Figure 15.1). In the diet, vitamin A is available in two forms, i.e. preformed vitamin A which occurs naturally only in animals and provitamin A carotenoids of plant origin. Preformed vitamin consists primarily of retinol and retinyl esters which are obtained from animal food products. Fish liver oils most notably those of halibut, cod and shark are the most concentrated sources of preformed vitamin A and are often used medicinally. Liver (goat, sheep or ox), egg yolk, butter and whole milk are good dietary sources of preformed retinol. However, synthetic vitamin is used in almost all vitamin A supplements and fortification of processed foods like sugar, cereals, condiments, fats and oils. The major commercial forms are acetate and palmitate esters which are relatively stable.

Provitamin A carotenoids are present in dark green vegetables and yellow and orange fruits as well as vegetables. Dark green leafy vegetables, mangoes, carrots, papaya and red palm oil are some rich dietary sources of provitamin A carotenoids. Of more than 600 carotenoids which have been identified in nature, more than 50 possess vitamin A activity. Of these, all-trans β-carotene makes the largest contribution to vitamin A activity in foodstuffs. Others like α-carotene, γ-carotene and β-cryptoxanthin contribute to a lesser extent. These provitamin A carotenoids make up 80% of all dietary vitamin A intake consumed by most people in Asia and Africa where vitamin A deficiency is a public health concern [8]. These provitamin A carotenoids are first cleaved to retinol and then converted to other vitamin A metabolites in the body.

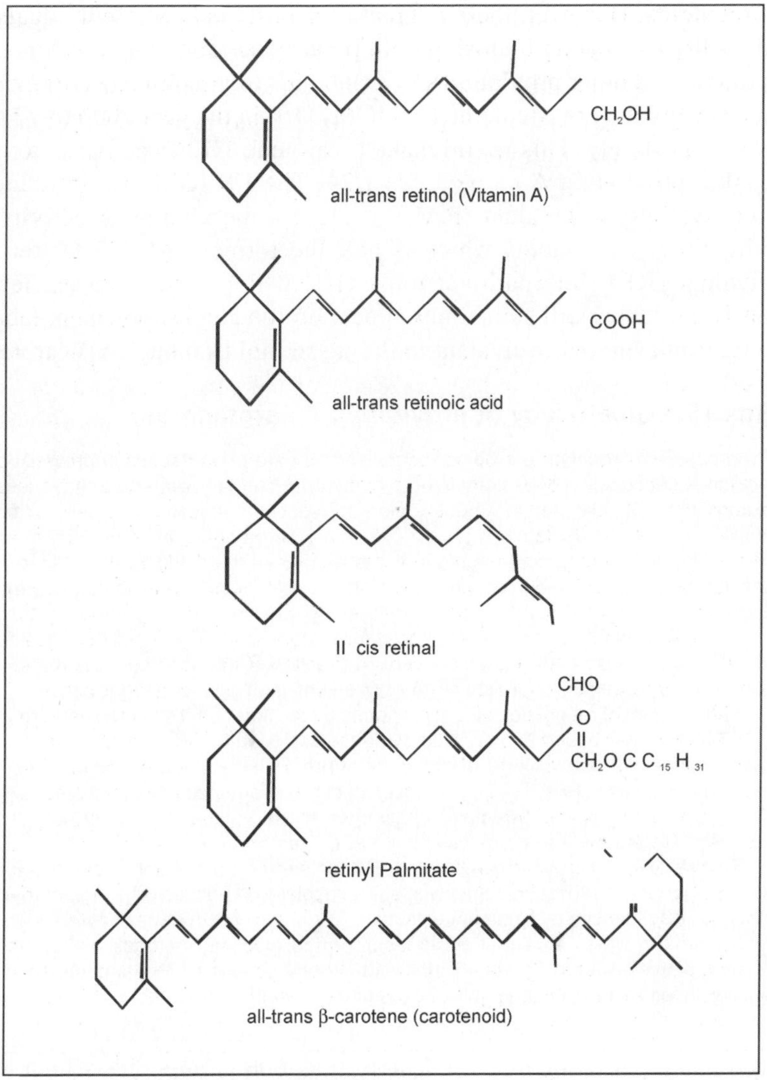

CH_2OH

all-trans retinol (Vitamin A)

COOH

all-trans retinoic acid

II cis retinal

CHO

O

II

$CH_2OCC_{15}H_{31}$

retinyl Palmitate

all-trans β-carotene (carotenoid)

15.1 Structures of vitamin A and some related compounds

To express the vitamin A activity of different food sources, the term retinol equivalent (RE) is used. On equal weight basis β-carotene has less vitamin A activity than preformed vitamin A (retinol). Other provitamin A carotenoids, like α-carotene, γ-carotene and crypotoxanthin, have only about half the activity of β-carotene. Thus, on the basis of the recommendation of FAO/WHO (1967) [9], 1 μg RE is equal to 1 μg retinol, 6 μg β-carotene and 12 μg of other carotenoids. The total amount of vitamin A in foods is expressed as μg retinol equivalents, calculated from the sum of μg preformed vitamin A + 1/6 × μg β-carotene + 1/12 × μg other provitamin

A carotenoids. However, there is great variability between individuals in their ability to respond to dosing with β-carotene. The bioequivalence of β-carotene and other provitamin A carotenoids to vitamin A were revised by the US Institute of Medicine (US IOM) [10] in the year 2000 to 12 and 24 μg, respectively. This would make β-carotene 1/12 as active as retinol and other provitamin A carotenoids 1/24. The US IOM also introduced Retinol Activity Equivalent (RAE) to express the vitamin A activity of provitamin A carotenoids which is half the former FAO/WHO Retinol Equivalent (RE). International units (IU) which were used earlier to quantify carotenes still sometimes appear on food and supplement labels. One IU is considered equivalent to 0.3 μg retinol or 0.6μg of β-carotene.

Box 15.1 Bioefficacy of provitamin A carotenoids

Food-based approaches are being recognized as safe and effective in preventing vitamin A deficiency. Foods containing provitamin A carotenoids tend to have less biologically available vitamin A but are more affordable than animal products which are rich in preformed vitamin A. The provitamin A carotenoids make up 80% of all dietary vitamin among most people in those regions of the world where vitamin A deficiency is a public health concern. Also strict vegetarians of any society depend upon the provitamin A carotenoids for their entire vitamin A intake. In this context, the issue of the bioefficacy which encompasses bioavailability (fraction of the ingested amount that is absorbed) and bioconversion (fraction of the absorbed amount that is converted to retinol) of provitamin A carotenoids is of profound significance.

The concept of retinol equivalent proposed by the Joint FAO/WHO Expert group (1967) which was based on very little evidence assigned β-carotene 1/6 and other provitamin A carotenoids 1/12 of the value of preformed vitamin A. Nevertheless, it was useful in assessing the equivalences of different sources of vitamin A activity. Research since the mid-90s have challenged these values and many complex factors that determine the bioavailability have been brought to light.

Bioavailability of provitamin A carotenoids and also non-provitamin A carotenoids such as lycopene, lutein and others with possible role in prevention of several chronic diseases is influenced by a number of factors. The chemical structure of carotenoids, food matrix in which a carotenoid is incorporated, cooking methods, dietary fat, nutrient status (Vitamin A, protein, zinc) of the host, genetic factors and interaction among those factors influence bioefficacy of carotenoids. The effect of food matrix and processing on bioavailability of carotenoids is depicted in Figure 15.2.

Very high bioavailability ↑	Synthetic carotenoids in oil
	Carptempodes oil form (Red palm oil)
	Yellow or green fruits
	Yellow or green tubers
	Lightly cooked yellow, orange or green vegetables or fruit juices
	Fresh vegetables juices (without fat)
	Raw yellow/orange vegetables
Very low bioavailability	Raw Green leafy vegetables

15.2 Bioavailability of carotenoids [11]

Dietary intervention studies from Indonesia, Vietnam and China have suggested that one retinol equivalent is derived from either 26–28 μg of β carotene in vegetables or 12 μg of β Carotene in fruits. Based on research evidence from developing countries, US IOM recommended in the year 2000 that 1 μg of retinol is equal to 12 μg of dietary b-carotene or 24 μg of dietary α-carotene or β-cryptoxanthin. These revised conversion factors have serious implications on food based approaches to control vitamin A deficiency as rich sources of provitamin A carotenoids are needed to improve the dietary adequacy of vitamin A among vast section of population in the developing regions. However, the methodology for the accurate determination of provitamin A carotenoid bioactivity in man is still evolving and more data are needed to substantiate the present recommendations.

15.4 Metabolism and storage of vitamin A

Vitamin A available from the diet in the intestinal lumen in two forms: preformed vitamin A as retinol and retinyl esters and provitamin A carotenoids. Retinol is absorbed as such from the intestinal lumen into the mucosal cells, whereas retinyl esters are hydrolysed to retinol prior to intestinal absorption. The uptake of provitamin A carotenoids occurs via passive diffusion similar to other dietary lipids and some is possibly mediated by certain membrane transporters. The physiological processing of vitamin A is discussed in this section. The whole body vitamin A metabolism is also illustrated in Figure 15.3.

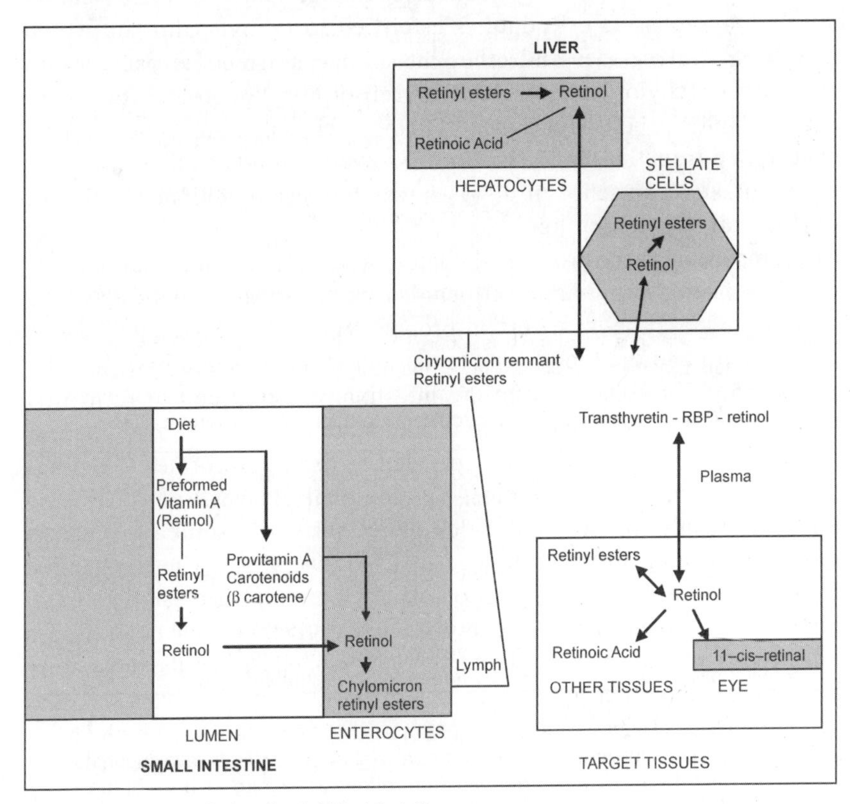

15.3 Metabolism of vitamin A [12, 13, 14]

(a) Digestion and absorption

Dietary vitamin A and its precursors are released from protein in the stomach by proteolysis. Thorough cooking and mastication facilitates the release of provitamin A carotenoids, especially in case of green leaves in which carotenoids exist within chloroplasts as pigment – protein complexes. It is important that carotenoids are released from the cellulose structures so that they are available for absorption. Released vitamin A and carotenoids aggregate with lipids and pass into the upper part of the small intestine. Dietary fat and protein and their hydrolytic products stimulate the secretion of bile which emulsifies the contents of the gut lumen and promotes the formation of lipid micelles. These micelles have lipophilic groups on their inside and hydrophilic groups on their outside which facilitates fat absorption. Bile salts stimulate pancreatic lipase and other esterases that hydrolyze retinyl esters in the enterocytes (intestinal mucosal cells). On hydrolysis, retinol is formed which is well absorbed (70–90%) by intestinal mucosal cells. In the mucosal cells, a specific cellular binding protein (CRBPII) carries the retinol to the enzyme lecithin-retinol acyltransferase (LRAT) which esterifies retinol before incorporation into chylomicrons [15]. Retinol is esterified to retinyl palmitate which along with triglycerides and other fat soluble nutrients is packed into chylomicrons (chylo-the triglyceride rich absorptive lipoproteins that carry dietary fat into the body) for transport to the liver. Both retinol and carotene are absorbed from the small intestine dissolved in lipid and therefore very low fat intake or presence of diseases which interfere with absorption of lipids impair this absorption.

In comparison to the preformed vitamin A, the provitamin A carotenoids as well as the non-provitamin carotenoids are absorbed unmodified by the intestinal mucosal cells. A certain proportion of these passes unchanged into the lymp and the blood. The remaining is metabolized by a specific enzyme 15, 15′-dioxygenase in the intestinal mucosal cell to form first retinal which is mostly reduced to retinol palmitate. At the stage, there is no difference between the retinol provided by diet as preformed vitamin A and as provitamin A carotenoids. Symmetrical cleavage of β-carotene molecules results in two molecules of retinal while some cleavage is asymmetrical and produces less retinal (Figure 15.4). The unchanged carotene which enters the circulation via chylomicrons is cleared by liver. Some of it is cleaved by carotene dioxygenase in liver or some other tissues giving rise to retinal and retinyl esters. As mentioned earlier, the bioactivity of â carotene and other provitamin A carotenoids is much lower than that of retinol. This is because the absorption of dietary carotene (which varies between 5% and 60%) and its conversion to retinol is not a very efficient process.

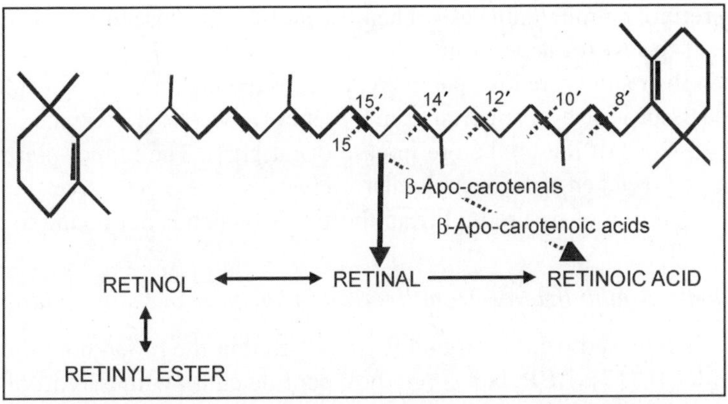

15.4 Conversation of b-carotene into vitamin A via central and excentric cleavage [13]

The absorption of dietary carotene depends to a great extent on the nature of the food ingested, whether cooked or raw, the amount of fat in the meal and also the presence of intestinal parasites such as ascaris lumbricoides and giardia lamblia. Deficiencies of protein, zinc or presence of higher amounts of other carotenoids such as lutein in diet depress the dioxygenase activity. Further, asymmetric or excentric cleavage of β-carotene which also occurs, results in formation of certain apo-carotenals (derivatives of β-carotene) which are oxidized to retinoic acid but cannot be used as sources of retinol.

(b) Metabolism of vitamin A in liver

The chylomicrons carry retinol esters and carotenoids from the gut via lymph into the general circulation where they are broken to some extent to form chylomicron remnants. These remnants have most of the retinyl esters which are taken up by the liver's parenchymal cells (hepatocytes) when they reach liver which is the major organ for vitamin A storage (>80%) in the body. There is evidence that extra-hepatic cells (in lung, intestine and kidney) take up some retinyl esters from the circulation, which are converted to retinoic acid and can be used for regulation of gene expression.

In the parenchymal cells, retinyl esters are hydrolysed and much of the retinol is secreted from the cells after binding with retinol binding protein (RBP or RBP_4). (The vitamin A binding protein, referred to as RBP so far is now referred by investigators by its generic nomenclature, RBP_4). Most of the retinol bound to the protein is transferred to specialized liver cells called stellate cells. These cells which comprise 7% of the liver cell numbers are mainly responsible for storage of vitamin A as retinyl esters mostly retinol palmitate. In case of healthy individuals this store is generally sufficient to last for several months.

When liver stores are low, parenchymal cells are the major site of storage. Adipose tissue is also an important site for retinol as well as β-carotene storage (about 15–20% of the total store in case of rat [16]). The retinol present in adipose cells is taken up from chylomicron esters as in case of the liver. Further, there is secretion of free retinol from these cells which is not bound to RBP.

(c) Vitamin A mobilization from liver and transport in the circulation

Retinol is released from liver and is transported in the blood bound to the protein RBP_4 [17]. RBP_4 is a single polypeptide chain with a hydrophobic pocket within which the fat soluble retinol fits. It protects retinol against oxidation and delivers it to target tissues. RBP is mainly synthesized and secreted from liver and to a lesser extent by adipose tissue [18, 19]. The RBP – retinol complex also referred to as holo-RBP is released from liver bound to another blood protein, transthyretin (TTR) which increases its size as well as molecular weight. This is important to prevent the loss of retinol in glomerular filtrate in the kidney.

RBP concentration in the plasma of well-nourished adults is 1.9–2.4 μmol / l (40–50 μg/ml) [20]. In children the value is 60% of that of adults. Certain condition such as protein-energy malnutrition, infections and parasitic infestations lower plasma RBP concentration. If retinol reserves in liver have been exhausted as is the case in vitamin A deficiency, the holo RBP cannot be formed resulting in the rise in liver apo-RBP (RBP unbound to retinol) content and fall in plasma concentration of RBP. This serves as the basis of relative-dose response test (RDR) of vitamin A status discussed in the section on assessment of vitamin A status.

The specific membrane RBP receptors on target tissues take up retinol from the holo RBP complex and transfer it to an intracellular RBP. The apo-RBP (the free protein) is then released from the receptor some of which may be excreted by the kidney and the remaining is hydrolysed after re-absorption in the proximal renal tubules. Inside the cells there are many intracellular retinol binding proteins which protect retinol within the cell and direct them to specific enzymes.

In the circulation, vitamin A is present in different forms. After a vitamin A rich meal a very high concentration of vitamin A can be present as retinyl esters in chylomicrons. However, in the fasting state most of the retinol present in the circulation is bound in retinol–RBP–TTR complex. In addition to this, low amounts of retinyl esters bound to either very low density lipoproteins (VLDL) or low density lipoproteins (LDL), low amounts of retinoic acid bound to albumin as well as water soluble complexes of retinol and retinoic acid are present. Provitamin A carotenoids may also be present in the circulation mainly bound to LDL. There are no specific carrier proteins for carotenoids. Provitamin A carotenoids such as β-carotene, α-carotene and cryptoxanthin and non-provitamin A carotenoids such as lycopene, lutein and zeaxanthin are the common carotenoids in plasma (Figure 15.5). Their concentrations in plasma depend largely on diet. Some cells can take up retinol palmitate from circulating chylomicrons via lipoprotein receptors and some retinol may enter cells by diffusion. However, cellular uptake of retinol is mainly via membrane RBP receptors. Circulating carotenoids bound to LDLs enter cells having the LDL receptors. Even though, a very small proportion of vitamin A is present in the fasting circulation of well nourished adults as all-trans and 13-cis-retinoic acid bound to albumin

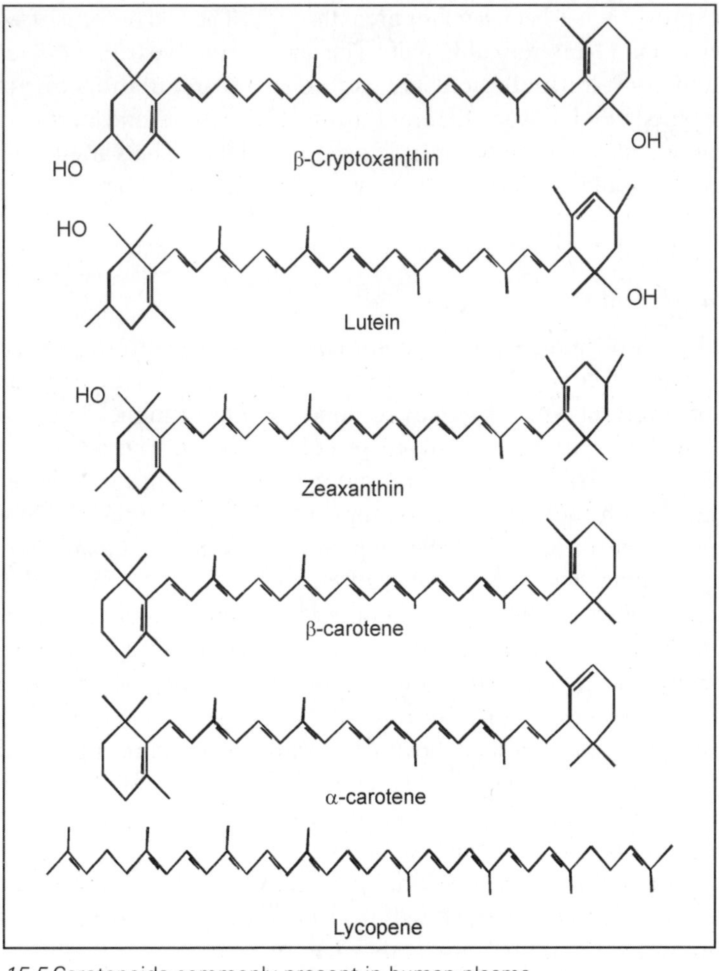

15.5 Carotenoids commonly present in human plasma

(0.1–0.4% of retinol-RBP), it contributes significantly to tissue pools of retinoic acid[21]. These acid derivatives of vitamin A bind to various nuclear receptors in cells and are responsible for increase or decrease in the level of expression of several genes.

15.5 Functions of vitamin A and carotenoids

Vitamin A activity is very important for maintaining human health. The most well-known function of vitamin A is in vision. Historically the requirement of vitamin A for normal functioning of the visual processes was known long before the vitamin was actually discovered. However, the knowledge of functions of vitamin A has advanced dramatically in the recent years. The discovery of nuclear retinoid receptors that regulates gene expression has been a major breakthrough. The active form of vitamin A in vision is 11-cis-retinaldehyde. The acid derivatives all-trans-retinoic acid and 9-cis-retinoic acid are active in the regulation of growth, development and tissue differentiation. β-carotene and certain other carotenoids have an important role as antioxidants. The varied functions of vitamin A and its derivatives as well as of carotenes are discussed in this section.

(a)Vitamin A in vision

In the retina of human eye there are two types of photo (light) receptor cells – rods and cones. The rods are responsible for vision in long intensity light or dim light whereas cones respond to light of higher intensities or bright light and are also involved in colour vision. The active form of vitamin A in vision is 11-cis-retinaldehyde. In retina it is reversibly associated with the light-sensitive opsin proteins, forming rhodopsin in rods and iodopsin in cones. The number of rods in the human eyes is far more (>30 times) than the number of cones.

When light strikes the retina, a number of complex biochemical changes take place, resulting in the generation of a nerve impulse. This process is referred to as phototransduction whereby the energy of photons (light energy) is converted in photoreceptor cells into a nerve signal for transmission of the message onwards towards the brain for interpretation. The retina of mammalian eye has ten layers and the photoreceptors form the outermost of these. Light has to pass through all other nine layers before phototransduction can begin.

In the retinal pigment epithelium, all-trans retinol is isomerized to 11-cis retinol which is then oxidized to 11-cis retinal. This is transported to the photoreceptor rod or cone cells where it reacts with protein opsin to form light sensitive rhodopsin or iodopsin respectively. When exposed to light, 11-cis retinal is isomerized back to all-trans retinal. This conformational change results in release of retinal from the protein and generates a nerve impulse. This process is known as bleaching as it results in the loss of colour of rhodopsin. The released all-trans retinal is then reduced to all – trans-retinol and joins the pool of retinol in the pigment epithelium to complete the cycle. The all-trans retinol is then isomerized to 11-cis-retinol for regeneration of rhodopsin. The availability of the isomer 11-cis retinal of vitamin A is important for initiation of the visual cycle (Figure 15.6).

In vitamin A deficiency the ability to see in dim light and the time taken to adapt to darkness are impaired. Failure to see in dim light, known as night blindness, is one of the earliest symptoms of vitamin A deficiency. Besides retinol, retinoic acid also has a role in the maintenance of a healthy eye. The pathological changes in the surface of the eye such as xerosis or Bitot's spots are early signs of vitamin A deficiency which can be reversed by vitamin A. Vitamin A, mainly as retinoic acid, is required to maintain the surface epithelium of the eye.

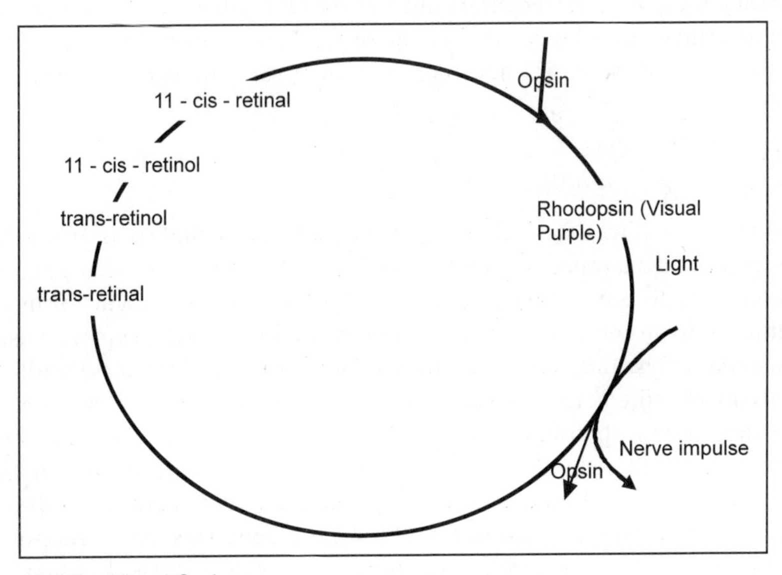

15.6 The Visual Cycle

(b) Regulation of gene expression

Most functions of vitamin A in the body with the exception of the visual process are under genetic control and are mediated by its acid derivatives. Control of cellular growth and differentiation is a major function of vitamin A which is regulated by all-trans retinoic acid and 9-cis-retinoic acid. These active retinoic acid isomers bind to nuclear receptors that bind to response elements on specific genes (nucleotide sequences in the DNA) to increase or decrease the level of expression of the gene. Many of these genes are involved in growth and differentiation, such as those involved in differentiation of the three germ layers, organogenesis and limbs development during embryogenesis. Therefore, both deficiency or excess of the vitamin during early fetal life can cause malformations in various systems of the body.

There are two families of nuclear retinoid receptors: the retinoic acid receptors (RAR) bind all-trans retinoic acid or 9-cis-retinoic acid and the retinoid X receptors (RXR) bind 9-cis-retinoic acid. Each family of receptors has three major subtypes: α, β, and γ. Most, if not all, cells express at least one of these six receptors. There are several hundred genes in different tissues which have been shown to be sensitive to control by retinoids. The retinoid receptors are recognized as part of hormone receptor super family called the Steroid–Thyroid–Retinoid Superfamily with a number of receptors such as vitamin D receptor, thyroid hormone, estrogen receptor progesterone receptor and many more. To recognize response elements, these nuclear receptors must act in pairs (dimers) and a member of RXR family must be present as one of the partners for the dimer to be functional. Thus, retinoids act as regulators of several hormone response systems.

(c) Cellular differentiation

Vitamin A is required for maintenance of healthy epithelial tissue. Cellular differentiation is a process whereby mature epithelium is formed. Vitamin A is required to prevent the synthesis of high molecular weight forms of keratin and to promote the synthesis of glycoproteins which is an important component of the mucous secreted by many epithelial tissues. Vitamin A mainly as retinoic acid regulates cellular differentiation.

In deficiency of vitamin A keratin producing cells replace mucous secreting cells in several epithelial tissues. The results in drying of the cells due to impaired mucous secretion, and the excess keratin synthesis makes the epithelial surface horny and keratinized. The same process is responsible for xerosis and keratinization of conjunctiva and cornea of the eye.

(d) Immune response

Once known as the “anti-infective vitamin”, vitamin A is now recognized as an important determinant of immune status. It is required for maintenance of the skin and mucosal cells which act as barrier against infection. In vitamin A deficiency, epithelial tissues loose their specialized function of mucous production and invasion by bacteria becomes easier. Besides this, vitamin A is involved in the development of white blood cells which play an important role in immune response. Further, vitamin A functions in T-cell mediated responses and may be involved in immunoglobulin production. Lack of vitamin A decreases resistance to infection and can increase the severity of infection as in case of measles, a common childhood infection, which becomes more serious in vitamin A deficient children. There is evidence to suggest that an oxidized retinol metabolite 14-hydroxy-4, 14-retroretinol is the active molecule in the immune system but its mechanism of action is not well defined [22].

(e) Growth

Vitamin A is involved in the growth of the musculo-skeletal system by modulating the growth of bones through remodeling. It has been demonstrated that both vitamin A and retinoic acid produce rapid release of cyclic AMP (adenosine monophosphate) and human growth hormone secretion [23]. A correlation between fasting plasma retinol and nocturnal growth hormone has been observed. The secretion of nocturnal growth hormone has been observed to increase after vitamin A supplementation among a group of short prepubertal children with low level of the hormone. These observations point towards the possible mechanism of the influence of vitamin A on growth. However, studies on the effect of vitamin A supplementation on early child growth in communities with widespread vitamin A deficiency have been inconsequential. The probable explanation of the negative results or lack of evidence of vitamin A supplement on growth in most studies is that growth is dependent on many nutrients, and providing only one of those may not be enough to demonstrate significant effect on growth.

(f) Hemopoiesis

The observations on humans and in experimental animals have repeatedly shown that iron deficiency anemia responds more completely if vitamin A is included along with iron therapy. Vitamin A deficiency might interfere with the absorption, transport or storage of iron. However, the role of vitamin A in hemopoiesis is not completely understood. There is evidence that retinoic acid is involved in the production of RBCs which are derived from stem cells after proper differentiation. This implies that vitamin A possibly controls the utilization of iron. Further, vitamin A appears to facilitate mobilization of iron stores to develop red blood cells. Studies have consistently shown that vitamin A deficiency restricts the release of iron from the stores which results in iron overload and, in the absence of increased absorption of iron in anemia. This can occur even in the absence of any infection. Research evidence also suggests that infection and inflammation depress iron absorption and mobilization, therefore, vitamin A supplementation improves hematological response due to reduced level of infection or improvement in health. The significance of improving vitamin A status in anemia control programme is evident.

(g) Reproduction

Retinol, as well as retinoic acid, is needed for successful reproduction but the precise mechanism of action is not known with certainty. Studies in animals show the requirement of vitamin A for normal spermatogenesis in male and in the prevention of placental necrosis and fetal resorption in the female. In addition, the deposition of substantial amount of β-carotene in corpus luteum also points towards its role in reproduction. There is increasing evidence that vitamin A is required for every stage in the reproductive process in the female.

In experimental animals, vitamin A deficiency as well as excess has been known to induce congenital malformations. In humans it has not been demonstrated conclusively that vitamin A deficiency causes congenital malformations. However, high incidence of fetal anamolies and poor reproductive outcomes have been reported among women ingesting therapeutic doses during early stages of gestation. In communities where vitamin A deficiency is widely prevalent, there is a consensus that, vitamin A supplementation throughout pregnancy should not exceed 10,000 IU per day.

(h) Carotenoids as antioxidants

Historically, the biological activity of a carotene has been considered synonymous with its corresponding vitamin A activity. Of the several provitamin A carotenoids, β-carotene is described as the most active because of its higher provitamin A activity. However, research in the recent years has identified many other activities of carotenoids, of which their role as antioxidants has received special attention. Under conditions of low oxygen availability, carotenes act as antioxidants by trapping singlet-state oxygen. The excessive amount of these reactive oxygen species in vivo can cause oxidative damage of lipids, proteins and DNA. It is accepted that imbalance between oxidative DNA damage and repair contribute to the risk of cancer development. Epidemiological evidence suggests an association between intake of diets rich in β-carotene and vitamin A and a lower risk of many types of cancers [24].

However, intervention trials with β-carotene supplements have not demonstrated its cancer prevention activity. On the contrary, increased incidence of lung cancer was observed among subjects receiving supplements [25, 26]. Thus, supplementation with large doses of specific nutrients is not advisable as it could disturb the finely balanced in vivo antioxidant system which possibly requires an optimal range of various antioxidants to ensure a balanced antioxidant status. A higher intake of fruits and vegetables provides a variety of antioxidants and other beneficial substances [27].

The non-provitamin A carotenoids viz. zeaxanthin, mesozeaxanthin and lutein are concentrated in the macula lutea in the centre of retina and are responsible for its yellow colour. The concentration of this pigment in the eyes of patients of age related macular degeneration disease is lower than those without disease [28]. This degenerative disease is responsible for loss of vision in the elderly. In the macula, lutien and zeaxanthin filter out the short wavelength blue light thereby limiting damage to the retina. Further, they have antioxidant potential and can quench reactive oxygen species generated in retina. These properties of the carotenoids form basis for their possible role in reducing the risk of macular degeneration. Dark green leafy vegetables are the richest source of dietary lutein and zeaxanthin. These carotenoids are also present in egg yolk. However, relation between the disease and dietary intake of the two macular pigments – lutein and zeaxanthin has not been clearly demonstrated.

Research has shown that lutein and zeaxanthin supplementation could improve visual performance in healthy people, particularly in situations of low light intensity. The preliminary findings indicate that macular pigment is important not only in reducing risk of age-related macular degeneration but could also improve the vision of healthy people.

Another non-provitamin A carotenoid, lycopene, the dominating red pigment in tomatoes, is also an antioxidant like β-carotene. Epidemiological evidence suggests that tomato products and lycopene consumption reduce the risk of prostrate cancer [29]. Clinical human trials with short term tomato product or lycopene feeding have indicated reduction in the levels of oxidative damage in prostrate cancer patients as well as in smokers. However, evidence from experimental models suggests that tomato powder, but not lycopene, significantly inhibited cancer growth. This suggests that lycopene is not the only anticancer factor in tomatoes. Further research is needed to clearly understand the protective role of various components within tomatoes in reducing the risk of prostrate cancer.

Box 15.2 Lycopene–the red pigment in tomatoes

Lycopene comprises 60–64% of the total carotenoids found in raw or ripe tomatoes. Other important carotenoids are phytoene, phytofluene, neurosporene and γ carotene. β-carotene constitutes only 1–2% of the total carotenoids. Lycopene is also found in pink grape fruit, guava, papaya and water melon.

All-trans lycopene is the predominant isomer present in plants, but in human tissues cis-isomers are mostly found. On heating and processing tomato products, the cis-isomers of lycopene increase thereby increasing its bioavailability. Besides lycopene, polyphenols especially quercetin and kaempferol which are also potentially beneficial anti-cancer compounds, are present in tomato products, mainly in the skin and seeds.

15.6 Recommended Dietary Allowances (RDA)

Requirements of vitamin A like those of other nutrients vary with age and physiological states such as pregnancy and lactation. The RDA are meant to prevent deficiency and to provide safe intake for majority of the population (97–98%). RDAs for vitamin A are expressed in terms of retinol equivalents (RE) per day which account for different biological activities of retinol and provitamin carotenoids.

The estimates of requirements are based on the minimum level of vitamin A required to reverse completely dark adaptation failure and abnormal retinogram and to maintain adequate stores.

The vitamin A intake for Indians recommended in 1989 and as proposed recently by the Expert Committee is presented in Table 15.1 along with recommended vitamin A intakes from different countries and sources.

The vitamin A intake of 600 RE/day or 9.3 RE/kg for Indian adult was recommended by Indian Council of Medical Research (ICMR) (1989) [30]. Requirements for the other age groups have been established by the factorial method and body weight. The recommendations on retinol requirements for all age groups, except pregnant women, have been retained by the ICMR Expert Group (2008) constituted to revise RDAs of nutrients for Indians. The requirement during pregnancy was established on the basis of studies on vitamin A supplementation required to prevent the fall of plasma vitamin A during last few weeks of pregnancy and which also associated with improved feto-placental function. The Expert Committee proposed a requirement of 800 RE/day on this basis. The additional needs during lactation have been estimated on the basis of vitamin A secreted in breast milk of well nourished mothers.

An additional intake of 350 RE/day during lactation has been recommended which is in line with the intake allowance of 50 μg/kg for infants. The vitamin A requirements of children have been derived from the requirement figures for infants (50 μg/kg) and adults (9.3 μg/kg) considering the growth rates at different ages.

Table 15.1 Recommended dietary intakes of vitamin A (μg RE/day)

Age group (years)	*FAO/WHO* [31]	*Age group (years)*	*NRC [32]*	*Age group (years)*	*UK [33]*	*Age group (years)*	*WHO [34]*	*Age group (years)*	*ICMR expert group* [30]*
0–1	350	0–1	375	0–1	350	0–6	375	0–1	350
1–6	400	1–3	400	1–3	400	months	400	1–6	400
						6–12			
						months			
6–10	400	4–6	500	4–6	500	1–6	400/450	7–9	600
10–12	500	7–10	700	7–10	500	7–9	500	10–18	600
12–15	600	Male		Male		10–18	600	Adult man	600
		11–51 +	1000	11–14	600			18+	
Male		Female		15–50 +	700	Adult man	600	Adult woman	600
15–18+	600	11–51 +	800			18 +		18 +	
Female		Pregnancy	800	Female		Adult	500	Pregnancy	800
15–18 +	500			11—51	600	woman 18+			
Pregnancy	600	Lactation	1300	Pregnancy	700	Pregnancy	800	Lactation	950
		first half yr.							
Lactation	850	second half yr.	1200	Lactation	950	Lactation	850	–	–

* Proposed 2008–2009. The Expert Committee recommended that a minimum of 50% RE be drawn from animal sources to ensure adequacy among vulnerable groups like pregnant and lactating women.

The ICMR Expert Committee (2008) has proposed a revision in the conversion factor of dietary β-carotene to retinol based on many controversial evidences in this regard. For β-carotene, a conversion ratio of 1:8 has been proposed by the committee on the basis of evidence from developing countries on bioequivalence of β-carotene and retinol as well as best association and compatibility of subclinical and dietary deficiency in different regions of the world. The earlier ratio of 1:4 was considered to be too high by the Committee and the ratio of 1:12 proposed by IOM (US) too low to correlate with deficiency reported in different regions. Thus, the proposed intake of β-carotene is on the basis of 1 μg of β-carotene = 0.125 μg of retinol.

No separate RDA has been proposed for β-carotene or other provitamin A carotenoids. According to IOM [10], daily consumption of 3–6 μg of β-carotene would maintain blood levels of β-carotene in the range which is associated with a low risk of chronic diseases. It is therefore advised to consume five or more servings of fruits and vegetables in the daily diet with some green leafy vegetables and deep yellow or orange vegetables and fruits to obtain sufficient amount of β-carotene and other carotenoids.

15.7 Assessment of vitamin A status

Nutritional status concerns some aspect of the state of the body as influenced by the intake and utilization of nutrients. An array of methods have been developed over the years for assessment of vitamin A status which are appropriate for detecting varying degrees of vitamin A deficiency. Measurement of reserves of vitamin A by liver biopsy is the only direct method of assessment of vitamin A status. However, this method is invasive and cannot be considered appropriate for routine assessment. There are several indicators which are used for assessment of vitamin A status at clinical and subclinical level of vitamin A deficiency [35]. An overview of these indicators is included in this section.

Vitamin A deficiency reflects the state of inadequate vitamin A nutriture which begins when liver stores of vitamin A fall below 20 μg/g (0.07 μmol/g). Historically, the recognition of eye lesions attributable to severe form of vitamin A deficiency formed the basis of xerophthalmia classification by ocular signs in 1976 by the first WHO Expert Group on assessment of vitamin A status (Table 15.2).

The term xerophthalmia includes all signs and symptoms affecting the eye that can be attributed to vitamin A deficiency. The second WHO Expert Group (1982) on the control of vitamin A deficiency and xerophthalmia revised the classification and established the criteria for assessing the public health significance of xerophthalmia and vitamin A deficiency based on the prevalence among children less than 6 years old in the community

Table 15.2 Xerophthalmia classification by ocular signs [36, 37]

X N	Night blindness
XI A	Conjunctival xerosis
XI B	Bitot's spots
X 2	Corneal xerosis
X3 A	Corneal ulceration / keratomalacia (involving less than one third of the corneal area
X 3 B	Corneal ulceration / keratomalacia (involving one third or more of the corneal area
X S	Corneal scar (from X 3)
X F	Xerophthalmic Fundus

(Table 15.3). In population surveys the purpose is to determine the magnitude and severity of vitamin A deficiency in the population. Thus, clinical signs of Vitamin A deficiency, viz Bitot's spots, corneal xerosis, keratomalacia /corneal ulceration which reflect the progressive changes due to keratinization of conjunctiva and cornea can be used for identification of those deficient in vitamin A.

Table 15.3 Prevalence criteria indicating vitamin A deficiency of public health significance in a population [37, 38].

Criteria	Minimum prevalence %)
Clinical (primary)	
Children 2–5 years old	
Night blindness (X N)	>1.0
Bitot's Spots (XIB)	> 0.5
Corneal Xerosis (X2) and Corneal Ulcers (X3)	> 0.01
Corneal Scars (XS)	> 0.05
Women of child bearing age	
XN during recent pregnancy	> 5.0
Biochemical (Supportive)	
serum retinol <0.70 μmol/L(20 μg/dL)	>15.0

The changes in the eye as a result of xerosis due to vitamin A deficiency which lead to development of conjunctival xerosis and Bitot's spots are preceded by changes of lesser degree which can be detected by the conjunctival impression cytology (CIC) technique. The technique involves microscopic examination of the impressions of conjunctival cells taken on cellulose acetate strips. The normal cells when stained show sheets of small regular epithelial cells and numerous mucin secreting goblet cells. In vitamin A deficiency, epithelial cells become enlarged, separated and reduced in number. There is marked decline in goblet cells or they may be totally absent [39]. Though it is simple, relatively less invasive and inexpensive technique, the difficulty in standardization of the interpretation of conjunctival impressions has presented its wide adoption for vitamin A status assessment. Further, the results of CIC do not correspond very well with the results of biochemical tests of vitamin A status [40, 41]. Another limitation of CIC is that it is unsuitable for younger children (<3 years) and is unreliable in the presence of eye infections such as acute conjunctivitis and trachoma [42].

As mentioned earlier, the vision in dim light which is dependent on the availability of vitamin A to the rod cells of the retina is impaired in early deficiency. There are methods to test rod function which can be used to assess vitamin A status but they require extremely cooperative subject and are unsuitable for young children who are most at risk of the deficiency. Thus, in deficient populations a brief questionnaire on using child's inability to see adequately in poor illumination such as at dusk using locally appropriate term(s) for night blindness is a simple method to know about the vitamin A status of a community. A dark adaptometer may be used for investigation of night blindness in the children over 2 years and among pregnant women. However, conventional laboratory based testing of dark adaptation is time consuming as a fully light adapted eye takes at least 30 minutes to become completely dark adapted. In this process, the eye becomes more sensitive to low light levels, largely because of shift from photopic vision based on cones to scotopic vision based on rods [43]. Several rapid dark adaptation tests which take 2–3 minutes have been developed which require subjects to identify a letter or to sort discs of different colors [44–47]. These are inherently less sensitive indicators of vitamin A deficiency as in all these rapid tests measurements carried out during the first few minutes of dark adaptation mainly rely on cones instead of rods in the retina.

Night blindness during the latter part of pregnancy is common among vitamin A deficient population and correlates well with other biochemical and functional indicators of vitamin A deficiency [48]. In community surveys eliciting history of night blindness is simple and the response is reliable. A cut-off of ≥ 5 % prevalence of maternal night blindness has been suggested as indicative of community vitamin A deficiency problem [49]. Further, it has been recommended that night blindness history be elicited for a previous pregnancy that ended in a live birth in past 3 years using preferably the local term for night blindness.

Pupillary dark adaptation is a completely different non-invasive technique the basis of which is that, the intensity of light needed to cause pupillary contraction indicates the subject's threshold of light visible in the dark adapted state. The pupils do not respond or constrict normally in low illumination among those who are night blind. The test required minimum cooperation from the subjects and has been successfully used for young children and pregnant women [50, 51]. The dark adaptation scores based on pupillary response respond to vitamin A supplementation and a close association has been demonstrated with serum retinol and RDR

[50–52]. The technique is useful in correctly identifying populations having normal or deficient Vitamin a status. However, the improvement in pupillary response among vitamin A deficient individual takes upto 4–6 weeks after dosing with vitamin A [43]. Thus, its use as an indicator for assessment of interventions designed to improve vitamin A status is constrained by this long waiting period. This technique requires preparation of an area that is sufficiently dark and approximately 20 minutes are needed per individual for testing. Despite these limitations, it has advantages of being non-invasive, acceptable to target populations and is able to detect subclinical vitamin A deficiency.

Serum retinol levels are homeostatically regulated and do not drop until body stores are significantly compromised. Thus, serum retinol concentration reflects on individual's vitamin A status especially when there are limited reserves of vitamin A in the body. Serum retinol level <20 μg/dl (0.7 μmol/L) are considered deficient although the average retinol levels in well nourished populations generally exceed 30 μg/dL (1.05 μmol/L) [53]. It is now known that factors such as presence of PEM as well as infection, inflammation or trauma result in lowering of serum retinol levels due to the acute phase response to such stressful situations. However, serum retinol is the most widely used indicator for population level assessment of vitamin A deficiency as it can be analyzed by many laboratories. For accurate estimation of serum retinol, high pressure liquid chromatography (HPLC) technique is preferred.

Serum retinol-binding protein (RBP) is another biochemical indicator recommended for determining whether vitamin A deficiency is a public health problem. Serum RBP is easier to measure than serum retinol as RBP can be detected with an immunologic assay which is simpler and expensive compared to HPLC analysis of serum retinol, requires very small amount of serum (10–20 μL) which can be obtained from a finger prick and serum handling is simpler as it is more stable than retinol with respect to light and temperature. However, serum RBP is also lowered in the acute phase response, protein energy malnutrition and conditions such as liver diseases and chronic renal failure. Further, the immunologic assays cannot differentiate between RBP in serum which is complexed with retinol (holo-RBP) and that which is not (apo-RBP). Though, serum RBP correlates well with serum retinol concentration, no universally applicable cut-offs have been suggested. Serum RBP can therefore only be used for those populations for which the relationship with serum retinol concentration has been determined in a sub sample.

The indirect methods of assessment of liver stores such as Relative Dose Response (RDR), Modified Relative Dose Response (MRDR), Serum 30-day response and deuterated retinol dilution technique are a true reflection of vitamin A status than serum retinol. As mentioned earlier, when retinol is in shot supply, apo-RBP accumulates in the liver. As retinol becomes available, holo-RBP is released into the circulation. The amount of retinol released from liver is proportional to the extent of depletion of liver. The relative dose-response tests are based on this phenomenon.

In the isotope dilution technique, a dose of vitamin A labeled with stable isotope deuterium is given. A blood sample is taken after a period of three weeks which is the time allowed for equilibration with the body reserves. The extent of dilution of the labeled tracer reflects the amount of body reserves.

When the deficiency sets in, liver vitamin A levels fall over a considerable period of time before the serum retinol levels fall and much before any functional or histological changes begin to occur. Thus, these tests are useful measures of vitamin A deficiency before any clinical lesions are evident. However, the logistics of employing these techniques for vitamin A status assessment limit their use as research tests.

Breast milk retinol concentration provides information about the vitamin A status of lactating mothers as well as exclusively breast fed infants. Since vitamin A is mostly present in the fat globules of milk, the concentration of vitamin A in milk is expressed per gram of fat. The borderline of deficiency in a population is suggested to be ≤1.05 μmol/L or ≤8 μg/g milk fat. The average breast milk vitamin A concentrations range from 1.75 to 2.45 μmol/L in vitamin A sufficient populations whereas in vitamin A deficient populations the average population values are below 1.4 μmol/L [54, 55]. Analysis of retinol in casual samples of milk is difficult and is considered less reliable except under ideal laboratory conditions. However, it has been used successfully to evaluate the effect of interventions to improve the vitamin A status of lactating mothers [56].

The tentative ranking of some of these biological indicators was proposed by WHO (1996) [57] for usefulness in various activities (Table 15.4). It was recommended that biological indicators are essential for evaluating the vitamin A status of a population. They are the most specific and useful for determining risk assessment, targeting programmes and evaluating their effectiveness. Wherever, it is not feasible to obtain biological indicators, demographic or ecologic indicators may be used to define whether vitamin A deficiency is a problem of public health significance in a population. Some of the most relevant of these indirect risk indicators proposed by WHO are presented in Table 15.5. A public health problem exists when the prevalence in a population of atleast two of the biological indicators of vitamin A status is below the cut-off or when one biological indicator is supported by atleast four ecological indicators (two of which are nutrition and diet related). Though dietary intake of vitamin A does not directly indicate vitamin A status, it provides useful information on the utilization of available vitamin A rich sources in a population group. However, none of the ecological indicators are sufficient to determine if the problem of vitamin A deficiency exists in a population.

Table 15.4 Relative ranking on a population base of some biological indicators useful for various surveillance purposes [57]

Indicator	*Risk assessment*	*Targeting programmes*	*Evaluating effectiveness*
Night Blindness	+++	+++	+++
Breast milk retinol (lactating mothers and breast fed infants)	++	+++	++
Serum retinol	++	+	++
RDR / MRDR	+++	+++	+++
CIC	+	–	–

Table 15.5 Ecological indicators of areas/populations at risk of vitamin A deficiency – nutrition and diet related indicators [57]

Indicator	*Suggested Prevalence*
Breastfeeding pattern	
<6 months of age	< 50% receiving breast milk
≥6–18 months of age	< 75% receiving vitamin A containing foods in addition to breast milk, 3 times/week
Nutritional status (< -2SD from WHO/NCHS reference for children <5 years of age)	
Stunting	≥ 30%
Wasting	≥ 10 %
Low birth weight (<2500 g)	≥ 15%
Food availability	
Market	DGLV* unavailable ≥6 months/year
Household	<75% households consume vitamin A – rich foods 3 times/week
Dietary patterns	
6–71 months old children, pregnant /lactating women	< 75% consume vitamin A rich foods at least 3 times/week
Semi-quantitative/qualitative food frequency	Foods of high vitamin A content eaten <3 times/week by ≥75% vulnerable groups

* DGLV – Dark green leafy vegetable

Table 15.6 Illness related indicators in children of 6–71 months

Indicator	*Suggested prevalence*
Immunization coverage at 12–23 months of age	<50% fully immunized or <50% immunized for measles
Measles CFR	≥1%
Reported diarrhea disease rate (2 week period prevalence)	≥20%
Reported fever rates (2 week period prevalence)	≥20%
Helminthic infection rates, particularly ascaris	≥50%

The suggested prevalence are arbitrary, and are suggested only to assist in the relative ranking of population vulnerability.

The Global Vitamin A Initiative report had suggested under-five mortality rate (U5MR) as a surrogate indicator to know whether the problem of vitamin A deficiency is likely in a population and full-scale assessment is necessary [58]. Based on the existing data it was proposed that a country with U5MR >50 is very likely to have vitamin A deficiency as a public health problem that requires immediate action [59]. Countries with U5MR between 20 and 50 may have a problem until surveys prove otherwise. Though the ecological indicators are useful in suggesting the likelihood of vitamin A deficiency as a public health problem for formal assessment of vitamin A status of the population, biological indicators must be used as they directly reflect vitamin A status.

References

1. MCCOLLUM EV AND DAVIS M (1913). The necessity of certain lipins in the diet during growth. *J Biol Chem* **15**, p. 167.
2. MCCOLLUM EV AND DAVIS M (1915). The essential factors in the diet during growth. *J Biol Chem* **23**, p. 231.
3. OSBORNE TB AND MENDEL LB (1919). The vitamins in green foods. *J Biol Chem* **37**, p. 187.
4. STEENBOCK H (1919). White corn vs. yellow corn and probable relationship between the fat soluble vitamin and yellow plant pigments. *Science* **50**, p. 352.
5. MOORE T (1930). Vitamin A and carotene. VI. The conversion of â carotene to vitamin A, in vivo. *Biochem J* **24**, p. 692.
6. KARRER P, HELFENSTEIN A, WEHRLI H AND WETTSTEIN A (1930). Pflanzenfarbstoffe. XXV. uber die konstitution des lycopins and carotins. *Helv Chim Aeta* **13**, p. 1084.
7. KARRER P, MORF R AND SCHOPP K (1931). Zur kenntnis des vitamin A aus Fischtranen II. *Helv Chim Aeta* **14**, p. 1431.
8. FAO/WHO EXPERT CONSULTATION (1988). Requirements of vitamin A, iron, folate and vitamin B_{12}. Food and Nutrition Series No. 23, FAO, Rome.
9. FAO/WHO (1967). Requirements of vitamin A. thiamine, riboflavin and niacin. WHO Tech. Rep. Ser. No. 362.
10. US INSTITUTE OF MEDICINE (2001). Dietary reference intakes for vitamin A, vitamin K, arsenic, boron, chromium, copper, iodine, iron, manganese, molybdenum, nickel, silicon, vanadium and zinc. US Institute of Medicine, Food and Nutrition Board, Standing Committee on the Scientific Evaluation of Dietary Intakes. Washington: National Academic Press.
11. BOILEAU TWM, MOORE AC, ERDMAN JW JR (1999). Carotenoids and vitamin A. In: Papas AM (ed). *Antioxidant Status, Diet, Nutrition and Health.* Boca Raton: CRC Press, pp. 133–158.
12. BLOMHOFF R, GREEN MH, GREEN JB, BERG T, NORUM KR (1991). Vitamin A metabolism: new perspectives on absorption, transport and storage.

13. BLOMHOFF R (1994). Introduction: Overview of vitamin A metabolism and function. In : BLOMHOFF R (ed). *Vitamin A in Health and Disease*. New York: Marcel Dekker, pp. 1–35.
14. GREEN MH and GREEN JB (2005). Contributions of mathematical modeling to understanding whole-body vitamin A metabolism and to the assessment of vitamin A status. *Sight and Life Newsletter*, **2**, pp. 4–10.
15. WONGSIRIROJ N and BLANER WS (2007). Recent advances in vitamin A absorption and transport. *Sight and Life Magazine* **3**, pp. 32–37.
16. WEIS S, LAI K, PATEL S et al (1997). Retinyl ester hydrolysis and retinol efflux from BFC – I B adipocytes. *J Biol Chem* **272**, pp. 1459–1465.
17. KANAI M, RAZ A, GOODMAN DS (1968). Retinol-binding protein: The transport protein for vitamin A in human plasma. *J Clin Invest* **47**, pp. 2025–2044.
18. BLANER WS, HENDRIKS HF, BROUWER A et al (1985). Retinoids, retinoid-binding proteins and retinyl palmitate hydrolase distributions in different types of rat liver cells. *J Lipid Res* **26**, pp. 1241–1251.
19. SOPARNO DR, BLANER WS (1994). Retinol-binding protein. In: SPORN MB, ROBERT AB, GOODMAN DS (eds). *The Retinoids: Biology, Chemistry, and Medicine*. 2nd edition. New York: Raven Press.
20. SIVAPRASADARAO A, FINDLAY JBC (1994). The retinol-binding protein superfamily. In: BLOMHOFF R (ed). *Vitamin A in Health and Disease*. New York: Marcel Dekker, pp. 87–117.
21. BLANER WS and OLSON JA (1994). Retinol and retinoic acid metabolism. In: Sporn MB, Robert AB, Goodman DS (eds). The Retinoids: Biology, Chemistry and Medicine. 2nd edition. New York: Raven Press.
22. BUCK J, RITTER G, DANNECKER L et al (1991). Intracellular signaling by 14-hydroxy – 4, 14 – retroretinol. *Science* **254**, pp. 1654–1655.
23. DJAKOURE C, GUIBOURDEUCHE J, PORQUET D et al (1996). Vitamin A and retinoic acid stimulate within minutes cAMP release and growth hormone secretion in human pituitary cells. *J Clin Endo Metab* **81**, pp. 3123–3126.
24. FONTHAM ETH (1990). Protective dietary factors and lung cancer. *Int J Epidemiol* **19**, pp. S32–S42.
25. The Alpha – Tocopherol, Beta-carotene Cancer Prevention Study Group (1994). The effect of Vitamin E and â Carotene on the incidence of lung cancer and other cancers in male smokers. *N Eng J Med* **330**, pp. 1029–1035.
26. OMENN GS, GOODMAN GE, THORNQUIST MD et al (1996). Risk factors for lung cancer and for intervention effects in CARET, the â Carotene and Retinol Efficacy Trial. *J Natl Cancer Inst* **88**, pp. 1550–1559.
27. ORFANOS CE, BRAUN-FALCO O, FARBER EM et al (eds) (1981). Retinoids: Advances in Basic Research and Therapy. Berlin: Springer-Verlag.
28. SCHALCH W (2004). Lutein and Zeaxanthin supplementation improves visual performance: Report on a recent DSM R&D Colloquium. *Sight and Life Newsletter* **3**, pp. 4–7.
29. FORD NA AND ERDMAN JR JW (2006). Lycopene intake and prostrate cancer risk. *Sight and Life Newsletter* **1**, pp. 4–9.
30. INDIAN COUNCIL OF MEDICAL RESEARCH (1989). Nutrient Requirements and Recommended Dietary Allowances for Indians. Report of Expert Group, 1989. Proposed 2008/2009.
31. FAO/WHO EXPERT CONSULTATION (1988). Requirements of Vitamin A, iron, folate and vitamin B_{12}. Food and Nutrition Series No. 23, FAO, Rome.

32. National Research Council, Recommended Dietary Allowances (1989). 10th Edition. Washington DC: National Academy Press.
33. Panel on Dietary Reference Values (1991). Dietary reference values for food energy and nutrients for the United Kingdom. HMSO, London.
34. WHO/FAO (2004). Vitamin and mineral requirements in human nutrition. 2nd Edition, WHO, Geneva.
35. MACLAREN DS AND FRIGG M (2001). Sight and Life Manual on Vitamin A deficiency Disorders (VADD). Assessment of Vitamin A status. 2nd edition. Chapter 4, pp. 37–50.
36. WHO/USAID (1976). Vitamin A deficiency and xerophthalmia: report of joint WHO/USAID meeting. WHO Technical Report Series 590: World Health Organization, Geneva, Switzerland.
37. WHO/UNICEF/USAID/HELEN KELLER INTERNATIONAL/IVACG (1982). Control of vitamin A deficiency and xerophthalmia: report of joint WHO/UNICEF/USAID/Helen Keller International/IVACG meeting. WHO Technical Report Series 672: World Health Organization, Geneva, Switzerland.
38. SOMMER A AND DAVIDSON FR (2002). Assessment and control of vitamin A deficiency: The Annecy Accords. *J Nutr* **132**, pp. 2845S–2850S.
39. WITTPENN JR, TSENG SCG, SOMMER A (1986). Detection of early xerophthialmia by impression cytology. *Arch Ophthal* **104**, pp. 237–239.
40. TANUMIHARDJO SA, PERMAESIH D, DAHRO AM et al (1994). Comparison of vitamin A status assessment techniques in children from two Indonesian villages. *Am J Clin Nutr* **60**, pp. 136–141.
41. MAKDANI D, SOWELL AL, NELSON JD et al (1996). Comparison of methods of assessing vitamin A status in children. *J Am Coll Nutr* **15**, pp. 439–449.
42. LIETMAN TM, DHITAL SP, DEAN D (1998). Conjunctival impression cytology for vitamin A deficiency in the presence of infectious trachoma. *Br J Ophthalmol* **82**, pp. 1139–1142.
43. CONGDON NG AND WEST KP Jr (2002). Physiologic indicators of vitamin A status. *J Nutr* **132**, pp. 2889S–2894S.
44. VILLARD L AND BATES CJ (1986). Dark adaptation in pregnant and lactating Gambain women: feasibility of measurement and relation with vitamin A status. *Hum Nutr Clin Nutr* **40**C, pp. 349–357.
45. THORNTON SP (1977). A rapid test for dark adaptation. *Ann Ophthalmol* **9**, pp. 731–734.
46. FAVARO RM, DE SOUZA NV, VANNUCCHI H, DESAI ID and DE OLIVEIRA JED (1986). Evaluation of rose bengal staining test and rapid dark-adaptation test for the field assessment of vitamin A status of preschool children in Southern Brazil. *Am J Clin Nutr* **43**, pp. 940–945.
47. SOLOMONS NW, RUSSELL RM, VINTON E, GUERRERO AM and MEJIA L (1982). Application of a rapid dark adaptation test in children. *J Pediatr Gastroenterol Nutr* **1**, pp. 571–574.
48. CHRISTIAN P, WEST KP JR, KHATRY SK, KATZ J, SHRESTHA SR, PRADHAN EK, LE CLERQ SC and POKHRAL RP (1998). Night blindness of pregnancy in rural Nepal: nutritional and health risks. *Int J Epidemiol* **27**, pp. 231–237.
49. CHRISTIAN P (2002). Recommendations for indicators: Night blindness during pregnancy – A simple tool to assess vitamin A deficiency in a population. *J Nutr* **132**, pp. 2884S–2888S.

50. CONGDON N, SOMMER A, SEVERNS M, HUMPHREY J, FRIEDMAN D, CLEMENT L, WU LS AND NATADISASTRA G (1995). Pupillary and visual thresholds in young children as an index of vitamin A status. *Am J Clin Nutr* **61**, pp. 1076–1082.
51. CONGDON N, DREYFUSS M, CHRISTIAN P, NAVITSKY R, SANCHEZ A, WEST KP JR and THAPA M (2000). Dark adaptation thresholds as an indicator of vitamin A status among pregnant and lactating women in Nepal. *Am J Clin Nutr* **72**, pp. 1004–1009.
52. SANCHEZ A, CONGDON N, SOMMER A, RAHMATHULLAH L, VENKATASWAMY PG, CHANDRAVATHI PS and CLEMENT L (1997). Pupillary threshold as an index of population vitamin A status among children in India. *Am J Clin Nutr* **65**, pp. 61–66.
53. DE PEE S and DARY O (2002). Biochemical indicators of vitamin A deficiency: Serum retinol and serum retinol binding protein. *J Nutr* **132**, pp. 2895S–2901S.
54. World Health Organization (1985). The quantity and quality of breast milk. Geneva.
55. NEWMAN V (1992). Vitamin A and breastfeeding: a comparison of data from developed and developing countries. Wellstrart International, San Diego, CA.
56. RICE AL, STOLTZFUS RJ, DE FRANCISCO A et al (2000). Evaluation of serum retinol, the modified relative–dose response ratio and breastmilk vitamin A as indicators of response to postpartum maternal vitamin A supplementation. *Am J Clin Nutr* **71**, pp. 799–806.
57. WHO (1996). Indicators for assessing vitamin A deficiency and their application in monitoring and evaluating intervention programmes. WHO, Geneva.
58. Vitamin A Global Initiative (1998). A strategy for acceleration of progress in combating vitamin A deficiency: consensus of an informal technical consultation, 18–19 December 1997. UNICEF, New York.
59. SCHULTINK W (2002). Use of under-five mortality rate as an indictor for vitamin A deficiency in a population. *J Nutr* **132**, pp. 2881S–2883S.

16

Vitamin A deficiency: prevention and control

Sheila C. Vir

Sheila C Vir, MSc, PhD, is a senior nutrition consultant and Director of Public Health Nutrition and Development Centre, New Delhi. Following MSc (Food and Nutrition) from University of Delhi, Dr Vir was awarded PhD by the Queen's University of Belfast, United Kingdom. Dr. Vir, a past secretary of the Nutrition Society of India, is a recipient of the fellowship of the Department of Health and Social Services, UK, and Commonwealth Van den Bergh Nutrition Award. Dr Vir worked briefly with the Aga Khan Foundation (India) and later with UNICEF. As a Nutrition Programme Officer with UNICEF for twenty years, Dr. Vir provided strategic and technical leadership for policy formulation and implementation of nutrition programmes in India.

16.1 Vitamin A – an essential micronutrient

Vitamin A is essential for regulating a number of key biological processes in the body and contributes to the normal functioning of the visual system, growth and development, maintenance of epithelial cellular integrity, immune function, and reproduction [1]. Vitamin A is known to be involved in maintaining immuno-competence by helping to maintain the lymphocyte pool and playing a role in T-cell-mediated responses [2, 3]. Neither humans nor animals can synthesize or survive without vitamin A. It is therefore vital that the micronutrient vitamin A is provided in the diet in sufficient amounts to meet all the physiological needs. Key functions of vitamin A are summarized in Table 16.1.

Table 16.1 Functions of vitamin A [4]

Vision	Photopic and colour, scotopic
Cellular differentiation and morphogenesis	Gene, transcription
Immune response	Non-specific, cell-mediated
Haemopoiesis	Iron metabolism
Growth	Skeletal
Fertility	Male and female

16.2 Consequences of vitamin A deficiency

Dietary vitamin A is consumed from animal sources or fortified food items as preformed retinyl esters or from plant sources as provitamin A carotenoids. Vitamin A and its precursor carotenoids are fat-soluble compounds.

Approximately, 5–10 g of fat in a meal is sufficient to ensure absorption of vitamin A and its precursor [5, 6]. Vitamin A (retinol) being fat soluble is stored in body organs when intake is in excess of physiological need – 90% of stored vitamin A is in liver [1]. From liver, vitamin A is released into circulation in association with retinol binding protein (RBP) and transthyretin, a protein complex that transfers vitamin A to tissues sites and becomes available for use by cells throughout the body, including those of the eye.

Liver stores form an important buffer against variations in the intake of vitamin A and its precursors. When intake surpasses physiological requirements, the excess vitamin A is stored and liver reserves increase. On the other hand, when dietary vitamin A intake is less compared to body requirements, liver stores are drained to maintain serum retinol at the normal level of above 0.7 μmol/l [6, 7]. Because of prolonged periods of low intake of vitamin A, and its usage by tissues or breastfeed, liver stores get depleted of the vitamin. With such depletion, the vitamin is actively recycled through the liver and among specific tissues and results in partially adapting to the diminishing availability. This adaptation and recycling mechanism maintain relatively constant blood levels until body stores become depleted below a critical point. The level of depletion at which physiological functions begin to be impaired is not entirely clear [1].

The time required for vitamin A deficiency to precipitate depends on the amount of vitamin A (or precursor) ingested, the extent of pre-existing liver stores, and the rate at which vitamin A is being utilized by the body. A child who routinely consumes marginal or poor intake of vitamin A will have very limited stores. In such children, any further reduction in intake of vitamin A, either as a result of a change in diet or because of impaired absorption (as in gastroenteritis), or a sudden increase in metabolic demand (febrile state notably measles or growth spurt) will cause rapid use of limited reserves of vitamin A resulting in depletion of the vitamin. Additionally, reduced synthesis of retinol binding proteins (RBP) in protein-deficient or severely malnourished children impairs vitamin A utilization of the available stored vitamin A, even when liver stores are high [7].

In vitamin A deficiency, keratin-producing cells replace mucus-secreting cells in many epithelial tissues of the body. The integrity of epithelial barriers and the immune system are compromised before the visual system is impaired. This is the basis of the pathological process termed xerosis that leads to the drying of the conjunctiva and cornea of the eye followed by destruction of the cornea and blindness. As indicated in Fig. 16.1, with a decline in vitamin A status, systemic consequences of vitamin A deficiency (VAD), including increased mortality, begin to occur even before the appearance of appreciable rates of clinical xerophthalmia [6].

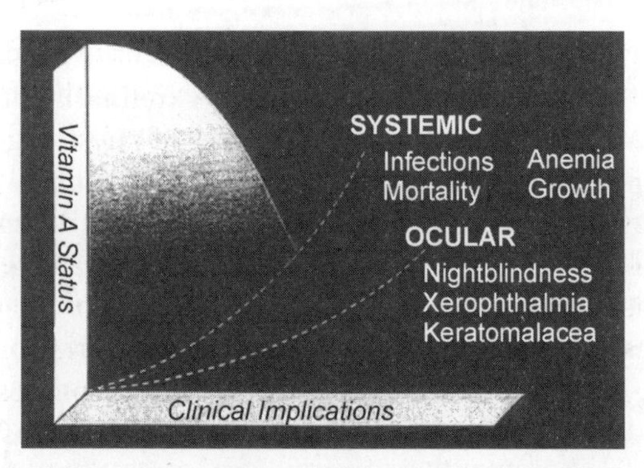

16.1 Vitamin A status and clinical implications [6]

Public health consequences that can be attributed to vitamin A deficiency are defined as vitamin A deficiency disorders or VAD disorders (VADD). The term VAD disorders was introduced in 2002 at the XX International Vitamin A Consultative Group (IVACG) meeting and is defined as health or physiological consequences attributable to VAD, whether clinically evident (e.g., xerophthalmia, anemia, growth retardation, increased infectious morbidity and mortality) or not (e.g., impaired iron mobilization, disturbed cellular differentiation and depressed immune response) [6]. The mortality risks increases from the stage when vitamin A is depleted in tissues and plasma but there is no clinical sign of deficiency. The spectrum of vitamin A deficiency disorders (VADD) has been diagrammatically presented as in Fig. 16.2 [8]. In children, vitamin A deficiency causes xerophthalmia and results in blindness. Xerophthalmia is the general term applied to all ocular manifestations of impaired vitamin A metabolism, from night blindness through complete corneal distribution. VADD therefore covers what was previously referred to as "subclinical manifestations".

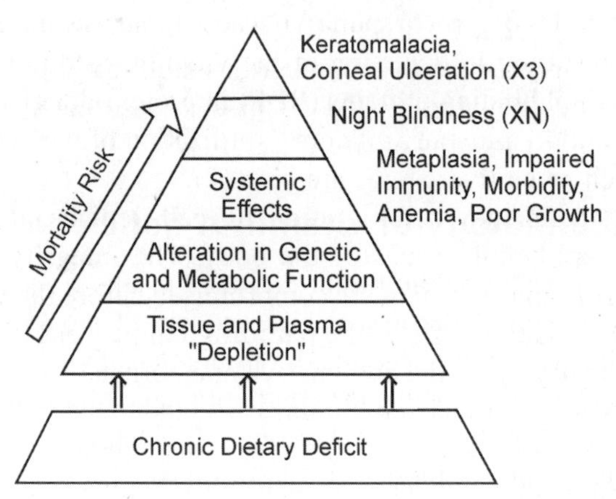

16.2 Spectrum of vitamin A deficiency disorders [8]

Xerophthalmia remains the most specific and readily recognized clinical manifestation of vitamin A deficiency, and has served as the definitive criterion for assessing vitamin A status. Ocular manifestations are the most easily identifiable signs of an overt vitamin A deficiency. Table 16.2 presents the xerophthalmia classification [8]. The stage XIB (Bitot's spot) is not always responsive to improvement in vitamin A status. However, up to the stage of corneal xerosis (X2) prompt treatment with large doses of vitamin A can result in full restoration of sight without any residual impairment [4]. Ulceration/ keratomalacia marks progression of the disease. Ulceration which involves less than one-third of the corneal surface (X3A) generally spares the central pupillary zone, and prompt therapy ordinarily preserves useful vision. More widespread involvement (X3B), usually results in perforation, and loss of eye globe and prompt therapy may still save the other eye and the child's life.

Table 16.2 Xerophthalmia classification [8]

XN	Night blindness
X1A	Conjunctival xerosis
X1B	Bitot's spot
X2	Corneal xerosis
X3A	Corneal ulceration / keratomalacia (involving less than one third of the corneal area)
X3B	Corneal ulceration / keratomalacia (involving one third or more of the corneal area)
XS	Corneal scar (from X3)
XF	Xerophthalmic fundus

Vitamin A deficiency in children also limits growth, weakens innate and acquires host defenses, exacerbates infection and increases the risk of death [9]. The health consequences of vitamin A deficiency in women of reproductive age contributes to increase in morbidity and mortality during pregnancy and early post-partum. Vitamin deficient night-blind women in pregnancy are associated with higher risks of severe anemia, wasting malnutrition, and reproductive and infectious morbidity [10]. Severe VAD during pregnancy or maternal VAD is also associated with increase in mortality in the first months of life [9].

16.3 Epidemiology of vitamin A deficiency

Vitamin A deficiency, a public health problem, results from a chronic low dietary intake of vitamin A due to social and economic factors which adversely influence regular availability, access and consumption of vitamin A rich foods. Table 16.3 presents the recommended nutrient intake of vitamin A.

In addition to low dietary intake, other factors which contribute to and exacerbate VAD are increased requirements for vitamin A during infections or malabsorption due to the absence of fat in the diet [12].

The type and amount of vitamin and pro-vitamin ingested, absorbed, transported, stored and metabolized determines the extent of inadequacy of vitamin A [7]. Unrelated disease states can also sometimes dramatically alter each of these factors and, in turn, the individual's vitamin A balance. For example, gastroenteritis affects both the types and amount of food given and the child's appetite while the shortened transit time in this diseased situation further decreases absorption of any vitamin A that is

Table 16.3 Dietary vitamin A reference intakes for children from birth to 6 years of age[(a)]

	Age groups < *1 year* *µg*	*1–3 years* *(µg)*	*4–6 years* *(µg)*
FAO			
Basal requirement	180	200	200
Safe intake	350	400	400
Estimated average requirement (EAR)[(b)]	–	210	275
RDA[(c)]	–	300	400

[(a)] Basal requirement is defined as the minimum daily intake of vitamin A needed to prevent the appearance of clinical signs of vitamin A deficiency (xerophthalmia) and to permit normal growth. Safe intake is defined as the amount of vitamin A needed to meet basal needs and other vitamin A dependent functions and maintain a minimally adequate liver vitamin A store of 20 µg/g for the median person plus 2 sd; thus safe intake meets needs for 97–98% of all healthy people.

[(b)] EAR is defined as the amount of vitamin A needed to meet basal needs and other vitamin A dependent functions and maintain a minimally adequate liver vitamin A store of 20 µg/g in half of all healthy people.

[(c)] RDA is defined as the EAR + 2 sd; thus, the RDA meets the needs for 97–98% of all healthy people.

ingested. If a child is already protein-deficient, transport and storage could decrease while fever could result in increasing the metabolic needs. The key underlying epidemiological traits that tend to characterize most situations where vitamin A deficiency occurs as a public health problem are as follows [1, 7].

16.3.1 Ecological, social and economic factors

Consumption of vitamin A and duration of consumption is influenced by the availability of foods rich in vitamin A activity that are grown and available in specific seasons at a reasonable cost. Fruits and vegetables are sources of vitamin A which are in the form of provitamin A carotenoids and represent the major source dietary vitamin A in the developing world, among which β-carotene is the most bioavailable. Food sources of provitamin A carotenoids include dark green leafy vegetables such as spinach and amaranth, yellow and deeply coloured orange vegetables and fruits such as carrot, ripe mango, papaya, yellow sweet potato, pumpkin, chillies. These need to be converted into retinol before they can provide protection from vitamin A deficiency. Carotene needs dietary fat or oil to be absorbed. On the other hand, vitamin A from animal foods such as milk, cheese, yogurt, butter, eggs, liver and small fishes are rich sources of retinol and can be directly used by the body.

A number of process steps, dependent on normal physiological functions, convert provitamin A forms to retinol. Absorption and bioconversion of dietary β-carotene and other provitamin A carotenoids into retinol are a part of a complex process which is influenced not only by the amount of carotenoid consumed in a meal but a number of factors – these factors are incorporated into the mnemonic SLAMENGHI: species of carotenoid, molecular linkage, amount of carotene consumed in a meal, matrix in which carotenoid is incorporated, effectors of absorption and bioconversion, nutrient status of the host, genetic factors, host related factors and interaction between the other factors [13–15]. Therefore in addition to availability of fruits and vegetables, the actual conversion to retinol is critical. In the past, the molar retinol equivalency of dietary β-carotene and other pro-vitamin A carotenoids was assumed to be 6:1 and 12:1, respectively [15]. The food composition and database in meals and food supplies was accordingly calculated. Further evidence from research findings resulted in increasing the ratios to 12:1 for dietary β-carotene and 24:1 for other pro-vitamin A carotenoids [16, 17]. It has been estimated that in the undernourished populations, carotenoid bio-conversion may be even less efficient from mixture of vegetables and fruits and the rate of conversion may be very poor with a high conversion ratio of about 21:1. [15]. The implications of such poor ratio of conversion imply a significant increase in the requirements of fruits and vegetables to meet the dietary vitamin A requirement of population who are dependent on these sources.

Vegetables and fruits are often seasonal and require abundant water supplies and/or moderate temperature to grow. In regions and countries, with long periods of water shortage and relatively constant hot temperatures, regular food sources of vitamin A are often inadequate resulting in higher possibility of having high prevalence of vitamin A deficiency.

16.3.2 Child feeding practices

Child feeding practices play an important role in the epidemiology of vitamin A deficiency. Children of both well-nourished and poorly nourished populations are born with limited hepatic store of vitamin A at birth. Liver stores at birth are sufficient to supply the infant's vitamin A requirements for only a few days, even when mother is well nourished during pregnancy [18]. Breast milk provides retinol in a readily absorbable form. Clinical symptoms of vitamin A deficiency rarely occur in breastfed infants during the first year of life in populations with endemic vitamin A deficiency [9]. It is well-documented that breast milk affords protection against VAD in infants who are predominantly breastfed even in situations when breast milk vitamin A content is low. The concentration of vitamin A in breast milk is influenced by maternal vitamin A intake and status as well as the fat content and stage of lactation [18]. Colostrum secreted in the first 4–6 days post-partum and transitional milk from about 7–21 days of lactation contain much higher concentration of vitamin A than mature breast milk. The practice of discarding of colostrum in some developing countries therefore deprives the newborns of concentrated source of vitamin A. In situations, when a mother is deficient in vitamin A or the child is bottle fed or the child is given skimmed milk or whole milk diluted with water, deficiency of vitamin A often results since the body stores of vitamin A in infant gets depleted resulting in subclinical vitamin A deficiency and consequent health risks.

Discontinuation of breast milk or introduction of complementary feed at six months with poor content of vitamin A as well as reduction in breast milk fed deteriorate vitamin A status of young children. Low routine consumption of milk, egg, yellow fruits and vegetables, dark green leaves or meat/fish in the first 12 months of complementary feeding have been reported to be three times more likely to be xerophthalmic than matched control given these foods [19].

The problem of subclinical depletion therefore has been observed to increase significantly between 6 months and 3 years of age when a child is introduced to complementary food and the breast milk quantity gradually continues to diminish. Unless special effort is made, family diet often do not contain adequate vitamin A to meet the demands of growing child and for adequately replacing the amount that was provided by breast milk in early part of infancy. The situation is further worsened by the fact that the diet of young children is often small in quantity and frequently contains less fat resulting in dietary fat being not available for the absorption of vegetable source of provitamin A. Additionally, vitamin A status of children in developing countries is often adversely influenced by the poor vitamin A status of mother who produces breast milk low in vitamin A.

16.3.3 Infection and worm infestation

Infants in developing countries are often exposed to conditions of frequent infections or disease and increased catabolism which deteriorate vitamin

A status. In young children, the frequency, duration and severity of infections contribute directly or indirectly to vulnerability to vitamin A deficiency. Infection induces vitamin A deficiency through a variety of ways depending on the vitamin A status of the host at onset, cause, duration and severity of infection. Infections not only lessen appetite but adversely influence absorption, conservation and utilization of vitamin A. Frequent acute bacterial infections damage mucosal surface required for absorption. Infectious illness, such as diarrhoea, measles or severe respiratory infections result in increased demands and urinary losses of vitamin A. Serum retinol levels therefore may reduce as a result of infection resulting in malabsorption due to diarrhoea or intestinal pathogens, impaired release or accelerated depletion of hepatic retinol reserves, increased retinol utilization by target tissues or increased urinary losses. Lowered levels of retinol or hyporetinolemia may adversely affect immune competence, which could exacerbate or predispose children to infection [20].

In situations of disease, vitamin A deficiency tends to precipitate significantly following the peak prevalence of diarrhoeal and respiratory diseases. Measles is reported to severely deplete vitamin A stores, leaving a child more vulnerable to disease such as pneumonia, diarrhoea and xerophthalmia. Frequency of diarrhoeal and respiratory infections is therefore associated with vulnerability to vitamin A deficiency [21]. Measles is estimated to precipitate as much as 25–50% of cases of blinding xerophthalmia in Asia and Africa [7]. Low availability of vitamin A from milk combined with higher requirement due to chronic infection in infants contributes to lowering liver stores, especially failing to accumulate beyond early infancy [11].

Protein energy malnutrition is an important contributory cause of VAD since it interferes with storage, transport and utilization of vitamin A [7].

Intestinal worms, soil transmitted helminthes (STHs), i.e. round worm, hook worm and whipworm in pre-school children directly compete for vitamin A intake and contribute to VAD [22]. It is estimated that 230 million children of 0–4 years globally are infected with STHs. Roundworms are the most prevalent STH reported in preschool children and cause significant vitamin A malabsorption [23]. Roundworms live in the gut and need vitamin A to grow and this results in competition for the nutrient resulting in VAD. In Nepal where prevalence of both VAD and STH is high, children with xerophthalmia are reported to have three times the load of roundworm infection compared to uninfected control group [24].

16.3.4 Age

VAD can occur in individuals of any age. However, it is a disabling and a potentially fatal public health problem for preschool children. Clinical symptoms of vitamin A deficiency rarely occur in predominantly breastfed infants during the first year of life even in populations with endemic vitamin A deficiency [9]. VAD affects children of the preschool age group because of low intake of vitamin A and great susceptibility to infections as well as due to an increased requirement for the micronutrient vitamin A to support the rapid growth during this period. VAD related blindness is most prevalent in children under 3 years of age and is associated with Protein energy malnutrition or PEM [1].

The prevalence of mild xerophthalmia (XN, XIB) has been found to increase with age through the fifth year of life and possibly beyond, since children in high risk population continue to be exposed to diet lacking vitamin A or pro-vitamin A rich food items. No estimates for school aged children exist. In older children of school age, the prevalence of mild xerophthalmia, notably Bitot's spots, may be highest, although this is considered to possibly be a reflection of past rather than current vitamin A status [1].

16.3.5 Sex

There is no consistent, clear indication in humans of a sex differential in vitamin A requirements during childhood [1]. In most societies or cultures, the risk of severe blinding xerophthalmia (corneal ulceration and keratomalacia) is equal in both sexes; moreover, improvement in vitamin A status generally reduces mortality equally in both sexes.

16.3.6 Season

In many areas of the world sources of vitamin A (and of food in general) are in short supply during the hot and dry season. During such specific seasons, high rate of infections such as measles and diarrhoea are reported. Both these factors are important seasonal aspects influencing vitamin A status.

16.3.7 Cluster

Vitamin A deficiency and xerophthalmia tend to cluster within countries and within specific families and neighborhoods possibly since the dietary and health practices responsible for vitamin A deficiency are shared by most members of the same community [1, 7]. Clustering of risks appears to intensify within smaller disadvantaged groupings. Survey findings from Africa, South and South-East Asia reveal a consistent 1.5- to 2.0-fold risk of xerophthalmia among children in villages where other children have the condition [25, 26]. There is a 7-

to 13-fold higher risk of xerophthalmia in families where siblings have clinical signs of deficiency compared to children of those families where siblings present with no such signs of VAD [25]. The occurrence of clinical vitamin A deficiency tends to cluster rather than being evenly distributed and such clustering of vitamin A deficiency cases primarily applies to clinical eye signs. Such clustering is also a reflection of convergence of a number of risk factors that lead to depletion of vitamin A stores in the surrounding child population and of these a few individuals who are exposed to additional causal factors possibly develop clinical deficiency of vitamin A. These factors responsible for clustering are important with reference to prioritizing families and communities for implementing treatment and preventive actions.

16.4 Vitamin A deficiency (VAD) – a public health problem

Table 16.4 presents details of the prevalence criteria indicating VAD to be a public health problem within a defined population. Vitamin A status of preschool children is particularly crucial and ideally childhood prevalence criteria are recommended to be restricted to children 2–5 years of age. There has been a review and modifications suggested in the level of cut-off presented earlier [6, 27]. The revised proposed criterion of IVACG 2001 includes a clinical prevalence criterion of the prevalence of night blindness during pregnancy in the past three years. This information has been observed to be simple and practical to collect [6, 28].

Table 16.4 Prevalence criteria indicating VAD within a defined population [6]

Criteria	Prevalence (%)
Clinical	
Children 2–5 years old	
Night blindness (XN)	>1.0
Bitot's spots (X1B)	>0.5
Corneal xerosis (X2)	
and corneal ulcers (X3)	>0.01
Corneal scars (XS)	>0.05
Women of childbearing age	
XN during most recent pregnancy	>5.0
Biochemical	
Serum retinol <0.70 μmol/L (20 μg/dL)	>15

The status of VAD can be assessed by two biochemical measure such as serum retinol concentrations and serum retinol binding protein or RBP [29]. Serum retinol concentration of <20 μg/dL (0.70 μmol/L) is an indicator of subclinical VAD and requires high precision analysis by high performance liquid chromatography (HPLC). Serum retinol concentration reflects an individual's vitamin A status, particularly when reserves of vitamin A are limited. However, the limitation of the indicator serum retinol level is that it is affected by infection and protein energy malnutrition. Prevalence of deficiency, assessed by serum retinol concentration below the conventional cut-off of 0.70 μmol/L, of more than 15% among preschool children 6–71 months of age is considered to represent a public health problem [6].

Table 16.5 Prevalence of VAD in children ≥1 year of age of serum values ≤0.70 μmol/L [1]

Level of public health problem	*Prevalence*
Mild	≥2 to <10%
Moderate	≥10 to <20%
Severe	≥20%

HPLC is considered the only laboratory technique that is reliable for routine measurement of serum retinol. When HPLC measurements are not available, assessment of VAD is recommended to be based on clinical criteria. The clinical signs of xerophthalmia (Greek term xeros meaning "drying" and ophthalmia meaning "of the eye") as well as the early stages of the condition such as squamous metaplasia can be measured by impression cytology or impaired dark adaptation that precedes complaints of night blindness (poor vision at dusk). XN is often difficult to detect in younger children while Bitot's spot (X1B) in older children are often remnants of earlier deficiency. In assessing the presence or absence of XN in a child, it is recommended to use one or more locally appropriate terms (often translated as chicken eyes or chicken blindness). In northern India and Nepal, the term commonly used is *rathondi* meaning *blindness of night* while in South East Asia, terms used are *matang manak, kurap, harapan,* etc.

In well-nourished populations, history of night blindness during pregnancy is consistently reported to be below 3%. As indicated in Table 16.4, a minimal prevalence of 5% XN in these women is the cut-off value recommended for labelling presence of VAD in the population [28].

Maternal night blindness or a woman's history of experiencing night blindness (XN) at some point during last live-birth pregnancy is a good indicator of VAD in the wider population. As indicated in Table 16.6, in poor rural regions, where xerophthalmia in children constitutes a public health problem, night blindness in women during pregnancy is also commonly reported [28]. It is therefore recommended to study the prevalence of night blindness in women of reproductive age who have had a live birth in the past three years [29]. This indicator is proposed to be even more accurate than questioning parents about XN in their preschool-age children [6].

Table 16.6 Prevalence estimates of xerophthalmia in preschool children and maternal night blindness during pregnancy by country

Country	*Xerophthalmia in children (%)*	*Blindness during pregnancy (%)*
Nepal[(a)]	3[30]	16.2[31]
India	1.1[32]	12.1[32]
Philippines	0.4–0.7[33]	8.6[34]
Zambia	6.2[35]	11.6[35]

[(a)] pre-national vitamin A program

The clinical and biochemical indicators for assessing VAD presented in Table 16.4 are subject to limitations. WHO therefore recommends that at least two indicators be used for assessing the vitamin A status of a population [1, 27]. In the absence of direct clinical and biochemical criteria to assess VAD, it is proposed that under-5-year mortality rate (U5MR) be used as a "surrogate" indicator for VAD in a population. Population of countries with high U5MR invariably has been proven to have significant VAD [30–36]. Any country or localized population with U5MR >50 is likely to have vitamin A problem unless proven otherwise and therefore this indicator is used for screening VAD as a public health problem at the national level and for ensuring actions are taken immediately for addressing vitamin A deficiency.

16.5 Public health significance of vitamin A deficiency disorders

Vitamin A deficiency is a major public health nutrition problem in the developing world. It is among the "top ten" health problems contributing to the global burden of disease and childhood mortality [31–36].

In 1995, VAD was reported to be a public health problem in 78 developing countries [1], and VAD was reported to be widespread in peri-equatorial regions of the world. In 2000, VAD was considered to be a public health problem in 118 countries [32–37]. The extent and severity of VAD is most widespread across large areas of south and south-east Asia and Sahelian and sub-Saharan Africa. The highest prevalence of clinical VAD occurs in Africa, while south East Asia has the highest number of children affected.

In early 1990s, it was estimated that VAD causes blindness in 250,000–500,000 children [33–38] and was a major factor contributing to 1–3 million child deaths [34–39]. A region wise global data on prevalence of VAD (Table 16.7), reported in 2002, estimates that 127.2 million preschool children are vitamin A deficient and of these about 4.4 million children under the age of five are affected by clinical xerophthalmia [8]. This global estimate excludes a number of countries who were unable to assess the true level of deficiency due to technical and financial constraints.

Table 16.7 Global prevalence of preschool child vitamin A deficiency and xerophthalmia, with numbers of cases, by region [8]

Region	*Population <5 years (× 10³)*	*Vitamin A deficient[(a)]*		*Xeropthalmia*	
		%	*No (× 10³)*	*%*	*No (× 10³)*
Africa	103,934	32.1	33,406	1.53	1,593
Eastern Mediterranean	59,818	21.2	12,664	0.85	510
South/Southeast Asia	169,009	33.0	55,812	1.20	2,026
Western Pacific	122,006	14.0	17,128	0.18	220
Region of the Americas	47,575	17.3	8,218	0.16	75
Total	502,494	25.3	127,273	0.88	4,424

[(a)] Defined by serum retinol <0.70 μmol/L or, occasionally, abnormal conjunctival impression cytology

As presented in Table 16.7, 33.0% of VAD children live in South and South East Asia, 32.1% in Africa and 21.2% in eastern Mediterranean region. Table 16.8 indicates that the largest number of vitamin A deficient children are estimated to live in India (35.3 million) followed by Indonesia (12.6 million) and China (11.4 million). The geographical distribution roughly matches with ecological indices of poverty and undernutrition. As is evident from the data, a far greater numbers of children show no external signs of VAD, but live with dangerously low vitamin A stores, which indicate that the child population is vulnerable to infection and reduced immunity to fight

Table 16.8 Prevalence of preschool child vitamin A deficiency and xerophthalmia, with numbers of cases, in selected countries of the six regions [8]

Region	*Population <5 years (× 10³)*	*Vitamin A deficient[(a)]*		*Xeropthalmia*	
		%	*No (× 10³)*	*%*	*No (× 10³)*
Africa					
Ethiopia	11,032	4,462	61.2	40.6	6,752
Kenya	1,812	4.80	2.00	530	89
Eastern Mediterranean					
Pakistan	23,793	24.0	5,710	0.24	57
South/Southeast Asia					
Bangladesh	15,120	30.8	4,649	0.62	94
India	114,976	30.8	35,355	1.56	1790
Indonesia	22,006	57.5	12,653	0.34	75
Western Pacific					
China	97,793	11.7	11, 442	0.17	170
Philippines	9,800	38.0	3,724	0.07	7
Other countries	5,959	16.2	964	0.44	26
Region of the Americas					
Brazil	15,993	13.7	2,187	0.13	20
Gautemala	1,816	13.4	244	0.00	0
European Region					
Macedonia	152	29.5	45	0	0

[(a)] Defined by serum retinol < 0.70 μmol/L or, occasionally, abnormal conjunctival impression cytology.

common childhood diseases. These children have a markedly increased risk of illness and death, particularly from measles and diarrhoea. VAD is estimated to be an underlying cause of at least 650,000 early childhood deaths due to diarrhoea, measles, malaria and other infections each year [8].

Besides children, there is increasing evidence that VAD is a problem among women in the reproductive age group. Night blindness is common among women in the latter half of pregnancy, affecting 10–20% of pregnant women in South and Southeast Asia. The condition appears to be 25 times more prevalent in pregnant women than in preschool children [10]. It has been estimated that nearly 20 million pregnant women in the developing world have low vitamin status and almost 6.2 million are clinically night blind [8].

In the past VAD was viewed as a public health concern primarily for addressing preventable blindness, and therefore earlier in many countries actions for improving vitamin A status was a part of blindness prevention programme. Since 1982, research findings have increasingly stressed on the significance of vitamin A in the broader context of child health and survival. These were based on the results of epidemiological investigations and community-based studies launched in late 1970s into the role of VAD in child mortality. One of the earliest study was from Indonesian where children with mild xerophthalmia, but no other obvious nutrition stress, were reported to be 2–3 times more likely to develop respiratory infections or diarrhoea and more likely to die than children without eye signs [41, 42]. Between the period 1986 and 1993, eight population-based intervention trials in South-East Asia, South Asia and Africa further supported this finding. It was found that vitamin A supplementation, achieved by periodic high potency dosing (200,000 IU for over 12 months children and lower dose IU for 6–12 months), weekly low potency dosing (15,000 IU) or food fortification could reduce child mortality by 6–54% [43–51].

Meta-analyses of the findings of the study concluded that in areas where vitamin A deficiency is prevalent, child mortality is reduced by 23–34% after vitamin A intervention [52–55]. The pooled estimate is 23% reduction in the risk of all cause mortality in children 6–59 months with vitamin A supplements [53]. The impact of vitamin A on lowering case fatality by measles was estimated to be about 50% [8], while the risk of fatality from diarrhoea and dysentery was lower at about 40%. A recent analysis has estimated about 50% reduction in case fatality from diarrhoea and measles among vitamin A recipients [56]. The impact of vitamin A supplementation on risk of mortality from respiratory infections, unrelated to measles, is reported to have no significant influence [57, 58]. The effect of vitamin A on infant and child morbidity is not conclusive. It has, however, been indicated that vitamin A possibly benefits infant survival in undernourished populations depending on the age of administering the dose, supplementation method used, nutritional status and dominant disease pattern [51]. Three reported trials of vitamin A supplementation in the neo-natal period in low-income countries indicates that neonatal vitamin A supplementation is associated with reduced mortality. A pooled analysis of all studies from South Asia indicates 21% reduction in mortality in babies younger than 6 months [37]. Similarly, in chronically undernourished population, vitamin A deficiency is considered to pose a health risk to women during pregnancy and lactation. VAD during pregnancy is associated with anemia, wasting, undernutrition and other morbid symptoms [29, 59, 60].

The risk groups are therefore children from age of six months to six years, pregnant and lactating women while high priority risk groups are children with xerophthalmia, measles, diarrhoea, severe protein–energy malnutrition, children with acute or prolonged diarrhoea and with acute lower respiratory infection.

16.6 International focus on prevention of vitamin A deficiency

A number of events since 1970 drew attention to the problem of vitamin A deficiency [61]. Recognizing the gravity of the situation of xerophthalmia, the 25th World Health Assembly urged intensification of activities in 1972 to prevent needless loss of sight. Xerophthalmia was recognised as one of the three important causes of preventable blindness [62]. This was followed by a WHO meeting at Hyderabad, India and World Food Conference on the subject [61], which resulted in recommendations and commitment of the participating governments to reduce the problem of vitamin A deficiency. From 1974 to 1990, a committed scientific community worked extensively to remove existing gaps in knowledge related to addressing vitamin A deficiency through public health interventions [2, 61].

In 1980s, the focus was on VAD and its serious impact on xerophthalmia. It was reported that at least 5 million children in Asia develop xerophthalmia and every year 250,000 of them go blind [63]. In 1984, the emerging evidence of protective role of vitamin A in child health and survival was followed by the resolution of the 37th World Assembly (WHA 37.18) for prevention and control of vitamin A deficiency and xerophthalmia. The wording of this resolution is of historical significance since in the political arena vitamin A deficiency was for the first time recognised to result in health consequences beyond xerophthalmia and blindness [61]. The overall strategy proposed included long-, medium- and short-term measures. New impetus for reduction of VAD was provided by results of intervention trials which had indicated the relationship of vitamin A status with child survival [53]. The remarkable impact of vitamin A supplement on child mortality increased the significance of prevention of vitamin A deficiency at the World Summit for Children in 1990 and at the follow-up International Conference of Nutrition in 1992. The significance of vitamin A was recognised in 1992 by the Fifty-fifth World Health Assemblies which directed WHO to intensify its efforts to control the impact of vitamin A deficiency on child health, blindness and survival since the problem of vitamin A deficiency was estimated to be responsible for as many as one out of every four child deaths in regions and countries.

The experiences from different countries proved that long-term goal of VAD prevention programme should be to ensure adequate dietary intake of vitamin A and elimination of all form of vitamin A deficiency in children between six months to five years who are at the greatest risk of deficiency. The most cost-effective child health and child survival strategies for vitamin A elimination included a combination of strategies – comprising breast feeding, dietary diversification, food fortification and vitamin A supplementation.

WHO-UNICEF established a "Mid Decade Goal" to be achieved by the end of 1995: to ensure that at least 80% of all children under 24 months living in areas with inadequate vitamin A received adequate vitamin A through a combination of breastfeeding, dietary improvement, fortification and supplementation. As part of the global call to action, the UN Special Session on Children in 2002 set as one of its goals the elimination of vitamin A deficiency and its consequences by the year 2010 [64]. Universal supplementation of children 6–59 months with vitamin A is recommended to be included in the health package in all countries where U5MR exceeds was 70 deaths per 1,000 live births, an internationally accepted proxy indicating a high risk of deficiency among children under five [65].

16.7 Intervention strategies for preventing vitamin A deficiency disorders (VADD)

Vitamin A supplementation and vitamin A fortification have been recognised to have robust evidence to improve child nutritional status and recommended to be included in the package of nutrition interventions in countries with high burden of undernutrition [37]. With emerging information, it is evident that elimination of VAD as a public health problem is one of the major interventions for improved child survival.

To successfully combat VAD, WHO recommends vitamin A supplement intervention as a short-term measure and establishment of proper infant feeding practices as a long-term sustainable solution [1]. The strategy to achieve the goal of elimination of VAD is to ensure that young children living in areas where the intake of vitamin A is inadequate receive the vitamin through a combination of breastfeeding, dietary improvement, food fortification, and supplementation.

16.7.1 Promotion of breastfeeding

Promotion of breastfeeding is an integral component of a comprehensive strategy to combat VAD. Colostrum and early breast milk are concentrated sources of vitamin A and for the first 6–12 months infants depend on readily absorbable vitamin A provided in breast milk. Mothers whose vitamin A intake is adequate produces breast milk with vitamin A concentration that meets their infants' needs for at least the first six months of life [66]. Breast milk is a critical dietary source of vitamin A and therefore is important in the protection of xerophthalmia in children. Mature breast milk of healthy women contains 600–700 μg of vitamin A per litre [18]. Over 90% of vitamin A content is derived from highly bioavailable esters. A breastfed infant of a vitamin A adequate mother, with an intake of about 725 ml milk per day, consumes about 435–500 μg dietary vitamin A [67]. In developing countries with high prevalence of malnutrition, vitamin A concentration in milk has often been reported to be half of that reported from well-nourished population of women [67]. In well-nourished societies, therefore, body vitamin A stores of children continue to improve with age while in situations where mother is deficient in vitamin A, the amount provided through breast milk is reduced. However, despite reduction in concentration of vitamin A in developing countries, breast milk provides clinically protective amounts to infants especially when exclusively breastfed for the first 6 months. The significance of breast milk in protecting infants from xerophthalmia is evident from studies in situations of early cessation of breastfeeding.

The concentration of vitamin A in milk is influenced by the vitamin A status of the mother, stage of lactation and fat content of milk [68]. The average vitamin A concentration in mature breast milk of women in developing countries is much lower—about 300 μg/L and colostrum concentration of vitamin A is 50 μg/dL [11]. In well-nourished women, the concentration of vitamin A tends to decrease in the first month and remains relatively stable during the remaining period of lactation in well-nourished women [69]. In case of women in developing countries with marginal intakes of vitamin A, milk vitamin A concentration shows a progressive decrease with the lowest levels at three months [70, 71].

The extent to which infants are estimated to meet their vitamin A requirements from breast milk is presented in Table 16.9 [18]. Although these are approximate estimates, the information reveals that in "high" milk intake group, exclusive breastfeeding is enough to result in vitamin A stores to accumulate even if the breast milk concentration is low (<30 μg/dl) or adequate (50 μg/day) but not if deficient with less than 20 μg/dl.

Table 16.9 Estimated vitamin A intakes compared with requirements assuming different values for breast milk volume and vitamin A concentration [18]

Age (month)	*Breast milk retinol*[(a)]	**Low breast milk intake**[(b)]			**Average breast milk intake**[(b)]			**High breast milk intake**[(b)]		
		Milk volume (ml)	*Vitamin A intake (μg)*	*% of requirements*[(c)]	*Milk volume (ml)*	*Vitamin A intake (μg)*	*% of requirements*[(c)]	*Milk volume (ml)*	*Vitamin A intake (μg)*	*% of requirements*[(c)]
0–2	Def.	457	91	30/73	714	143	48/114	959	191	64/153
	Low		137	46/110		214	71/171		288	96/230
	Adeq.	228	76/182			357	119/286		479	160/383
3–5	Def.	515	103	34/82	784	157	52/126	1, 022	204	68/163
	Low		154	51/123		235	78/188		307	102/246
	Adeq.		257	86/206		392	131/314		511	170/409
6–8	Def.	355	71	24/57	776	155	52/124	982	196	65/157
	Low		106	35/85		233	78/186		295	98/236
	Adeq.		177	59/142		388	129/425		491	163/392

(a) Deficient (Def.) <20 μg/dl, Low <30 μg/dl, Adequate (Adeq.) ≥50 μg/dl
(b) Low intake −2 sd below mean; average intake, mean intake in developing countries; high intake +2 sd above mean
(c) Requirement to build stores (300 μg/day)/basal requirement (125 μg/day)

It is evident that along with promotion of breastfeeding, effort needs to be directed to increase the consumption of foods rich in vitamin A by mothers in developing countries who are reported to be often deficient in vitamin A due to consuming diets low in vitamin A during periods of high requirements. High fertility with prolonged breastfeeding further reduces vitamin A stores in mothers [11].

16.7.2 Dietary diversification

Promoting consumption of food rich in vitamin A is the long-term solution to address vitamin A deficiency. Local foods rich in vitamin A need to be identified and effort needs to be made to promote consumption of vitamin A rich food items to build stores in infants, young children and women in the pre-pregnancy or pregnant stage since this population group is at the highest risk of VAD and implications of deficiency are serious at this stage. The richest source of vitamin A is found in foods of animal origin such as liver, meat, eggs and dairy products. Vitamin A is also found in plants. The best dietary sources are dark green leafy vegetables (DGLV) including spinach, cassava leaves, amaranth, baobab leaves and red sorrel. Equally rich are deep yellow and orange fruits such as carrot, sweet potato, pumpkin, mango and papaya. Red palm oil, widely used in plants in Africa, is another good source of vitamin A. A certain amount of fat and protein is also necessary in the diet for the body to be able to absorb and transport the vitamin A in these foods.

Improved dietary intake of vitamin A rich food requires an adequate, affordable and diverse supply of food sources of vitamin A through out the year. A number of efforts made in the past have demonstrated positive impact on increasing market availability and affordability of inexpensive source of fruits and vegetables through introduction of horticultural activities at micro level. Such actions at household or community level are feasible in situations of adequate water availability and suitable humidity and land fertility. Animal foods, though excellent sources of vitamin A, are not available to the population at risk in developing countries due to economic and social constraints.

Introduction of foods rich in vitamin A in the complementary feed of a child is critical for preventing VAD. Soft yellow fruits and vegetables, dark green leaves, eggs and other food sources of vitamin A need to be routinely fed to children after 6 months, along with continuation of breastfeeding. In many developing countries, a regular supply of such food items at an affordable cost is not feasible. Moreover, availability and accessibility to vitamin A rich food items at family level is constrained not only by cost but poor availability of vitamin A rich foods in certain seasons and the effort required to clean and cook dark green leafy vegetables (DGLV).

A number of countries have experimented with innovative approaches to increase production and consumption of foods rich in vitamin A activity. Increase in production and consumption of vitamin A rich foods has been demonstrated through introduction of home or community gardening complemented with intensive nutrition education and social marketing [72, 73]. Social marketing project of Thailand concentrated on promoting one single vitamin A rich source vegetable – the ivy gourd [74]. Promotion of ivy gourd in Thailand was used as an image representing other vitamin A rich vegetables. Lessons learnt from these projects emphasized the need to focus efforts to identify and selectively propagate DGLV and other B-carotene rich foods, promote acceptability of such foods as well as influence use of such food items in family diet practices. Additionally, it is important to promote appropriate cooking methods in the traditional diets to ensure maximal retention of nutritive value [74, 75].

Changes in food consumption patterns require complex efforts to influence deeply ingrained family habits and cultural norms. An effective communication strategy to achieve the long-term goal of sustained behaviour change is critical. Messages and communication strategy, specially designed to address mother's specific concern about feeding selected vitamin A rich foods to children, is crucial. Long-term shift in fact requires consistent efforts and monitoring of impact over several years.

Demonstration sessions have been shown to be effective for convincing community regarding how to prepare local foods with inclusion of vitamin A rich food, especially for children. As a rough guide, a handful of fresh green or red varieties of amaranth (40 g) or drumstick leaves (35 g) or a medium-sized mango (100 g) provides the daily requirements for toddlers and preschool children [7]. A study undertaken in India [76] indicated that using a conversion ratio of 1:6 for β-carotene to retinol, a child less than 2 years needed about one table spoon of cooked dark green leafy vegetables (DGLV) per day to meet daily vitamin A requirements. Similarly, it has been estimated that a pregnant woman/nursing mother required about 3 table spoon of cooked DGLV per day for meeting the recommended dietary allowance for vitamin A. According to this study, it has been recommended that a family of five persons needs to procure and cook about 250 g of DGLV (cooked one cup) on a daily basis for the entire family. Based on the revised proposed factor for converting carotenoids into retinol of 12 or 21 μg of β-carotene to 1 μg of retinol for a mixed fruit and vegetable diet [11], the estimated amount of DGLV required to meet the RDA will increase at least two- to threefolds.

Biotechnology approach is being increasingly used to increase β-carotene and/or increase bioavailability of vitamin A and pro-vitamin A carotenoids from plant foods comprising commonly eaten cereals and vegetables such as rice, sweet potato, corn etc. New technologies are being introduced for processing red palm oil, a rich source of carotenoids, so that over 80% of the carotenes present in crude palm oil is retained [77].

16.7.3 Fortification of food with vitamin A

Food fortification is a highly effective strategy to correct low intake of vitamin A in daily diet. Food fortification is being introduced in increasing number of countries, and holds great hope for long-term control of vitamin A deficiency. Fortification of commonly consumed foods such as sugar, cereals, oils, milk, margarine, infant food and various types of flour is being implemented in a number of countries [78]. Oil is considered an ideal food for vitamin A fortification for two primary reasons – fats in oil assists in the absorption of vitamin A and oil fortification process is relatively inexpensive. In Brazil, vitamin A added to oil is well absorbed and has been demonstrated to significantly increase plasma retinol and liver vitamin A stores [79]. A model for oil fortification is expected to emerge from the ongoing efforts in West Africa [80]. The technology for fortifying sugar with vitamin A, developed in Guatemala in mid-1970s, is now well established and the technology of fortification of sugar with vitamin A as well as iron has also been successful. An effectiveness study has demonstrated improved vitamin A status with fortification of sugar in Guatemala and other Central American countries [81]. Guatemala cost-analysis study revealed that critical targeting and central processing conditions contributed in making fortification two to four times more cost-effective in reaching beneficiaries with adequate amounts of vitamin A than vitamin A capsule distribution or efforts to promote dietary diversification [82]. Sugar fortified with vitamin A, zinc, and iron either alone or in combination is being marketed in Brazil. In South-East Asia, vitamin A fortified monosodium glutamate (MSG) is widely promoted and is reported to improve breast milk and serum retinol concentrations as well as growth and survival of preschool children in Indonesia and Philippines [83, 44]. Despite successful biological impact, MSG fortification is not a national programme [81].

Fortification initiatives in any country are dictated by the cost, expertise, infrastructure, policies and political will. Development and marketing of finished products sometimes takes several years to reach all at-risk children and their families. It has been recommended that successful fortification programmes in a country should be complemented with administration of vitamin A supplements to the high-risk population group. It is estimated that in approximately 40 of the vitamin A supplementation priority countries, vitamin A fortified foods are available but the extent of its usage is not known [80].

16.7.4 Provision of high dose vitamin A supplement

High dose Vitamin A supplement (VAS)

While dietary and food-fortification strategies are essential, it is not feasible to implement such interventions quickly or widely in those developing countries where VAD is most severe. Administration of routine vitamin A supplements is critical to prevent occurrence of vitamin A deficiency in situations where dietary intake of vitamin A is inadequate and the scope for rapidly improving the situation through dietary means is low for many years, e.g. in situations of chronic poverty, chronic shortage of food including food sources of vitamin A or fat [7]. Periodic high-dose vitamin A supplement (VAS) is intended to protect against VAD and its consequences by immediately improving the body reserves of vitamin A. As a result, efforts directed to eliminate VAD have turned to regular administration of supplement as a low cost, highly effective means of rapidly and sustainably improving the vitamin A status and health of children [38].

For children living in deficient population, the periodic supply of high-dose vitamin A supplement (VAS) has been accepted as a swift, simple, low-cost, high-benefit intervention. VAS has produced remarkable results, reducing mortality by 23% overall and by up to 50% for acute measles sufferers and that of diarrhoeal disease mortality by about 33% [9, 46, 84, 85, 86]. Administration of vitamin A supplement is also recommended to be used in conditions for treatment of those with signs of acute xerophthalmia as well as in situations where high-risk individuals need to rapidly improve vitamin A status, e.g. children with infections such as diarrhoea or measles or in emergency situations such as drought or feeding of refugees who are dependent on relief rations. The administration of vitamin A supplement along with measles vaccine to infants has been reported not only in improving serum retinol levels but also to result in improving sero conversion of measles [87].

High potency vitamin A supplement has been introduced as a child survival tool since 1990s. At the global level, vitamin A supplement programme was accelerated in 1993. Two forms of vitamin A supplement preparations of high potency, oil based and water miscible, are used (Box 16.1). Water miscible VAS preparations are not recommended for public health programmes.

Vitamin A supplementation has been listed among the key interventions achievable on a large scale that have proven potential to reduce the number of preventable child deaths each year [37] and is therefore recognised as a critical intervention for achieving the Millennium Development Goal 4 (MDG-4) pertaining to child survival, particularly in countries with high under-five mortality and /or vitamin A deficiency prevalence rates. In order to have substantial impact on child survival, all children between the ages of six and 59 months in the target countries are recommended to receive high dose vitamin A supplements every 4–6 months.

Box 16.1 Vitamin A supplement high dose preparations

Preparations of high-dose vitamin A supplement are supplied as retinyl palmitate, retinyl acetate or retinol. The most widely available commercial form is retinyl palmitate [66–72]. A dose of 200,000 IU is equivalent to 110 mg of retinyl palmitate, 69 mg retinyl acetate, or 60 mg retinol. As long as recommended doses are administered, the chemical form is not important. Vitamin A preparations for supplementation programme are diluted with high-quality vegetable oil, usually peanut oil. Addition of vitamin E (40 mg) for 200,000 IU of vitamin A acts as an antioxidant to stabilize the product and to enhance the absorption and storage of vitamin A by the body.

Water-miscible preparations of vitamin A high-dose supplement are not considered suitable [88, 89]. Water-miscible emulsified and dry preparation of retinol are reported to be ≥ 10 times more toxic as compared to oil-based preparations of retinol. Oil-based preparations are preferred for oral administration of vitamin A.

Vitamin A supplement preparations, especially in liquid form, are recommended to be stored in a dark bottle (or an aluminium container) to shield from light since the chemical stability and therefore the biological activity of vitamin A is affected by temperature and sunlight and other sources of ultra violet light. Vitamin A supplement preparation is sufficiently stable and requires no cold chain. The estimated shelf-life of oil-based solution of vitamin A properly stored in unopened opaque container is estimated to be at least 2 years. Once a container has been opened, potency is gradually reduced. Liquid vitamin A preparations from properly stored containers should be used within 6–8 weeks of opening. Although such preparations beyond the designated periods are less potent, they remain safe and often contain adequate vitamin A for therapeutic use [66].

Partial protection against the loss of potency is acquired when the oil-based VAS solution is formulated in capsules. VAS is available as gelatin capsules which can be swallowed by children at least 36 months of age or adults. For younger children, the nipple on the capsule is cut off or the capsule pricked with a pin, and the contents squeezed into child's mouth. The high dose retinol gel capsules (in single doses of 200,000 IU or lower dose capsules of 100,000, 50,000, 25,000 and 10,000 IU) are available for public health programme [65]. The cost of a single capsule is US$0.02 and US$0.04 per child can prevent and correct the deficiency.

Vitamin A is used as oily solution rather than in form of capsules in only 9 countries – India, Nigeria, Mali, Brazil, Bangladesh, Iran, Mexico, Guatemala, Nicaragua and Iran [65]. Indian government procures vitamin A supplement in flavoured syrup form mixed with Arachidonic oil [90]. Vitamin A is supplied in India as oil-based syrup in dark brown coloured bottles of 100 ml. The concentration of supplement is 100,000 IU/ml. A spoon measuring 2 ml is supplied with each bottle. A spoon to the upper level measures 2 ml (200,000 IU) while the half level marking measures up to 1 ml (100,000 IU). The cost of 100 ml or 50 doses of VAS of 200,000 IU is approximately one US dollar or each dose of vitamin A supplement costs 2 US cents.

The timely distribution of vitamin A preparation to field requires a well-functioning storage system at central warehouse. Linking with supply of primary health care and maternal and child health services is practical. Unopened containers of both liquid and capsules retain over 90% activity for six months at 30°C. Vitamin A supplement preparation is recommended NOT to be kept below zero degree centrigrade [66]. Vitamin A supplement storage does not require any special storage measures such as cold chain. It should be stored in a cool dark room protected from sunlight.

For individuals one year of age and older, administration of 200,000 IU of vitamin A supplement (VAS) provides adequate protection for 4–6 months, the exact interval depending on the vitamin A content of the diet and rate of utilization by the body. The recommended appropriate dose interval for high dose VAS is 4–6 months, although it is indicated that 3-month interval is safe [66]. The recommendation is to scale up twice yearly vitamin A supplementation for children aged between six months and five years to achieve at least 70% coverage on a recurrent basis [80].

The VAS doses for various age groups recommended in the IVACG meet 2001 are presented in Table 16.10.

Table 16.10 Recommended schedule for routine prophylactic high-dose vitamin A supplementation in vitamin A deficient populations [91, 92]

Population	*Amount of vitamin A to be administered*	*Time of administration*
Infants 0–5 months	150,000 IU as three doses of 50,000 IU with at least a 1-month interval between doses	At each DTP contact (6, 10, and 14 weeks) (otherwise at other opportunities)
Infants 6–11 months	100,000 IU as a single dose every 4–6 months	At any opportunity (e.g., measles immunization)
Children 12 months and older	200,000 IU as a single dose every 4–6 months	At any opportunity
Postpartum women	400, 000 IU as two doses of 200, 000 IU at least 1 dose apart And / or 10, 000 IU daily or 25,000 IU weekly	As soon after delivery as possible and not more than 6 weeks later And / or during the first 6 month after delivery

Additional dosage is required for children with clinical signs of vitamin A deficiency as a part of treatment package for those children suffering with severe acute malnutrition or infection such as measles and diarrhoea (Table 16.11). Children with concurrent vitamin A deficiency and measles can suffer serious complications and immediate vitamin A therapy is therefore recommended to reduce the risk of excessive measles case fatality. Similarly in situations of diarrhoea episode or severe acute malnutrition, additional vitamin A supplement dose administration is recommended. Table 16.11 presents the recommended treatment dosage for children and women 13–49 years [92].

Recent studies report that pregnant and breastfeeding women in a poor population have high prevalence of night blindness and biochemical vitamin A deficiency and likely adverse impact on both mother and her infant [92–96]. Prophylactic doses of vitamin A supplement for lactating women have been recommended [86]. Earlier the VAS dose recommended was a single dose to mothers in the first 4–6 weeks postpartum. WHO

Table 16.11 Vitamin A treatment regimens [92]

Infants and children[(a)]	*Vitamin A dose (IU)*
Young infants (0–5 months)	50,000
Older infants (6–11 months)	100,000
Children (males: 12 months or more; females 12 months to 12 year and ≥ 50 years)	200,000
Women (13–49 years)	10,000 every day or 25,000 every week
Xerophthalmia: night blindness and/or Bitot's spot	for at least 3 months
Active corneal lesions (rare)	200,000 on days 1, 2 and 14

[(a)] Schedule – severe malnutrition, day 1; measles, days 1 and 2; xerophthalmia, days 1, 2 and 14. Severe malnutrition: kwashiorkor or weight for height below –3 sd (NCHS)

recommended revised dosage for women in vitamin A deficient areas to be increased to two doses of 200,000 IU vitamin A – first dose of 200,000 IU at delivery and the next dose within 6 weeks postpartum [92, 97]. This recommendation ensures that infants receive the necessary immune boosting protection of vitamin A for the first six months of life. For fertile woman, independent of the vitamin A status, 10,000 IU is the maximum daily supplement recommended at any time during pregnancy [92–97]. For women with xerophthalmia, a treatment dosage of 10,000 IU every day or 25,000 IU every week for at least 3 months is recommended [98].

The efficacy of VAS appears to be 90% in preventing any stage of xerophthalmia for six months in children [9] despite projected dosage absorption of only 30–50% in developing countries. During periods of reduced dietary intake or increased need, a gap of 4–6 months is estimated to provide nutrition reserve for use. Protection with massive dose of VAS against hyporetinolemia (serum retinol <20 μg/dL or <0.70 μmol/L) may be less sustained as serum retinol remains elevated for only up to 2 months following high-potency VAS [9].

Vitamin A supplement (VAS) – delivery strategy

The goal of VAS is universal coverage of children 6–59 months [65]. "Adequate coverage" in a country is defined as reaching ≥ 70% of children age 6–59 months with VAS on two occasions, 4–6 months apart while "insufficient coverage" is defined as countries reaching ≥70% of children ages 6–59 on one occasion while poor coverage is defined as countries reaching <70% children with VAS on any occasion [99]. The coverage threshold of 70 percent represents "the minimal coverage at which countries can expect to observe reductions in child mortality comparable to those measured in large scale vitamin A supplementation trials in the community" [65]. Administering vitamin A supplement is a simple action, especially in situations where vitamin A capsules (VAC) are used. One of the greatest challenges for vitamin A programme is to find sustainable cost-effective mechanisms for delivery to achieve the goal of adequate VAS coverage.

Innovative ways of VAS administration strategy was launched in 1988 when the 41st World Health Assembly committed WHO to the goal of global eradication of poliomyelitis by 2000 in ways *"which strengthen national immunisation programmes and health infrastructure"* [100]. Linking provision of vitamin A supplement during National Immunisation Day (NID) along with polio vaccine was considered a cost-effective delivery system since target group of children for polio were the same and the nation wide campaign aimed to reach the unreached that were also at risk of vitamin A deficiency. Moreover, it was apparent that it was logistically easy to introduce VAS during NIDs since no refrigeration or special storage effort was required and training involved was relatively simple. VAS administration was piggybacked to the ongoing national NID programme and a field guideline on distribution of vitamin A supplements with NID was developed [101, 102], which facilitated a number of countries to link vitamin A supplement administration to Polio NIDS towards achieving the goal of elimination of vitamin A deficiency by 2000 which was one of the goals committed by member countries at the World Summit for Children in 1990 and the International Nutrition Conference in 1992 [103, 104].

In 1998, 75 percent of 118 countries where VAD is a known or suspected public health problem conducted NIDs and of these 89 countries (75%) included vitamin A supplementation in their NIDs [38]. Moreover, administration of VAS along with polio vaccine during NIDs was valued and welcomed by community. VAS was found to act as incentive to mothers and care-givers to take children to immunization sites. However, based on country-programme experiences, linking VAS administration with polio vaccine administration also was of concern to public-health experts since it was observed that the extra planning and management support that was required for VAS possibly compromised the performance of Polio NIDS [105, 106]. Moreover, since NID was organised normally only once annually, a special strategy for the additional dose or second dose was required. Several countries, including Bangladesh and Myanmar, took the lead and organised additional specific periods such as "vitamin A week" or "vitamin A months" when high dose vitamin A supplements were distributed. This resulted in organization of "Micronutrient day" or "Vitamin A days" six months after the annual NID in various countries including Bangladesh, Nepal, Niger and the Philippines [38].

Following Polio NIDS being gradually discontinued in many countries, the lessons learnt were applied to link VAS with routine immunisation with high degree of success. In fact, WHO strategy which was introduced in 1988 for integration of delivering vitamin A supplement through Expanded Programme on Immunisation (EPI), as a cost-effective strategy for the control of vitamin A deficiency in a community, was revived [91]. Providing the doses of VAS to children on the days of routine immunisation services offered a long-term solution and this was the strategic shift made by many countries. Box 16.2 presents details of emergence of such a strategy in Cambodia [107].

Box 16.2 Cambodia experience – linking vitamin A and immunisation programme [107]

The national vitamin A program was initiated in Cambodia in 1994; in 1995 National Immunisation Days (NIDs) for polio began. While NIDs were being organised, it was recognised early on that it would be good for vitamin A capsule (VAC) distribution to "piggy back" on to the NIDs. The National Vitamin A Working Group, consisting of members from Ministry of Health / Departments of Nutrition, Polio Eradication and Expanded Program for Immunisation (EPI), UNICEF, WHO and HKI agreed to conduct a pilot to see how well-distribution of vitamin A high dose capsules (VACs) with NIDS would work. Results of the pilot were very promising and led to the country adopting VAC distribution linked to NIDs as one of the main strategies for distribution of VAC. By 1996 VAC distribution became fully integrated into NIDs.

Distribution of VACs through NID-linked strategy continued until the end of 1997 after which the NIDs for polio ended. It was then decided that VACs would be distributed through routine immunisation services. In 1998, Cambodian government took steps to distribute vitamin A capsules (VACs) to children aged 6–59 months through the following channels:

- Routine immunisation outreach activities – this was carried out by health-centre staff who visited 10–20 villages, approximately three to four times per year for immunization services. The outreach team was expected to carry supply of VACs at least twice yearly, around the months of March and November.
- VAC distribution on sub-national immunisation days (SNIDs): special supplemental campaigns such as SNIDS.
- Measles outbreak response.

Following the success of this strategy, VAC distribution was integrated into the National Immunisation Program (NIP) and is currently being distributed twice a year to children 6–59 month of age through routine immunisation outreach.

Like Cambodia, many other countries such as Thailand, Bhutan and Afghanistan adopted the sustainable approach of integrating vitamin A supplement administration with the ongoing routine child immunisation programmes or to the routine Maternal Child Health (MCH) programmes [108]. However, in many countries immunisation contact was suitable to reach only under ones and the first opportunity to administer VAS along with measles vaccine at around 9 months of age was found to be effective [65]. The delivery system, however, was not adequate to reach children 12–59 months twice annually. Overall coverage achieved through, traditional VAS linked to immunization sessions routine services, remained low due to poor access and utilization of services and an inability to reach older children. It was recognised that regular outreach and events were required to be organised to protect children from the life-threatening effects of VAD. In 1997, a consultation of experts was organised to discuss ways to rapidly increase acceptance and adoption of countries of VAS as a critical child survival intervention [65, 109]. A number of delivery strategies emerged and innovative approaches were launched for vitamin A programmes such as Child Health Days or Child Health Nutrition biannual months. The experiences of West and Central Africa have demonstrated that VAS to children is effectively delivered by institutionalization of Child Survival/Health Days. The twice yearly distribution of VAS through existing permanent institutions in the region is considered sustainable [110].

Figure 16.3 indicates that by 2004, the strategy of Child Health Days were used by 23% of the countries, 15% organised special micronutrient events while 26% administered VAS on polio national or sub-national immunisation days [65].

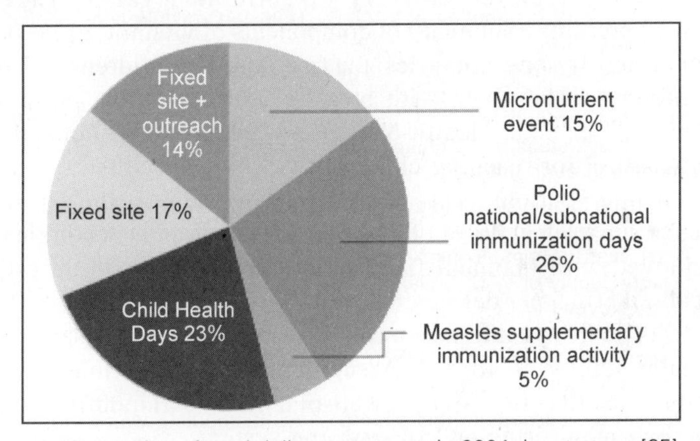

16.3 Proportion of total delivery attempts in 2004, by strategy [65]

VAS administration events required significant planning, strong logistical support and special allocation of resources and it was considered cost-effective to add additional important child-health activities linked to vitamin A administration. Deworming of preschool children was often linked to vitamin A administration (Box 16.3).

Box 16.3 Vitamin A plus programme – integrating vitamin A distribution with deworming [22]

It is estimated that as many as 230 million children aged 0–4 years are infected with soil-transmitted helminthes (STHs). Roundworms are the most prevalent STH infection in preschool children and cause significant vitamin A malabsorption. Worm infections contribute to vitamin A deficiency. Worm infections and vitamin A deficiency are public health problems in the same geographical areas. The target groups for vitamin A and deworming are very similar. Both VAS and deworming is administered twice a year. However, the main difference in the target age group is important. Vitamin A supplements are given from age of six months while deworming tablets are given from age of one year, i.e. the target group for vitamin A supplement is 6–59 months whereas the target group for deworming is 12–59 months. One of the two following deworming drugs are recommended – Albendazole (400 mg tablet – half tablet for 12–23 months and one tablet for 24 months and older) or Mebendazole (500 mg tablet – one tablet for 12 months and older children). Integrating administration of deworming and VAS programme is not only effective in terms of impact and increasing coverage of both supplements and deworming drug but is also noted to result in increasing community's trust in health personnel since deworming is extremely popular due to its immediate and highly visible effect. Such vitamin A plus programme has been successfully implemented in Nepal, DPR Korea and Cambodia.

The integrated programme concept resulted in the intervention package of health services termed as "vitamin A plus" package and efforts were made for the integrated delivery of child survival package [65]. Table 16.12 presents a summary of components of vitamin A plus package of 15 countries. In some countries, the first dose for children 6–12 months was continued to be given with measles administration and a special period was allocated as Health-Nutrition week or fixed biannual "Child Health Months" for reaching children twice a year with VAS and other additional interventions [111]. Rapid improvement in the coverage of second and subsequent doses of massive dose of vitamin A administration was achieved with biannual fixed month approach, with an estimated cost of about $0.25 per delivered dose [112, 113]. The success, to a large extent, was achieved due to appropriate strategies for ensuring timely and regular supply of vitamin A supplements, integrating distribution with public health care system, a well-planned social mobilisation effort and a strong monitoring and supervision system.

Vitamin A supplement promotion and training

For the sucess of VAS programme, communication and social mobilisation is essential. An effective communication strategy with rigorous audience focus, with consistent message across the entire broad geographic areas, is critical for improvements in VAS coverage. Communication efforts must be complemented with an appropriate delivery system, which takes into consideration consumer perspective for distribution such as timing and location, information on product advantages and on the simple "where"

Table 16.12 Components of child health day packages in recent years [65]

Country	*Under-5 supplementation*	*Deworming*	*Immunisation*	*Mosquito nets*	*TT vaccination (mothers)*	*Growth monitoring*	*IEC*	*Iron supplementation (pregnant women)*	*Iron supplementation (LBW infants)*	*Ivermectin treatment (onchocerciasis)*
Bangladesh	X	X								
Cambodia	X	X	X					X		
Congo, Democratic Republic of the	X	X	X							
Ethiopia	X	X	X	X		X				
Ghana	X		X	X		X				
Korea, Democratic People's Republic of	X	X					X			
Lao People's Democratic Republic	X	X	X							
Nepal	X	X								
Nigeria	X	X	X							X
Philippines	X	X	X			X	X		X	
Swaziland	X	X	X			X		X		
Tanzania, United Rep. of	X	X	X	X						
Uganda	X	X	X		X					
Zambia	X	X	X	X		X	X			

TT = tetanus toxoid; IEC = information, education and communication; IEC focuses on infant and young child feeding and the promotion/testing of iodised salt in the cited countries. Bangladesh plans to pilot the inclusion of birth registration in upcoming child health packages. Mosquito net distribution in the Philippines is limited to remote areas where malaria is endemic.

and "when" of distribution is useful when built in as part of the message. Additionally, commitment by service providers is critical for program success. Special effort needs to be made to address concern and fear of frontline workers of the safety of distribution of high dose vitamin A supplement. The communication strategy needs to address the issue of the serious consequences of children administered extra doses of VAS and the significance of adhering to the dosage schedule.

It is important to set up a monitoring and feedback mechanism for communication strategy and actions at the smallest administrative level. Such a strategy is crucial not only for fixing problems but in keeping the providers motivated. In case of VAS administration programme, simple rapid household survey could be useful to get information on the knowledge of five "Ws" at family level – what are the vitamin A supplements, where and when do you get them, who are they for and why do you want them. Moreover, feedback on the sources of information about vitamin A as well as whose opinion on VAS administration is of significance to the family has been proposed to be useful for re-visiting and modifying communication strategy [120].

For effective implementation of VAS administration, training of health persons and other stakeholders is critical. Training needs to stress on the significance of VAD on child survival, the methods to be adopted for identifying and enlisting all beneficiaries at risk of VAD, understanding of comprehensive strategy comprising breastfeed, dietary diversification, fortification and supplementation, treatment and prevention protocol of the supplement for preschool children and mothers, recognizing signs and symptoms of deficiency, treatment schedule to be followed for children with xerophthalmia, diarrhoea, measles and severe malnutrition. In addition, training needs to address programme issues with reference to logistics management, communication strategy and monitoring, as well as recording mechanism to be followed. It is critical that training emphasizes on the safety of VAS and the importance of adhering to the recommended doses of VAS as well as the need to take cautions for preventing over dosage which could cause toxicity (see Box 16.4).

Monitoring VAS programme

The system for monitoring of administration of VAS needs to be designed with the objective to provide information on the "effective coverage", i.e. the proportion of children receiving two annual doses of vitamin A [65]. Recording of VAS in special tally sheets or within the maternal and child health or immunization programme has been streamlined in many countries by recording the information in the existing health or nutrition record systems such as growth charts,

Box 16.4 Safety of administration of vitamin A supplements to infants and children

The recommended high doses of vitamin A supplements for children and mothers are perfectly safe [97]. Clinical Toxicity due to hypervitaminosis does not result from public health intervention programmes [114]. Virtually no risk has been observed when prophylactic vitamin A doses, two doses of 200,000 IU separated at least by one month interval is administered to 1–6 years old. About 200 cases of hypervitaminosis are estimated to occur annually compared to an estimated 3 million preschool children who develop VAD each year and are exposed to an increased risk of morbidity, mortality with 250,000–300,000 becoming blind [115].

Administration of excessive amount of vitamin A supplement can lead to toxicity or hypervitaminosis. The manifestations of toxicity depend on age of the individual, hepatic function, dose and duration of vitamin A administration and the vitamin A status. The adverse effects of periodical vitamin A supplementation are occasional in the range of 1.5–7.0% [114]. The symptoms reported are mild and transient [114]. The side effects experienced are loose stools, headache, irritability, fever, nausea, vomiting which disappear practically in all children within 24–48 hours. In neonates and young infants under the age of six months, vitamin A supplementation has been associated with an increased incidence of transient bulging of fontanelle that resolves within 24–72 hours. The recommended postpartum two doses of vitamin A of 200,000 IU are reported to be well tolerated [97].

Toxicity, acute or chronic, has been reported with the abuse of vitamin A supplements. Signs and symptoms of acute vitamin A toxicity (single ingestion of 25,000 IU per kg body weight or 500,000 IU consumed over a short time-appear within 8–24 hours after ingestion and include manifestations such as nausea, vomiting, diarrhoea, changes in behaviour, increased intracranial pressure causing headache, diplopia, papilloedema and bulged fontanelle in infants and skin changes etc [116–118].

Chronic hyper vitaminosis A results from long term intake of moderate vitamin A doses (about 4000 IU/kg body weight or over >18000 IU) daily for 6–15 months. The symptoms are low grade fever, headache, fatigue, irritability, anorexia, loss of weight, gastrointestinal disturbances, hapatosplenomegaly, skin changes, anemia, hypercalcemia, pseudotumor cerebri, etc [58–60]. Toxicity is reversible by discontinuing vitamin A but may take several weeks.

During pregnancy, the recommended vitamin A supplement is recommended to be limited to 10,000 IU .This level of daily consumption is safe and beneficial. Vitamin A supplement exceeding 10,000 IU/day, especially in early pregnancy, may cause major birth defects and are considered harmful [119].

family-held immunisation cards and health records. Record keeping of VAS administered is considered essential not only for monitoring coverage but also for serving as an effective tool to intensify efforts to ensure full coverage as well as for avoiding dose duplication and potential side effects. Box 16.4 presents details regarding the issues pertaining to safety of administration of vitamin A supplements to infants and children.

For measuring progress of vitamin A supplementation programme, indicator used is the percentage of children between the ages of 6 and 59 months receiving two annual doses of vitamin A, 4–6 months apart. Only a few countries carry out coverage surveys immediately following VAS distribution using methods similar to those developed to track immunisation coverage [65]. Data on number of children receiving vitamin A distribution from one distribution to the next is more easily available than information on specific children receiving two doses per year which denotes "effective coverage" or full protection to children. In the absence of such data, assumptions for two doses of vitamin A administered are being derived from the information available regarding percentage coverage of children in a population for at least one high dose of VAS in the past six months. Efforts are ongoing to improve the recording system with a view to overcome the constraint and facilitate direct monitoring of two dose coverage [56].

Progress in vitamin A supplementation coverage

Assessment has been undertaken in a total of 103 countries [66]. These countries were identified as priority countries for vitamin A supplementation – 61 countries with high U5MR, 35 additional countries with relatively low U5MR but elevated prevalence of VAD and another seven countries which continued to consider vitamin A deficiency as a public health problem. It was estimated that only 26 of the 103 priority countries attained effective coverage levels in 2004, i.e. reached at least 70 percent children with two rounds of VAS. There was a sharp increase reported in the global coverage with two doses of VAS during the years 1999–2004. In 1999, globally only 16% of children were fully protected with two annual doses which increased to 58% in 2004, 72% in 2005 and a drop to 62% was observed in 2007. The reduction in overall percentage coverage observed in 2007 was attributed to the drop in percentage coverage reported from India with the introduction of policy in the year to extend VAS coverage to children over 3–6 years in the national VAS programme instead of focusing on only 6 months to three years (Fig. 16.4). It is evident from reported data that despite such an accelerated progress since 1999, further effort is required to reach every child with VAS twice a year and sustain universal coverage for as long as the need is evident.

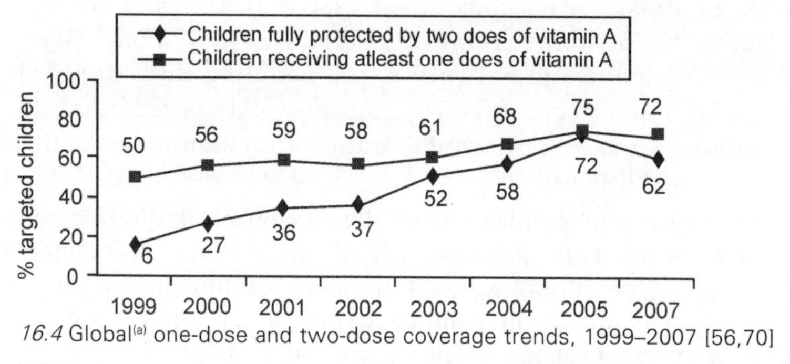

16.4 Global[(a)] one-dose and two-dose coverage trends, 1999–2007 [56,70]

[(a)] Global coverage calculations exclude China

Administration of VAS to women at the contact during delivery or at the contact with mother during newborn's first immunization with BCG has been reported to be rather low. By 2004, post-partum administration of VAS has been reported to be operational in only two-thirds of the 103 countries identified as priority countries for addressing VAD [56] and only 12 countries exceeded 50% coverage: Azerbaijan, Benin, Cape Verde, Egypt, Honduras, Marshall Islands, Morocco, Myanmar, Oman, Sao Tome and Principe, Tajikistan and Vietnam.

Analysis of success of VAS programme reveals that the success and continuity of the programme depends greatly on political commitment, vitamin A supplies being available regularly at peripheral level, community awareness and demand. Timely procurement and distribution of VAS supply is critical. Procurement involves adequate resources, timely purchase of appropriate quantities of VAS supplies according to the size of the target population and appropriate logistic system for effective distribution. Determination of supply requirement needs to be assessed on the basis of population age group and percentage coverage planned with preventive dosage of VAS. An additional supply of VAS is required for special conditions such as xerophthalmia or clinical VAD, measles, diarrhoea, severe protein–energy malnutrition.

Indicators for assessment – elimination of vitamin A deficiency.

For assessing, the virtual elimination of VAD, the following indicators have been proposed (Table 16.13).

Table 16.13 Core indicators for assessing progress towards the goal of virtual elimination of VAD [6, 92–96, 98]

Functional indicator[(a)]	*Prevalence goal*
Night blindness (children 24–71 months of age)	< 1%
Biochemical indicators	
Serum retinol ≤0.70 μmol/L (children 6–71 months of age) or	<15%[(b)]
Breast milk retinol ≤1.05 μmol/L or ≤8 μg/g milk fat	< 10%

(a) Other clinical indicators of xerophthalmia, i.e. conjunctival xerosis with Bitot's spots (X1 B) <0.5%; corneal xerosis/ulceration/keratomalacia (X2, X3A, X3B) <0.01%; corneal scars (XS) <0.05%, where known to occur can also be used to assess progress towards eliminating VAD and especially towards eliminating vitamin A.

(b) The prevalence criteria in 2001 was proposed to be raised from >5% to >15%.

The big challenge for prevention and control of VAD is to effectively implement the well-integrated mix of interventions that including food-based approach to improve overall dietary supply and quality, improving infant and young child feeding practices, ensuring food fortification reaching the most deprived population section and universal coverage of young children with vitamin A supplementation for prevention of VAD. For elimination of VAD, integrated efforts for VAD control need to be combined with overall maternal and child public health measures to reduce infections and improve mother's nutritional status.

References

1. WHO (1995). MDIS – Micronutrient Deficiency Information System, World Health Organisation. MDIS Working paper # 2. Global prevalence of vitamin A deficiency.
2. UNDERWOOD BA (2004). Vitamin A deficiency disorders: international efforts to control a preventable "pox". *J Nutr* **134**, pp 231S–236S.
3. SEMBA RD (1999). Vitamin A as "anti-infective" therapy 1920–1940. *J Nutr* vol 129, pp 783–791.
4. MCLAREN DS, FRIGGY M (2001). Sight and life manual on vitamin A deficiency disorders (VADD), 2nd edition. Basel: Task Force Sight and Life.
5. BLOMHAFF R, BLOMHAFF HK (2006). Overview of retinoid metabolism and functions. *J Neurobiol* **66**, pp 601–630.
6. SOMMER A, DAVIDSON FR (2002). Assessment and control of vitamin A deficiency. *J Nutr* **132**, no. 9S, pp 2845S–2849S.
7. SOMMER A (1995). Vitamin A deficiency and its consequences, 3rd edition. A field guide to detect and control, WHO, Geneva.
8. WEST KP JR. (2002). Extent of vitamin A deficiency among preschool children and women of reproductive age. *J Nutr* **132**, pp 2857S–2866S.
9. SOMMER A, WEST KP JR. (1996). *Vitamin A Deficiency: Health, Survival and Vision.* New York, Oxford University Press.
10. IVACG (1997). IVACG statement – Maternal Nightblindness: extent and associated factors.
11. MILLER M, HUMPREY J, JOHNSON E, MARINDA E, BROOKMEYER R, KATZ J (2002). Why children do became vitamin A deficient. *J Nutr supplement* **132**, no. 9S, pp 2867.
12. WORLD BANK (2004). Vitamin A – At a glance.
13. DE PEE S, WEST CE (1996). Dietary carotenoids and their role in combating vitamin A deficiency: a review of literature. *Eur J Clin Nutr* **50**, pp S38–S53.
14. CASTENMILLER JJM, WEST CE (1998). Bioavailability and bioconversion of carotenoids. *Ann Rev Nutr* **18**, pp 19–38.
15. WEST CE, EILANDER, A, LIESHOUT VAN M (2002). Consequences of reused estimated of carotenoids bio-efficiency for dietary control of vitamin A deficiency in developing countries. *J Nutr* **132**, no. 9S, pp 2920S.
16. OTTEN JJ, HELLWIG JP, MEYERS LD (eds). Dietary reference intakes: the essential guide to nutrient requirements: Institute of Medicine of the National Academy of Sciences. Washington DC National Academies 2006, 170–181.
17. Dietary reference intakes for vitamin A, vitamin K, arsenic, boron, chromium, copper, iodine, iron, manganese, molybdenum, nickel, silicon, vanadium and zinc (2001). Institute of Medicine, Washington DC. National Academy 2001, pp 82–161.
18. ALLEN LH, HASKELL M (2001). Vitamin A requirements in infants under six months of age. *Food and Nutrition Bulletin* **22**, no. 31, pp 214–234.

19. MCLE L, WEST K P JR, KUSDIIONO, PANDJI A, NENDRAWAT H, TILDEN, R. L. et al (1991). Nutritional and household risk factors for xerophthalmia in Aceh, Indonesia: a casê control study. *Am J Clin Nutr* **53**, pp. 1460–1465.
20. SEMBA RD (1994). Vitamin A, Immunity and Infection. *Clin Infect Dis* **19**, pp 489–499.
21. SOMMER A, TARWOTJO J, KATZ J (1987). Increase risk of xerophthalmia following diarrhoea and respiratory diseases. *Am J Clin Nutr* **45**, pp 977–980.
22. WHO and UNICEF (2004). How to add deworming to vitamin A distribution.
23. STOLTZFUS, R. et al (1996). Hemoquant determination of hookworm – related blood loss and its role in iron deficiency in African children.
24. MAHALANABIS D et al (1976). Vitamin A absorption in ascariasis. *Am J Clin Nutr* **29**, pp. 1372–1375.
25. KATZ J, ZEGER SL, TIELSCH JM (1988). Village and household clusters of xerophthalmia and trachoma. *Int J Epidemiol* **17**, pp 865–869.
26. KATZ J, ZEGER SL, WEST KP JR, TIELSCH JM, SOMMER A (1993). Clustering of xerophthalmia within households and villages. *Int J Epidemiol* **22**, pp. 709-715.
27. WHO (1996). Indicators for assessing vitamin A deficiency and their application in monitoring and evaluating intervention programme. WHO (1996), Geneva. WHO / NUTR 96.10.
28. CHRISTIAN P (2002). Recommendation for indicators: nightblindness during pregnancy – a simple tool to assess vitamin A deficiency in a population. *J Nutr* **132**, no. 9S, pp 2884S–2888S.
29. DE PEE S, DARY O (2002). Biochemical indicators of vitamin A deficiency: serum retinol and serum binding protein. *J Nutr* **132**, no.9S, pp 2895S–2901S.
30. MDIS (1995). Global prevalence of vitamin A deficiency. Information system paper no. 2, WHO, Geneva, Switzerland.
31. KATZ J, KHATRY SK, WEST KP, HUMPHREY JH, LECLERQ SC, KIMBROUGH E, POHKREL PR, SOMMER A (1995). Night blindness is prevalent during pregnancy and lactation in rural Nepal. *J Nutr* **125**, pp 2122–2127.
32. USAID MISSION OFFICE INDIA (2000). Benefits and safety of administration of synthetic vitamin to children. Background document for national consultation on vitamin A, Sept 29–30, 2000, New Delhi, India.
33. HKI, INDIA (1999). Vitamin A status throughout the lifecycle. Vitamin A survey, 1997–1998.
34. VILLAVIEJA GM, PALAFOX EF, CERDENA CM, LANA RD, DE LOS REYES M, SHEKAR M (1998). Maternal night blindness in selected areas of the Philippines: Initial results of the 5th national survey. Government of The Philippines, The Philippines.
35. LUO C, MWELA C, FOOTE D, KAFWIMBE E, SCHULTZ, K (1999). The national vitamin A deficiency prevalence survey in Zambia (abstract). XIX International vitamin A Consultative group meeting, Durban, South Africa.
36. SCHULTINK W (2002). Use of under-five mortality rate as an indicator of vitamin A deficiency in a population. *J Nutr* **132**, no. 9S, pp 281S–288S.
37. BHUTTA ZA, AHMED T, BLACK RE, COUSENS S, DEWEY K, GUGLIANI E, HAIDER BA, KIRKWOOD B, MORRIS SS, SACHDEV HPS, SHEKHAR M (2008). Maternal and Child Undernutrition Study Group. What works? Intervention for maternal and child nutrition and Survival. *Lancet* **371**, no. 9610, pp. 417–440.
38. GOODMAN T, DALMIYA N, DE BENOIST B, SCHULTINK W (2000). Polio as platform: using national immunisation days to deliver vitamin A supplements. *Bulletin of World Health Organisation* **78**, pp 305.

39. THYLEFORS B, NÉGREL AD, PARARAJASEGARAM R, DADZIE KY (1995). Global data on blindness. *Bull World Health Organ* **73**, pp 115–121.
40. HUMPHREY JH, WEST KP, SOMMER A (1992). Vitamin A deficiency and attributable mortality among children – 5-year olds. *Bulletin of World Health Organisation* **70**, pp 225–232.
41. SOMMER A, KATZ J, TARWOJO I (1984). Increased risk of respiratory disease and diarrhoea in children with pre-existing mild vitamin A deficiency. *Am J Clin Nutr* **40**, pp 1090–1099.
42. SOMMER A, TARWOTJO I, HUSSAINI G, SUSANTO S (1983). Increased mortality in children with mild vitamin A deficiency. *Lancet* **2**, pp 585–588.
43. SOMMER A, TARWOTJO I, DJUNAEDI E, WEST KP JR, LOEDEN A, TILDEN R, MELE L (1986). Impact of vitamin A supplementation on childhood mortality. A randomised controlled community trial. *Lancet* **1**, pp 1169–1173.
44. MUHILAL, PERMEISIH D, IDJRADINATA Y R, MUHERDIYANTININGSIH, KARYADI D (1988). Vitamin A fortified monosodium glutamate and health, growth and survival of children: a controlled field trail. *Am J Clin nutr* **48**, pp 1271–1276.
45. RAHMATHULLAH L, UNDERWOOD BA, THULASIRAJ RD, MILTON RC, RAMASWAMY K, RAHMATHULLAH R, BABU G (1990). Reduced mortality among children in southern India receiving a small weekly dose of vitamin A. *N Engl J Med* **323**, pp 929–935.
46. VIJAYARAGHAVAN K, RADHAIAH G, PRAKASAM BS, SARMA KVR, REDDY V (1990). Effect of massive dose of vitamin A on morbidity and mortality in Indian children. *Lancet* **336**, pp 342–345.
47. WEST KP JR, POKHREL RP, KATZ J, LECLERQ SC, KHATRY SK, SHRESTHA SR, PRADHAN, EK, TIELSCH JM, PANDEY MR, SOMMER A (1991). Efficacy of vitamin A in reducing preschool child mortality in Nepal. *Lancet* **338**, pp 67–71.
48. DAULAIRE NMP, STARBUCK ES, HOUSTON RM, CHURCH MS, STUKEL TA, PANDEY MR (1992). Childhood mortality after a high dose of vitamin A in a high risk population. *BMJ* **304**, pp 207–210.
49. Ghana VAST Study Team (1993). Vitamin A supplementation in northern Ghana: effects on clinic attendances and hospital admissions, and child mortality. *Lancet* **342**, pp 7–12.
50. HERRERA MG, NESTEL P, EL AMIN A, FAWZI WW, MOHAMED KA, WELD L (1992). Vitamin A supplementation and child survival. *Lancet* **340**, pp 267–271.
51. WEST KP JR, IAN DARNTIN-HILL (2008). Vitamin A deficiency. *Nutrition and Health in Developing Countries*, 2nd edition. Richard D. Semba and Martin W. Bloem (eds), New Jersey, Humana Press, p 377.
52. TONASCIA JA (1993). Meta-analysis of published community trials: impact of vitamin A on mortality. Proceedings of the Bellagio meeting on vitamin A deficiency and childhood mortality. New York, Helen Keller International.
53. BEATON GH, MARTORELL R, ARONSON KJ, EDMONSTON B, MCCABE G, ROSS AC et al (1993). Effectiveness of vitamin A supplementation in the control of young child morbidity and mortality in developing countries. Geneva: Administrative Committee on Coordination – Sub Committee on Nutrition (ACC / SCN). ACC / SCN State of the Art Series Nutrition Policy Discussion Paper No. 13.
54. FAWZI WW, CHALMERS TC, HERRERA MG, MOSTELLAR E (1983). Vitamin A supplementation and child marketing – a meta-analysis. *JAMA* **269,** pp 898–903.
55. GLASZIOU PP, MACKERRAS DEM (1993). Vitamin A supplementation in infectious diseases: a meat analysis. *BMJ* **306**, pp 366–370.

56. RICE AL, WEST KP JR, BLACK RE. Vitamin A deficiency. In: *Comparative quantification of health risks. Global and regional burden of disease attributable to selected major risk factors*, vol 1. EZZATI M, LOPEZ AD, RODGERS A, MURRAY CJL (eds.). Geneva, World Health organisation **4**, pp 211–256.
57. Vitamin A and Pneumonia Working Group (1993). Potential interventions for the prevention of childhood pneumonia in developing countries: a meta-analysis of data from field trials to assess the impact of vitamin A supplementation on pneumonia morbidity and mortality. *Bulletin of World Health Organisation* **73**, pp 609–619.
58. GROTTO J, MIMOUNI M, GDALEVICH M, MIMOUNI D (2003). Vitamin A supplementation and childhood mortality from diarrhoea and respiratory infections: a meta analysis. *J Paed* **142**, pp 297–304.
59. CHRISTIAN P, WEST KP JR, KHATRY SK, KATZ J, SHRESHTHA SR, PRADHAN EK, LECLERQ SC, POKHREL RP (1998). Nightblindness of pregnancy in rural Nepal – nutritional and health risks. *Int J Epidemiol* **27**, pp 231–237.
60. SEMBA RD, DE PEE S, PANAGIDES D, POLY O, BLOEM MW (2003). Risk factors for night blindness among women of child bearing age in Cambodia. *Eur J Clin Nutr* **57**, pp 1627–1632.
61. UNDERWOOD BA (1990). Vitamin A prophylaxis programs in developing countries: past experiences and future prospects. *Nut Rev* **48**, pp 265–273.
62. SOMMER A, (1982). A field guide to detection and control of xerophthalmia.
63. SOMMER A, TARWOTJO I, HUSSAINI G, SUSANTO D, SOEGIHARTO T (1981). Incidence, prevalence and scale of blinding malnutrition. *Lancet* **1**, no. 8235, pp 1407–1408.
64. IVACG (2002). The Annecy Accords to assess and control Vitamin A deficiency. Summary of Recommendations and Clarifications. Washington, DC, IVACG Secretariat, c/o ILSI Research Foundation (available at: http://ivacg.ilsi.org/).
65. UNICEF (2007). Vitamin A supplementation – a decade of progress. 2007, New York.
66. WHO / UNICEF / IVACG (TASK FORCE), 1997. Vitamin A supplements – a guide to their use in the treatment and prevention of vitamin A deficiency and xerophthalmia, 2nd edition. WHO, Geneva.
67. HASKELL MJ, BROWN KH (1999). Maternal vitamin A nutriture and the vitamin A content of human milk. *J Mammary Gland Biol Neoplasia* **4**, pp 243–257.
68. REDDY V (2001). Benefits and safety of vitamin A supplementation during pregnancy and lactation in preschool children and pregnant and lactating women. Edited by U. Kapil and Srivastava, V.K., Ministry of Health and Family Welfare and All India Institute of Medical Sciences.
69. NEWMAN V. (1994). Vitamin A and breastfeeding: a comparison of data from developed and developing countries. *FNB* **15**, pp 161.
70. BHASKARAN P (2000). Vitamin A deficiency in infants: Effects of Postnatal maternal vitamin A supplement on growth and vitamin A status. *Nutr Res* **20**, pp 769.
71. STOLFUZ RJ, HAKIMI M, MILLER KW, RASMUSSEN KM, DAWIESAH S, HABICHT JP, DIBLEY MJ (1993). High dose vitamin A supplement of breast feeding Indonesian mothers: effects on vitamin A status of mother and infant. *J Nutr* **23**, pp 666.
72. TALUKDE A, ISLAM N, KLEMM R, BLOEM M (1993). Home gardening in South Asia. The complete handbook. HKI, Bangladesh.

73. SMITASIRI S, ATTIG GA, VALVASEVI A, DHANAMITTA S AND TONTISIRIN K (1992). Social marketing, vitamin A rich foods in Thailand, Institute of Mahidol University, ISBN 974-587-516-3.
74. NARASINGA RAO BS (1996). Bioavailability of â carotene from plant foods, *NFI Bulletin* **17**, no. 4, p. 1.
75. ZEITLIN MF, MEGAWANGI R, KRAMER EM and ARMSTRONG HC (1992). Mothers and children's intake of vitamin A in rural Bangladesh. *Am J Clin Nutr* **56**, pp. 136–147.
76. MINISTRY OF AGRICULTURE, GOVERNMENT OF INDIA, 1996. Increasing production of vitamin A rich horticulture crops – a long term solution to combat vitamin A deficiency, 1996, Department of Agriculture and Cooperation.
77. CHANDRASHEKHARAN N. Red palm oil for the prevention of vitamin A deficiency. Palm Oil Developments, 27.
78. LINDSAY A. et al (2006). Guidelines on food fortification with micronutrients, WHO, 2006, page 1122.
79. FAVARO RMD (1992). Evaluation of the effect of heat treatment on the biological value of vitamin A fortified soyabean oil, *Nutr Res* **12**, pp. 1357–1363.
80. Micronutrient Initiative (2009), Investing in the Future: A United Call to action on vitamin and mineral deficiencies, Global Report.
81. DARY O AND MARA JO (2002). Food fortification to reduce vitamin A deficiency. *J of Nutr* **132**, no. 9S, pp. 2927S–2933S.
82. PHILLIPS M, SANGHVI T, SUAREZ R, MCKIGNEY J, FIDLER J (1996). The cost of effectiveness of three vitamin A interventions in Guatemala. *Soc Sci Med* **42**, pp. 1661–1668.
83. SOLON FS, LATHAM MC, GUIRRIEC R, FLORENTINO R, WILLIAMSON DF AND AGUILAR J (1985). Fortification of MSG with vitamin A: the Philippines experience. *Food Technology* **39**, pp. 71–79.
84. BEATON, G. H., et al (1994). Vitamin A supplementation and child morbidity and mortality in developing countries. *Food and Nutr Bulletin* **15**, pp. 282–289.
85. IVACG Policy statement on vitamin A, diarrhoea and measles. Washington, Int Vitamin A consultation Group, 1996.
86. HUTTLY SRS, MORRIS SS, PISSANI V (1997). Prevention of diarrhoea in young children in developing countries. *Bulletin of the World Health Organisation* **75**, pp. 163–174.
87. BHASKARAN P AND VISWESWARA RK (1997). Enhancement in sero conversion on simultaneous administration of measles vaccine and vitamin A at 9 months old Indian infants. *Ind J. Paed* **54**, p. 234.
88. SRIKANTIA SG AND REDDY V (1970). Effect of a single massive dose of vitamin A on serum and liver levels of vitamin. *Amer J. Clin. Nutr* **23**, pp. 114–118.
89. MYHRE AM, CARLSEN MH, BOHN SK, WOLD HL, LAAKE P and BLOMHOFF R (2003). Water miscible, emulsified and solid forms of retinol supplements are more toxic than oil based preparations. *Am J Clin Nutr* **78**, pp. 1152–1159.
90. Ministry of Health (2001). Policy on Management of Vitamin A deficiency, Ministry of Health and Family Welfare, Government of India.
91. WHO/OMS (Dec 1988). Expanded programme on immunisation and vitamin A deficiency: time for action. Immunisation services can help.
92. ROSS DA (2002). Recommendations for vitamin A supplementation. *J of Nutr* **132**, no. 9S, pp. 2902.
93. DIXIT DT (1966). Night blindness in third trimester of pregnancy. *Ind J Med Res* **54**, pp. 791–795.

94. KATZ J, KHTATRY SK, WEST KP JR, HUMPHREY JH, LECLARQ SC, KIMBOROUGH E, POHKREL PR and SOMMER A (1995). Nightblindness is prevalent during pregnancy and lactation in rural Nepal. *J of Nutr* **125**, pp. 2122–2127.
95. CHRISTIAN P, SCHULTZEK K, STOLZFUS RJ and WEST KP JR (1998). Hypretinolemia, illness symptoms and acute phase protein responses in pregnant women with and without night blindness. *Am J Clin Nutr* **67**, pp. 1237–1243.
96. CHRISTIAN P, WEST KP JR, KHATRY SK, KIMBOROUGH-PRADHAN E, LECLERQ SC, KATZ J, SHRESHTHA SR, DAL SM and SOMMER A (2000). Night blindness during pregnancy and subsequent mortality among women in Nepal effects of vitamin A and â carotene supplementation. *Am J Epidemiol* **152**, pp. 542–547.
97. LINDSAY HA AND HASKELL M (2002). Estimating the potential for vitamin A toxicity in women and young children. *J Nutr* **132**, no. 9S, pp. 2907S–2919S.
98. WHO AND MICRONUTRIENT INITIATIVE (1998). Safe vitamin A dosage during pregnancy and lactation. Recommendation and report of a consultation. WHO, 1998.
99. UNICEF (2005). Vitamin A supplementation: progress for child survival. Working paper prepared by the nutrition section, UNICEF, HQ (2005).
100. Global eradication of poliomyelitis by the year 2000. Geneva, World Health Organisation, 1988, 41st World Health assembly, Resolution WHA 41.28.
101. Distribution of vitamin A' during national immunisation days: a "generic" addendum to the field guide for supplementary activities aimed at achieving polio eradication, 1996 revision. Geneva, WHO (1998), vaccines and Biological, WHO, 1211, Geneva 27, Switzerland.
102. WHO (1998). Expanded programme on immunisation – using national immunisation day to deliver vitamin A. Global programme for vaccines and immunisation, WHO, Geneva.
103. WORLD SUMMIT FOR CHILDREN (1990). World Declaration on the survival, protection and development of children and plan of action for implementing the World Declaration on the survival, protection and development of children in the 1990s. World Summit for children, United Nations. New York, 30th Sept, UN, 1990.
104. World Declaration and Plan of Action for Nutrition, International Conference on Nutrition, Rome, Dec 1992. Geneva, World Health Organisation, 1992.
105. Joint statement: Policy and operational questions relating to vitamin A and EPI/NIDs, Geneva, WHO/UNICEF, 1998.
106. VIR SC (2001). Linkage of vitamin A massive dose supplements administration with pulse polio immunisation – an overview (2001). In benefits and safety of administration of vitamin A to pre school children and pregnant and lactating women. Edited by U. Kapil and Srivastava, V.K. Ministry of Health and Family Welfare and All India Institute of Medical Sciences, New Delhi.
107. HKI (2000). Linking vitamin A and immunisation programme. *HKI Cambodia Bulletin* **2**, no. 3.
108. MI/UNICEF/TULANE UNIVERSITY. Progress in controlling vitamin A deficiency, 1998, Ottawa, Canada.
109. Vitamin A Global Initiative (1998). A strategy for acceleration of progress in combating vitamin A deficiency: consensus of an informal technical consultation, New York, 18-19th Dec 1998.
110. AGUAYO VM, GARNIER D AND BAKER SK (2007). Drops of life. Vitamin A supplementation for child survival. Progress and lessons learned in West and Central Africa.

111. VIR SC, PRASAD LB, JAIN A, SINGH R, ATEGBO EA, HETTIARATCHY N AND SCHULTINK W (2007). Vitamin A Supplementation Programme an effective entry point for addressing Malnutrition in the State of Uttar Pradesh, India. Abstract In Consequences and Control of Micronutrient Deficiencies – Science, Policy and programme – Defining the Issues, 16–18th April, 2007, Istanbul, Turkey.
112. WEST KP JR, SOMMER A. Delivery of oral doses of vitamin A to prevent vitamin A deficiency and nutritional blindness, Rome. United Nations Administration Committee on Coordination, Subcommittee on Nutrition, 1993, State of the Art Series, Nutrition Policy Discussion Paper No. 2.
113. LOEVINSOHN BP, SUTLER RN, COSTALES MO (1993). Using cost-effectiveness analysis to evaluate targeting strategies: the case of vitamin A supplementation. *Health Policy Plan* **12**, pp. 29–37.
114. BHASKARAN P, KRISHNASWAMY K (2000). Vitamin A Supplementation Strategies – Indian Status. In Benefits and Safety of Administration of Vitamin A to preschool children and pregnant and Lactating Women edited by Kapil U and Srivastava VK, pp. 45–58.
115. BAUERNFEIND JC, The Safe use of vitamin A: A report of the international Consultative Group (IVACG), Washington DC, The Nutrition Foundation, 1980.
116. MILLER DR and HAYES KC (1982). Vitamin excess and toxicity. In: *Nutritional Toxicity*, vol 1, JN Hathcock (ed.), New York: Academic press, pp. 81–133, 1982.
117. BENEDICH A and LANGSETH L (1989). Safety of Vitamin A. *Am J. Clin Nutr* **49**, pp. 358–371.
118. HATHCOCK JN (1990). Evaluation of vitamin a toxicity. *Amer J. Clin. Nutr* **52**, pp. 183–202.
119. NALUBOLA R and NESTEL P (1999). The Effect of vitamin A Nutriture on Health-A Review. ILSI Press.
120. MOST, the USAID Micronutrient Program, Vitamin A Capsule Distribution: Key Behavioral and Communication Issues.

17

Vitamin A prevention and control programme in India – past efforts and current status

Sheila C. Vir and *Richa Singh Pandey*

Sheila C Vir, MSc, PhD, is a senior nutrition consultant and Director of Public Health Nutrition and Development Centre, New Delhi. Following MSc (Food and Nutrition) from University of Delhi, Dr Vir was awarded PhD by the Queen's University of Belfast, United Kingdom. Dr. Vir, a past secretary of the Nutrition Society of India, is a recipient of the fellowship of the Department of Health and Social Services, UK, and Commonwealth Van den Bergh Nutrition Award. Dr Vir worked briefly with the Aga Khan Foundation (India) and later with UNICEF. As a Nutrition Programme Officer with UNICEF for twenty years, Dr. Vir provided strategic and technical leadership for policy formulation and implementation of nutrition programmes in India.

Richa Singh Pandey, MD (Community Medicine), has several years of experience in the field of public health and nutrition. Dr. Singh is currently a nutrition specialist with UNICEF (India). Prior to joining UNICEF, she worked on an important newborn care project with Saksham Study group of Johns Hopkins–King George Medical College Collaborative Centre and as a consultant with UNICEF on maternal child health and nutrition issues.

17.1 Vitamin A deficiency status in India

Vitamin A deficiency (VAD) has been recognised as a major public health problem in India since 1960s. Surveys carried out in the southern and eastern parts of the country during this period had revealed that at least 30–50% of all children in the preschool age group suffered from eye manifestations as a result of deficiency of vitamin A [1]. It was estimated that about 12,000–14,000 children became blind in the country as result of keratomalacia caused due to severe deficiency of vitamin A. Studies of the past two decades indicate a substantial reduction in severe VAD problem and a reduction in ocular signs caused due to deficiency of vitamin A (Table 17.1). Such a decreasing trend observed in the

Table 17.1 Reported prevalence of VAD in India

Year	*Prevalence (%)*	*Criteria*
1971–74	2.0	Nutritional blindness(a) [2]
1975–79	2.0	Bitot's spot(c) [3]
1988–90	0.7	Bitot's spot(c) [4]
1995	1.4	Bitot's spot(a) [5]
1998	0.21	Bitot's spot(b) [6]
1998	0.11	Corneal xerosis(b) [6]
1998	0.05	Keratomalacia(b) [6]
1998	0.05	Corneal opacity(b) [6]
2000	0.7–2.2	Bitot's spot [7]
2000	1.2–4.0	Night blindness [7]

prevalence of VAD coincides with the implementation of the National Vitamin A Prophylaxis Programme in the entire country in the early 1970s under the Fourth Five Year Plan [1].

No national survey on prevalence of VAD has been undertaken in the country. The Ministry of Human Resource, however, has compiled data of three major surveys and developed a national database on clinical signs of xerophthalmia [6]. The emerging national profile on prevalence of VAD indicates a wide variation in VAD prevalence in 26 states/union territories (Table 17.2).VAD surveys within a state report a wide intra-district and cluster to cluster variation in VAD prevalence in preschool children [8].

Despite reduction in clinical signs of VAD, subclinical deficiency of vitamin A continues to be widespread. This is evident from the data presented in Table 17.3 [9–11]. Subclinical VAD as measured by serum retinol levels, below 0.7 μg/dl [9–11], in children below 6 years is reported to be between 34% and 60% while the corresponding clinical VAD prevalence is found to be rather low. The data available from the Indian Council of Medical Research (1999) from 5 districts indicate an average prevalence rate of 1.84% night blindness, 1.12% Bitot's spot and 0.15% corneal scars [12]. These survey findings confirm vitamin A deficiency disorders (VADD) is a public health problem in India.

The primary cause of widespread VADD in preschool children is low dietary intake of vitamin A and carotenoids by infants and children (Table 17.4) [6, 13, 14]. The average intake of vitamin A by preschool children is reported to range between 106 and 214 mg with almost 80 percent have intakes less than 50 percent of the recommended dietary allowance (RDA). Such low intake of vitamin A combined with recurrent infection result in poor vitamin A status of preschool children.

Table 17.2 Prevalence (%) of vitamin A deficiency signs in 26 states/union territories (UTs) of India [6]

State/UT	*Bitot's spot*
Haryana	0.04
Mizoram	2.97
Himachal Pradesh	0.01
Nagaland	0.35
Punjab	0.12
Tripura	0.02
Rajasthan	0.22
Dadra Nagar Haveli	0.38
Chandigarh	0
Daman & Diu	0.05
Delhi	0.05
Goa	0
Bihar	0.14
Gujarat	0.20
Sikkim	0.19
Maharashtra	0.72
Orissa	0.86
Kerala	0.25
Arunachal Pradesh	0.34
Karnataka	0.77
Assam	0.45
Tamil Nadu	3.11
Manipur	0.14
Andhra Pradesh	0.79
Meghalaya	0.18
Madhya Pradesh	2.62

Table 17.3 Prevalence of vitamin A deficiency in children in the state of UP [9–11]

Districts	*Prevalence of Bitot's spot (%)*	*Plasma retinol (% <0.07 μg/dl)*	*Plasma retinol (% <0.35 μg/dl)*
Dehradun	0.02	–	–
Badaun	0.0	–	–
Mainpuri	0.96	–	–
L.Kheri	0.46	55.8	4.2
Bahraich	5.6	–	–
Hardoi	–	38.8	4.1
Sitapur	–	50.0	3.0
Rai Bareilly	–	33.8	4.2
Unnao	–	44.8	12.7
Lucknow	–	59.7	12.6

Table 17.4 Intake of vitamin A (IU/day) [6,13,14]

Vitamin A intake (IU/day)		*1-3 years*	*4-6 years*
RDA		400	400
(1998)	intake	201	214
	% RDA	50	60
2002	intake	106	127
	% RDA	26.5	31.8
2006	intake	129	166
	% RDA	32.3	41.5

Maternal VAD is reported to be common in India. Clinical reports published during 1960s indicated problem of night blindness in pregnant and lactating women [15, 16, 17]. Night blindness during pregnancy has also been reported in the nutritional surveys undertaken in India in the last decade [6, 18, 19]. Studies from the National Institute of Nutrition indicated 4% of pregnant women belonging to low socio-economic status had night blindness during the third trimester while all the pregnant women surveyed had low serum retinol levels <30 g/dl [19]. The data of the DWCD and the National Family Health Surveys 2 [6, 18] confirm that maternal night blindness (Table 17.5) is prevalent and that there is wide variation from state to state [7, 18]. Nutrition survey among tea estate women workers in Assam state in 2008 also reveals that 16.3 percent women during the last pregnancy had a history of night blindness [20]. The high prevalence of maternal night blindness is a proxy indicator of vitamin A deficiency in a community. A percentage prevalence rate of over 5 percent maternal night blindness indicates VAD to be a public health problem in the population surveyed [21].

17.2 Measures taken for prevention and control of VAD

Recognizing vitamin A deficiency to be a public health problem, efforts have been made in India since 1970s to control the deficiency. Promotion of diets rich in vitamin A including promotion of exclusive breastfeeding to infants in the first six months and appropriate complementary feeding from six months onwards have been recognised to be the long-term solution to overcome VAD. Role of food fortification of dairy products and fats and oils in controlling VAD has been considered important. Efforts are being directed to identify suitable food vehicles for vitamin A fortification. Higher priority is being accorded for ensuring access to vitamin A fortified foods by economically deprived population. Appreciating the slow progress in dietary intervention measures, intensive efforts are continuously being made to strengthen the vitamin A supplement (VAS) administration programme for preschool children and establish a suitable VAS delivery

Table 17.5 Prevalence of clinical vitamin A deficiency [6, 18]

State/UT	*Bitot's spot (%) [7]*	*Maternalnightblindness opacity [18]*
Delhi	0.05	3.8
Haryana	0.04	1
Himachal Pradesh	0.01	3.8
Chandigarh	0	
Jammu & Kashmir		18.5
Punjab	0.12	0.8
Rajasthan	0.22	14.7
Madhya Pradesh	2.62	19.7
Uttar Pradesh		14
Bihar	0.14	19.4
Orissa	0.86	18.7
West Bengal		11.6
Arunachal Pradesh	0.34	20.2
Assam	0.45	6.9
Manipur	0.14	8.5
Meghalaya	0.18	23.9
Mizoram	2.97	14.6
Nagaland	0.35	21.1
Sikkim	0.19	21.6
Goa	0	2.2
Gujarat	0.20	10.9
Maharashtra	0.72	9.7
Andhra Pradesh	0.79	5.3
Dadra & Nagar Haveli	0.38	
Daman & Diu	0	
Karnataka	0.77	6.3
Kerala	0.25	2.1
Tamil Nadu	3.11	3.7
Tripura	0.02	
WHO cut-off for public health problem	> 0.5%	Do not exist

mechanism to ensure each preschool child receives at least two doses of VAS six months apart in a year. This chapter primarily focuses on the vitamin A supplementation component of the VAD programme.

17.3 Vitamin A supplementation programme

In India VAS programme implementation commenced in 1970 and it was the first country to launch the VAS administration programme. The evolvement of the VAS programme in the last three decades, with reference to policy and delivery mechanism model, can be broadly divided into the following three phases:

- Phase I – Launch of Vitamin A Prophylaxis Programme for Prevention of Nutritional Blindness, 1971
- Phase II – Revision of Policy in 1991 and Integration of Vitamin A Programme with the child survival efforts

- Phase III – Acceleration of vitamin A programme — establishing effective biannual VAS Delivery Model, 2000

(a) Phase I – National Vitamin A Prophylaxis Programme for Prevention of Blindness

In India, the National Programme for Prevention of Vitamin A Deficiency was launched by the Ministry of Health and Family Welfare in 1971 as nutritional blindness prevention programme under the Fourth Five Year Plan [1, 22]. It was estimated that such a programme will prevent vitamin A deficiency which was contributing to about 20% of all cases of blindness [23]. The most important rational approach to address the problem of VAD was to increase the dietary intake of vitamin A. Such an approach was viewed as a time-consuming complex process which would delay in preventing children from going blind. Urgent measures were required. Administration of massive dose of vitamin A supplementation (VAS) was the solution proposed to prevent VAD and associated blindness [1].

The national programme initially focused on children residing in only seven states of the country where VAD prevalence was considered high [22]. Later, the programme was extended to all other states. Under the programme children 1–5 years received 2 ml of syrup providing 200,000 IU of vitamin A, once in six months. The dosage and frequency was based on clinic-based studies by Srikantia and Reddy in 1969 and 1970 [24, 25]. These studies concluded that oral administration of 300,000 IU of oil soluble preparation of vitamin A was associated with less toxicity and also sustained normal serum retinol levels for a period of six months. It was observed that in situation where dietary intakes were very poor, the levels were maintained for a period of 3–4 months [26]. Extensive field trials were undertaken involving 2500 preschool rural children who were administered 300,000 IU vitamin A in oil once a year over a period of five years. The prevalence of ocular signs of vitamin A deficiency was reduced by 75% from a baseline of 10%. No new cases of corneal lesions were reported during the study period [27]. Based on these trials, it was recommended that all children at risk be given vitamin A supplement of 200,000 IU biannually to prevent blindness. Such a dose was considered appropriate to prevent blindness and was not expected to completely build up the stores and prevent vitamin A deficiency. Based on these recommendations of the dosage, a meeting of state officers was organised in June 1970 and an operational plan for the national VAS programme was developed.

The vitamin A programme was launched in 1971. In view of the limited resources, the programme was initially confined to such areas where prevalence of vitamin A deficiency was believed to be high. The programme in the first year aimed at covering all children 1–3 years. Later under the programme, all children of 1–5 years were recommended to be provided with six monthly dosage of 200,000 IU vitamin A. Initially 1.6 million children in 7 states of the country were covered [22]. The technical information issued by the Maternal Child Health (MCH : No.2) stated "As coverage of the entire age group and avoidance of any repeated administration of the drug are of great importance, it is desirable to fix a specified period for administering the programme. For example, the primary health centre/urban MCH centre may decide to cover all eligible children during the month of September 1970 and complete the administration of the drug during the period of one month; the administration of the next dose to these children as well as new children to be included, would then have to be done in March 1971 only" [1].

Vitamin A, specially prepared for the programme, contained 100,000 IU per ml of syrup. A spoon of 2 ml was supplied with each 100 cc bottle of vitamin A solution .The Maternal and Child Health and Family Welfare Organization was responsible for the implementation of the programme through the primary health centres. The Auxiliary Nurse Midwife (ANM) and other paramedical working in primary health centres were responsible for administering the VAS concentrate to children in rural centres, under the supervision of medical officers. In urban areas, the programme was instructed to be administered at child welfare clinics of urban family planning centres. For effective coverage and to avoid repeated administration, it was recommended that the distribution be done during a fixed time period, on a "crash" basis instead of spreading it over prolonged periods.

An interim evaluation was undertaken in two states, Karnataka and Kerala, after the children had received at least two massive doses of vitamin A. The coverage was 75–90% of the expected number of children and there was 75% reduction in the prevalence of conjunctiva signs of vitamin A deficiency in children who had received two doses of vitamin A [22]. The results demonstrated the administration feasibility of VAS on large scale and indicated that massive dose of vitamin A could be administered as a public health programme without requiring any significant additional inputs. On the basis of these findings, the vitamin A programme was later extended to several states.

In 1975, the Department of Family Welfare of the Government of India assigned the task of a comprehensive evaluation of the vitamin A massive dose programme to the National Institute of Nutrition in 1975 [3]. The programme was evaluated in 1976. Thirteen states where the programme was in operation for a minimum period of two years at the time of evaluation in 1978 were selected [22]. These 13 states were Andhra Pradesh, Bihar, Gujarat, Haryana, Karnataka, Kerala, Orissa, Madhya Pradesh, Maharashtra, Rajasthan, Tamil Nadu, Uttar Pradesh and West Bengal. The evaluation was finally conducted in only 8 states between January and July 1978 and the 5 states that were excluded for various reasons were Bihar, Madhya Pradesh, Haryana, Tamil Nadu and Uttar Pradesh. About 69,000 children were covered and the incidence of Bitot's spot was assessed age-wise to study the impact of the massive dose of vitamin A and to evaluate the operational aspects. The findings revealed that the programme guidelines of "crash programme approach", particularly with respect to administering VAS during the fixed months of the year, were not followed in many primary health centres, except in two of the eight states, i.e. Andhra Pradesh and Karnataka. Vomiting was reported to be the side effect of commonly encountered by almost all 33 workers of 42 sub-centres interviewed while diarrhoea and fever were reported occasionally. All workers mentioned such side effects were observed in children under two years and were transitory. These symptoms "subsided by itself" [3]. Recording of information on vitamin A dose administered was poor except in Karnataka where separate record registers were provided. Massive dose of vitamin A supplements were reported to be well accepted by community and effort to create awareness was considered essential. The study identified several operational problems including problems in supply of vitamin A, poor knowledge of the programme amongst functionaries, reliance on clinic rather than extension approach and low community awareness.

(b) Phase II – Reformulation of policy and its implementation

The Government of India in September 1988 constituted a Task Force [28] to study various operational issues of the National Prophylaxis Programme for Prevention of Blindness Due to Vitamin A deficiency (NPPVAD) and propose measures for increasing VAS coverage. It was observed by the Task Force that NPPVAD was implemented as a part of the Maternal and Child Health (MCH) programme of the health sector but was a low priority programme. It was estimated that only 30-million or 30% of the children in the vulnerable age group of 1–5 years were being covered under the programme.

For improving VAS coverage, as per the direction of the Task Force, a study on the supply stock situation of vitamin A concentrate dose manufactured and supplied under the NPPVAD was undertaken [29]. The supply study reported that in 1985, the projected consumption of vitamin A in the country was 90 million mega units (MMU) and of this only 11.76 MMU was for vitamin A prophylaxis programme while the rest was allocated for use as additive to vanaspati, cattle and poultry feed and other pharmaceutical uses. Following report of the production and supply of vitamin A in India, it was proposed by the Task Force on 8th May 1989 to link VAS administration with Universal Immunisation Programme or UIP (including the first dose of vitamin A administered at the time of measles vaccine and the second with DPT booster). It was envisaged that such a system for VAS delivery would result in achieving a high coverage with VAS in preschool children without causing any additional pressure on the existing infrastructural and operational costs. With such a strategy of linking VAS with UIP, it was projected that by 1995, the requirement for vitamin A supplement would increase significantly to 25 MMU from 10 MMU. It was recommended that the existing technology for the production of vitamin A supplement therefore be updated to meet the increase in supply requirement and VAS be made available at a reasonable controlled price. The price of syrup was then estimated to be Rs 28 per 100 ml or about 56 paise (1.2 US cents) for one mega dose of 200,000 IU (equivalent to 110 mg vitamin A Palmitate or 66 mg of vitamin A acetate). The guidelines issued by WHO in 1988 for improving coverage of vitamin A dosage by linking with Expanded Programme Immunisation or EPI [30] gave an impetus to the decision of the Task Force of the Ministry of Health and Family Welfare, Government of India to consider linking vitamin A massive dose programme with the Universal Immunisation Programme (UIP).

The World Summit for Children in 1991 drew the attention of global leaders for urgently addressing the problem of VAD and for directing efforts to rapidly improve the vitamin A supplement coverage of preschool children for reducing child mortality and improving child survival [31]. The Government of India revisited the NPPVAD which had been in operation in the entire country since the Fourth Five Year Maternal Child Health (MCH) Plan. The Ministry of Health and Family Welfare in 1990, in collaboration with UNICEF, constituted an expert Task Force under the chairmanship of Commissioner MCH [33]. The Task Force primarily debated on the issue of inclusion of infants 6–12 months as beneficiaries of VAS programme, proposing a suitable delivery system for administering VAS to infants, overall management of NPPVAD and proposing the treatment dosage for clinical cases of VAD. The Task Force took into consideration the increasing evidence that vitamin A supplement administration (VAS) influenced child survival and that the impact of VAS was not limited to mere prevention of nutritional blindness. The protective effect of vitamin A supplement during episodes of measles and the advantages of administering massive dose of vitamin A supplement at 9 months along with measles vaccine was reviewed [30]. The Task Force agreed to include children 6–11 months in the vitamin A programme and administer VAS dose of 100,000 IU. For administering VAS to infants, the contact with infants during measles vaccination at 9 months was considered practical. The combined VAS-measles vaccine administration policy was further supported and influenced by the findings of the National Institute of Nutrition (NIN) which observed that seroconversion rates of measles vaccine were significantly improved (84%) when vitamin A supplement was co-administered with vaccine compared to low rate (63%) under routine field conditions of immunization. This combined schedule was reported to be effective in improving serum retinol levels [33]. Such a strategy was found to be beneficial, safe and feasible. In 1991, based on the recommendations of the Task Force, a new revised "Policy on Management of Vitamin A Deficiency" was formulated [34] and issued by the Ministry of Health and Family Welfare of the Government of India (Box 17.1).

Box 17.1 Policy on management of vitamin A deficiency 1991 [34]

"Administration of massive dose of vitamin A to preschool children at periodic intervals is a simple, effective and most direct intervention strategy. This is a short term strategy.

Under the massive dose programme every infant 6–11 months and children 1–5 years is to be administered vitamin A every 6 months. Priority is to be given for coverage of children 6 months – 3 years since the highest prevalence of clinical signs of vitamin A deficiency is reported in these age group. The recommended schedule is as follows:

6-11 months – 1 dose of 100, 000 IU

1-5 years – 200, 000 / 6 months

A child must receive a total of 9 oral doses of vitamin A by its 5th birthday.

The contact with an infant during administration of measles vaccine between the age of 9–12 months is considered a practical time for administrating the vitamin A supplement – 100, 000 IU for infants. A camp approach may be used for administering vitamin A to children 1–3 years and 3–5 years. However, the DPT /OPV booster in mid 2nd year to a child is a suitable time for the 2nd dose of vitamin A. Wherever ICDS programme is functioning, AWW should be involved in the distribution and administration of vitamin A.

Treatment dose – all children with clinical signs of vitamin A deficiency must be treated as early as possible. Treatment schedule is to administer 200,000 IU of vitamin A immediately after diagnosis. This must be followed by another dose of 200,000 IU 1–4 weeks later. Children with eye lesions must be treated immediately with vitamin A even if they are being refereed for special care.

Vitamin A syrup concentrate, as per the Policy, be made available at primary health centres and sub-health centres in the form of flavoured syrup at a concentration of 100,000 IU/ml or 100,000 IU capsule only for 6-11 months (fixed dose 100,000 IU vitamin A capsules is referred in the Policy). For children 1–5, vitamin A only in syrup form is recommended. Vitamin A solution bottle, once opened, is advised to be utilized within 6–8 weeks.

The Policy also focuses on promoting consumption of vitamin A rich food. Breastfeeding, including feeding of colostrum is emphasized. Feeding of locally available β-carotene (precursor of vitamin A) rich food such as green leafy vegetables and yellow and orange vegetables and fruits like pumpkin, carrots, papaya, mango, oranges etc along with cereal and pulse to a weaning child is stressed and should be promoted. In addition, whenever economically feasible consumption of milk, cheese, paneer, yogurt, ghee, eggs, liver, etc. is advised to be promoted.

The Policy emphasizes on the dietary measures – promotion of breastfeeding, including feeding of colostrum, and foods rich in vitamin A as well as recommends universal coverage of children 6 months to 5 years with six monthly high dose vitamin A supplements (Box 17.1). A total of nine doses of VAS are instructed to be administered by the fifth birthday while priority for administration of VAS is instructed to be given to children between 6 months and 3 years. The Policy recognizes that the contact with infants during measles immunization is a practical approach for providing the first dose of vitamin A to a large number of children 6–11 months. The policy also defines the vitamin A supplementation schedule for treatment of VAD cases.

India VAD programme Policy does not include prophylactic VAS administration for women in the reproductive age. During pregnancy and lactation, the need for regular dietary intake of vitamin A rich foods by pregnant and lactating mothers in mproving diet is emphasized. The public health strategy focuses on bringing about changes in dietary practices of the population through education and horticultural interventions. The Policy does not refer to any interventions even for treatment of maternal VAD. However, treatment of individual women with night blindness and Bitot's spot is addressed by daily supplements of a much smaller dose of VAS of 5000–10,000 IU vitamin A per day a period of 4–6 weeks. With the emerging evidence that vitamin A content of breast milk is influenced by the maternal vitamin A status, it has been proposed that diagnosis and management of VAD be considered to be a part of routine antenatal care [35].

In 1992, the Policy guidelines for the administration of VAS to preschool children, including infants at nine months, were incorporated as one of the major activities of the Child Survival & Safe Motherhood (CSSM) Programme [36]. The VAS administration under the CSSM Programme focused only on children of 9 months to 3 years and children over 3–5 years were excluded in the operational plan. The CSSM Programme guidelines emphasized that the first dose of vitamin A (100,000 IU) be administered at nine months along with measles vaccine while contacts with children at 18 months for the DPT/OPV booster dose was considered an appropriate time for the second dose (200,000 IU). Remaining 3 doses of VAS of 200,000 IU each were to be given at six monthly intervals to children 18 months to 3 years. Treatment dose recommended in the Policy was included in the CSSM Programme. Additionally, therapeutic doses of VAS were recommended to be administered to those suffering from diarrhoea, measles and acute respiratory infections presenting with signs of vitamin A deficiency. Later, these guidelines on VAS administration that were issued under the CSSM Programme continued to be implemented under the Reproductive and

Child Health (RCH) programme which was launched with the modification of the CSSM programme [8].

Under the CSSM and later under the RCH programme, six bottles of vitamin A supplement (VAS) syrup of 100 cc were supplied for a population of 5000, as part of "drug kit A" of the government. This was supplied every six months i.e. a total of 12 bottles of 100 cc per 5000 population per year using the following calculation (Box 17.2). The VAS supply projection was based on the assumption that a subcentre would have an average population of 5000. The supply estimated was inadequate since the population covered by the subcentre was often as high as 7000–8000 for the high population states of Uttar Pradesh, Bihar, Madhya Pradesh, Orissa, Rajasthan, etc. The VAS programme implementation was monitored as a part of the RCH programme monitoring system. However, it was observed that the record of VAS administration was maintained for only the first dose of VAS which was administered to infants along with measles vaccine.

Box 17.2 Estimation of Vitamin A supplement supplied in Kit A under CSSM/RCH programmes

1. Subcentre population = 5000
2. Birth rate (BR) = 25/1000 live births
3. Infants born per year = BR × subcentre population = 25/1000 × 5000 = 125
4. Children between 1–2 year = 125
5. Children between 2–3 years = 125
6. Requirement of 100 cc VAS Syrup bottles
   (a) Requirement of doses for children 9-12 months = 125 × 1 ml = 125 ml
   (b) Requirement of vitamin A doses for children 1–2 yrs = 125 X 2 ml × 2 times a year = 500 ml
   (c) Requirement of vitamin A doses for children > 2–3 yrs = 125 × 2 ml × 2 times a year = 500 ml
   (d) Total requirement = 125 + 500 + 500 = 1125 ml
7. Total bottles required = 1125/100 ml = 11.25 = 12 bottles

The strategy of linking first dose of VAS with measles vaccine administration proved practical [8, 38]. The national coverage for VAS increased to 48.9% as against the all India measles coverage of 55.2% [37]. Sixteen states reported the coverage of over 55% for both measles vaccine and vitamin A administration indicating that the linkage of administrating VAS with measles vaccine was effective in reaching children 6–12 months. On the other hand, coverage of children 1–3 years with the second and third dose continued to be as low as 3 percent – in fact the drop out rate from the first to the third dose was reported to be 91% [7]. In 1998, studies conducted in Madhya Pradesh and West Bengal highlighted the constraints in vitamin A programme with regard to inadequate and irregular supply of VAS, poor logistics management and monitoring. The study of Madhya Pradesh also reported that only 28% children had ever received vitamin A syrup [39].

The findings of national and state surveys revealed that the strategy of integrating vitamin A supplementation into routine health services of RCH had improved the coverage of children only within the first year of life .Once children were immunized, there was no contact of children with the health system except when children were sick. It was therefore evident that a mechanism was required to reach children with VAS during the critical years of preschool children. A delivery approach for VAS that would reach out to a much larger number of children under 5 years was apparently essential to attain the levels of population coverage that would result in achieving the full potential of benefits of vitamin A supplement on child survival [8, 9, 39]. A need for an establishment of a reliable delivery mechanism to reach children with the six monthly dosage of VAS was considered critical. The challenge for the success of VAS programme was to address programme issues such as irregularity in supply of vitamin A, poor orientation of the functionaries who were providing the services to the population, lack of supervision and lack of inter-sector coordination between the health functionaries and the Integrated Child Development Services (ICDS) functionaries.

(c) Phase III – Emergence of VAS Delivery System Models

In mid 1990s, there was a global level effort to revive the VAS programme by linking VAS administration with polio NIDs (National Immunisation Days). In July 1998, a Joint WHO /UNICEF statement [40] encouraged all countries where VAD was a public health problem to include policy of administration of age appropriate VAS dosage to children during NIDs – an integration of "two powerful child survival tools". Between October 1999 to March 2000, VAS administration linkage with polio vaccine was administered in two states, Orissa and Uttar Pradesh [41, 42]. Linking vitamin A with Pulse Polio Immunization (PPI) provided different experiences. In Orissa, where a systematic effort was made to link VAS administration with PPI, the coverage rates were high. The risk of immediate side effects such as fever, nausea and vomiting reported from Orissa was about 3% for children administered vitamin A dose along with oral polio vaccine. This incidence of illness reported in children with combined VAS and polio administration was similar to those who received only vitamin A or received neither VAS nor OPV [8, 41]. In the state of Uttar Pradesh, the coverage of VAS showed a wide variation and the poor coverage was attributed to poor logistic support as well as poor organization, training and absence of monitoring mechanism [8]. The

National Consultation on vitamin A held in September 2000 recommended not linking VAS administration with polio vaccine administration in the country and alternative strategies to be explored for improving VAS coverage [43].The strategy of administering VAS along with measles vaccine at 9 months was recommended to be continued. The significance of ensuring VAS supplementation during the second half of infancy was considered critical for the reported benefits on child health [35].

In early 2000, a number of delivery strategies were experimented for vitamin A supplement (VAS) administration such as intensive campaign approach as well as the biannual delivery strategy [8]. The early trials of the biannual strategy in the two fixed months of the year (June and December), undertaken in the state of Uttar Pradesh, were reviewed by the expert working group of the Tenth Five Year Plan. The biannual strategy model was considered appropriate for up scaling the vitamin A programme in the country under the Tenth Five Year Plan [44]. It was stated in the Plan that the administration of 2nd to 5th doses of vitamin A be linked to routine immunization days in the two fixed months of the year.

A number of states launched the biannual strategy with modifications introduced by the state governments in the operational plan. Between 2001 and 2008, the fixed month biannual strategy programme was reported to have been established in at least 10 states – Assam, Bihar, Chattisgarh, Gujrat, Jharkhand, Karnatka, Madhya Pradesh, Orissa, Tamil Nadu, Uttar Pradesh. In September 2007, all children upto 5 years and not only upto 3 years were instructed by the Government of India to be covered under the VAS Programme in the entire country [45]. The instruction of the government to include children over 3–5 years under the RCH-2 was revived (earlier also stated in the Vitamin A Management Policy of 1991 of the Government of India [34] which included all children 6 months to 5 years) since reaching all preschool children was considered critical for improving child survival.

The biannual strategy of vitamin A programme emphasizes on the organization of six-monthly VAS administration sessions in fixed period of the year along with community mobilization. As per the biannual strategy, two months, six months apart are identified as VAS months, when vitamin A doses are to be administered. All states follow the RCH guidelines and administer the first dose to infants only at nine months. However, the strategy for administering the first dose differs. Some states continue to administer the first dose along with measles vaccine while others adopt the strategy of giving all the nine doses to children 9 months to 5 years in the fixed designated months. Vitamin A supplementation is administered through the existing network of primary health centres and sub-centres under the Reproductive and Child Health Programme 2 [46–48]. The female multipurpose worker (Auxillary Nurse Mid-wife or ANM) and other paramedics of the health centres are responsible for administering vitamin A concentrates universally to children in the 9–59 months of age. The services of frontline workers of Health and ICDS (ASHAs or Accredited Social Health Activist who is a community volunteer under the National Rural Health Mission and anganwadi workers or AWW of ICDS) are utilized for the implementation of the programme. In some states, the VAS programme has been successfully used as a stand alone programme while in a few as an entry point to address other important child nutrition issues such as iodised salt promotion, campaign for identifying severely undernourished etc [46–48].

The bi-annual events require a significant amount of planning, logistical support, training, monitoring and coordination with other sectors to enable health systems to reach marginalized communities at least twice a year with VAS and a basic package of services. Effective district planning and implementation include defining roles of the primary stakeholders and developing their capacity to execute their roles, ensuring timely supply of VAS, effective communication and social mobilisation, establishing a monitoring mechanism.

The Tenth Plan recommendations that the two months (pre-summer/ pre-winter period) in a year, 6 months apart should be taken up for VAS distribution for coverage of children has resulted in accelerating the adoption of the biannual strategy. The state implementation plans focus on the enumeration of children under five years, ensuring VAS supply and appropriate logistic management, publicity of VAS distribution during the specific months through mass media as well as peripheral health workers, organization of regular training and orientation sessions and establishing a system for the maintenance of records of VAS coverage. Successful demonstration of biannual VAS in various states has resulted in incorporation of this strategy in the ongoing Eleventh Five Year Plan by the Government of India [49]. Details of the process and impact of establishment of a biannual strategy VAS Programme are evident from the details presented for a state of northern India, Uttar Pradesh.

17.4 Establishment of the biannual fixed month strategy – an overview of a state initiative

The efforts made to accelerate the vitamin A supplementation (VAS) programme through the launch of the biannual strategy in the state of Uttar Pradesh is presented at the time of launch of the biannual strategy, Uttar Pradesh, the largest state in India had a population of approximately 190 m, a high infant mortality rate (67/1000 live births), under-five mortality rate (96/1000 live births) and a very high incidence of malnutrition (>42% in <3 years children). Poor infant feeding practices, frequent infections like diarrhoea and acute respiratory infections (ARI) and micronutrient deficiency (vitamin A, iron, iodine) contribute significantly to malnutrition, morbidity and mortality in children.

For evidence-based planning of VAD elimination programme in the state as well as for seeking high political support, a survey was undertaken in 1999 in the four regions of the state to estimate the prevalence of vitamin A deficiency [50]. A total of 46,544 children between 2 and 6 years were surveyed for night blindness and 58,216 children 6 months to 6 years were examined for the assessment of Bitot's spot. The study revealed a very high presence of clinical vitamin A deficiency in the state as indicated in the Table 17.6 below. The incidence of Bitot's spot with conjunctival xerosis was reported to be much higher than the public health level cut off of 0.5%. The survey findings confirmed that VAD is an important public health problem in the state (Table 17.6). The coverage of children who were reported to have received vitamin A supplementation (VAS) was reported to be one of the poorest in the country – only 14.3 % of the population ever receiving the first dose. Coverage with subsequent 2nd to 5th dose was extremely low with dropout for 3rd dose being 91% [51]. The national survey findings of 1998–99 [18] also revealed that the supplementation with vitamin A doses was very low with only 10% children reported to have received at least one dose of vitamin A supplement. It was noted that the primary coverage was in the age group of 9–12 months with estimated 68.1% infants receiving VAS during measles vaccination. Coverage with 2nd to 5th dose was reported to be almost negligible.

Table 17.6 Prevalence of Bitot's spot and night blindness in children in the state of Uttar Pradesh [6]

District	*Year when study was conducted*	*No. of children surveyed*		*Prevalence of Bitot's spot (6 months to 6 years)*	*Prevalence of night blindness (2–6 years)*	*Prevalence of malnutrition (weight/age)*
		2–6 years	6 moths to 6 years			
Bahraich	1999	11989	14250	5.6%	3.4%	–
Badayun	2001	11509	14686	9.17%	4.7%	74.9%
Mirzapur	2001	12120	14940	10.5%	9.7%	56.7%
Etawah	2001	10926	14340	1.9%	7.1%	49.4%

The high prevalence of clinical vitamin A deficiency and low coverage with VAS led to the launch of a pilot project in one of the districts – Bahraich district [51]. Twice yearly administration of VAS in a campaign mode was considered appropriate. The biannual strategy model focused on a one week intensive drive for improving vitamin A coverage of children 9 months to 3 years. The intervention package, besides VAS administration, focused on the administration of measles vaccines to infants 9–12 months and promoting appropriate complementary feeding practices. For promotion of complementary feeding, ANMs of health system were trained to check and record the practice of feeding semi-solid food to infants that was being followed by caregivers or mothers at the time of VAS and measles vaccine administration. Using a standardized recording registers, the mothers were also questioned regarding the composition and frequency of feeds and breastfeeding practices being followed. Following the analysis of this information, ANM was advised to counsel the caregivers on appropriate infant and child feeding practices along with advice to incorporate vitamin A rich food and additional 1–2 tea spoon of fat in the portion of diet being fed to a child.

For launching the pilot project, children 9–36 months were enumerated by ANMs in the special registers provided for the project. A district operational plan for one week drive was developed with travel plans of each ANM to visit the 4–7 sub-centre villages with a population of about 6000–7000. In addition, VAS administration plans to reach urban children through the staff of district hospital was also worked out. Supply requirements of vitamin A, measles vaccine, etc were estimated and supplied. For measles vaccine, appropriate actions were taken for the cold chain. Social mobilisation drive for informing community of the importance of VAS and measles and the system to be adopted for monitoring vitamin A administration was planned by the health department [52]. This was followed by imparting training to ANMs and supervisors of the health department of the district. Training focused on creating data base of beneficiaries, calculating supply requirements (VAS, measles vaccine, monitoring registers and counselling printed materials), logistic management and skills in counseling on feeding and administrating VAS and measles vaccine. The health staff was also trained for organising community mobilisation drives. Community participation was ensured by undertaking intensive awareness generation activities in the district.

A week long campaign, six months apart, in the months of December 2000 and June 2001 was organised. Technical, financial and logistic support for the above campaign was provided by UNICEF. The first round in December 2000 was carried out only in rural areas while the second round in June 2001 was organized both in rural and urban areas. As a result of the biannual strategy, vitamin A supplementation coverage increased from 10% in 1998–99 to 83.5% in December 2001 and measles vaccine coverage increased from 23% to 43.5% in two rounds in the district [52].

The lessons learned from the pilot project were synthesized. The campaign approach was found effective but not considered a sustainable approach for the state since the health sector manpower was occupied most of the time with pulse polio campaigns. The campaign mode for VAS administration was therefore dropped and a shift was made in the strategy [53]. The two fixed months – June and December, six months apart, were designated as the child health and nutrition months (in local language *Bal*

Swasthya Poshan Mah or BSPM). The VAS programme was referred as the BSPM programme. Administration of VAS was spread out in the entire month and not limited to a week. The VAS administration was linked to the routine immunizations plans of these two months. The first dose of VAS of 9–12 months was administered along with measles vaccine throughout the year while vitamin A supplement to children >1–3 years was administered only in the two fixed BSPM months in the outreach immunisation sessions as per the routine immunisation (RI) micro-plans. Effort was also made to cover all children 9–12 month of age in these BSPM months if they had missed their first dose of vitamin A supplement during the RI sessions in the preceding six months. The biannual BSPMs were also viewed as opportunity to deliver a package of the following set of interventions for improving child health and nutrition.

- Management of severely malnourished children (grade III and grade IV)
- Promotion of Infant and Young Child Feeding (IYCF)
- Promotion of consumption of iodised salt and organizing salt testing events at community level

The BSPM programme in the state was launched in December 2003.The two years gap in implementation of the programme, following completion of the pilot project, was due to frequent intensive pulse polio drives in the state during this period. Between 2003 and 2005, the biannual BSPM was implemented in only 18 of the 70 districts of the state with the support of UNICEF, MI and USAID/MOST. These districts were located in three distinct regions of the state comprising 180 administrative blocks with a population of 37 m and 2.5 m children (between 9 and 36 months). The programme was taken to scale in 2006 in the entire state and was included in the State Plan of Implementation of the National Rural Health Mission (NRHM) from 2007 onwards.

Health and Integrated Child Development Services (ICDS) programme of district, block and village level were responsible for implementation of the BSPM activities. For maximising reach and increasing VAS coverage, an operational plan was developed using the strategy diagrammatically presented in Figure 17.1.

The health sector was assigned the task of administering VAS to children while the ICDS sector with responsible for identification, listing and mobilization of beneficiaries to the VAS-immunization site. The job responsibilities of each of the two primary sectors for performing the following primary actions for the implementation of the BSPM activities was clearly defined (Box 17.3).

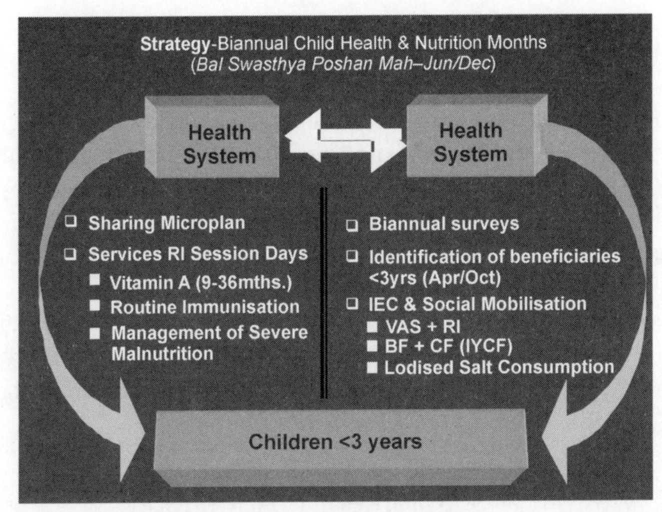

17.1 Biannual child health and nutrition strategy

Box 17.3 Role of the two primary departments

Health department

- Block medical officer to prepare and share a copy of the RI microplan with the Block ICDS officer.
- Health Supervisors to ensure that ANMs visits RI session sites as per her microplan.
- ANMs to supplement first dose of vitamin A along with measles vaccine to all the children who have missed it during the routine immunization sessions through out the year.
- ANMs to administer second to fifth dose of vitamin A to >12-36 months children during the biannual months only (since 2007, children up to five years are reached with VAS).
- Compilation of ANMs report at block and further compilation of block reports at district level after completion of biannual rounds. District data to reach Directorate within one month following BSPM month (i.e. in first week of February and August).

Role of ICDS during BSPM months

- Survey and identification of children under three and pregnant mothers by AWW
- Listing of under threes by AWW for following health services
  - Vitamin A supplementation
  - Routine Immunization and
  - Referral of severely malnourished children.
- Block ICDS officer to share the list of enumerated beneficiaries with Block Medical Officer
- AWW to undertake social mobilization and IEC activities for increasing VAS coverage. AWW to intensively promote exclusive breastfeeding for six months, introduction of complementary feeding after six months and consumption of iodised salt during the biannual rounds.
- AWW to support ANM on outreach immunization days for administration of vitamin A supplementation and routine immunization to children 9 months to 3 years (since 2007 up to 5 years).

17.4.1 Identification and listing of beneficiaries through conducting biannual survey

ICDS is the largest programme in the country having a village based worker for providing essential nutrition and health services to the community with support of health department. Under the ICDS programme, community surveys are expected to be undertaken twice a year. For identification of VAS beneficiaries, the timings of the biannual surveys were reorganized to April and October of the year to proceed the fixed months of the BSPM. The list of beneficiaries of each village was prepared and shared by block (about 100–125 villages per block) officer of ICDS (Child Development Project Officer – CDPO) with the Block Medical Officer of the Health sector.

17.4.2 Vitamin A supplement (VAS) supply

VAS supply requirement based on population estimates was calculated using a bottom-up approach for district and (average 10–12 blocks per district) the state (Box 17.4). VAS supply distribution from district level to block primary health centre (about 1,00,000 population) and to the health subcentres was undertaken at least 2–4 weeks prior to the BSPM months. Each ANM was advised to carry at least two bottles of vitamin A supplement to the village on the administration day. VAS supply from 2003 to 2007 was entirely supported by UNICEF and MI.

17.4.3 Microplan development and sharing

The health subcentre in India caters to a population of 5000 (5–6 villages with about 1000 persons/village) and is the smallest administrative unit of the health infrastructure. The subcentre is manned by an auxillary nurse mid-wife (ANM), a female health worker, who provides a gamut of preventive and curative services to the community residing within the subcentre area. As per the visit plan, the health worker visits each of the sub-centre villages at least once in a month for provision of health services, including routine immunization.

In the state of Uttar Pradesh, Wednesday of every week is fixed for RI and the Wednesdays are known as the "RI days" of the state. The RI micro-plans present field visit plan on RI day for each of the ANMs of the block. The RI micro-plans at the block level is a therefore a compilation of field visit plans of each of the ANMs (about 20–30 ANMs in each block) for conducting RI sessions in the assigned sub-health centre area comprising 5–7 villages/hamlets (population 5000–7000). The RI micro plans present details of the specific outreach areas being visited by ANM for undertaking

Box 17.4 Vitamin A supply estimation for a district with population of 1,00,000

1. Total population	100,000
2. Birth rate	25/1000 live births
3. Total no. of infants (0–1 year)	2500
4. Total no. of 9 months–12 months (25% of total infants)	625
5. Total no. of children in age groups 1–2 year, 2–3 year, 3-4 year and 4-5 year	2500 (for each of the four age groups)
6. Vitamin A supply calculation (in ml)	
(a) 9 months-12 months requiring first dose (1 ml/child × 625 children)	625
(b) 1-2 years requiring 2nd–3rd dose (2ml/child/dose × 2500 children × 2 doses)	10000 ml
(c) 2-3 years requiring 4th and 5th dose (2 ml/child/dose × 2500 children × 2 doses)	10000 ml
(d) 3-4 years requiring 6th and 7th dose (2 ml/child/dose × 2500 children × 2 doses)	10000 ml
(e) 4-5 years requiring 8th and 9th dose (2 ml/child/dose × 2500 children × 2 doses)	10000 ml
(f) Total volume of vitamin A required for children 9 months-5 years (625 ml + 10000 ml + 10000 ml + 10000 ml + 10000 ml)	40625 ml
(g) Adding wastage of 10% to the total requirement (10% × 40625 ml)	4063 ml
(h) Total requirement of VAS for 9 months-5 years (40625 + 4063)	44687 ml
7. Therefore, total number of 100 cc vitamin A bottles required for a district with population of 100,000 (44687/100)	447 bottles

primary health care activities, including RI activities, on each of the Wednesdays and Saturdays of the months. The plan includes the details of sites within a village/hamlet being used as "immunisation sites" for administering vaccines. The RI plan also includes information on the link ICDS frontline worker who coordinates with ANM and community for execution of the RI activities, population of the village and date of immunization. The RI microplan for the biannual BSPM months forms the basis for administration of VAS on the RI days (Figure 17.2). It is therefore critical that the RI micro plans of the BSPM months are shared with the ICDS sector for effective coordination and management of the BSPM Programme.

17.4.4 Communication and social mobilisation

An effective, well defined, sustainable and replicable communication and social mobilisation strategy is pre-requisite for improving vitamin A coverage and influencing correct dietary and feeding practices. Education and social mobilisation activities are an integral component of the BSPM

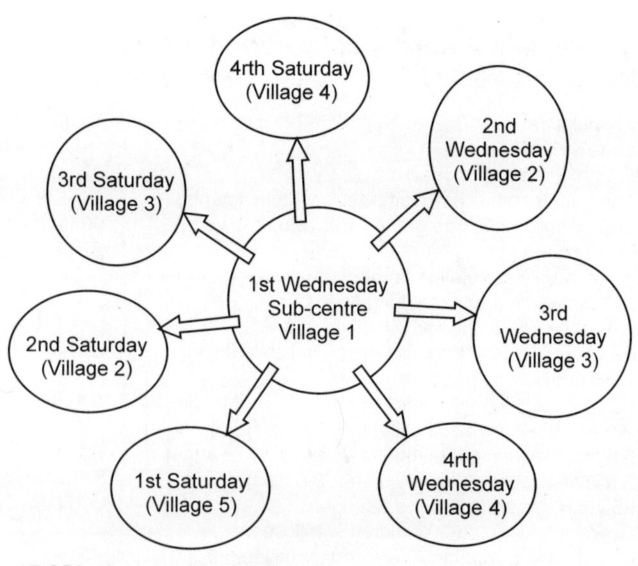

17.2 RI microplan for a sub-centre

programme. Communication and social mobilization activities were planned to be undertaken by the ICDS system throughout the fixed biannual BSPM months of June and December. In the BSPM programme, ICDS frontline worker were entrusted with the responsibility of mobilizing beneficiaries to the RI site for administration of VAS and immunisation. The communication messages focused on creating demands for services as well as promotion of infant and young child feeding. Standardized messages on vitamin A, iodised salt and Infant & Young Child Feeding were displayed at the selected sites. Rallies by school children, wall painted slogans, placards, banners and posters were used for these communication and social mobilisation activities. Two days prior to the VAS administration on RI days, intensive social mobilisation activities were conducted by organising rallies in the village or organising public announcements as well announcements in primary schools, ICDS centres etc (Figure 17.3). The pulse polio programmes had demonstrated that such intensive social mobilisation actions, 1–2 days prior to the vaccination days were important actions for timely creation of awareness and mobilizing community to visit the vaccination sites. A set of information and communication materials (posters, banners, folders, inserts, calendar) containing technical details about biannual strategy, vitamin A supplementation, iodised salt, infant and young child feeding were developed and distributed in the entire state. These proved to be extremely useful in disseminating correct standardized messages in the community.

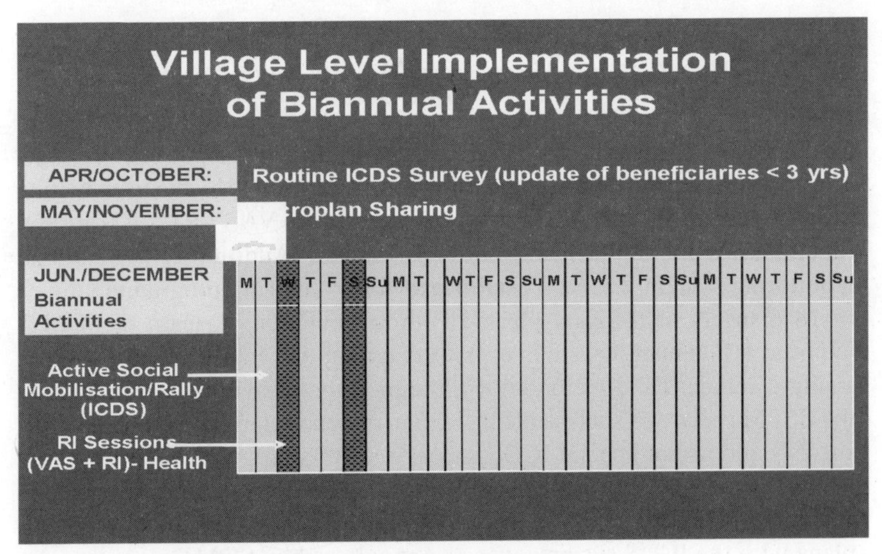

17.3 Village-level implementation of biannual activities

17.4.5 Capacity building health and ICDS staff

For execution of the BSPM activities, a joint training of health and ICDS sectors was considered critical. Intensive training was undertaken for state, district, block and village functionaries of joint health and ICDS teams. Faculty members of the departments of Community Medicine of the nine State Medical Colleges were designated "State Observer-cum-Monitoring Trainers" or (SOMTs) and were trained as master trainers for the state level BSPM activities. SOMTS in turn selected eight persons as "Block Core Trainers" from the health and ICDS sectors at block level. These block trainers undertook the joint training health and ICDS functionaries (ANM and ICDS Anganwari Worker or AWWs) with supervision support of SOMTs. Prior to the BSPM months, a rapid re-orientation training was undertaken for the managers and functionaries of both the sectors.

Training materials were developed by the State Government. Important amongst these was a joint training module which was used for training programme managers as well as functionaries. Based on the performance and feedback, training content was continuously modified. Special effort was made to train all functionaries on the importance of following the VAS recommended age-wise schedule and cautions to be taken for preventing overdose administration. Management of side effects, if any, formed part of the training. During 2006, the training on biannual strategy was taken to scale in the entire state. Approximately 1650 Health & ICDS district and block programme mangers and approximately 6500 block health and ICDS functionaries were trained for implementation of the BSPM strategy.

17.4.6 Supervision and monitoring

The activities during the biannual rounds were monitored by the introduction of a supervision format for monitoring joint VAS -RI sessions by functionaries of both the health and ICDS sectors. Additionally, an external monitoring system was also established for monitoring programme inputs in 18 districts of the first phase of implementation. A team of SOMTs monitored biannual activities at both planning and implementation stage. Using a standardized methodology, the monitors provided information on the BSPM processes such as identification of beneficiaries through biannual surveys and use of special ICDS survey registers provided, administration of VAS as per the schedule. In addition, status of the availability of health sub-centre RI micro-plans for the BSPM months and sharing of these micro-plans with the ICDS systems was also monitored by SOMTs.

17.4.7 Establishment of VAS Coverage Record System

In December 2004, effort to institutionalize an effective monitoring system was made by introducing child centered recording and monitoring system for the biannual VAS administration. A total of 25,000 special biannual child centered registers were supplied for recording data by health workers at the village level on VAS, treatment doses for clinical VAD cases, administration of measles vaccine, and for recording status of introduction of complementary foods at nine months. Data was planned to be computed in specially developed block and district level formats. Training on developing skills for completing these registers and formats was imparted not only to district managers and programme functionaries but to the data computing persons attached to the 70 districts of the state. The impact of using such a system had a positive impact on the VAS coverage in June 2005 but the child-centered recording system was not considered sustainable. Experimenting with an alternative monitoring mechanism was considered essential.

17.4.8 Impact of the programme in selected districts

The impact of the biannual BSPM programme on VAS coverage in the first two years, December 2003 to December 2005, was evaluated by an external agency [54]. The intensive programme inputs in 18 districts resulted in increasing the coverage of vitamin A supplements of children 9–12 months to 63% while the coverage of 2nd to 5th dose increased from almost nil to 62% (Figure 17.4). The process of evaluation also presented a very significant positive impact on skills for undertaking village survey and identifying beneficiaries and knowledge of health and ICDS functionaries regarding age-wise correct doses of vitamin A supplements for preschool children. The BSPM strategy, with defined responsibilities of health and ICDS sectors, resulted in appreciating their roles in complementing the efforts for achieving the common objective of improving child nutrition, survival and development. This was reflected in improvement in functional collaboration between health and ICDS sectors. BSPM was also demonstrated to be a good example of using VAS administration as an entry point for operationalising a comprehensive child health and nutrition programme.

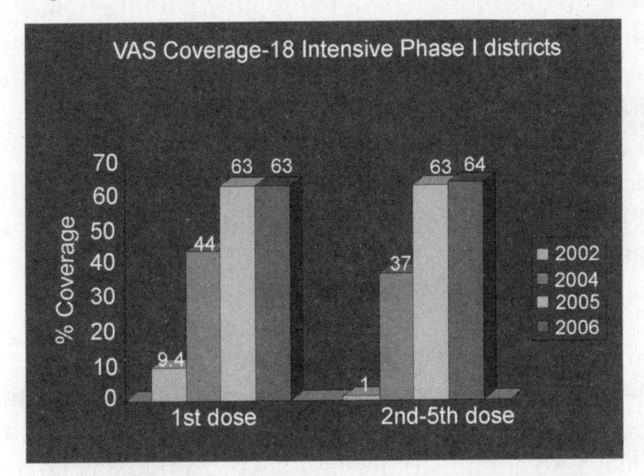

17.4 VAS coverage-18 intensive Phase I districts

The VAS programme strategy linked to RI was reported to result in improving not only VAS but improving RI coverage and streamlining RI sessions. The development and availability of RI micro-plans at block level steadily increased and by the fourth BSPM round, 94% blocks were reported to have RI micro-plans as compared to 65.1% at the beginning of BSPM activities in 18 districts of the first phase (Figure 17.5). The percentage of immunisation/ outreach session held increased from 60% to 82%. Iodised salt consumption increased from 6% to 49%. A total of 59,889 children were identified as severely undernourished and were followed up for management.

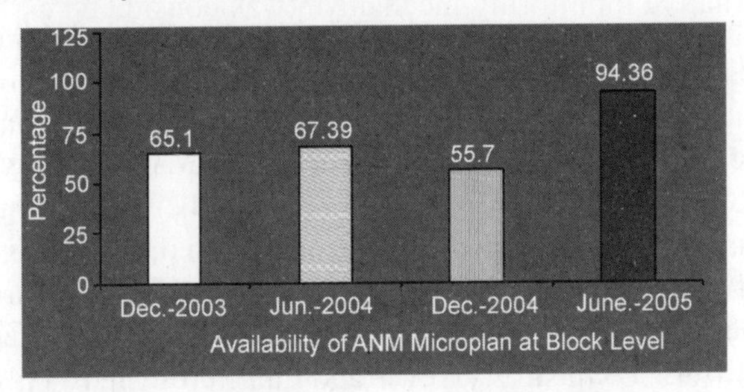

17.5 Impact of BSPM on RI microplan availability between 2003 and 2005

17.4.9 Scaling up the biannual VAS delivery system in the entire state

Based on the experience and positive outcome of the implementation in 18 districts, the BSPM initiative was taken to scale in the entire state in 2006 of over 190 million population comprising 70 districts with estimated 12 million children <3 years. The coverage of infants with the first dose of VAS in the state increased from 9.4% to 43% and of 2nd to 5th dose from nil to 37% (Figure 17.6). In 2007 the BSPM strategy was included in the State Programme Implementation Plan for the Rural Health Mission (State PIP–NRHM).

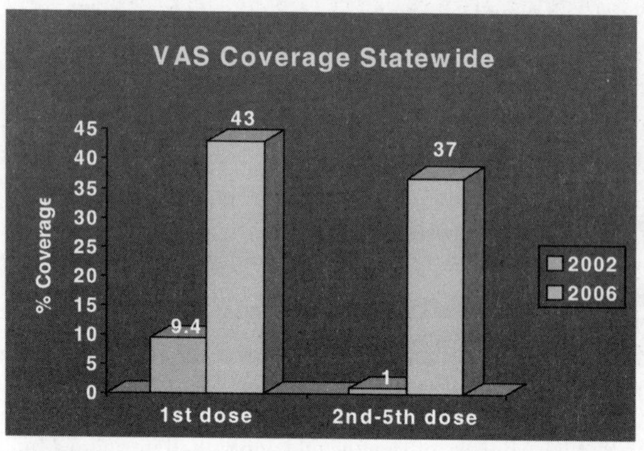

17.6 VAS coverage statewide

17.5 Elimination of vitamin A deficiency – future direction

VAS Programme is an integral part of the RCH-2 Programme of the National Rural Health Mission (NRHM) 2005–2011. The biannual strategy for improving coverage of VAS is a sustainable model which can be effectively taken to scale. Reaching preschool children in both rural as well as urban regions is crucial and a suitable sustainable VAS programme design needs to evolve to reach the unreached urban children. For the implementation of VAS administration in rural and urban regions, streamlining of the procurement of adequate quantity of VAS supply remains a challenge. Higher priority and political commitment for implementation of the vitamin A supplementation programme, along with commitment to improve production and access to vitamin A fortified foods is essential to eliminate vitamin A deficiency in India and making a significant difference in survival rate and quality of life of children in the country.

References

1. Fourth Five Year Plan, Family Planning programme. Technical information: MCH No. 2. Maternal and Child health Scheme for Prophylaxis against Blindness in Children caused by Vitamin A Deficiency. Indian Council of Medical Research (1971–74).
2. Text Book of Human Nutrition (1996). Oxford and IBH Publishing Company, New Delhi.
3. National Nutrition monitoring Bureau Report (1991). National institute of Nutrition, Hyderabad.
4. BAGCHI K (2001). In: Benefits and safety of administration of vitamin A to pre school children and pregnant and lactating women. Kapil, U and Srivastava VK (eds), Ministry of Health and Family Welfare and All India Institute of Medical Sciences, New Delhi; p 67.
5. WHO (1995). MDIS-Micronutrient Deficiency information System, World Health organization. MDIS Working Paper # 2. Global Prevalence of Vitamin A Deficiency.
6. Department of Women and Child Development, Government of India, India, Nutrition Profile, 1998.
7. CHAKRAVARTHY I (2001). Indian Scenario of Prevalence of Vitamin A Deficiency. In: Benefits and safety of administration of vitamin A to pre school children and pregnant and lactating women. Kapil U and Srivastava VK (eds), Ministry of Health and Family Welfare and All India Institute of Medical Sciences, New Delhi; p 100.
8. VIR S. Linkage of vitamin A massive dose supplement administration with pulse polio immunization – an overview. In: Benefits and safety of administration of vitamin A to pre school children and pregnant and lactating women. KAPIL U AND SRIVASTAVA VK (eds), Ministry of Health and Family Welfare and All India Institute of Medical Sciences, New Delhi; pp. 60–68.
9. AWASTHI S (2000). DEVTA project. Uttar Pradesh – Personal Communication.
10. Draft report of District nutrition Project, ICMR 1998–99.
11. SRIVASTAVA VK (1999). Vitamin A status of preschool children in Baharaich district, Uttar Pradesh, Study for Government of UP.
12. Indian Council of medical research (1999). District nutrition Project, draft report (1).
13. National Nutrition monitoring Bureau Report (2002). National institute of Nutrition, Hyderabad.
14. National Nutrition monitoring Bureau Report (2006). National institute of Nutrition, Hyderabad.
15. DIXIT DT (1966). Nightblindness in third trimester of pregnancy. *Ind J Med Res u*, pp. 791–795.
16. MANDAL GS, NANDA KN and BOSE J (1969). Nightblindness in Pregnancy. *J. Obstet Gynecol.* **19**, pp. 453–458.
17. VENKATACHALAN PS (1962). Maternal nutritional status and its effects on the newborn. *Bull. World Health Organ* **26**, pp. 193–201.
18. National Family Health Survey (NFHS) 2, 1998–99. International Institute of Population Sciences, Mumbai.
19. BHASKARAN P and KRISHNASWAMY K (2002). Vitamin A supplementation strategies – India status. In: Benefits and safety of administration of vitamin A to pre school children and pregnant and lactating women. Eds Kapil, U and Srivastava

VK, Ministry of Health and Family Welfare and All India Institute of Medical Sciences, New Delhi, pp. 45–58.

20. VIR S (2008). Addressing child malnutrition in tea gardens of Dibrugarh district, Assam. UNICEF consultancy report.
21. SOMMER A and DAVIDSON FR (2002). Assessment and control of vitamin A deficiency: the Annecy Accords. *J Nutr* **132**, no. 9S, pp. 2845S–2849S.
22. VIJAYARAGHAVAN K and N PRAHLAD RAO (1978). National Programme for the Prevention of Vitamin A Deficiency – An evaluation. National institute of Nutrition, Indian Council of Medical research, Hyderabad.
23. Indian Council of Medical Research (1974). Annual Report, p 75.
24. SRIKANTIA SG and REDDY V (1970). Effect of a single massive dose of vitamin A on serum and liver levels of the vitamin. *Amer J Clin Nutr* **23**, pp. 114–118.
25. SRIKANTIA SG (1969). Prevention of vitamin A deficiency, world. *Rev Nutr Diet* **31**, pp. 95–99.
26. PREIRA SM and BEGUM A (1969). Prevention of vitamin A deficiency. *Amer J Clin Nutr* **22**, pp. 858–862.
27. SUSHEELA TP (1969). Studies on serum vitamin A levels after a single massive oral dose. *Ind. J med Res.* **57**, pp. 2151–2152.
28. Task force, Government of India (1988) constituted by the Ministry of Health and Family Welfare, government of India, New Delhi. National prophylaxis programme for prevention of blindness due to vitamin A deficiency.
29. MANNAR MGV (1989). Production and supply of vitamin A in India. Report prepared for the Ministry of Health and family Welfare, Government of India, 1989.
30. WHO (1988). Expanded programme on immunisation update - vitamin A: Time for action.
31. World Summit for Children (1990). World Declaration on the survival, protection and development of children and plan of action for implementing the World Declaration on the survival, protection and development of children in the 1990s. World Summit for children, United Nations. New York, 30th Sept, UN, 1990.
32. Ministry of Health and Family Welfare (GoI). Communication No. M 12015/6188-MCH III. 9th March 1990. Task force on vitamin A programme, Minutes of the Task Force (1990). Chaired by Deputy Commissioner MCH.
33. BHASKARAN P and VISWESWARA RAO K (1997). Enhancement in seroconversion on simultaneous administration of measles vaccine and vitamin A in 9 months old Indian infants. *Ind. J. Paed.* **54**.
34. Ministry of Health and Family Welfare, Government of India (1991). Policy on Management of Vitamin A Deficiency.
35. REDDY V (2002). Benefits and safety of vitamin A supplementation during pregnancy and lactation page 16-25. In: Benefits and safety of administration of vitamin A to pre school children and pregnant and lactating women. Eds KAPIL, U and SRIVASTAVA VK, Ministry of Health and Family Welfare and All India Institute of Medical Sciences, New Delhi.
36. Ministry of Health and Family Welfare, Government of India. Child Survival and safe Motherhood Programme, 1992.
37. Ministry of Health and Family Welfare, Government of India. Evaluation of Immunization 1998–1999, 2000.
38. UNICEF (1998). Integration of vitamin A supplements with immunization policy and programme implementation: report of a meeting, UNICEF, New York, 12–13 Jan 1998.

39. VIJAYARAGHAVAN K, BRAHMAM GNV, REDDY G, REDDY V (1996). Linking periodic dosage of vitamin A with universal immunization programme – An Evaluation. National Institute of Nutrition, Indian Council of Medical Research, Jamai Osmania PO, Hyderabad 500007.
40. WHO / UNICEF (1998). Joint Policy and Operational Questioning relating to vitamin A and EPI / NIDs. Joint statement, WHO / UNICEF, Geneva, 1998.
41. National institute of Nutrition (2000). Impact of vitamin A supplementation delivered with OPV as a part of immunization campaign in Orissa, India. ICMR/ WHO/UNICEF and MI.
42. Directorate of Family Welfare, government of UP (2000). Vitamin A given during pulse polio immunization campaign. Dec 1999 to Jan 2000.
43. KAPIL U and SRIVASTAVA V (2002). Benefits and safety of administration of vitamin A to pre school children and pregnant and lactating women. Ministry of Health and Family Welfare and All India Institute of Medical Sciences, New Delhi.
44. 10th Five Year Plan. Planning Commission, Government of India, 2002–2007.
45. Policy on Management of Vitamin A Deficiency 1991(No Z 28020/30/2003-CH,Government of India, Ministry of Health and Family Welfare, Child Health Division dated 2nd Nov 2006).
46. VIR S, PRASAD LB, JAIN A, SINGH R, ATEGBO EA, HETTIARATCHY N AND SCHULTINK W (2007). Vitamin A Supplementation Programme an effective entry point for addressing Malnutrition in the State of Uttar Pradesh, India. Abstract – Consequences and Control of Micronutrient Deficiencies – Science, Policy and Programme – Defining the Issues, 16–18 April, 2007, Istanbul, Turkey.
47. G SINGH, S VIR, V AGUAYO, U NARAYAN. Child health and nutrition months significantly improve vitamin A supplementation coverage in Uttar Pradesh, India (TU 33) in program/abstracts. Micronutrients, health and development: evidence based programme, 12–15 May 2009, Beijing, china, micronutrient Forum.
48. SAXENA S, SAXENA V AND NAMSHUM N. Challenges of addressing vitamin A deficiency in India (TU 40), in program / abstracts. Micronutrients, health and development: evidence based programme, 12-15th May 2009, Beijing, china, micronutrient Forum.
49. Government of India, Ministry of Women and Child Development (2006). Report of the working group on integrating nutrition with health, 11th five year plan (2002–2012).
50. SRIVASTAVA VK (1999). Vitamin A status of preschool children in selected districts in UP. Report submitted to UNICEF.
51. Department of Women and Child Development, Government of Uttar Pradesh and UNICEF, 1997. Nutritional Profile of Women and Children in Uttar Pradesh.
52. GUPTA SB, SALUJA DBS, VIR S, SAXENA V, HASAN MZ, SRIVASTAVA VK (2001). Child Health and Nutrition week: Intervention coverage with vitamin A supplement and measles vaccination. Training manual. Department of Health and Family Welfare, Government of UP and UNICEF (Lucknow Field Office).
53. Government of Uttar Pradesh and UNICEF (2003). Biannual vitamin A supplementation programme in Uttar Pradesh, Bal Swasthya Poshan Mah.
54. MOST, India (2004). Coverage evaluation of vitamin A supplementation in Uttar Pradesh, Academy of Management Studies.
55. Department of Health and Family Welfare (2008). State Programme Implementation Plan, National Rural Health Mission (NRHM).

18

Iodine metabolism and indicators of iodine status

Madan M. Godbole and *Rajan Sankar*

Madan M. Godbole is Professor and Head of the Department of Endocrinology at Sanjay Gandhi Postgraduate Institute of Medical Sciences, Lucknow. Research fields including brain development, breast cancer and stroke in relation to iodine/thyroid hormone. He is a Fellow at National Academy of Medical Sciences.

Rajan Sankar is the Regional Manager and Special Adviser in South Asia for the Global Alliance for Improved Nutrition (GAIN). Prior to this, he was a Project Officer in UNICEF, India Country Office and Regional Technical Advisor of the Micronutrient Initiative. Dr. Shankar was the Head of Thyroid Research Centre at the Defence Research and Development Organisation in Delhi.

18.1 Introduction

Iodine is a constituent of thyroid hormone (TH) and is an essential micronutrient for normal growth, development and function. Iodine deficiency (ID) causes an enlargement of the thyroid gland, physical function and mental retardation. Mild to moderate ID results in loss of intelligence points, learning disabilities and poor human resource development. The former being the tip of the iceberg and latter constitutes the invisible bulk of the pyramid [1].

National governments are putting in place universal salt iodization (USI) as a major vehicle to prevent the problem of IDD [2]. Salt-iodization levels and urinary iodine excretion are the most commonly used parameters for process and impact assessment of USI and IDD elimination. The serum thyroid stimulating hormone (TSH), thyroglobulin (Tg) and ultrasound measurement of thyroid gland volume have been validated as secondary parameters for monitoring the success of the salt iodization program and elimination of IDD [3–4]. Countries with strong monitoring and evaluation machinery in place have been able to overcome the problems pertaining to major obstacles of USI such as poor quality of salt, inadequate iodization, losses during transportation, humidity, logistic problems and poor public and administrative awareness [5]. The understanding and choice of impact assessment parameters is governed not only by administrative decisions and economics of scale, but also by the choice of survey methodology and selection of target groups like school children, pregnant and lactating mothers. The clear understanding of iodine metabolism through the human-life cycle and various factors that may affect iodine metabolism and thyroid hormone synthesis during pregnancy, neonatal, childhood, adolescence and adult life is of prime importance.

18.2 Metabolism – iodine absorption and transport

Iodine present in foods as iodides is readily absorbed from the gastro-intestinal tract. Other forms of iodine in food is converted into the iodide ion in the gut lumen, and >90% is rapidly absorbed in the upper-small intestine. Fifteen percent of ingested iodine is taken up by the thyroid gland within 24 hours of ingestion, and the excess is excreted by the kidneys in urine [6]. Urinary-iodine excretion per day reflects the iodine-nutrition status of a population and is the most widely used parameter for monitoring the impact assessment of intervention protocols. However, it is not used to assess an individual's iodine-nutrition status. The only direct test of thyroid function employs a radioactive isotope of iodine as a tag for the body's stable form of iodine. Most often the test involves the measurement of the fractional uptake by thyroid of a tracer dose of radio iodine. The isotope quickly mixes with stable endogenous pool of body iodine in the extracellular fluid and begins to be removed by two major organs thyroid and kidneys. As this process continues the plasma levels of tracer iodine decreases exponentially. The low levels are reached by 24 hours and inorganic radioactive iodine becomes virtually undetectable in plasma after 72 hours of administration.

In contrast, thyroid content of radioactive iodine increases rapidly in early hours, and then decreases until a plateau is reached. The proportion of administered radioactive iodine ultimately accumulated by thyroid is a reflection of the clearance of iodine by thyroid and kidney. The normal *thyroid clearance rate* (TCR) is approximately 0.4 L/h and the *renal clearance rate* (RCR) is 2.0 L/h, so that radio iodine uptake (RAIU) generally approximates 20% of the administered dose and indicates the rate of thyroid hormone synthesis and by inference the rate of thyroid hormone releases into the blood [7]. These considerations of iodine metabolism make the measurements of these parameters of value for assessment of iodine nutrition status of an individual. Several factors have made many of these tests, except measurement of urinary iodine, less frequently used. However, understanding the measurement of iodine status using these methods is important since these various methods are valuable in the interpretation of the situational analysis of iodine deficiency and its correction due to many confounding factors that clinicians and epidemiologist may confront in management of regular program monitoring and evaluation [6–7].

18.3 Iodine requirement and intake

The daily dietary intake of iodine varies widely throughout the world, depending on the iodine content of soil and water and on dietary practices. Even in a single area, iodine intake varies among different individuals and in the same individual from day to day. Availability of adequate amount of exogenous iodine to allow sufficient thyroidal uptake for formation of normal quantities of thyroid hormone is a pre-requisite for normal growth and development and maintenance of good health in adults. Taking into account daily loss of about 10–20 μg and 100–150 μg through fecal and urinary routes, at least 100 μg is required daily to eliminate any signs of iodine deficiency. This requirement is enhanced during pregnancy and growth, as indicated in Table 18.1.

Table 18.1 Recommended daily intake (μg/day)

Adult	150
During pregnancy	250
children	90–120

18.4 Iodide trapping, organification, coupling, TH synthesis and release (Figure 18.1)

Iodine ingested in inorganic and organic forms from dietary sources is rapidly and efficiently absorbed by the gastrointestinal tract. In the body, iodine remains in the form of iodide (I^-) that is confined largely to extracellular compartment. Iodide concentration in plasma is very low and is completely filterable, reabsorbed passively and a specialized mechanism is required for its uptake by thyroid cells. This process called iodide trapping is accomplished by a membrane protein, the sodium-iodide symporter (NIS). The transport of iodide is an active process dependent on the presence of sodium gradient across the basal membrane of the thyroid cells. Update of $2Na^+$ ions result in the entry of one iodide atom against an electrochemical gradient. The iodide transport system generates an iodine gradient of 20–40 over the cell membrane.

Iodide from both intracellular and extracellular pools within thyroid gland participates in series of reactions that lead to the synthesis of thyroid hormones. Iodide get oxidized to produce intermediates that get rapidly incorporated in tyrosine moieties of thyroglobulin, a matrix protein to form hormonally inactive monoiodotyrosines (MITs) and diiodotyrosines (DITs), by a process termed as *organification*. Oxidation of thyroidal iodide is mediated by the heme containing protein *thyroid peroxidase* (TPO). Iodotyrosines formed by oxidation and organic binding are precursor of hormonally active iodothyronines namely Triodothyronine (T_3) and Tetraiodothyronine (Thyroxine; T_4). The coupling reaction that catalyzed by TPO either two DITs or one MIT and one DIT through an ether linkage to produce T_4 and T_3. Thyroglobulin (T_g) is required for TH synthesis and is considered a sensitive indicator for measuring iodine status. This matrix protein is required for the efficient formation of T_4 and T_3 and is found in a ratio of 20:1 in human T_g molecule and alterations indicate a disease state making Tg as an attractive biomarker.

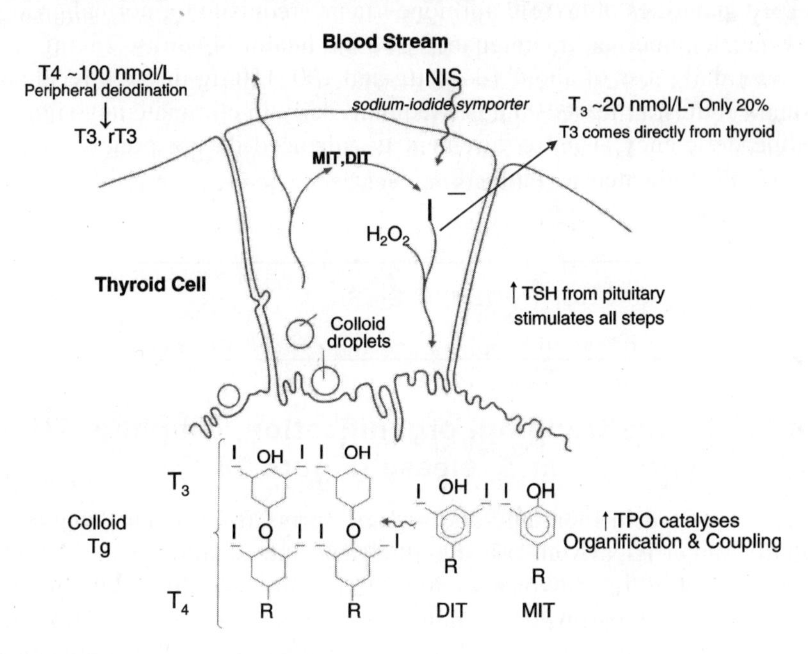

18.1 Synthesis and release of thyroid hormone, T4-Thyrroxine, T3-Tetraiodothyronine, DIT-Diiodotyrosine, MIT-Monoiodotyrosine, TSH-Thyroid-stimulating hormone, T_g-Thyroglobulin, TPO-thyroid peroxidase

18.5 Storage and availability of throid hormones (TH)

The high homeostatic value of thyroid hormone economy relates to large storage capacity of hormones and extremely restricted turnover of ~1% per day in thyroid gland. This large reservoir provides long-term protection against cessation of TH synthesis and sporadic iodine deficiency. Considering that normal thyroid gland weighing 20 g contains approximately 5 mg of T_4, the protection offered can be sufficient to maintain euthyroidism for at least 50 day period [16]. Thus low-circulating levels of T_g indicates long-term depletion of iodine. The value of circulating levels of T_g as biomarker is still to be validated with adequately large sample size in view of questionable contribution of peripheral hydrolysis of T_g.

18.5.1 Thyroid hormone release

The higher T_4/T_3 ratio in T_g compared to thyroidal secretion indicates that in addition to synthetic mode, T_3 is also produced by T_4 deiodination by two enzymes type 1 and 2 deiodinases. Because of the decreased iodine supply and in the DIT/MIT ratio, the T_4/T_3 ratio decreases in human T_g molecules in thyroid glands of operated iodine-deficient subjects. Excess amount of iodide first increases and then decreases the organification within thyroid cells resulting in reduction in yield of organic iodine with increasing doses of iodide. This effect known as *Wolff-Chaikoff Effect,* has been used to treat the hyperthyroid patients and has been cited in support of so-called ill effects of excess iodine [8].

18.5.2 Thyroid hormones in plasma

A wide variety of iodothyronines and their derivatives exist in plasma. The iodine economy is closely related to metabolic transformation of thyroid hormone in peripheral tissues. The levels in peripheral tissues determine the biologic potency and effects. The knowledge of pathways of thyroid-hormone metabolism is fundamental to understand the physiopathology of iodine-deficiency disorders and consequences for impact assessment of intervention programs.

Of the thyroid hormones, T_4 is highest in circulation and is the only hormone solely synthesized by thyroid gland. On the other hand, 80% of T_3 comes from the peripheral tissues and only 20% comes from synthesis in thyroid gland. Only trace amount of other iodothyronines, iodotyrosines and conjugated products are found in plasma and the released iodine from deiodination is recycled to maintain iodine economy. Iodotyronines remain in circulation bound to thyroid binding globulin (TBG) (80%), transthyretin (TTR), thyroid binding per-albumin (TBPA) and albumin.

Maintenance of large quantity of major Iodothyronines in circulation in spite of poor solubility in water is possible due to their association with high capacity-low affinity thyroid binding globulin (TBG), transthyretin (TTR) and thyroid binding per-albumin (TBPA) and albumin with 75–80% THs binding to TBG [17, 18]. These binding proteins provide a large capacity reservoir for release of free TH to meet the day-to-day energy demands of the body as well as to meet the sporadic iodine deficiency situation.

18.6 Iodine metabolism and their mechanism of action

18.6.1 Thyroid stimulating hormone (TSH)

Thyroid stimulating hormone, a major regulator of the morphologic and functional status of the thyroid gland circulation of α-subunit of 14 kD (92 amino acids) is common to leutanizing hormone (LH), follicle-stimulating hormone (FSH) and chrionic gonadotrophin (CG) and a specific β-subunit (112 amino acid) that is a glycoprotein produced in the pituitary gland by thyrotrophs under the influence of thyrotrophin-releasing hormone (TRH) secreted by hypothalamus. It displays both pulsatile and circadian variations. The linear inverse relationship between serum-free T4 concentration and TSH makes it a sensitive indicator of thyroid status of patients with intact hypothalamic-pituitary axis. All steps in the formation of and release of thyroid hormones are stimulated by Thyroid Stimulating Hormone (Thyrotrophin; TSH) [19].

18.6.2 Thyroid peroxidase (TPO)

The synthesis of T_4 and T_3 from DITs and MITs requires the TPO-catalysed coupling of two iodotyrosine moieties. TPO is a microsomal antigen whose recombinant form is used for detection of anti-thyroid microsomal antibodies commonly present in the serum of patients with Hashimoto's disease. Some of such abnormalities have been reported to be present in subjects with history of iodine deficiency and administered excess iodine. Though such cases are rare, the advent of the same has been used as an argument against universal salt iodization programs [13, 14, 20, 21]. Side-effects of excess iodine in general include: (1) Iodine-induced hyperthyroidism. An increase in toxic nodular goitre is probably transient and eventually its incidence is expected to decrease. However, an increased incidence of autoimmune Graves' disease is probably permanent. (2) Iodine-induced hypothyroidism. (3) Iodine-induced autoimmunity, both of the Hashimoto and of the Graves types. (4) An increase in the incidence of papillary cancers, probably with a decrease in the more aggressive types. In any case, the benefits of iodisation programs far outweigh the risks, provided they are implemented and monitored carefully.

18.6.3 Response of thyroid-pituitary-hypothalamic axis to iodine deficiency

Iodine, being a limited resource, thyroid-pituitary-hypothalamic axis is designed to conserve this scarce micronutrient and improve the efficacy of its proper utilization. The severe decrease in dietary iodine supply over a prolong period of time results in fall of T_4 and simultaneous increase in circulating TSH. Human body tries to meet the moderate to mild iodine shortfall in several ways that involves adjustments occurring at hypothalamic-pituitary-thyroid axis and peripheral tissue levels. Surprisingly, majority of goitreous population in iodine deficiency areas are euthyroid (normal thyroid function). This condition is maintained through the adaptive response that involves TSH-mediated increase in thyroid gland size, T_g synthesis, etc. [22–23]. The adaptive response is also the result of economical use of iodine by the thyroid gland by enhancement of DIT–MIT coupling to produce T_3 (a more active thyroid hormone). *The TSH-mediated increase in thyroid-gland size in populations is indicated by goitre prevalence rate that constitutes the primary impact assessment of iodine deficiency and its correction.* Although thyroid size changes inversely in response to alterations in iodine intake, there is a lag before the goitre rate normalizes after iodine repletion. The duration of this lag period is unclear, with experts suggesting it may last from months to years [2]. During this period, the GR is a poor indicator of effect because it reflects a population's history of iodine nutrition but not its present iodine status. Cross-sectional studies have reported a discrepancy between the UI and the GR in the immediate post–USI introduction period [3–4]. *The lower excretion of iodine through urine is the most apparent indicator of such an adaptive response and constitutes the most important impact assessment indicator of iodine deficiency.* The severe iodine deficiency however produces hypothyroidism (less than normal Thyroid function), with abnormally high circulating TSH, that results in majority of symptoms of poor-mental development and cretinism including stunted physical and mental growth, sluggishness, deaf-mutism and defective gait. The extent of symptomology and their manifestation depends on the time of insult of iodine deficiency that is encountered by an individual [24–28]. The in-utero deficiency occurring to fetus in early period (up to second trimester) leads to more neurological damage and the late deficiency results in myxedematous manifestations. It is interesting to note that it is not uncommon to find a full grown neurological cretin with normal physical growth and a normal size functioning thyroid gland and also a myxedematous cretin with signs of neurological deficits; however, it is more common to find cretins with mixed variety of symptoms [26, 29].

The elevated TSH among many functions primarily serves to stimulate the cell division and enlargement of thyroid cells and thyroid gland leading to goitre. Secondly, undetectable decrease in circulating T_3 in iodine-deficient subjects indicates that reduced intra-pituitary conversion of T_4 to T_3 acts as a signal of increased TSH synthesis/secretion from pituitary gland. TSH also helps to maintain the increased T_3 residence time in CNS. *Thus the multifactor highly sensitive response of TSH to iodine deficiency makes it an ideal biomarker for impact assessment of correction of iodine deficiency* [29].

18.7 Role of iodine in biological functions

Severe degree of iodine deficiency disorders (IDD) includes goitre, spastic dilplegia, squint, deaf-mutism and physical (myxedematous) and mental (neurological) retardation termed as endemic cretinism. Most abnormalities with iodine metabolism in patients with endemic goitre are consistent with iodine deficiency [30, 31]. Thyroid iodine clearance and radio iodine uptake (RAIU) are increased in proportion with decrease in urinary iodine excretion of stable iodine. The absolute iodine uptake is normal or low. In areas of moderate iodine deficiency, the serum T_4 concentration is generally in the lower range of the normal. However, areas of severe iodine deficiency the T_4 values are decreased. Nevertheless, most subjects in these areas do not appear to be in hypothyroid state because of an increase in the synthesis of T_3 at the expense of T_4 and because of the increase in activity of thyroidal deiodinases. In such situations, TSH levels are typically in the upper range of normal. However, persistent severe iodine deficiency in sub-set of population leads to hypothyroidism or myxedema with significant increase in TSH levels which is the most important clinical consequence of iodine deficiency [30, 31]. The reduced production of thyroid hormone is the central feature of the clinical state termed hypothyroidism. The symptoms include coarse or dry skin, periorbital puffiness, cold skin and delayed ankle reflex relaxation, reduced pulse rate, weight gain and general lethargy to perform routine tasks. The basal metabolic rate shows a significant decrease in hypothyroid state. The low circulating T_4, T_3 and high TSH provide characteristic biochemical profile of hypothyroid state [31]. The immune manifestations do not come into play in the absence of hypothyroidism and the effects of goitre are only cosmetic. Chronic changes with reference to inadequate iodine intake as well as continuous; the changing thyroid hormonal status eventually leads to alternating enlargement and size reduction of the thyroid follicles. This results in an enlarged thyroid gland with nodules (classic multinodular goitre). However, a haemorrhage in one of the nodules can cause pain and a swelling, mimicking sub-acute thyroiditis. Susceptibility to excess iodine in a miniscule of iodine deficient individuals is also known to lead to immune response.

18.8 Importance of iodine nutrition for human populations

The populations at large require proper iodine nutrition for their development and achievement of their full potential. The vulnerability of human subjects to iodine deficiency depends not only on the extent but also on the timing of iodine deficiency. The iodine requirement also varies according to age as well as the physiological state of human being. Iodine requirement is highest during growth period and pregnancy, stabilizes during adulthood, and declines with advancement of age. This is borne out by the fact that neurological deficits constitute the most serious consequence of iodine deficiency resulting in socio-economic burden of bringing up a cretin and compromised human potential of large number of school children due to learning disabilities, impaired memory, and inability to perform abstract mathematical and other skills. Combination of factors like road connectivity, measures to reduce floods, better land and water management with or without salt iodization program in place is known to introduce incremental iodine correction [25]. This is exemplified in insufficient penetration of adequate iodine supply in far flung rural areas reported from countries like India [32–33]. Unfortunately, dramatic disappearance of cretinism and reduced goitre rate with incremental iodine correction though to desirable strategy of universal iodised salt consumption, masks the subtle and clinically not visible ill effects of persisting iodine deficiency of moderate to mild grade leading to complacency among health planners.

Persistence of subtle deficits on much wider scale than perceived at present can lead to great mass of populations in developing economies remaining away from achieving their full human potential [1]. Monitoring of impact assessment of intervention or corrective programs and appropriate choice of indicators is therefore of great importance for achieving the goal of Universal Salt Iodization (USI) and sustaining measures to ensure access to iodised salt by the entire population. WHO estimates that 54 countries out of 126 still have inadequate iodine nutrition (i.e., median UI <100 μg/l), and 16 countries globally need to rapidly accelerate and sustain USI programme (Table 18.2).

Table 18.2 2006 UNICEF/Network high-priority countries for IDD control

Country	*Total population (thousands)*	*Annual births (thousands)*	*Households using adequately iodized salt (%)*	*Infants unprotected from IDD (thousands)*
Russia	143,899	1,511	35	982
Ukraine	46,989	391	32	266
Indonesia	220,077	4,513	73	1,219
China	1,307,989	17,372	93	1,216
Philippines	81,617	2,026	56	891
Ethiopia	75,600	3,064	28	2,206
Angola	15,490	749	35	487
Sudan	35,523	1,163	1	1,151
Egypt	72,642	1,890	56	832
India	1,087,124	26,000	50	13,000
Pakistan	154,794	4,729	17	3,925
Bangladesh	139,215	3,738	70	1,121
Afghanistan	28,574	1,395	28	1,004
Niger	13,499	734	15	624
Ghana	21,664	679	28	489
Senegal	11,386	419	16	352

Source: Adapted from Zimmerman MB (2007) – www.a2zproject.org

18.9 Iodine requirement

Iodine turnover, thyroidal radioiodine uptake, and balance studies suggest that the average daily requirement for iodine in non-pregnant women is 91–96 μg/d [41]. The US Estimated Average Requirement (EAR) for iodine for non-pregnant, non-lactating women aged 14 years is 95 μg/d, and the Recommended Dietary Allowance – defined as the EAR plus twice the coefficient of variation (CV) in the population—is 150 μg/d [41–42]. This agrees with the WHO/ICCIDD/UNICEF recommended nutrient intake for iodine 150 μg/d for non-pregnant women [2].

18.9.1 Iodine requirements in pregnancy and lactation

The iodine requirement during pregnancy [31, 34–36] is sharply elevated because of (1) an increase by 50% in maternal thyroxine (T_4) production to maintain maternal euthyroidism and to transfer thyroid hormone to the fetus; (2) need for iodine to be transferred to the fetus for fetal thyroid hormone production, particularly in later gestation; and (3) probable increase in renal iodine clearance (RIC). The US EAR is 160 μg/d for pregnancy in women of age 14 years, and the Recommended Dietary Allowance, set at 140% of the EAR rounded to the nearest 10 μg, is 220 μg/d [31, 34–36]. Recently, an increase in the nutrient intake for iodine during pregnancy from 200 to 250 μg/d has been recommended [34–36]. This implies the need for more data on the level of iodine intake and the corresponding urinary iodine (UI) concentration that ensures maternal and newborn euthyroidism.

Pregnancy is associated with profound changes in thyroid function and iodine metabolism to meet the increased demand of hormone production by the maternal thyroid gland (Tables 18.3 and 18.4). The events associated events constitute a transition from a preconception steady-state thyroid gland to a pregnancy steady-state thyroid gland. Once the new equilibrium has been reached, the increased demand for hormones during pregnancy is sustained until full term [36]. Calculation of estimated average requirement (EAR) of 115–120 μg/day for pregnant women based on balance studies indicating retention 20–25 μg of iodine per day by full-term fetus have been flawed. The error has crept in due to not taking in to consideration the need for increased maternal T4 production and higher urinary iodine losses. Studies seeking correlation between thyroid volume and iodine supplementation in pregnant women have also suggested increased need of iodine in the range of 200–250 μg per day during pregnancy [56–57].

During lactation, the physiology of thyroid function and urinary iodine excretion returns to normal. Iodine during lactation is concentrated in mammary gland for excretion in breast milk. The mean breast milk concentration in iodine-sufficient women has been found to be 146 μg/l and average daily loss of iodine through breast milk has been estimated to be 115 μg/day [34]. Addition of EAR for non-pregnant women the EAR for lactating women works out to be 210 mg/day [34]. The WHO recommended daily intake of 250 μg of iodine is found to be sufficient to take care needs of both pregnant and lactating women [3].

When diet lacks iodine, adequate physiological adaptation is difficult to achieve and is progressively replaced by pathological alterations occurring in parallel with the degree and duration of iodine deprivation which leads to maternal hypothyroxinaemia. Pregnancy typically acts to reveal an underlying iodine deficiency even in conditions with only a marginally poor intake, a state that is observed in many countries [3]. The borderline supply of iodine in many areas of mild iodine deficiency is also exemplified of compensatory maternal and fetal goitre during pregnancy and adolescence girls due to the increased requirement of thyroid hormone during gestation and adolescence.

Table 18.3 Pregnancy is associated with profound changes in thyroid function and iodine metabolism

Parameters	*Preconception steady-state iodine sufficient state ~150 µg per day*	*Pregnancy steady-state iodine sufficient state ~150 µg per day*
Oestrogens	Normal	Elevated
Thyroxine binding globulin	Normal	Elevated in first trimester reaches plateau in second that is maintained in third trimester
Renal blood flow	Normal	Elevated
Glomerular filtration	Normal	Elevated
Iodine clearance with obligatory loss of iodine	Normal	Enhanced
Thyroid gland stimulation	Normal through TSH	Enhanced through elevated HCG (Chorionic gonadotrophins)
Free T4	Normal	Slight elevation
Peripheral metabolism	Unaltered	Alters in second half of gestation under the placental type 3 iodothyronine deiodinase
Iodine metabolism	Thyroid gland metabolism unaltered	Thyroid gland requires 50% increase in TH production by maternal thyroid gland (physiological adaptation).

Table 18.4 Higher iodine requirement in pregnant women accentuates the deficiency [36]

Preconception steady-state iodine sufficient state(a)	*Pregnancy steady-state iodine sufficient state*	*Pregnancy in Iodine deficient state(b)*
50% is used by thyroid gland for TH production by ~35% uptake of available iodine Of daily intake, one-tenth is lost through faeces and one-third is distributed among thyroid and irreversible urinary loss. Metabolic balance remains positive and ample thyroid stores of iodine are maintained in range of 10–20 mg.	Metabolic balance is maintained in equilibrium mainly through; (a) 30–50% increase in renal iodine clearance; (b) sustained increase in TH production by 50%; (c) lowered circulating plasma inorganic iodine is accompanied by compensatory increase in thyroidal clearance. This is reflected in increased physiological state of thyroid gland. Thyroid stores of iodine are adequately maintained.	Body increases iodide trapping through pituitary-thyroid feedback to maintain necessary absolute iodine intake. A shortfall of 10–20 µg per day occurs. Thyroid gland is forced to use stored iodine that progressively falls to 2–5 µg in continuous deficient state. Metabolic balance becomes negative. In iodine-deficient healthy pregnant women physiological adaptation changes to pathological alterations.

(a) Iodine sufficient ~150–200 µg per day
(b) Iodine deficient ~50–75 µg per day

Epidemiological studies have shown that children born to women with mild to moderate hypothyroxinemia exhibit neurological alterations and reduced IQ scores, as well as an increased incidence of attention problems [25]. Although, a study of children with mild to moderate ID reported an association between first trimester ID and reduced IQ in as many as two-thirds of the children [37] confirming the findings reviewed earlier [38], most studies were carried out in the context of maternal hypothyroidism or isolated hypothyroxinemia. A conclusive proof of deficient iodine status in each trimester causing subtle neuro-psychiatric and intellectual deficits in infants/children born to mothers residing in conditions with mild to moderate ID was lacking.

The results of a very well-designed study indicate that a brief delay of just a few weeks during early gestation in initiating iodine fortification increases the risk of neuro-developmental delays in the offspring and to almost the same level as in those whose mothers were not iodine-supplemented until term [39]. The fascinating aspects of reported results and its clever study design, unique among all other studies published so far on the consequences of iodine deficiency (ID) during pregnancy have been brought about by equally absorbing editorial [40]. This work not only conveys the message that dietary iodine fortification is important throughout pregnancy, especially at the beginning, but also supports the recommendation of an urgent-daily supplement of iodine to all women when considering conception. The present study confirms that earlier recommendation, based on the randomized clinical trial carried out, was justified not only for maternal health, but also for the offspring [41]. The report gains in importance if one looks at the number of unprotected infants from IDD all over the world (Table 18.2).

18.10 Assessment of iodine status (Impact indicator)

18.10.1 Goitre surveys

Thyroid size enlargement has been one of the signs of glandular disease that accompanied stunted growth and occurrence of deaf-mutes in mountain ranges all over the world. Recognition that a visible enlargement indicates severity and decrease in thyroid swelling indicates effective correction of iodine deficiency made the size measurement an important tool for clinicians and epidemiologists to make a situation analysis of extent of problem before and after the intervention programs in place. Assessment of goitre size by palpation by trained observers as per criteria's laid down by WHO–UNICEF from time to time has served the purpose of large scale surveys and national correction program implementation assessment [2–3]. However, subjectivity in size assessment, lack of understanding of criteria's and training, over-burdened health system compounded with compromise in designing and implementation of survey tools more often leads to erroneous data collection and interpretation. Thyroid-size assessment still remains an instrument of choice for majority of national surveys at least in developing nations due to economic and logistic constraints.

In last decade the improvisation in thyroid size measurement by ultrasonography has been validated in most of the western countries especially of Europe [42–43]. Though the technique has the desirable component of accuracy, in terms of training and technical competence at primary health care system, it is still beyond the affordability of developing economies.

18.10.2 Urinary iodine concentration

The approximate thyroid clearance rate (TCR) of 0.4 L/h and renal clearance rate (RCR) of 2.0 L/h of a euthyroid normal individual indicate that thyroid gland and kidneys are two major competing organs for the amount of iodine ingested daily. The low TCR of thyroid indirectly reflects daily synthetic output of TH and increased TCR reflects the thyroidal hunger for iodine in a deficient individual [6]. This hunger is directly reflected in lowering of urinary iodine excretion (UIE) making it an exceptionally good marker of very recent dietary-iodine intake. Many studies have convincingly shown that profile of iodine concentration in even a casual urine sample provides an adequate assessment of population's iodine nutrition provided a sufficient number of samples are collected representing the population group to surmount the day to day and within a particular day variations. It should be borne in mind that UI test done in an individual's casual sample and its expression in terms of creatinine can further lead to erroneous conclusions. Iodine/Creatinine ratio is of little clinical value due to ignorance of protein intake of the individuals and often leads a unreliable estimates especially in populations suffering from malnutrition

Acceptance of urinary iodine (UI) indicator is very high due to ease of collection of a casual urine sample, minimum need of storage like refrigeration and preservatives and simple assay method based on iodine's catalytic activity in reduction of ceric ammonium sulfate (yellow color) to cerous form (colorless). A digestion/purification step using ammonium persufate or chloric acid is necessary to get rid of interfering substances prior to catalytic reaction [44]. The method is amenable for automation and large-scale analysis and availability of quality control and reference material allows for inter-laboratory comparisons [45]. The median UI concentration is recommended by the WHO [2–3] for assessing iodine intake in populations with cut-off levels defined separately for pregnant women.

More reference data on UI concentrations in chronically iodine-sufficient pregnant women, including trimester-specific values, would be valuable. The WHO[8] recommends that a median UI concentration in a population of pregnant women of 150–249 μg/l indicates adequate iodine intake (Table 18.5).

Table 18.5 Epidemiologic criteria for assessing iodine nutrition in a population of pregnant women based on median urinary iodine concentrations [8]

Median urinary iodine	*Iodine intake*
<150 μg/l	Insufficient
150–249 μg/l	Adequate
250–499 μg/l	Excessive

The median urinary iodine concentration (UI) in school-aged children is recommended for assessment of iodine nutrition in populations. If the median UI is adequate in school-aged children, it is usually assumed that iodine intakes are also adequate in the remaining population, including pregnant women. The data suggest the median UI in school-aged children should not be used as a surrogate for monitoring iodine status in pregnancy; pregnant women should be directly monitored [47]. The meta-analysis of samples of 6 study sites included 3529 children evenly divided between boys and girls at each year (Mean ± SD age: 9.3 ± 1.9 years) showed a range of median urinary iodine concentrations 118–288 μg/L [48].

18.10.3 Blood constituents as impact assessment indicators: TSH and T_g

In spite of the fact that hypothyroidism in an iodine-deficient subject is accompanied by increase in TSH in the measurement of TSH is not recommended for monitoring iodine nutrition for school-based or adult-based surveys due to large amount of overlap.

TSH estimations in neonates, however, are a valuable indicator of iodine sufficiency. The neonatal thyroid has a low-iodine content compared to that of an adult, and hence iodine turnover is much higher. This high turnover is exaggerated in iodine deficiency and requires increased stimulation by TSH. Hence, TSH levels are increased the neonates in the first week of life in iodine-deficient populations for first week of life. The prevalence of neonates with elevated TSH levels is therefore a valuable indicator of the severity of iodine deficiency in a given population. Recent data from a large-representative Swiss study suggest that newborn thyrotropin concentrations, obtained with the use of a sensitive assay from blood samples collected 3–4 days after birth, is a sensitive indicator of even mild iodine deficiency in pregnancy [50]. These findings support the WHO recommendation that a <3% frequency of thyrotropin values >5 μ/l indicates iodine sufficiency in a population. This finding should be confirmed in other iodine-sufficient countries with newborn-screening programs. For UI, the WHO states that a median 100 μg/l in infants is sufficient [3]. The median UI concentration during infancy that indicates optimal iodine nutrition is estimated to be = 100 μg/l. In iodine-sufficient countries, the median-UI concentration in infants ranges from 90–170 μg/l, suggesting adequate iodine intake in infancy.

Nevertheless, TSH screening is inappropriate for developing countries where health budgets are low- and high-infant mortality due to nutritional deficiencies and infections makes the whole exercise cost-ineffective.

Thyroglobulin (T_g)

In contrast T_g, a thyroid protein that acts as a matrix for TH synthesis, is found to be increased in circulation as a result of thyroid hyperplasia and goiter a characteristic of iodine deficiency. In this setting serum T_g reflects iodine nutrition over a period of months or years. This contrasts to urinary iodine concentration which assesses more immediate iodine intake. A serum T_g assay has recently been adapted for use on dried blood spots and makes sampling practical even in remote areas [54]. Measurement of Dried blood spot (DBS) T_g in school age children is a sensitive indicator of iodine status in a population and can be used to monitor improving thyroid function after iodine repletion. The international reference range of 4-14 μg /L for DBS T_g assays has been established for iodine sufficient five to fourteen year children. DBS T_g correlates well with urinary iodine and thyroid size and complements these tests and can be used in conjunction with UI to measure recent iodine intake and thyroid volume to assess long-term anatomic response [55].

18.10.4 Assessment of iodine status during pregnancy

The median-UI concentration is recommendations by the WHO (2–3) for assessing iodine intake in populations with cut-off levels defined separatcly for pregnant women have been recently reviewed. Traditionally, the median UI in school-going children is recommended for assessment of iodine nutrition in population. If median UI is adequate in school children, it is usually assumed that iodine intake is also adequate in rest of the population, including pregnant women. A recent study carried out within family eating from the same food supply showed that while children had adequate median UI their pregnant mothers had significantly low-median UI [47]. Daily iodine intake can be extrapolated from the UI concentration assuming 24 hours urine volumes and iodine bioavailability of 92% using the formula: urinary iodine (μg/l) × 0.0235 × body weight (kg) daily iodine intake [6, 7, and 34]. Using this formula, a median UI of 100 μg/l corresponds roughly to daily iodine intake of 150 g per day. The pregnancy often occurs in adolescence in developing countries; in a 15 year girl weighing approximately 50 kg, daily iodine intake of 200 to 250 μg would correspond to median UI of 185–215 μ/l. The recommended daily iodine intake during pregnancy of 220–250 μg [31, 35] would correspond to a median UI concentration of 135–155 μg/l during pregnancy. However, during pregnancy this extrapolation of iodine intake from the UI concentration may be less valid because of an increase in RIC [31, 46]. If RIC increases in pregnancy, the daily-iodine intake extrapolated from the UI concentration in pregnancy would be lower than that in non-pregnancy.

Table 18.6 Usefulness of impact-assessment indicators of iodine insufficiency are influenced by pregnancy

S. no.	*Effects on indicators*	*Usefulness of indicator*
1.	Hypothyroxinemia (low T_4)	Non-usable due to changes sometimes within normal range
2.	Preferential secretion of tri-iodothyronine (T_3)	Non-usable due to changes sometimes within normal range
3.	High TSH	Useful indicator (invasive) cost and feasibility makes its use difficult for populations
4.	Enhanced thyroid volume	Good indicator, physical grading is subjective, ultrasound measurement requires trained personal, costly equipment and validation (non-invasive)
5.	Low urinary iodine	Useful indicator for short-term iodine deficiency in populations (non-invasive)
6.	Increased serum thyroglobulin	Useful indicator for long-term iodine deficiency in populations (invasive), amenable to blood spot collection and analysis

18.11 Conclusion

Iodine deficiency disorders have multiple adverse effects in humans, most serious being the compromised mental and physical development of progeny. The adequate iodine intake during pregnancy and infancy is essential for prevention of impairment of growth and development of the offspring. Assessment methods including urinary-iodine concentration, goitre, and blood thyroglobulin carried out in school-going children frequently overlook the prevailing iodine deficiency during pregnancy and lactation. The monitoring of universal salt iodization programs to assess the impact often does not take into account the need of additional iodine requirement of pregnant and lactating women due to incomplete understanding of iodine metabolism and difficulties in carrying out the metabolic balance studies during pregnancy and lactation. The median UI in school-aged children may not always be a good substitute for monitoring iodine status in pregnancy; it may be sensible to monitor pregnant women directly. The recommended iodine intake in pregnant women by WHO needs further proving by additional scientific evidence to clarify the issue.

References

1. HETZEL BS (1988). Iodine-deficiency disorders. *Lancet* **1**, no. 8599, pp 1386–1387.
2. WHO, UNICEF, ICCIDD (2007). Assessment of iodine deficiency disorders and monitoring their elimination. Geneva, Switzerland: WHO.
3. WHO (2007). Technical consultation for the prevention and control of iodine deficiency in pregnant and lactating women and in children less than two years old. 2nd ed. Geneva, Switzerland: WHO.
4. RISTIC-MEDIC D, PISKACKOVA Z, HOOPER L, RUPRICH J, CASGRAIN A, ASHTON K, PAVLOVIC M, GLIBETIC M (2009). Methods of assessment of iodine status in humans: a systematic review. *Am J Clin Nutr* **89**, no. 6, pp 2052S–2069S.
5. YADAV S, GUPTA SK, GODBOLE MM, JAIN M, SINGH U, V PAVITHRAN P, BODDULA R, MISHRA A, SHRIVASTAVA A, TANDON A, ORA M, CHOWHAN A, SHUKLA M, YADAV N, BABU S, DUBEY M, AWASTHI PK (2009). Persistence of severe iodine-deficiency disorders despite universal salt iodization in an iodine-deficient area in northern India. *Public Health Nutr* **11**, pp 1–6.
6. DUNN JT, DUNN AD (2001). Update on intrathyroidal iodine metabolism. *Thyroid* **11**, no. 5, pp 407–414.
7. ALEXANDER WD, KOUTRAS DA, CROOKS J, BUCHANAN WW, MACDONALD EM, RICHMOND MH, WAYNE EJ (1962). Quantitative studies of iodine metabolism in thyroid disease. *Q J Med* **31**, pp 281–305.
8. WOLFF J (1998). Perchlorate and the thyroid gland. Pharmacol Rev **50**, pp 89–105.
9. DAI G, LEVY O, CARRASCO N (1996). Cloning and characterization of the thyroid iodide transporter. *Nature* **379**, pp 458–460.
10. DOHAN O, DE LA VIEJA A, PARODER V (2003). The sodium iodide symporter (NIS): character, regulation and medical significance. *Endocrine Rev* **24**, pp 48–77.
11. SPITZWEG C, HEUFELDER AE, MORRIS JC (2000). Thyroid iodine transport. *Thyroid* **10**, pp. 321–330.
12. VAN SANDE J, MASSART C, BEAUWENS R, SCHOUTENS A, COSTAGLIOLA S, DUMONT JE, WOLFF J (2003). Anion selectivity by the sodium iodide symporter. *Endocrinology* **144**, pp. 247–252.
13. TAUROG A, DORRIS ML, DOERGE DR. Mechanism of simultaneous iodination and coupling catalysed by the thyroid peroxidase.
14. GERARD AC, DAUMERIE C, MESTDAGH C, GOHY S, DE BURBURE C, COSTAGLIOLA S, MIOT F, NOLLEVAUX MC, DENEF JF, RAHIER J, FRANC B, DE VIJLDER JJ, COLIN IM, MANY MC

(2003). Correlation between the loss of thyroglobulin iodination and the expression of the thyroid specific proteins involved in iodine metabolism in thyroid carcinomas. *J Clin Endocrinolo metab* **88**, pp 4977–4983.

15. OHMIYA Y, HAYASHI H, KONDO T, KONDO Y (1990). The location of dehydroalanine residues in the amino acid sequence of bovine thyroglobulin. Identification of "donor" tyrosine sites for hormonogenesis in thyroglobulin. *J Biol Chem* **265**, pp 9066–9071.
16. LARSEN PR (1975). Thyroidal triiodothyronine and thyroxine in Grave's disease: correlation with presurgical treatment, thyroid status and iodine content. *J Clin Endocrinolo Metab* **41**, pp 1098–1104.
17. BIANCO A, SALVATORE D, GEREBEN B, BERRY MJ, LARSEN PR (2002). Biochemistry, cellular and molecular biology and physiological roles of iodotyrosine deiodinases. *Endocr Rev* **23**, pp 38–89.
18. SCHUSSLER GC (2000). The thyroxine binding proteins. *Thyroid* **10**, pp 141–149.
19. MAGNER JA (1990). Thyroid-stimulating hormone: biosynthesis, cell biology and bioactivity. *Endocr Rev* **11**, pp. 354.
20. ST GERMAIN DL, GALTON VA (1997). The deiodinase family of selenoproteins. *Thyroid* **7**, pp 655–668.
21. BERRY MJ, LARSEN PR (1992). The role of selenium in thyroid hormone action. *Endocr Rev* **13**, pp 207–219. Nakabayashi K, Matsumi H, Bhalla A Thyrostimulin, a heterodimer of two new human glycoprotein hormone subunits, activates the thyroid-stimulating hormone receptor. *I Clin Invest.* **109**, pp. 1445–1452.
22. RIESCO G, TAURAG A, LARSEN PR (1997). Acute and chronic responses to iodine deficiency in rats Endocrinology **100**, pp. 303–313.
23. ZIMMERMANN MB, JOOSTE PL, PANDAV CS (2008). The iodine deficiency disorders. *Lancet* **372**, pp 1251–1262.
24. HALPERN JP (1994). The neuromotor deficit in endemic cretinism and its implications for the pathogenesis of the disorder. In: Stanbury, JB (ed). The damaged brain of iodine deficiency. New York, Cognizant Communication, pp 15–24.
25. HADDOW JE, PALOMAKI GE, ALLAN WC, WILLIAMS JR, KNIGHT GJ, GAGNON J, O'HEIR CE, MITCHELL ML, HERNOS RJ, WAISBREN SE, FAIX JD, KLEIN RZ (1999). Maternal thyroid deficiency during pregnancy and subsequent neuropsychological development of the child. *N Engl J Med* **341**, pp 549–555.
26. MORREALE DE ESCOBAR G, OBREGON MJ, ESCOBAR DEL REY F (2004). Role of thyroid hormone during early brain development. *Eur J Endocrinol* **151**, no. 3, pp U25–U37.
27. AUSO E, LAVADO-AUTRIC R, CUEVAS E, DEL REY FE, MORREALE DE ESCOBAR G, BERBEL P (2004). A moderate and transient deficiency of maternal thyroid function at the beginning of fetal neocorticogenesis alters neuronal migration. *Endocrinology* **145**, pp 4037–4047.
28. ZOELLER RT, ROVET J (2004). Timing of thyroid hormone action in the developing brain: clinical observations and experimental findings. *J Neuroendocrinol* **16**, pp 809–818.
29. ZIMMERMANN MB (2006). Iodine and the iodine deficiency disorders. *Present Knowledge in Nutrition.* Washington, DC: International Life Sciences Institute, ed. 1st, pp 471–479.
30. THILLY CH, DELANGE F, LAGASSE R, et al (1978). Fetal hypothyroidism and maternal thyroid status in severe endemic goitre. *J Clin Endocrinol Metab* **47**, pp 354–360.
31. GLINOER D (2004). The regulation of thyroid function during normal pregnancy: importance of the iodine nutrition status. *Best Pract Res Clin Endocrinol Metab* **18**, pp 133–152.

32. YADAV S, GUPTA SK, GODBOLE MM, JAIN M, SINGH U, V PAVITHRAN P, BODDULA R, MISHRA A, SHRIVASTAVA A, TANDON A, ORA M, CHOWHAN A, SHUKLA M, YADAV N, BABU S, DUBEY M, AWASTHI PK (2009). Persistence of severe iodine-deficiency disorders despite universal salt iodization in an iodine-deficient area in northern India. *Public Health Nutr* **11**, pp 1–6.
33. International Institute for Population Sciences & Macro International (2007) National Family Health Survey (NFHS-3), 2005–06: India, I. Mumbai: IIPS; available at http://www.nfhsindia.org/volume_1.html
34. Institute of Medicine, Academy of Sciences. Iodine. In: Dietary reference intakes for vitamin A, vitamin K, arsenic, boron, chromium, copper, iodine, iron, manganese, molybdenum, nickel, silicon, vanadium and zinc. Washington, DC: National Academy Press, 2001:258–89.
35. DELANGE F. Iodine requirements during pregnancy, lactation and the neonatal period and indicators of optimal iodine nutrition. *Public Health Nutr* **10**, no. 12A, pp 1571–1580.
36. GLIONER D (2007). The importance of iodine nutrition during pregnancy. *Public health Nutrition* **10**, no. 12A, pp 1542–1546.
37. VERMIGLIO F, LO PRESTI P, MOLETI M, SIDOTI M, TORTORELLA G, SCAFFIDI G, CASTAGNA MG, MATTINA F, VIOLI MA, CRISA A, ARTEMISIA A, TRIMARCHI F (2004). Attention deficit and hyperactivity disorders on the offspring of mothers exposed to mild-moderate iodine deficiency: a possible novel iodine deficiency disorder in developed countries. *J Clin Endocrinol Metab* **89**, pp 6054–6060.
38. GLINOER D, DELANGE F (2000). The potential repercussions of maternal, fetal, and neonatal hypothyroxinemia on the progeny. *Thyroid* **10**, pp 871–887.
39. BERBEL P, MESTRE JL, SANTAMARIA A, PALAZON I, FRANCO A, GRAELLS M, GONZALEZ-TORGA A, MORREALE DE ESCOBAR G (2009). Delayed neurobehavioral development in children born to pregnant women with mild hypothyroxinemia during the first month of gestation: the importance of early iodine supplementation. *Thyroid* **19**, pp 513–521.
40. GLINOER D, ROVET J (2009). Gestational hypothyroxinemia and the beneficial effects of early dietary iodine fortification thyroid **19**, no. 10, pp. 431–434.
41. GLINOER D, DE NAYER P, DELANGE F, LEMONE M, TOPPET V, SPEHL M, GRU¨ N JP, KINTHAERT J, LEJEUNE B (1995). A randomized trial for the treatment of mild iodine deficiency during pregnancy: maternal and neonatal effects. *J Clin Endocrinol Metab*, **80**, pp 258–269.
42. ZIMMERMANN, MB (2004). New reference values for thyroid volume by ultrasound in iodine sufficient school children. A world health organization/Nutrition form health and development iodine deficiency study group report. *Am J Clin Nutr* **79**, pp 231–237.
43. ZIMMERMANN, MB, ITO Y, HESS SY, FUJIEDA K, MOLINARI L (2005). High thyroid volume in children with excess iodine intakes. *Am J Clin Nutr* **81**, pp 840–844.
44. BOURDOUX P (1988). Measurement of iodine in the assessment of iodine deficiency. *IDD Newsletter* **4**, pp 8–12.
45. OHASHI T, YAMAKI M, PANDAV CS, KARMARKAR MG, IRIE M (2000). Simple microplate method for determination of urinary iodine. *Clin Chem* **46**, no. 4, pp 529–536.
46. ZIMMERMANN MB (2009). Iodine deficiency in pregnancy and the effects of maternal iodine supplementation on the offspring: a review. *Am J Clin Nutr* **89**, pp 668S–672S.
47. GOWACHIRAPANT S, WINICHAGOON P, WYSS L, TONG B, BAUMGARTNER J, MELSE-BOONSTRA A, ZIMMERMANN MB (2009). Urinary iodine concentrations indicate iodine

deficiency in pregnant Thai women but iodine sufficiency in their school-aged children. *J Nutr* **139**, no. 6, pp 1169–1172.

48. ZIMMERMANN MB, HESS SY, MOLINARI L, DE BENOIST B, DELANGE F, BRAVERMAN LE, FUJIEDA K, ITO Y, JOOSTE PL, MOOSA K, PEARCE EN, PRETELL EA, SHISHIBA Y (2004). New reference values for thyroid volume by ultrasound in iodine-sufficient schoolchildren: a World Health Organization/Nutrition for Health and Development Iodine Deficiency Study Group Report. *Am J Clin Nutr* **79**, no. 2, pp 231–237.
49. LARSEN PR, MERKER A, PARLOW AF (1976). Immunoassay of human TSH using dried blood samples. *J Clin Endocrinol Metab* **42**, pp 987–990.
50. ZIMMERMANN MB, AEBERI I, TORRESANI T AND BÜRGI H (2005). Increasing the iodine concentration in the Swiss iodized salt program markedly improves iodine status in pregnant women and children: a 5-year prospective national study. *Am J Clin Nutr* **82**, pp 388–392.
51. DOREY CM, ZIMMERMANN MB (2008). Reference values for spot urinary iodine concentrations in iodine-sufficient newborns using a new pad collection method. *Thyroid* **18**, pp 347–352.
52. ZIMMERMANN MB (2007). The impact of iodised salt or iodine supplements on iodine status during pregnancy, lactation and infancy. *Public Health Nutr* **10**, no. 12A, pp 1584–1595.
53. AZIZI F, SMYTH P (2008). Breastfeeding and maternal and infant iodine nutrition. *Clin Endocrinol* **70**, no. 5, pp 803–809.
54. ZIMMERMANN MB, MORETTI D, CHAOUKI N, TORRESANI T (2003). Development of a dried whole-blood spot thyroglobulin assay and its evaluation as an indicator of thyroid status in goitrous children receiving iodized salt. *Am J Clin Nutr* **77**, pp 1453–1458.
55. ZIMMERMANN MB, DE BENOIST B, CORIGLIANO S, JOOSTE PL, MOLINARI L, MOOSA K, PRETELL EA, AL-DALLAL ZS, WEI Y, ZU-PEI C, TORRESANI T (2006). Assessment of iodine status using dried blood spot thyroglobulin: development of reference material and establishment of an international reference range in iodine-sufficient children. *J Clin Endocrinol Metab* **91**, pp 4881–4887.
56. ROMANO R, JANNINI EA, PEPE M, GRIMALDI A, OLIVIERI M, SPENNATI P, CAPPA F, D' ARMIENTO M (1991). The effects of iodoprophylaxis on thyroid size during pregnancy. *Am J Obestet Gynecol* **164**, pp 428–485.
57. PEDERSON KM, LAURBURG P, IVERSON E, KNUDSEN PR, GREGERSON HE, RASMUSSEN OS, LARSEN KR, ERIKSEN GM, JOHANNESEN PL (1993). Variations in thyroid function by iodine supplementation. *J Clin Endocrinol Metab* **77**, pp 1078–1083.
58. ZIMMERMANN MB (2009). Iodine deficiency. *Endocrine Reviews* **30**, no. 4, pp 376–408.

19

Sustaining iodine deficiency disorders (IDD) control programme

Chandrakant S. Pandav

Chandrakant S. Pandav is a physician, medical scientist, public health specialist, epidemiologist & health economist. Currently, he is Professor and Head at the Centre for Community Medicine at All India Institute of Medical Sciences, New Delhi. Dr. Pandav completed his MBBS and MD (Community Medicine) from AIIMS; M.Sc (Health Economics, Clinical Epidemiology and Biostatistics) from the McMaster University, Hamilton, Canada. He has worked as a consultant for WHO, UNICEF, ICCIDD, PAMM & MI at the global and regional level in over sixty countries, and also in India for more than twenty five years.

19.1 Introduction

Only a few countries like the Scandinavian countries, Switzerland, Japan, Australia, the USA and Canada were completely iodine sufficient before 1990. Since then, globally, the number of households using iodized salt has risen from 20% to 68%, dramatically reducing iodine deficiency [1]. This effort has been spurred by UN agencies and International NGOs including WHO, UNICEF, MI and ICCIDD, working closely with national IDD control committees and the salt industry, and funded by Kiwanis International, the Gates Foundation and country aid programs. In 2007, WHO estimated that nearly two billion individuals have an insufficient iodine intake including 1/3 of all school-age children [2] (Table 19.1).

Achieving the Universal Salt Iodisation (USI) and thus ensuring that adequate iodine intake is only the first step towards the goal of elimination of IDD. Sustaining USI efforts and tracking progress of IDD elimination is of utmost importance to prevent recurrence of IDD. IDD cannot be eradicated in one great global effort like smallpox and, hopefully, poliomyelitis. Smallpox and poliomyelitis are infectious diseases with only one host, i.e. man. Once eliminated, they cannot come back. In contrast,

Table 19.1 Prevalence of iodine deficiency in WHO Regions (2007), total number (millions) and percentages, in general population (all age-groups,) in school-age children (6–12 years) in 2007 and the percentage of households with access to iodized salt.

WHO regions[a]	*Population with urinary iodine 100 μg/L*[b]		*% of households with access to iodized salt*[c]
	General population	*School-age children*	
Africa	312.9 (41.5%)	57.7 (40.8%)	66.6
Americas	98.6 (11.0%)	11.6 (10.6%)	86.8
Eastern Mediterranean	259.3 (47.2%)	43.3 (48.8%)	47.3
Europe	459.7 (52.0%)	38.7 (52.4%)	49.2
Southeast Asia	503.6 (30.0%)	73.1 (30.3%)	61.0
Western Pacific	374.7 (21.2%)	41.6 (22.7%)	89.5
Total	2000.0 (30.6%)	263.7 (31.5%)	70.0

[a] 193 WHO Member States.
[b] Based on population estimates for 2006 (United Nations, Population Division, World Population Prospects: the 2004 revision).
[c] These figures do not include data for non-UNICEF countries (e.g., the US and Western Europe).

IDD is a nutritional deficiency that is primarily the result of deficiency of iodine in soil and water. Although IDD can be eliminated with iodine supplementation, the iodine deficiency of soil and water would remain and persist with massive deforestation, flooding, and rivers changing its course. IDD can therefore return any time after elimination if there is slackening in iodine supplementation efforts. Thus regular monitoring of Iodine Deficiency Disorders Control Programmes is absolutely critical.

19.2 Controlling of IDD – a three prong strategy

The control of IDD is an essential "three-pronged" involving the following components:

- Correcting iodine deficiency
- Sustaining IDD elimination
- Tracking progress of sustainable elimination of IDD

19.2.1 Correcting iodine deficiency

Correcting iodine deficiency can be done through iodine supplementation or food fortification.

(a) Iodine supplementation

The first iodine supplements were in the form of an oral solution of iodine such as Lugol, which was given daily. In the original controlled trial in Ohio school children (1917–1922), Marine and Kimball used 200 mg sodium iodide in water daily for 10 days in the spring and repeated this in the autumn. Satisfactory regression of goiter was observed. After the Second World War, considerable progress was made in reducing IDD with iodized oil, initially using the intramuscular form and in the 1990s, using the oral form. For example, iodized oil was used with success in Papua New Guinea and thereafter in China, several countries in Africa and Latin America and in other severely endemic areas. The oral form of iodized oil has several advantages over the intramuscular form: it does not require special storage conditions or trained health personnel for the injection and it can be given once a year. Compared to iodized salt, however, it is more expensive and coverage can be limited since it requires direct contact with each person. With the introduction of iodized salt on a large scale, iodized oil is now only recommended for populations living in severely endemic areas with no access to iodized salt.

(b) Food fortification with iodine

Over the past century, many food vehicles have been fortified with iodine: bread, milk [3], water source [4] and salt. Salt is the most commonly used vehicle. It was first introduced in the 1920s in the United States [5] and in Switzerland [6]. However, this strategy was not widely replicated until the 1990s when the World Health Assembly adopted universal salt iodization (USI), for the iodization of salt meant for both human and livestock consumption, as the method of choice to eliminate IDD. As mentioned above, in 2002 at the Special Session on Children of the United Nations (UN) General Assembly, the goal to eliminate IDD by the year 2005 was set. USI was chosen as the best strategy based on the reasons presented below:

In order to meet the iodine requirements of a population it is recommended to add 20–40 parts per million (ppm) of iodine to salt (assuming an average salt intake of 10 g/capita/day) [7]. There are two forms of iodine fortificants, potassium iodate and potassium iodide. Since iodate is more stable under extreme climatic conditions it is preferred to iodide, especially in hot and humid climates such as in India where potassium iodate is used as a fortificant. For historical reasons such as high solubility and lower cost, North America and some European countries use potassium iodide whereas due to greater stability leading to decreased losses especially at high moisture and high temperature, most tropical countries use potassium iodate [8].

(c) Safety in approaches to control iodine deficiency

Iodine fortification and supplementation are safe if the amount of iodine administered is within the recommended range. Though the optimal requirement of iodine for adults is 150 μg many people are regularly exposed to huge amounts of iodine in the range of 10–200 mg/day without apparent adverse effects. The threshold upper limit of iodine intake (the intake beyond which thyroid function is inhibited) is not easy to define because it is affected by the level of iodine intake before exposure to iodine excess. The WHO stated in 1994 that, "Daily iodine intakes of up to 1 mg, i.e. 1000 μg, appear to be entirely safe" [9]. For more than 50 years, iodine has been added to salt and bread without noticeable toxic effects [10].

Iodine-induced hyperthyroidism (IIH) is the most common complication of iodine prophylaxis and it has been reported in almost all iodine supplementation programmes in their early phases [11]. IIH occurs in the early phase of the iodine intervention and primarily affects the elderly who have long-standing thyroid nodules. However, it is transient and its incidence reverts to normal after one to 10 years. The most well documented epidemic of IIH occurred in Tasmania in late 1960s following substitution of potassium iodate in place of potassium bromate as bread conditioner but increased cases were transient and lasted for only 5 years with only minor peaks following the 1960s epidemic [12]. Similar transient increases in thyrotoxicosis lasting for only a year were reported from Kivu, Zaire in 1990s [13]. Monitoring of salt quality and iodine status of populations and training of health staff in identification and treatment of IIH are the most effective means for preventing IIH and its health consequences [14].

19.2.2 Sustaining IDD elimination

Elimination of IDD from a population should always be coupled with mechanism to ensure the sustainability of the program. As has been borne out by numerous case studies across the globe, one time elimination of IDD is not the answer. By virtue of iodine deficiency being the inherent nature of the soil, IDD do recur when the IDD elimination efforts slacken. In several countries where IDD had been eliminated by IS programs – including Colombia, Guatemala, Azerbaijan, and other countries of the former Soviet Union – control programs faltered, and IDD recurred [15, 16, 17]. In Guatemala, a previously effective iodized salt program deteriorated, currently, only 46% of households are receiving iodized salt, the median UI is 72 μg/L, and new cases of cretinism have appeared [15]. In addition, IDD may be reemerging in industrialized countries previously thought to be iodine sufficient, such as Australia and New Zealand [18, 19].

The task of *sustaining* iodine deficiency elimination requires constant vigilance. As borne out by experience from both developing and developed countries across the globe in the absence of sustainable efforts, iodine deficiency can reoccur (backsliding). One of the models proposed for sustaining IDD elimination efforts is the Social Process Model.

There are three major components to consolidate and sustain the elimination of IDD:

(a) Sustained political support
(b) Effective administrative infrastructure
(c) On-going assessment and monitoring

(a) Sustained political support. Political support is essential for the passage of laws or regulations on salt iodization through the legislature. Since governments change, the mechanism to ensure continuity must be in place. The critical role of sustainable political support was highlighted by the removal of ban on sale of iodised salt in India in 2005 and subsequent set back to USI. The ban was reinstated after vigorous efforts by the various national and international agencies working for IDD elimination in the country and civil society at large.

(b) Effective administrative infrastructure. The National Body responsible for the management of IDD control programme should operate with a process model. A useful example of such a process model is known as the social process model [20] or the "wheel" described by Hetzel et al (Figure 19.1).

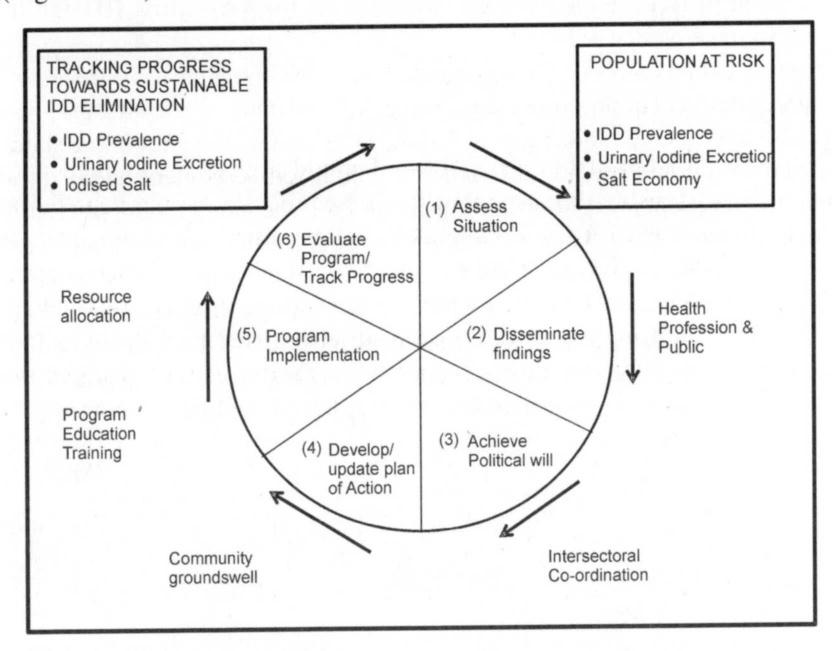

19.1 The social process model

The social process model for health care programmes may be represented by a six element circular model: Firstly, assess/reassess the situation epidemiologically.

1. Increase awareness of the situation through communication and dissemination of findings.
2. Develop and achieve political resolve and agreement at all levels (from national level to community level).
3. Create and update plans for infrastructure development and plan of action.
4. Vigorously implement the programme.
5. Assess/reassess the programme progress (viz. monitoring and evaluation) to track progress towards sustainable elimination of IDD.

(c) On-going assessment and monitoring. The effectiveness of a national programme is providing an adequate amount of iodine to the target population. This is reflected in measurements of salt iodine (at factory, retail and household level) and urine iodine (measured in casual samples from school children or households). Additional measures that would help in the assessment are estimation of thyroid size and blood tests. All these procedures require internal and external quality control in order to ensure reliability of the data collected.

19.2.3 Tracking progress towards sustainable elimination of IDD

Ensuring achievement of IDD elimination and sustaining the same thereafter requires tracking of progress made during both the phases. Tracking progress will broadly include indicators to monitor salt iodine content, iodine status of population and programme indicators. Salt iodine content needs to be monitored both at production and consumer level including the supply chain. The indicators short listed to monitor the iodine status of population are thyroid size by palpation and/or by ultrasonography, Urinary Iodine (UI), Thyroid Stimulating Hormone (TSH) and Thyroglobulin (TG). In Jan 2007 a joint WHO/UNICEF/ICCIDD Technical meeting (IDD Network Board Meeting, Atlanta, 22nd to 23rd February, 2007) looked at revising guidelines on IDD indicators. Changes agreed to include:

1. Introduction two new indicators: serum concentration of thyroglobulin and thyroid volume as measured by ultrasound.
2. Decision tree to facilitate choice of indicator (A decision tree would enable modeling of decisions taken to select a particular indicator and their possible consequences, including chance event outcomes, resource costs, and utility).
3. Inclusion of pregnant women among population to be surveyed.

(a) Three phases of IDD elimination programmes – relationship between laboratory and clinical indicators

Tracking progress towards sustainable elimination of IDD involves assessment of iodine status of the population. Iodine status can be done using a set of laboratory and clinical indicators which are closely related to each other. But the co-relation between these laboratory and clinical indicators is not a linear correlation and changes with the evolution of the IDD elimination programs. In general, the Iodine Deficiency Disorders Elimination Programmes in any region can be seen going through three phases. The three phases depict a gradual evolution from the .virgin state of iodine deficiency to the iodine replete state. The status of the indicators of assessment of Iodine Deficiency is variable from phase to phase (Figure 19.2). The three phases are given below:

1. Phase 1 – Community Diagnosis (Iodine deficiency)
2. Phase 2 – Community Intervention (Iodine deficiency to sufficiency)
3. Phase 3 – Sustainability (Ensuring optimum iodine intake)

Phase 1: Community diagnosis. This is the phase where the problem has been newly detected. Iodine deficiency exists as a public health problem and efforts to recognize it and measures to control it are yet to be initiated. In this case there is a good association between the Total Goitre Rate (TGR) and Urinary Iodine Excretion (UIE). This is because the thyroid gland, which has been starved of iodine, will take up as much of the iodine as it possibly can and the rest is excreted in the urine.

Phase 2: Community intervention. In this phase, the intervention has already begun and a mixed picture is often observed. The impact indicators are determined by environmental and community factors. Goitre is a historic marker of iodine deficiency. The inverse association between TGR and UIE is not seen. Even though the median urinary iodine values are on the increase, there is a time lag before the goiter prevalence also starts decreasing.

Phase 3: Sustainability. Control of iodine deficiency is the initial success that an effective programme will achieve. Soon after, there comes into play the need for sustainability of the control programme already in place. This is with the aim to ensure optimum iodine intake on a regular and continuous basis for all time to come. In this phase, once again, there is a good association between TGR and UIE.

The three indicators mentioned below in Fig. 19.2 assess different aspects of the IDD status in a community and thus help to track progress towards elimination of IDD. For example, iodine content of salt samples collected in a cross-sectional survey indicates the present level of iodine in salt, but gives no information about the variation occurring in the past.

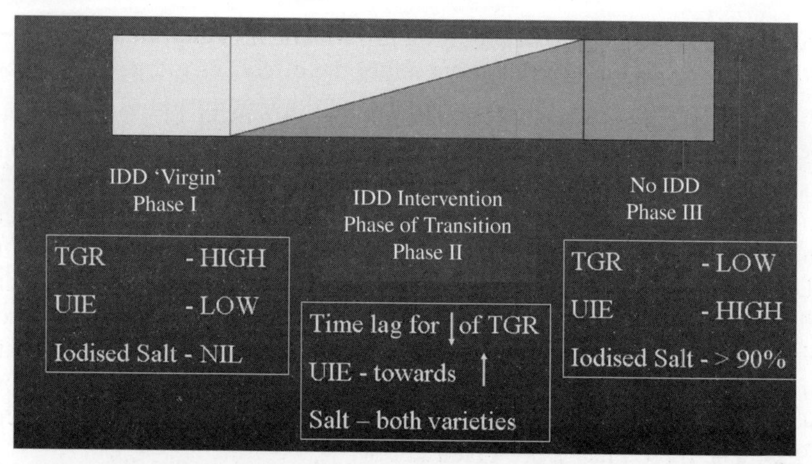

19.2 Relationship between laboratory and clinical indicators

Total goiter rates show long term effects of bioavailability of iodine and the urinary iodine excretion pattern reflects the existing levels of iodine intake and body iodine stores. To understand the status of IDD elimination programmes, the result of these indicators should be viewed in totality.

In addition there are various environmental and community factors that play a role in Phase 2 of the IDD Elimination Programme (Figure 19.3).

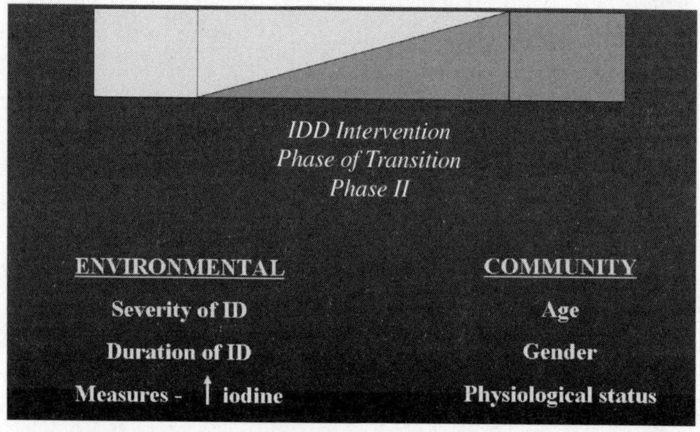

19.3 Factors influencing duration of phase of transition

The following three environmental factors play a role in the Phase 2 of the IDD Elimination Programme:

1. *Severity of iodine deficiency* – The severity of iodine deficiency plays an important part in the efforts to eliminate IDD. It is known that more severe the iodine deficiency, more intense efforts that are needed to bring the iodine deficiency under control.

2. *Duration of iodine deficiency* – To a part, it is also important how long the region/area has been under the effects of iodine deficiency.
3. *Control measure* – It is important that the monitoring of the control measure is in place. The persistence of goiter during Phase 2 can also be due to the consumption of non-iodized or inadequately iodized salt by part of the population. In case of iodized salt, one has to make sure that adequately iodized salt is consumed by the population on a regular basis. If it is not so, which is the case in most situations, a scenario emerges where there is no association between total goiter rate and urinary iodine excretion.

   The population factors that play a part in Phase 2 are age, gender and physiological status such as pregnancy and lactation. It is seen that the effects of iodine deficiency tends to show up more vividly in the younger age groups and in females whose physiological status such as pregnancy and lactation makes them vulnerable.

(b) Tracking progress towards sustainable IDD elimination

In order to achieve the failed global goal set for 2005, IDD control programmes and monitoring need to be constantly sustained due to the fact that IDD simply re-appears if salt iodization is interrupted. This may happen when the responsible public health authorities are demobilized or if the salt industry fails to effectively monitor iodine content. In order to assess the sustainability of control programmes and track their progress towards the IDD elimination WHO has established goals and indicators (Table 19.2).

Table 19.2 Criteria for monitoring progress towards sustainable IDD elimination

Indicators	*Goals*
Salt iodization coverage[(a)]	
• Proportion of households consuming adequately iodized salt	>90%
Urinary iodine	
• Proportion of population with urinary iodine levels below 100 μg/l	<50%
• Proportion of population with urinary iodine levels below 50 μg/l	<20%
Programmatic indicators	At least 8 of the 10
(i) National body responsible to the government for IDD elimination. It should be multidisciplinary, involving the relevant fields of nutrition, medicine, education, the salt industry, the media, and consumers, with a chairman appointed by the Minister of Health.	
(ii) Evidence of political commitment to USI and elimination of IDD;	

Indicators	Goals
(iii) Appointment of a responsible executive officer for the IDD elimination programme;	
(iv) Legislation or regulation of USI	
(v) Commitment to regular progress in IDD elimination, with access to laboratories able to provide accurate data on salt and urinary iodine	
(vi) A programme of public education and social mobilization on the importance of IDD and the consumption of iodized salt	
(vii) Regular data on iodized salt at the factory, retail and household levels;	
(viii) Regular laboratory data on urinary iodine in school-age children, with appropriate sampling for higher-risk areas;	
(ix) Co-operation from the salt industry in maintenance of quality control; and	
A database for recording results or regular-monitoring procedures particularly for salt iodine, urinary iodine and, if available, neonatal thyroid stimulating hormone (TSH), with mandatory public reporting.	

Source: WHO, UNICEF, ICCIDD. Assessment of iodine deficiency disorders and monitoring their elimination. Geneva, World Health Organization, 2001 (WHO/NHD/01.1)

[a] Adequately iodized salt refers to at least 15 ppm at household level

The problem of IDD is still largely perceived as equivalent to "Goiter". People consider it a cosmetic problem and hence a low priority issue. Focus should be more on the implications that iodine deficiency has on the Intelligence Quotient (IQ) of the child and the contribution of elimination of IDD to at least six of the Millenium Development Goals.

Iodized salt should be viewed as a vaccine to prevent brain damage. History teaches us that the sustained elimination of IDD requires constant vigilance of a range of professional and public interests.

Achieving elimination of IDD and thereafter sustaining it more to put it more aptly, tracking progress towards sustainable elimination of IDD should be the priority goal for national policy makers. The experience from both developed and developing countries across the globe and over a long period of time has shown the recurrent nature of IDD and thus underline the importance of sustained efforts to combat IDD.

The lessons learned from the more successful countries are

- Hold regular "National Advocacy" events to assure that all actors in the field are informed, active and participating.
- Hold regular "National and Sub National Monitoring Activities" and report them widely to demonstrate not only progress but where problems are difficult

- Maintain constant public information on the problems of iodine deficiency and the dangers of absence of iodine.
- Sustain high level national political commitment across the board.

There is a need for simple, operative, comparative and functional monitoring designs with a global oversight group not only to implement the 2005 World Health Assembly (WHA) Resolution of sustaining the elimination of IDD but to ensure that gains made are sustained thereafter. The control of IDD is essential a three pronged strategy involving correcting iodine deficiency, sustaining IDD elimination and tracking progress of sustainable elimination of IDD.

Databases are moving toward urinary iodine (UI) as a key indicator (because it tracks improvements in iodine intake more rapidly than goiter). This trend needs to be accelerated. The global databases on iodine nutrition need to be strengthened. There is need to learn from countries like China, Bolivia, Brazil, Ecuador and Bhutan, which have a sustainable IDD elimination program in place.

Sustainability requires national commitments. Sustained political support, effective administrative infrastructure and communication and on-going assessment and monitoring are essential components of proposed social process model of sustainable iodine deficiency disorders elimination. The country level policy maker need to short-list and arrive at a consensus on indicators to be used to track the progress of sustainable IDD elimination keeping in mind the relationship amongst the indicators changes with the phase of elimination and should be interpreted accordingly.

Countries should redouble their commitment to sustained elimination of IDD as a part of their regular public health programs and anti-poverty efforts through USI. A critical component of this is to establish multidisciplinary national coalitions that include salt producers and the education and media sectors, to monitor the state of iodine nutrition every three years and report to the WHA on their progress.

References

1. DELANGE F, BÜRGI H, CHEN ZP, DUNN JT, (2002). 'World status of monitoring iodine deficiency disorders control programs', *Thyroid*, **12**(10), pp. 915–924.
2. BENOIST B DE, MCLEAN E, ANDERSSON M (2007). Iodine deficiency in 2007: Global progress since 2003', *Food Nutr Bull* 2007 (in press).
3. PHILLIPS DIW (1997). 'Iodine, milk, and the elimination of endemic goitre in Britain: the story of an accidental public health triumph', *Journal of Epidemiology and Community Health,* **51**, pp. 391–393.
4. *Anonymous* (1997). 'Iodized water to eliminate iodine deficiency', *IDD Newsletter,* **13**, pp. 33–39.

5. MARINE D, KIMBALL OP (1920). 'Prevention of simple goiter in man', *Archives of Internal Medicine,* **5**, pp. 661–672.
6. BÜRGI H, SUPERSAXO Z, SELZ B (1990). 'Iodine deficiency diseases in Switzerland one hundred years after Theodor Kocher's survey: a historical review with some new goitre prevalence data', *Acta Endocrinology* (Copenhagen), **123**, pp. 577–590.
7. WHO, UNICEF, ICCIDD (1996). 'Recommended iodine levels in salt and guidelines for monitoring their adequacy and effectiveness', World Health Organization, Geneva (WHO/NUT/96.13).
8. Available at http://www.iccidd.org/pages/protecting-children/fortifying-salt/how-salt-is-iodized/iodate-or-iodide-more-detail.php
9. Iodine and health. Eliminating iodine deficiency disorders safely through salt iodization, Geneva, World Health Organization, 1994.
10. BÜRGI H, SCHAFFNER T, SEILER JP. (2001). The toxicology of iodate: A review of the literature. *Thyroid*, **11**, pp. 449–456.
11. STANBURY JB et al. (1998). Iodine-induced hyperthyroidism: occurrence and epidemiology. *Thyroid*, **8**, pp. 83–100.
12. CONNOLLY RJ (1971). An increase in thyrotoxicosis in southern Tasmania after an increase in dietary iodine, *Med J Austral* i: 1268.
13. BOURDOUX PP, ERMANS AM, MUKALAY WA MUKALAY A, FILETTI S, VIGNERI R (1996). Iodine-induced thyrotoxicosis in Kivu, Zaire. *Lancet*, **347**(9000), pp. 552–553.
14. TODD CH (1999). Hyperthyroidism and other thyroid disorders. A practical handbook for recognition and management. Geneva, World Health Organization, (WHO/AFRO/NUT/99.1, WHO/NUT/99.1).
15. Current IDD Status Database. International Council for the Control of Iodine Deficiency Disorders Website. Internet: http:/www. iccidd.org (accessed 11 September 2009).
16. MARKOU KB, et al. (2001). Iodine deficiency in Azerbaijan after the discontinuation of an iodine prophylaxis program: reassessment of iodine intake and goiter prevalence in schoolchildren. *Thyroid,*; **11**, pp. 1141–1146.
17. DUNN JT (2000). Complacency: the most dangerous enemy in the war against iodine deficiency. *Thyroid*, **10,** pp. 681–683.
18. LI M, MA G, BOYAGES SC and EASTMAN CJ (2001). Re-emergence of iodine deficiency in Australia. *Asia Pac J. Clin. Nutr.* **10**, pp. 200–203.
19. THOMSON CD, WOODRUFFE S, COLLS AJ, JOSEPH J and DOYLE TC (2001). Urinary iodine and thyroid status of New Zealand residents. *Eur J. Clin. Nutr.* **55**, pp. 387–392.
20. HETZEL BS (1987). An overview of the prevention and control of Iodine Deficiecncy Disorders. In: Prevention and Control of Iodine Deficiency Disorders (HETZEL BS, DUNN JT, STANBUIY JB, eds). Elseiver Science Publishers B.V. (biomedical Division), pp. 7–31.

20

Iodine deficiency and iodine deficiency disorders (IDD) control program

Sheila C. Vir

Sheila C Vir, MSc, PhD, is a senior nutrition consultant and Director of Public Health Nutrition and Development Centre, New Delhi. Following MSc (Food and Nutrition) from University of Delhi, Dr Vir was awarded PhD by the Queen's University of Belfast, United Kingdom. Dr. Vir, a past secretary of the Nutrition Society of India, is a recipient of the fellowship of the Department of Health and Social Services, UK, and Commonwealth Van den Bergh Nutrition Award. Dr Vir worked briefly with the Aga Khan Foundation (India) and later with UNICEF. As a Nutrition Programme Officer with UNICEF for twenty years, Dr. Vir provided strategic and technical leadership for policy formulation and implementation of nutrition programmes in India.

20.1 Epidemiology of iodine deficiency

Iodine, a micronutrient, is an essential element for normal growth and development in animals and men. Iodine is not synthesized by the body and is required to be provided through the daily diet in the recommended amounts. Iodine deficiency occurs when iodine intake falls below the recommended levels. Iodine requirements for various population groups range from 90 to 250 μg/day, the requirement being much higher during pregnancy and lactation (Table 20.1). During lactation, a higher level of iodine is required to meet the additional demands during the first six-month period of exclusive breastfeeding and for the maintenance of adequate level of iodine.

Table 20.1 Recommended daily intake of iodine [1, 2, 3]

Age/state	*Micrograms per day*
0–59 months	90
6–12 years	120
>12 years (adolescents) to adults	150
Pregnancy	250
lactation	250

Iodine deficiency in food occurs when crops are grown in iodine-deficient soils. Reduction of iodine in soil is a natural ecological phenomenon that occurs in many parts of the world. Iodine occurs in the form of iodide in soil and sea water. Iodide is oxidized by sunlight to elemental volatile iodine. The concentration of iodide in sea water is about 50–60 μg per litre while the concentration of iodine in the atmospheric air is much lower at approximately 0.7 $\mu g/m^3$. Iodine present in atmosphere is returned to the surface of earth by rain which has iodine concentration in the range of 1.8–8.5 μg/l. Iodine in soil is further reduced due to leaching by rain, flooding, deforestation and glaciations. This cycle of iodine in nature between the ocean, the atmosphere, and rainfall into streams, river, and soil is not maintained resulting in loss of balance in the iodine cycle in nature and depletion of iodine in soil. Persistent lower level of iodine in soil occurs when return of iodine to soil by rain is slow and small in amount compared to original big loss of iodine by floods or glacial. In fact, large loss of iodine from soil surface has been occurring for years with continuous leaching of iodine from the surface soil by glacial, snow and rain which are carried by wind, rivers and floods into sea. Iodine content of soil can be assessed by estimation of iodine levels in local drinking water – iodine-deficient areas have water-iodine levels below 2 μg/l [4]. Crops and animals raised on iodine-deficient soil have low-iodine content (Table 20.2).

Table 20.2 Iodine content of some common Indian foods [5]

Food item	*Iodine content (μg/1000 grams)**	
	Goitrous region	*Non-goitrous region*
Cereals		
Rice	10	40
Wheat	15	32
Pulses / oils		
Lentil	4	13
Soyabean	4	49
Groundnut	14	47
Vegetables / fruits		
Amaranth	8	15
Ladies finger / cabbage / onion	Nil	3–6
Fruits (apple, orange, banana, grapes, papaya)	Nil	5–16

Iodine deficiency results from geological rather than social and economic conditions [6]. The richest dietary source of iodine is seafood and seaweeds. Iodine in drinking water is usually a small part of total iodine intake, providing less than 10% iodine in the most iodine rich areas [7]. Low-iodine content in foods grown in soil deficient in iodine fails to meet the daily recommended intake of this essential micronutrient and results in iodine deficiency in diets of human beings and animals. Iodine content is further reduced in foods during the cooking process – the average iodine loss is estimated to be about 20%. Depending upon the method of cooking used, the loss of iodine could range between 6 and 70 percent [3, 5, 7, 8]. Iodine deficiency cannot be eliminated either by changing dietary habits or by growing and consuming specific types of foods which is primarily produced in iodine-deficient regions.

In the past, severe iodine-deficient environments were considered to commonly exist in only mountainous areas and in elevated regions with high rainfall as well as in regions with frequent flooding. The occurrence of iodine-deficiency disorders (IDD) was therefore primarily considered to be restricted to such specific geographic areas such as mountain ranges and alluvial plains. Goitre surveys, combined with increasing use of urinary iodine measurement and other methods for assessing iodine deficiency, have revealed that IDD has a much wider occurrence. Moreover, even those areas which are relatively free of IDD problem are at risk of becoming endemic because of intensive agricultural operations which can result in depletion of iodine in soil. Living on sea coast does not guarantee iodine sufficiency. In recognition of such wider occurrence of IDD than previously thought, the entire population of a region or a country is considered to be at risk of iodine deficiency. Iodine deficiency, when endemic, affects the entire population in various age groups and manifests different physiological and pathological consequences.

In addition to lack of iodine from food consumed, environmental goitrogens found in food and water interferes with iodine metabolism at various levels, from absorption of iodine to synthesis and utilization of thyroxin and in such situations exacerbates iodine deficiency. Some of these goitrogens are thiocyanates, iso-thiocyantes, thio-oxazolidone, flavanoids, disulphides, phenols, phthalates, biphenyles, lithium, etc. Food items such as jowar, finger millets, tapioca ,cassava, kale, cabbage, cauliflower, mustard seeds, ground nuts contain goitrogens and regular consumption of these foods reduce production of thyroid hormone through a variety of mechanisms and play an important role in the aetiology of endemic goitre. Iodized salt can overcome the negative effects of environmental goitrogens. However, it may be necessary to discourage consumption of goitrogenic foods or increase the level of iodine during salt iodization [9].

20.2 Iodine deficiency disorders – a public health problem

In mid 1990s, it was estimated that more than 2 billion people from 130 countries were at risk of IDD (Table 20.3). In 2006, it was estimated that there were only 47 countries where IDD continues to be a public-health problem compared to 54 in 2004 and 126 in 1993 [3].

The human body contains about 15–20 mg of iodine, of which 70–80%

is in thyroid gland. Iodine is an essential constituent of thyroid hormone thyroxine (T_4) and triiodothyronine (T_3). Thyroid hormones are involved in a wide range of biological functions and are also involved in the regulation of development and differentiation of nearly all organs and systems through their influence on gene expression. Iodine deficiency results in thyroid gland being not able to synthesize adequate amounts of thyroid hormone. In children, iodine deficiency is characteristically associated with goitre and the prevalence of goitre increases with age [9]. In adults, as in school children, the most common visible manifestation is a goitre – a mass in the neck that is consistent with an enlarged thyroid that is palpable. The enlargement may or may not be visible when neck is in a neutral position. Females from adolescence onwards have a higher prevalence of goitre than males and this is associated with difference in metabolism during the growth period. However, classical clinical hypothyroidism is characteristically absent in most adults suffering from endemic goitre, while sub-clinical hypothyroidism with reduced thyroxine (T_4) levels accompanied by normal triiodothyronine (T_3) levels is common. Adults do not reliably reflect the existing iodine status due to the fact that nodules and goitre could have occurred in childhood and iodine supplementation may only partially influence goitre size while thyroid stimulating hormones (TSH) levels would be normalized only in a fraction of population [9].

Table 20.3 Estimates of population at risk of IDD by WHO regions in 1997[(a)] [10]

WHO regions	*Countries with IDD*	*Total population in IDD countries*	*At risk population*[(b)]	
		Millions	*Millions*	*%*[(c)]
Africa	44	610	295	48
America	19	477	196	25
South-East Asia	9	1, 435	599	41
Eastern Mediterranean	17	468	348	74
Europe	32	670	275	32
Western Pacific	9	1, 436	513	31
TOTAL	130	5, 096	2, 226	38

(a) Based on UN population division (UN estimates 1997);
(b) The at risk population is the population living in iodine deficiency areas where total goiter rate (TGR) is more than 5%;
(c) Expressed as a percentage of the total population in the region (ICCIDD/WHO/UNICEF 1999).

The most important adverse effect of iodine deficiency is on foetal brain damage. Iodine deficiency is specially damaging during early pregnancy and childhood [15]. The most critical period is from the second trimester of pregnancy to the third year after birth since impaired synthesis of thyroid hormones by mother and foetus has serious implications on brain development [2]. A significant degree of neurological development occurs within weeks of conception and especially during the first month of foetal growth. An insufficient supply of thyroid hormones to the developing brain of foetus in early months of gestation adversely affects brain development and may result in mental retardation. In foetus, iodine deficiency affects neurological development and even mild deficiency of iodine in the mother has effects on rapidly growing foetal brain. The first three years of life is critical since 90 percent of human brain development occurs by the third year of life. Severe form of iodine deficiency causes cretinism [19, 20]. Cretinism is a syndrome of both neurological and physical parameters with mental and growth retardation resulting from the deficiency of thyroid hormones during foetal and early life. Endemic cretinism is usually found where the prevalence of endemic goitre is higher than 30% and median urinary iodine concentration is less than 25 μg/g of creatinine [7].

It is now well known that that cretin is the most extreme form of iodine deficiency while subtle degree of brain damage and reduced cognitive capacity affecting the population is often goes unnoticed and public-health significance of iodine deficiency is not well-appreciated. An association between iodine deficiency and brain damage was originally proposed after studies showed an association between goitre and endemic cretinism. A study with iodized oil in Papua New Guinea established the fact that cretinism could be prevented by correction of iodine deficiency before pregnancy [11]. This association was also reported from Europe where correction of iodine deficiency resulted in apparent spontaneous disappearance of cretinism in Europe [12]. Studies with animal models confirmed that iodine deficiency caused retardation of foetal brain development [13]. Studies of such animal models and controlled trials clearly established that prevention of brain damage could be achieved by correction of iodine deficiency before pregnancy [14].

The term iodine deficiency disorders (IDD) was proposed by Hetzel in 1983 [15]. "IDD refers to all the consequences of iodine deficiency in a population that can be prevented by ensuring that the population has an adequate intake of iodine" [3]. The adoption of the term emphasizes that the problem of iodine deficiency is extended far beyond simple goitre and cretinism (Table 20.4). These early effects are preventable but not reversible [4, 15]. Iodine deficiency is the world's single greatest cause of preventable mental retardation [14, 15]. Effects on brain damage occur at all stages of life [14, 15] from foetal damage to the effects of hypothyroidism in the neonate, child or adult (Table 20.4). Incidence of neonatal hypothyrodism and median urinary iodine levels of general population have been observed to be correlated.

Table 20.4 The spectrum of iodine deficiency disorders (IDD) [3]

All ages	*Goitre* Hypothyroidism Increased susceptibility to nuclear radiation
Foetus	Spontaneous abortions Still births Congenital anomalies Perinatal mortality
Neonate	Endemic cretinism including mental deficiency with a mixture of mutism, spastic diplegia, squint, hypothyroidism and short stature Infant mortality
Child and adolescent	Impaired mental function Delayed physical development Iodine induced hypothyroidism (IIH)
Adult	Impaired mental function Iodine induced hypothyroidism (IIH)

With acceleration of salt-iodization programme, the population at risk of iodine deficiency and risk of brain damage has been reduced. However, the magnitude of problem continues to remain a great concern to public-health experts. Annually, as presented in Fig. 20.1, it is estimated that 38 million newborns in developing countries where the goal of Universal Salt Iodization (USI) has not been achieved are at risk of life-long consequences of brain damage associated with iodine deficiency [16]. Of the overall 38 million newborns, 18 million are in South Asia and of these 13 million are estimated to be in India.

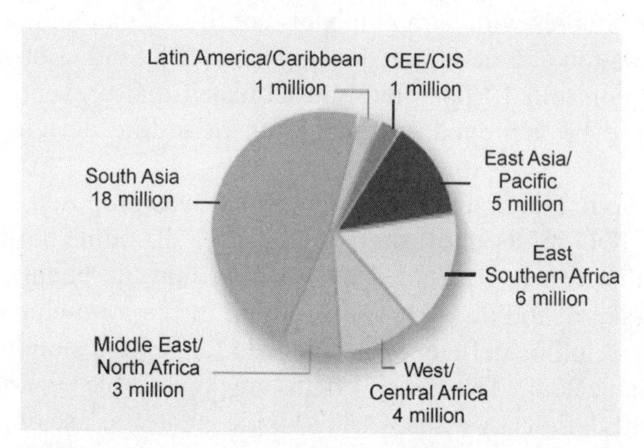

20.1 Distribution of infants born in developing countries annually who are unprotected against IDD, by region, 2000–2006 [16]

Other effects of iodine deficiency include impaired psychomotor and cognitive development. Neonatal hypothyroidism due to iodine deficiency may cause impaired mental and physical development and has been recorded in IDD endemic regions [9]. Lower school performance and significant difference in IQ have been reported in various studies comparing children from iodine deficient and iodine-sufficient areas. A meta-analysis of 18 studies comparing the performance of iodine-deficient children with iodine sufficient peers on a standardized intelligence quotient (IQ) concluded that iodine deficiency alone lowered the mean IQ scores by 13.5 points in school-aged children [17]. Lowering of mental performance due to iodine deficiency has an immediate effect on child-learning capacity and school performance. In addition, deficiency of iodine has adverse impact on women's health, the quality of life of communities and overall economic productivity with resulting adverse social and economic effects.

The primary clinical manifestations of iodine deficiency in adults are goitre (Table 20.4). In a person affected by iodine deficiency, thyroid gland makes an effort to increase the level of thyroid hormones in the blood and enlarges to form goitre. Goitre, an enlargement of thyroid gland, usually represents thyroid hyperplasia in response to insufficient iodine intake. Goitre is defined as enlargement of thyroid such that lateral lobes are larger than the terminal phalanx of the thumb of the person who is being examined by palpation on physical examination. The severity of goitre is usually proportional to the severity of iodine deficiency and with persistent enlargement of thyroid; nodules can form [7]. The status of IDD in general population is reflected by the total goitre rate in school children. However, it may be noted that in fact significant iodine deficiency has been found even in regions where the prevalence of goitre, based on palpation, is normal [18].

Iodine deficiency in women is associated with infertility and impaired fetal development [21]. From areas of iodine deficiency, higher rates of spontaneous abortions and still births have been reported. Improvement in iodine status with regular use of iodized salt is associated with reduction in stillbirths and congenital anomalies [22].

Higher perinatal mortality has been associated with goitre during pregnancy. Various controlled clinical trials of iodine supplementation, in the form of iodized oil injections, oral iodized oil or iodinated water undertaken in countries such as Zaire, Papua New Guinea, Indonesia and China have demonstrated 30–50% reduction in perinatal, infant and child mortality with improvement in iodine status [7].

The impact of iodine deficiency on animals is not well-recognised. Epidemiological and experimental studies indicate that reproductive, neurological and other defects are important effects of iodine deficiency in animal population. Reproductive failure, abortions and still births as well reduced milk and meat yields from animals and lower wool production from sheep has been reported [6, 23]. Milk production is positively correlated with iodine intake for many animals. Long-term deficiencies may result in decreased milk production that is important for the health of offspring as well as human consumption. Iodine supplementation has been reported to increase milk yield by 4–15%. Reproductive failure is the outstanding manifestation of iodine deficiency in farm animals. IDD in animals may also be more severe since animals are dependent on a relatively closed food chain compared to humans who have access to foods imported from non-deficient areas [24].

20.3 Elimination of iodine deficiency disorders (IDD) – international focus

At international level, a beginning was made in 1983 to address the problem of IDD [14]. In 1985, an international multidisciplinary network ICCIDD (International Council for Control of Iodine Deficiency Disorders) was formed to bridge the gap between research and its application in national programmes. The 1986 World Health Assembly (WHA), with representation of over 160 countries, passed a resolution which recognised the importance of iodine deficiency as a cause of brain damage and need for effective programmes of prevention and control [25]. This was followed by a WHA Resolution in 1990 [26] which adopted the goal of elimination of IDD as public-health problem by the year 2000. The goal for virtual elimination of IDD by the year 2000 was adopted by the World Summit for Children in September 1990 and was the part of action for child survival development and action – it was in fact one of the 27 goals accepted by the World Summit for Children [27]. In 1994, IDD prevention and control through universal salt iodization (USI) was endorsed as a safe, cost-effective and sustainable strategy to ensure adequate iodine consumption through achieving the USI goal. In 1996, there was an emphasis on significance of the sustainability of the programme through systematic monitoring [28]. The emphasis on sustainable elimination of IDD by 2005 was the goal adopted by the UN general Assembly in 2002. Table 20.5 presents the major milestones for elimination of IDD.

20.4 Fortification of salt with iodine

Unlike other nutrients such as iron, calcium or vitamins, the nutrient iodine does not occur naturally in specific foods but is in fact imbibed through foods grown on soil-containing iodine. Food grown in iodine-deficient regions can never provide enough iodine to the population or livestock living in the region. Daily dietary consumption of iodine through food fortification is essential. This led to efforts to experiment with fortification of selected food items as well as drinking water with iodine. Finally fortification of salt with iodine was considered the most suitable sustainable public health measure to ensure regular consumption of iodine.

Table 20.5 Major United Nations milestones for elimination of iodine deficiency [3, 16]

Year	*Milestone*	*Programme progress*
1990	Declaration of the World Summit for Children includes goal of virtual elimination of iodine deficiency disorders (IDD) 43rd World health Assembly accepts IDD elimination by 2000 as a major public health goal for all countries	Accelerated programme initiation and a shift from iodine supplementation to salt iodization
1993	WHO – UNICEF recommended universal salt iodization (USI) as the main strategy for elimination of IDD	
1994	UNICEF – WHO Joint Committee on Health Policy endorses universal salt iodization (USI) as a safe, cost-effective and sustainable strategy to ensure sufficient intake of iodine by all individuals	IDD prevention and control through expansion of salt-iodization programmes
2002	UN General Assembly Special Session on Children adopts "A World Fit for Children", the declaration that set the goal of sustainable elimination of IDD by 2005	Programme maturation with improvements in enforcement, public education and advocacy, monitoring and partnership with salt industry
2005	World Health Assembly adopts resolution committing reporting on the global IDD situation every three years.	
2007	"A World Fit for Children" commemorative session reviews progress in achieving and sustaining IDD elimination through universal salt-iodization programmes	Enhancements in programme sustainability

Iodization of salt was first suggested by Boussingault of Colombia, South America in 1883 for prevention of goitre since it was observed that local people benefited from salt containing large quantities of iodine, obtained from an abandoned mine in Guaca, Antioquia [29]. The first large scale trials with iodine were carried out between 1916 and 1920 by Marine and Kimball in Akron, Ohio, USA and this was followed with the introduction of mass prophylaxis of goitre with iodized salt on community scale in Michigan in 1924. The impact of iodized salt in control of goitre in Switzerland is well-documented. In Asia, actions for supply of iodized salt was initiated in the 1950s and 1960s but the progress was minimal until the late seventies [6].

Salt has been accepted to be the most appropriate food vehicle for fortification with iodine for the following reasons:

- Salt is universally consumed by almost all sections of a community irrespective of economic levels.

- Salt is consumed at approximately the same level through out the year in a region by all normal adults.
- Production of salt is limited to a few production centres and therefore processing on economic scale and under controlled conditions is feasible.
- The process of addition of iodine to salt is a simple technology and produces no adverse effect.
- The addition of iodine to salt does not impart any colour, taste or odour to the salt and iodized salt is indistinguishable from uniodized salt.
- The cost of iodization is low – on an average less than 5% of total cost at retail level.

The process of fortification with iodine or iodization consists of mixing salt with a determined quantity of a compound of iodine such as potassium iodide or potassium iodate. The iodine compound can be mixed with salt using the fortificant potassium iodide or potassium iodate in a dry form (dry method) or in solution form (wet method). Potassium iodate is more stable and therefore recommended for salt iodization in hot, humid environment where salt quality and packaging is less than ideal. Under proper iodization and packaging conditions (polyethylene bags of 75–80 micron thickness and containing 500 g salt), iodized salt has been found to retain at least 90% of iodine over 18-month period, irrespective of climatic conditions and textures [3]. Earlier it was estimated that iodized salt retained at least 75 percent of iodine after nine months of storage [5]. There is no universal global specifications for the level of iodine to be added to salt for iodization [30]. However, guidelines for estimating levels of iodine for salt at different salt consumption levels, environment and packaging conditions have been recommended [30, 31] as presented in Table 20.6.

Every country therefore based on local conditions must have regulations defining a minimum and maximum level of iodine at the point of production and consumption levels. As presented in Table 20.6, for recommending level of iodine for a given population, numerous factors need to be taken into consideration such as per capita consumption of salt in the region, degree of iodine deficiency, type of packaging, transit losses due to heat and humidity, shelf-life required. Per capita consumption of salt in different countries is estimated to range between 5 and 15 grams per day. For example, in India, the average consumption of salt is estimated to be 10 g/day and the cut-off level for minimum level of iodine in salt at production level is 30 ppm (50.6 mg potassium iodate) and at the consumption level 15 ppm. Most countries have fixed levels of 50 ppm (1 μg/g = 1 ppm) iodine at the time of production which corresponds to 85 mg potassium iodate. Global production and supply of iodine is derived from the nitrate deposits of Northern Chile, extraction of plants in Orient and North America and from brine wells in Japan as well as in North America.

Table 20.6 WHO/UNICEF/ICCIDD guidelines for recommended levels of iodine in salt[(a)] [30, 31]

Climate and average per capita salt intake (g/head)	*Parts of iodine per million (ppm) of salt (i.e., μg/g, mg/kg, g/tonne) for bulk and retail pack*						
	Required at factory outside the country		*Required at factory inside of country*		*Required at retail sale (shop/market)*		*Required at household*
	Bulk sacks	*Retail pack (<2 kg)*	*Bulk sacks*	*Retail pack (<2 kg)*	*Bulk sacks*	*Retail pack (<2 kg)*	
Warm moist							
5 g	100	80	90	70	80	60	50
10 g	50	40	45	35	40	30	25
Warm dry or cool moist							
5 g	90	70	80	60	70	50	45
10 g	45	35	40	30	35	25	22.5
Cool dry							
5 g	80	60	70	50	60	45	40
10 g	40	30	35	25	30	22.5	20

[(a)] 168.6 mg potassium iodate =100 mg iodine; 1 μg iodine/gram = 1 ppm

20.5 Universal salt iodization (USI)

Universal salt iodization (USI) has been recommended as a safe, cost-effective and sustainable strategy to ensure sufficient intake of iodine by all individuals in a region [27]. The policy of USI for sustained elimination of IDD was adopted by the joint UNICEF/WHO Committee on Health Policy 1994 with the goal to ensure that all salt for human and animal consumption, both locally produced and imported, is properly iodized, according to the national legislative and regulatory environment [32]. USI requires that all food grade salt for human and animal consumption be iodized including salt used by food industry [33]. The international goal for USI is achieved when over 90% of a representative sample of households is found to be using adequately iodized salt, defined as ≥15 ppm iodine [1]. Following 1994 Health Policy, USI was globally adopted as the main strategy to eliminate IDD. USI efforts were accelerated between 1995 and 2000 and countries were mobilized to introduce the policy of iodization of all edible salt regardless of having reported IDD problem.

The USI commitment was renewed at the UN General Assembly Special Session on Children (UNGASS) in 2002. In the declaration "World Fit for Children", 190 countries reinforced the need to sustain elimination of IDD [34]. By 2005, about 120 countries were implementing salt iodization programme compared to 90 in 2000 [35]. For the long-term success of the programme, all salt needs to be iodized to correct levels [36]. Iodized salt is the first global experience in national fortification of a food item to eliminate a public health problem [37]. Also USI is a unique successful example of public–private partnership for addressing a public health problem. China and Nigeria were the first countries to achieve USI.

In China, iodized salt intervention was first implemented in Chengde, Hebei Province and then expanded to the entire northern China after an important epidemiological survey, clinical investigation and intervention study was undertaken in 1960. The programme was later expanded to other IDD endemic areas in 1980s. In 1993, the Chinese Government made a political commitment for the elimination of IDD and achieved the goal of USI goal in the year 2000. Since 2000, the sustainability of USI has been maintained. China's success demonstrates that political commitment by the government and a strong alliance between the Ministry of Health and the Salt industry is a key factor for the success of achieving the USI goal [38].

Nigeria was the first country in Africa to achieve the USI compliance certification by the Network for Sustained Elimination of Iodine Deficiency in 2005. Nigeria initiated the USI programme in 1993 and within a period of five years access to adequately iodized salt had grown from zero base in 1993 to 98% consumption of iodized salt at household level in 1998 [39]. The key factors contributing to the success were political commitment by government, commitment by salt industry and effective multi-sectoral partnership. The salt industry of Nigeria has taken iodization programme as their social responsibility and the National Agency for Food and Drug Administration and Control (NFDAC) also encourages salt industries to have efficient in-house quality assurance (QA) and quality control (QC) systems which were and are continued to be duly certified by NFDAC. USI has been achieved and sustained through aggressive enforcement by government and compliance by salt industry. A ban on salt packaging in 25 kg sacs has been imposed by NFDAC and it is mandatory for all salt industries to pack salt for domestic use in small retail sizes (1 kg and less) to enhance retention of quality of iodine and content. With the introduction of iodized salt in Nigeria, the total goitre rate reduced to 6.2% in 2005 as compared to 20% in 1993. Median urinary iodine excretion has consistently been over 130 μg/dl since 1999. The USI programme in Nigeria operates with minimal domestic financing and donor investment and the incremental cost of potassium iodate is absorbed within the price of salt. NFDAC's high profile image and reputation for protecting rights of consumers continues to mobilise industry commitment and strengthens the confidence of consumers and other stakeholders.

According to UNICEF report [16], by 2006 more than 120 countries were reported to be implementing salt iodization programme. A total of 34 countries by this time had reached the USI goal and eliminated IDD as compared to 21 reported in 2001 (Figure 20.2). An additional 28 countries had greater than 70% household consuming iodized salt. WHO estimates that the number of countries where IDD is a public health problem has been reduced by half – from 110 countries in 1993 to 54 in 2003.

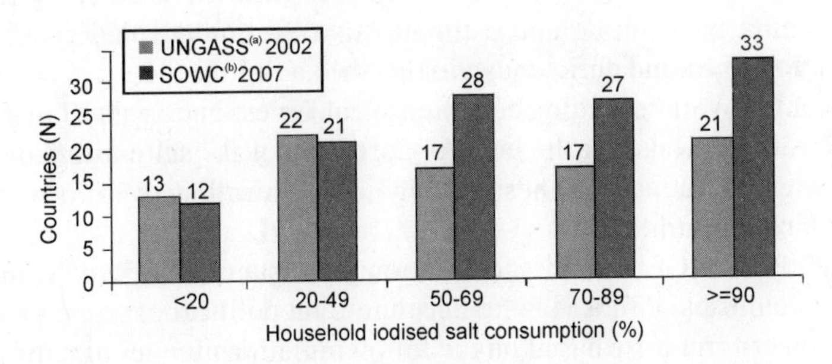

20.2 Countries (Numbers) by proportion of households consuming iodised salt in the last 5 years [35]

(a) UNGASS (UN General Assembly Special Session on Children)
(b) SOWC (State of the World's Children Report of UNICEF)

In 1990, less than one in five households in the world used iodized salt. In 2007, it was estimated 70% households have access to iodized salt [16, 35]. Table 20.7 presents the situation in six WHO regions with reference to proportion of population and estimated number of individuals in general population (all age groups) with inadequate iodine nutrition along with details on percentage of households consuming iodized salt. It is evident that there is a wide variation in the regions regarding percentage population having access to iodized salt – 47.3% in Eastern Mediterranean to 86.8% in Americas. In Europe, it was earlier estimated that only 27% salt was iodized while in 2007 it is reported to have increased to 49.2% [3, 16]. The significant progress in USI (Table 20.7) implies that every year 90 million newborn brains are protected against a significant loss of learning ability [40].

Table 20.7 Proportion of population and number of individuals in the general population (all age groups) with insufficient iodine intake by WHO regions during the period between 1994 and 2006, and proportion of households using iodized salt [3]

WHO regions	*Inadequate iodine nutrition*		*% households with access to iodized salt*
	Proportion (%)	*Total number (million)*	
Africa	41.5	312.9	66.6
Americas	11.0	98.6	86.8
South East Asia	30.0	503.6	61.0
Europe	52.0	459.7	49.2
Eastern Mediterranean	47.2	259.3	47.3
Western Pacific	21.2	374.7	89.5
Total	30.6	1900.9	70

Salt iodization has been recognised as the most successful public health effort in the past two decades. Salt iodization results in significantly decreasing risk of intellectual impairment caused by iodine deficiency [35]. World Bank 1994 [41] considers salt iodization as the most cost-effective intervention programme and estimates that each dollar dedicated to the prevention of iodine deficiency would yield a productivity gain of $28. A group of the World's leading economists confirmed during the Copenhegan Consensus meeting that the benefit–cost ratio of for salt iodization could be as high as 520, the highest among all interventions related to hunger and malnutrition [42].

In 2006, UNICEF with its international partners identified 16 "make or break" countries with a view to accelerate the USI programme [16]. The selection criteria were based on the following: high number of unprotected newborns, low level of salt iodization, large salt export activities as well as the need for special advocacy and professional support to renew strategies for the IDD-elimination programme. The countries identified were Afghanistan, Angola, Bangladesh, China, Egypt, Ethopia, Ghana, India, Indonesia, Niger, Pakistan, Philippines, Russian Federation, Senegal, Sudan and Ukraine. Efforts are being made to accelerate the USI programme in these countries. It is estimated that if these 16 critical countries achieve USI, the global coverage of iodized salt will increase from 70 percent in 2007 to about 85 percent.

An analysis of two decades of USI programme highlights the following lessons learned which are crucial for the success of USI:

- *Ensuring political commitment.* Political and government commitment along with continued motivation of industry is essential. The demand for iodized salt should be seen as a right of every person and access to iodized salt should be ensured by the state [40]. Periodic advocacy events are critical for renewed focus and political commitment. USI programme efforts not require one-time elimination of IDD but focus on sustainability. To sustain USI programme, it is of utmost importance to have political will and commitment to eliminate IDD.
- *Ensuring salt supply with adequate level of iodine.* Capacity for sustained production, availability and access to salt with adequate level of iodine. There is a need to focus on production of quality product and mechanisms for market penetration to reach each and every consumer. A high-level involvement and motivation of multiple players of the entire salt chain who produce, procure and sell iodized salt, i.e. producers of salt and iodized salt, packers, truckers and rail transporters, wholesalers, retailers and enforcement officers.
- *Consistent regulations which are effectively enforced.* A framework,

in the form of legislation and supportive regulations for mandatory iodization is critical with specific details on iodine content in salt at the production site for both human and animal consumption along with an outline of monitoring mechanisms and enforcement of agreed on actions.

- *Effective education and communication.* Sustained communication through mass media and in coordination with other ongoing health and education systems is important. Continued specific effort to reach and motivate salt producers and sellers network, including both wholesalers and retailers, is crucial. Additionally, health professionals need to work as a team with salt industry for IDD elimination since each has a very different professional orientation. The public needs to be made aware of the dangers associated with accepting and consuming non-iodized or inadequately iodized salt. The messages should focus on the impact of IDD on brain damage and the potential loss of IQ. It is also critical to keep in mind the cut-off level for usage of maximum recommended level of salt for cardiovascular health and ensuring communication on promotion of iodized salt is correctly positioned and does not create confusion regarding daily recommended amount of salt consumption.
- *Establishment of an effective system for monitoring.* Regular and effective monitoring system to check salt from production to household level. It is important that the reporting process is rapid, regular, well-supported, transparent and benefits people, process and policy makers.
- *Establishment of a multi-sector coordination and monitoring mechanisms for regular review of progress.* Review system to facilitate in planning and execution of roles identified for various sectors or professional groups. The multi-sector group ideally should involve representatives of all stakeholders – health, salt industry and food manufacturers/industry, veterinary sciences and agriculture, education, legislation and justice, communication, finance, consumer groups, scientists and professional groups.
- *Implementing USI as an integrated programme.* Salt-iodization programme efforts linked with broader health and nutrition programme and not as a vertical programme. Such integration is critical for effective sustained implementation of USI.

20.6 Monitoring IDD control programme

Indicators for monitoring IDD control programme need to be considered in the following three major groups – monitoring process, impact and sustainability [3].

(a) *Monitoring process* – This involves monitoring the salt-iodization programme and deals with the entire salt-trade chain from production, procurement to distribution and sale to consumers. Monitoring of salt-iodization programme process is critical to ensure that implementation is being undertaken as planned and information is available routinely to take corrective actions at the various points in the iodized salt trade chain. A monitoring mechanism involves setting up a system in a country to periodically check iodine levels in salt at production, distribution and consumption centres to ensure all edible salt is iodized to correct defined levels and to ensure that salt iodization is sustained. Such monitoring involves both governments and salt industry – a close collaboration between public and private sectors.

Salt testing should be done using valid and reliable methods. Testing of salt for iodine levels is done by both quantitative and semi-qualitative tests – the former refers to use of the titration method (Box 20.1) and the latter to the use of spot testing kits (Box 20.2) or commonly referred as Rapid Test Kits or Salt Testing Kits (STKs). These kits provide results of iodine levels in a few seconds. However, since the sensitivity and specificity of STKs can be low, samples of salt should be tested by titration method which is a reliable quantitative test [30]. In the recent past, quantitative testing using potentiometer or spectrophotometer has also been developed.

Figure 20.3 presents an overview of the monitoring and evaluation system for salt iodization as recommended by WHO/UNICEF/ICCIDD [3]. The most critical step in monitoring is "internal monitoring" by iodized salt producer at the site of iodization. Salt samples from the production line should be regularly analysed – checking each batch at least once – using the titration method. At production site, facilities and skills for titration should be ensured. Additionally, an "external monitoring" or quality-control mechanisms needs to be in place for monitoring iodine when importers, distributors or wholesalers receive salt. It is critical that iodine levels are checked prior to distributing edible salt further to retailers or consumers in order to take timely action when salt is found to be non-iodized or not meeting the prescribed standards. External monitoring is facilitated when a country has a legal framework and establishes a law which makes it mandatory for all edible salt to have specific level of iodine with iodine levels being defined in terms of amount and the specific form of the fortificant, i.e. potassium iodate or potassium iodide. In addition, for effective monitoring, regulations with details of approved packaging and labelling norms are critical. The packaging details must include specifications of polythene packaging that should be used. Additionally, for institutionalizing external monitoring, appropriate institutions with laboratory facilities for undertaking titration and external monitoring need to be designated.

Box 20.1 Titration method for estimating iodine content in salt [3, 30]

The iodometric titration method, as described by DeMaeyer, Lowenstein and Thilly (1979) has the following two major steps of reaction mechanism. At the level of iodized salt production, titration method is recommended. Use of the iodometric titration method by the quality control persons and food inspectors is recommended.

Step 1: Liberation of free iodine from salt. The method of liberating iodine from salt varies depending on whether salt is iodized with iodide or iodate.

- Addition of H_2SO_4 liberates free iodine from the iodate in the salt sample.
- Excess KI is added to help solubilise the free iodine, which is quite insoluble in pure water under normal conditions.

Step 2: Titration of free iodine with thiosulfate

- Sodium thiosulfate is used for titration. The amount of thiosulfate used is proportional to the amount of free iodine liberated from salt.
- Starch is added as an external (indirect) indicator in the titration and reacts with free iodine to produce a blue colour. Starch drops when added towards the end of the titration (that is, when only trace amount of free iodine is left) results in loss of blue colour, or endpoint, with further titration. The end point indicates that all remaining free iodine has been consumed by thiosulphate. The concentration of iodine in salt is calculated based on the titration volume of sodium thiosulphate using a standard formula [3].
- Reaction steps for iodometric titration of iodate

1.	IO_3^- +	$5I^-$ +	$6H^+$	$\rightarrow$	$3I_2$	+	$3H_2O$
	(from salt)	(from KI)	(from H_2SO_4)				
2.	$2Na_2SO_3$ Sodium Thiosulfate	+	I_2 Iodine	$\rightarrow$	2NaI Sodium Iodide	+	$Na_2S_4O_6$ Sodium Terathionate

Solutions can be kept for testing salt samples for 2–3 days, and the volume is sufficient for testing approximately 500 samples.

Box 20.2 Rapid-Testing Kits (RTK) / Salt-Testing Kits (STK)

Salt-testing kits – salt testing kits, manufactured by MBI (India) are used in India and many other countries. These kits are simple, handy, in-expensive, an ideal tool for monitoring at the field level and an excellent advocacy material for the USI programme. These STKs can be used by health and social workers, non-governmental organisations and even by school children. These are manufactured under strict quality control and all the raw materials and chemicals are thoroughly checked before use. These kits provide good semi-quantitative estimation of iodine in salt as they have sensitivity of 89.98%, specificity of 81.1%, positive predictive value of 80.9% and negative predictive value of 79.9%.

STKs are specific for iodate and not iodide. These kits come ready to use and provide all the necessary materials needed for the test, including the test solutions (2–3 ampoules of 10 ml each), 1 red ampoule containing recheck solution for alkaline salt samples (containing sodium carbonate), a detailed instruction sheet in local language and a colour chart with circular colour spots with defined iodine levels against each spot. All contents are packed in a small kit box that can fit into a shirt pocket. The cost of a kit, tests about 100 samples, is about one-third of one US dollar.

These kits have a shelf-life of 12–18 months when not opened and a reduced shelf–life of generally 3–6 months once opened. Kits which have outlasted their shelf-life should not be used.

Procedure

- A spoon of salt is spread flat.
- The test solution ampoule is opened and the test solution is dropped on the surface of salt.
- The spot of salt surface where the test is dropped will turn from light to dark violet depending on the iodine content.
- The colour formed should be instantly compared with the colour chart. If the colour is not interpreted straight away, colour fading may occur over time.
- In the absence of any colour formation, a few drops of the recheck solution are to be spread on the salt surface before using the test solution.

Reaction mechanism of the test kit is as follows:

IO_3^- + $5I^-$ + $6H^+$ → $3I_2$ + $3H_2O$

(from salt) (from KI) (from H_2SO_4)

I_2 + Starch → Blue colour

The reaction liberates the iodine and depending on the iodine content starch turns the salt blue. The intensity of colour varies with the amount of iodine in the salt sample.

Monitoring iodine levels in salt at household level is the critical indicator for measuring the success of the USI programme. Household-level monitoring, through national surveys or community-based methods, is recommended. It is recommended that the use of STK for checking iodine levels is complemented with the simultaneous use of titration method for checking iodine levels in sub-samples of salt. Testing of salt samples at household level can be rapidly and easily undertaken by working with school network and school children bringing salt samples from their homes for testing iodine adequacy in salt. Instant feed back to community, using school child to community approach, has also proven to be effective [43]. School-level monitoring combined with the establishment of a monitoring mechanism to test iodine levels in salt at wholesalers' levels has been demonstrated to be a useful strategy for positively influencing correct iodized salt-trade practices.

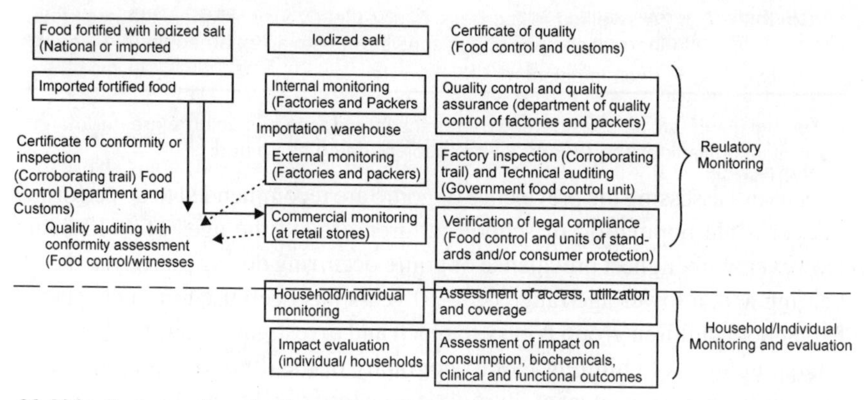

20.3 Monitoring and evaluation system for salt iodization [3]

20.6.1 Assessing iodine nutritional status – impact of IDD control programme

The following two methods are used for assessing impact of IDD control programme on iodine nutrition of the population: (a) assessment of thyroid size by palpation; and (b) urinary iodine excretion. The recommended sensitive methods are urinary iodine and the two recently added methods – measurement of thyroid stimulating hormone (TSH) levels in neonates and thyroglobulin (T_g) levels. Use of TSH and T_g have been proposed as indicators of iodine nutrition but their usefulness in assessing iodine status from cross-sectional surveys has variable results. However, the principal indicator of impact monitoring is urinary-iodine levels since the measurement of TSH and T_g is not feasible in public health programme situations of developing countries while measurement of thyroid size lacks sensitivity to acute changes in iodine intake resulting from introduction of salt-iodization programme. Measurement of thyroid size, however, is considered useful for baseline assessment of severity of IDD in a region and is also considered useful for the assessment of long-term impact of IDD control programme [3].

(a) *Assessment of thyroid size*. The term goitre refers to a thyroid gland that is enlarged. The grading classification adopted by WHO (Table 20.8) for the total goitre rate (TGR) is used for the assessment of iodine status in a population [3]. The goitre rate includes both visible and palpable goitre.

Table 20.8 Simplified classification of goitre[(a)] by palpation [3]

Grade 0	No palpable or visible goitre
Grade 1	A goitre that is palpable but not visible when the neck is in the normal position (i.e. the thyroid is not visibly enlarged). Thyroid nodules in a thyroid which are otherwise not enlarged fall into this category.
Grade 2	A swelling in the neck that is clearly visible when the neck is in a normal position and is consistent with an enlarged thyroid when the neck is palpated.

[(a)] Thyroid gland will be considered when each lateral lobe has volume greater than the terminal phalanx of the thumbs of the subject being examined.

Surveys assessing the prevalence of goitre are recommended to be performed in accessible population of school children around the ages of 6–12 years. However, with highest prevalence of goitre occurring during puberty and child bearing age, a lower age range of 8–10 years has been used in many studies [3]. School children group is easy to reach and investigators can easily palpate a large number of children. Ultrasonography of the thyroid gland provides a more precise measurement of thyroid size but the inter-observation are reported to be high and thyroid volume is slow to change in an evolving iodine-nutrition status [36]. Use of thyroid size or TGR for measuring impact is not recommended to assess impact once the salt-iodization programme has been introduced [3]. In fact, despite improvement in iodine-nutrition status of a population, it may take years for most palpable goitre to return to normal size. Goitre prevalence therefore has limitation to be used as a tool for assessment of iodine changes over a period of time [44].

Total goitre rate or TGR (number with goitres of grades 1 and 2 divided by total examined) of 5% or more in schoolchildren 6–12 years of age is recommended to indicate the presence of iodine deficiency as a public health problem [3]. This recommended cut-off on the TGR percentage is based on the observation that in normal, iodine-replete populations, the prevalence of goitre should be quite low. The cut-off point of 5% allows both for some margin of error of goitre assessment, and for goitre that may occur in iodine-replete populations due to other causes such as goitrogens and autoimmune thyroid diseases. Thyroid size is considered more useful in baseline assessments of the severity of IDD and is also useful for the assessment of the long-term impact of the programme.

(b) *Urinary iodine*. With the limitation in usefulness of thyroid size and biological markers for thyroid function, urinary iodine levels are used as the primary indicator for assessing iodine-nutrition status in representative group of subjects (Table 20.9). Urinary iodine reflects the recent intake of iodine and tends to vary within a day or day to day. However, this variation tends to even out among populations. Urinary iodine excretion provides an excellent indication of iodine intake of population [3]. Urinary iodine is not recommended to be used for the purpose of individual diagnosis and treatment. The median urinary iodine value for sampled population is the most commonly assessed indicator and can be easily assessed using the median level from only 40 subjects from each local community [3].

Taking into consideration the fact that developing foetus suffers the greatest damage as a result of iodine deficiency, two other potential targets have been recently proposed for urinary iodine estimations – women in the reproductive age group 15–49 years and pregnant women [3, 36]. As indicated in Table 20.9, in children and non-pregnant women, lower median urinary iodine concentrations of between 100 and 199 μg/l defines a population which has adequate iodine nutrition. In addition, not more than 20% samples in this population group should be below 50 μg/l in non-pregnant and non-lactating women [3]. During pregnancy, median urinary concentration between 150 and 249 μg/l defines a population which has no iodine deficiency.

Table 20.9 Epidemiological criteria for assessing iodine nutrition based on median urinary iodine concentrations of school age children (≥6 years)[a] and pregnant women [3]

Median urinary iodine (μg/l)	*Iodine intake*	*Iodine status*
Children ≥ 6 years		
<20	Insufficient	Severe iodine deficiency
20–49	Insufficient	Moderate iodine deficiency
50–99	Insufficient	Mild iodine deficiency
100–199	Adequate	Adequate iodine nutrition
200–299	Above requirements	Likely to provide adequate intake for pregnant/lactating women but may pose a slight risk of more than adequate intake in the overall population.
≥300	Excessive	Risk of adverse health consequences (iodine-induced hyperthyroidism, autoimmune thyroid diseases).
Pregnant women[b]		
<150	Insufficient	
150–249	Adequate	
250–499	Above requirements	
≥500	Excessive[c]	

[a] Applies to adults but not to pregnant and lactating women.

[b] For lactating women and children <2 years of age median urinary iodine concentration of 100 μg/l can be used to define adequate iodine intake, but no other categories of iodine are defined. Although lactating women have the same requirement as pregnant women, the median urinary iodine is lower because iodine is excreted in breast milk.

[c] The term "excessive" means in excess of the amount required to prevent and control iodine deficiency.

Box 20.3 Measuring urinary iodine [45]

Urinary iodine assay require total avoidance of contamination. Small amount of urine (0.5–1.0 ml) is required. Urine samples are recommended to be collected in small cups which are tightly sealed. No refrigeration is required. These samples can be stored for months, preferably in a refrigerator to avoid odour. Criteria for assessing urinary iodine methods are reliability, speed, technical demands, complexity of instrumentation, and availability of high quality reagents, safety and cost. Two methods are recommended – ammonium persulphate method and chloric acid methods [3]. These methods depend on iodine acting as a catalyst in the reduction of ceric ammonium sulphate (yellow colour) to the cerous form (colourless) in the presence of arsenious acid (the sandell-kolthoff reaction). Due to potential hazards of chloric acid method, ammonium persulphate is recommended [3]. Modification of these methods is commonly used for measuring urinary iodine [45]. Choice of methods depends on local resources and need. External quality control is essential since unrecognized iodine contamination is a common occurrence. To overcome this problem, an international network of resource laboratories has been established which collaborates with the Centers for Disease Control of USA.

Based on these facts, there is a proposal to examine urinary iodine levels not only in school children but also in pregnant women (sample pregnant women from prenatal clinics) for assessment of iodine nutrition status in a cross-sectional surveys, since information of school children alone is not adequate to reflect the urinary iodine status of women of child bearing age, pregnant or non-pregnant [36]. It is important that laboratories use recommended procedures for measuring iodine in urine and set-up mechanisms for internal quality control and also link up with recognised institute for external quality control programme [45].

20.7 Monitoring progress towards sustainable elimination of IDD as a public health problem

IDD is a nutritional deficiency and efforts for elimination through USI need to be sustained. Indicators for programme sustainability therefore comprise of (i) indicators to measure achievement of salt iodization and iodine status in population and (ii) indicators for measuring ongoing political support and programme strength [3]. Information about salt iodization is recommended to include measures of quality assurance at iodized salt production facilities as well as monitoring compliance of the requirements set by the country programme guidelines for imported iodized salt. Indicators for monitoring of political support and programme strength includes various elements of programme which are critical to sustainability such as multi-sector coalition, budget allocation, legislation and regulating mechanisms for monitoring of iodine levels in edible salt and iodine status, system for regular reporting of programme and updating of the national database.

The criteria for monitoring progress towards elimination of IDD as a public health problem were originally determined by a Joint WHO/UNICEF/ICCIDD working group on assessment and Monitoring of IDD in 1994 [46, 47] and was endorsed at the subsequent meeting in 2001 [1]. The sustainability criterion was introduced in 2007 and is presented in Table 20.10. This involves a combination of median urinary iodine levels in the population, availability of adequately iodized salt at the household level. Additionally, a set of programmatic indicators are recommended to be assessed as evidence of sustainability.

A network for sustained elimination of iodine deficiency has been launched by the Director General of WHO [47]. The network in a cost-effective manner is expected to provide USI / IDD review through use of simplified guidelines. The process is proposed to be initiated by the government who requests for such an external USI assessment through the country office of UNICEF or WHO. Such a process is viewed to be very important for national ownership of the situation and commitment to the process of sustained IDD elimination. The main objective of the review

Table 20.10 WHO / ICCIDD / UNICEF criteria for monitoring progress towards sustainable elimination of IDD as a public health problem [3, 48]

	Indicator	*Goal*
(1)	Salt iodization Availability and use of adequately iodized salt (over 15 ppm iodine and <40 ppm at household level)	>90% households
(2)	Urinary iodine – median in the general population – median in the pregnant women	 100–199 μg/l 150–249 μg/l
(3)	Programmatic indicators	Attainment of 8 out of 10 following indicators – National body appointed – Evidence of political commitment – Appointment of executive officer – Regulation of USI – Commitment to regular progress in IDD elimination – Public education and social mobilisation – Regular data on iodized salt at factory, retail and household level – Regular laboratory data on urinary iodine – Cooperation from salt industry – Data base (salt and urinary iodine, mandatory public reporting)

Box 20.4 Upper limit of iodine intake and iodine-induced hyperthyroidism

Excess of iodine ingestion can be harmful, which may inhibit the synthesis of thyroid hormones by the thyroid. This iodine-induced hypothyroidism is known as "Wolff-Chaikoff" effect, the manifestation of which depends on level of iodine intake before exposure to iodine excess. This is generally encountered among newborns as neonatal chemical hypothyroidism when women during pregnancy receive high doses of iodine, in the form of iodized oil injections.

When iodine is supplemented to severely iodine-deficient communities, even at the total daily intake level of 100–200 μg, hyperthyroidism may occur, mainly amongst middle-aged people. It is related probably to (i) relative increase and (ii) rapidity in increase of iodine intake consequent to iodine supplementation in iodine-deficient communities. With intensive efforts to address IDD, examples of iodine excess are being recognised in situations where iodine levels in salt are excessive due to poor monitoring. The major epidemiological consequence of iodine excess is iodine induced hyperthyroidism (IIH). IIH occurs in severe iodine deficiency of long duration and in situations of introduction of salt with high iodine content (100 ppm) in a short period of time. Increased incidence of IIH is transient, minimal and self-limiting [47]. It has been reported that IIH occurs more commonly in older subjects with pre-existing nodular goitres and commonly affects older age group of over 40 years [3].

by the network is to help governments and program managers to assess and verify the country achievement towards their goals to sustain elimination of iodine deficiency. The network proposes to facilitate progress comparisons across regions by means of standardized tools/ guidelines. Additionally, the review will also analyse and identify lessons learned and best practices of the country programs and identify ways to address bottlenecks to ensure USI and recommend steps to sustain USI.

20.8 Supplementation with iodised oil in special situations of insufficient access to iodized salt

As indicated in Table 20.11, a substantial increase in intake of iodine is recommended to meet the higher biological needs for iodine during pregnancy. It is crucial that women have adequate iodine stores during the first trimester of pregnancy and iodine nutriture of women of reproductive age is taken care of to meet the added needs of developing foetus. Efforts to improve salt iodization programme must continue and given the highest priority. However, for regions with poor household consumption of adequately iodized salt, special additional temporary measures such as administration of iodized oil supplement has been proposed to ensure optimal iodine nutrition in the vulnerable group comprising pregnant and lactating women and children below two years [2, 3]. It is important that countries assess the country situation of iodization programme at national and sub-national levels and consider introduction of temporary measures to address the risk of iodine deficiency to the vulnerable groups in specific identified regions. Such a situation is particularly applicable in countries which are often in conflict situations and have not succeeded to achieve salt-iodization coverage of over 20% due to a number of hindrances. In such conditions, additional temporary measures are recommended to be introduced to ensure that optimal critical nutrition at the highest risk period of life – pregnancy and under-2-year children – is addressed. It has been proposed that in situations of poor iodized salt programme, the most vulnerable groups, pregnant and lactating women, need to be considered for supplementation with iodine until salt-iodization programme improves (Table 20.11). For children of 7–24 months, either supplementation or use of fortified complementary food for 7–24 months has been proposed as a possible temporary public health measure [2, 3].

Table 20.11 Recommended dosages of daily and annual iodine supplementation [3]

Population group	*Daily dose of iodine supplement (μg/d)*	*Single annual dose of iodized oil supplement (μg/y)*
Pregnant women	250	400
Lactating women	250	400
Women of reproductive age (15–49 years)	150	400
Children < 2 years[a, b]	90	200

[a] For children 0–6 months of age, iodine supplementation should be given through breast milk. This implies that the child is exclusively breast fed and the lactating mother receives iodine supplementation as indicated above.

[b] These figures for iodine supplements are given in situations where complementary food fortified with iodine is not available, in which case iodine supplementation is required for children of 7–24 months of age

References

1. WORLD HEALTH ORGANISATION, UNITED NATIONS CHILDREN'S FUND, INTERNATIONAL COUNCIL FOR CONTROL OF IODINE DEFICIENCY DISORDERS (2001). Assessment of the iodine deficiency disorders and monitoring their elimination. Geneva. WHO, 2001, WHO / NHD / 01, **1**, pp. 1–107.
2. DE BENOIST B, DELANGE F (2007). Report of a WHO Technical Consultation on Prevention and Control of Iodine Deficiency in Pregnancy, lactation and Children less than 2 years of age. *Public Health Nutrition* **10** no. 1A, 1–167.
3. ICCIDD/UNICEF/WHO (2007). Assessment of iodine deficiency disorders and monitoring their elimination. A guide for programme managers. 3rd edition. Geneva, WHO.
4. HETZEL BS (1989). The biology of iodine. In: *The Story of Iodine Deficiency: An International Challenge in Nutrition*. New Delhi: Oxford University Press, pp. 22–35.
5. RANGANATHAN S (1995). Iodine is safe. *Ind J Public Health* **39**, pp. 164–171.
6. MANNAR VMG (1994). The iodization of salt for the elimination of iodine deficiency disorders. In: HETZEL BS, PANDAV CS (eds): *SOS for a Billion*. International Council for the Control of Iodine Deficiency Disorders.
7. SEMBA RD, DELANGE F (2008). *Nutrition and Health in Developing Countries*. In: Semba RD, Bloem MW (eds). New Jersey: Humana Press, pp. 507–529.
8. GOINDI G, KAMARAKAR MG, KAPIL U, JAGANNATHAN J (1995). Effect of losses of iodine during different cooking procedures. *Asia Pacific Journal of Clin Nutr* **4**, no. 2, pp. 225–227.
9. WHO/UNICEF/ICCIDD (1993). Global prevalence of iodine deficiency disorders, micronutrient deficiency information system (MDIS) working paper #1.

10. ICCIDD/WHO/UNICEF (1999). Progress towards elimination of iodine deficiency disorders. WHO/NHD/99.4.
11. PHAROAH POD, BUTTERFIELD IH, HETZEL BS (1971). Neurological damage to the foetus resulting from severe iodine deficiency in pregnancy. *Lancet* **1**, pp. 308–310.
12. BURH H, SUPERSAXO Z, SELZ B (1990). Iodine deficiency disease in Switzerland: historical review and some new goitre prevalence data. *Alta Endocrinologica* **123**, pp. 577–590.
13. HETZEL BS and MANO M (1989). A review of experimental studies of iodine deficiency during foetal development. *J Nutr* **119**, pp. 145–151.
14. HETZEL BS (2007). Global progress in addressing iodine deficiency through USI: the making of a global health success story – the first decade (1985–1995). SCN#35, pp. 5–11.
15. HETZEL BS (1983). Iodine deficiency disorders and their eradication. *Lancet* **2**, pp. 1126–1129.
16. UNICEF (2009). Sustainable Elimination of Iodine Deficiency. Progress since the 1990. World Summit for Children.
17. BLEICHRODT N and BORN M (1994). A meta-analysis of research into iodine and its relationship to cognitive development. In: Stanbury JB (ed): *The Damaged Brain of Iodine Deficiency*. New York: Communication Corporation, pp. 195–200.
18. ICCIDD/UNICEF/WHO (2001). Assessment of iodine deficiency disorders and monitoring their elimination. A guide for programme managers. 2nd edition. WHO/NHD/01.1, Geneva, WHO.
19. DELANGE F (1994). The disorders induced by iodine deficiency. *Thyroid* **4**, pp. 107–128.
20. DELANGE F (1999). What do we call a goitre? *Eur J. Endocrinol* **140**, pp. 486–488.
21. PHARAOH POD, ELLIS SM, WILLIAMS ES (1976). Maternal thyroid function, iodine deficiency and foetal development. *Clin Endocrinol* **5**, pp. 159–166.
22. POTTER JD, MC MIACHAEL AJ, HETZEL BS (1979). Iodisation and thyroid status in relation to still births and congenital anomalies. *Int J Epidemiol* **8**, pp. 137–144.
23. HETZEL, BS (1996). The nature and magnitude of iodine deficiency disorders in SOS for a billion. In: HETZEL BS and PANDAV CS (eds): *SOS for a Billion*. International Council for the Control of Iodine Deficiency Disorders.
24. PANDAV CS and MANNAR VMG (1996). IDD in livestock population. In: HETZEL BS and PANDAV CS (eds): *SOS for a Billion*. Oxford University Press.
25. WHO (1986). Prevention and control of iodine deficiency disorders. Report to 39th World HEALTH ASSEMBLY, GENEVA, WHA 39.6.
26. WHO (1990). Prevention and control of iodine deficiency disorders. Report of 43rd World HEALTH ASSEMBLY. GENEVA WHA 43.2.
27. WORLD SUMMIT FOR CHILDREN (1990), United Nations, New York.
28. WHO (1996). Prevention and control of iodine deficiency disorders. Report of 49th World HEALTH ASSEMBLY, GENEVA WHA 49.13.
29. HETZEL BS (1989). History of goitre and cretinism. *The Story of Iodine Deficiency*. Oxford University Press.
30. SULLIVAN KM, HOUSTON R, GORSTEIN J, CERVINSKAS J (1995). Monitoring Salt Iodization Programme UNICEF/ICCIDD/PAMM/WHO/MI.
31. WHO (1994). Iodine and Health; eliminating iodine deficiency disorders solely through salt iodization. WHO/NUT/94.4, WHO, Geneva.
32. NATHAN R (1999). Regulation of Fortified Foods to Address Micronutrient Malnutrition: Legislation, Regulations and Enforcement, Micronutrient Initiative: Ottawa.

33. WHO/UNICEF/ICCIDD (1996). Recommended iodine levels in salt and guidelines for monitoring their adequacy and effectiveness. WHO / NUT 96.13. WHO. Geneva.
34. UNICEF (2002). A world fit for children, UNICEF, New York (online).
35. GAUTAM K (2007). Global progress in addressing iodine deficiency through universal salt iodization: the making of global public health success story – the second decade (1995–2007). SCN Newsletter # 35, p. 12.
36. SULLIVAN KM, SACHDEV PS, GRUMMA-STRAUUS L (2007). Achieving and sustaining USI: doing it well through quality assurance, monitoring and impact evaluation. *SCN News*, pp. 48–52.
37. UNICEF (2006). The state of the World's children. 2007. UNICEF online.
38. CHEN Z, DANG Z, LIN, J (2007). Effective programme development and management. Lessons learnt from USI in China. *SCN News*, pp. 33–36.
39. AKUNYLLI DN (2007). Achieving and sustaining universal salt iodization. Doing it well through regulation and regulation enforcement, lessons learned from USI in Nigeria. *SCN News*, pp. 43–47.
40. MANNAR V (2007). Guest editorial, SCN News, p 3.
41. WORLD BANK (1994). Enriching lives, overcoming mineral and vitamin malnutrition in developing countries. World Bank, Washington DC.
42. BEHRMAN JR, ALDERMAN H, HODDINOTT J (2004). Hunger and malnutrition. Copenhagen Consensus – Challenges and Opportunities, Copenhagen.
43. VIR SC, DWIVEDI S, SINGH R, MUKHERJEE A (2007). Reaching the goal of Universal Salt Iodisation: Experience of Uttar Pradesh, India. *Food and nutrition Bulletin* **28**, no. 4, p. 384.
44. GORSTEIN J, SULLIVAN KM, HOSUTON R (2001). Goitre assessment: help or hindrance in tracking progress in iodine deficiency programme? *Thyroid* **11**, pp. 1201–1202.
45. CALDWELL KL, MAKHMUDOVA JR, HOLLOWELL JG (2005). EQUIP: A world wide programme to ensure the quality of urinary iodine procedures. *Accreditation and Quality Assurance* **10**, pp. 356–361.
46. WHO/UNICEF/ICCIDD. Indicators for assessing iodine deficiency disorders and their control through salt iodization. Geneva, WHO, 1994.
47. UNICEF (2006). Network for sustained elimination of iodine deficiency. Review guidelines New York, UNICEF, 2006.
48. PANDAV CS, CHAKRABORTY A, SUNDARESHAN S, ANSARI MA, JAIN P, AGUAYO V, AG AYOYA M and KARMARKAR MG (2008). Salt for freedom and iodized salt for freedom from preventable brain damage. All India Institute of Medical Sciences.

21

Universal salt iodization (USI)

M. G. Venkatesh Mannar

M. G. Venkatesh Mannar is a leader in global health with thirty five years experience in pioneering effective international nutrition and development initiatives, focused on the world's most vulnerable citizens. Currently, he is the President of the Ottawa-based Micronutrient Initiative (MI), and oversees the organization's mission to develop, implement and monitor cost-effective and sustainable solutions for micronutrient deficiencies in more than 75 countries.

21.1 Introduction

Iodine is an essential nutrient for humans and animals. A deficiency of this mineral has a wide range of negative consequences such as still births, congenital abnormalities and decreased cognitive capacity.

The food supply of more than 2 billion people is lacking in adequate levels of iodine, resulting in the widespread prevalence of a spectrum of iodine deficiency disorders (IDD) [1]. This public health problem can be corrected by the regular delivery of small doses of iodine to the population through commonly eaten foods or condiments. Salt is an excellent carrier for iodine and other nutrients as it is consumed at relatively constant, well-definable levels by all people within a society, independent of the economic status.

Universal Salt Iodization (USI), which intends that all salt for human and animal consumption be iodized thus ensuring adequate iodine nutrition, was identified as the global strategy for the elimination of iodine deficiency. Salt is an excellent carrier for iodine and other nutrients as it is safe, consumed at relatively constant, well-definable levels by all people within a society, independently of economic status [2]. WHO provides guidelines as to the recommended prescribed levels of iodization as well as the recommended urinary iodine excretion levels for specific population groups.

In 1990, seventy Heads of State gathered at the World Summit for Children in New York and pledged to eliminate iodine deficiency disorders (IDD) as one of the health and social development goals to reach by the year 2000. Salt iodization was identified as the main intervention to deliver iodine on a continuous and self-sustaining basis to populations around the world. Governments working with the salt industry and supported by international agencies and expert groups then set to plan and implement programmes that would enable this measure. Over the past two decades, as part of the Universal Salt Iodization (USI) initiative, a large number of developing countries have taken steps to ensure that all salt produced for human and livestock consumption is iodized.

Once established in a country, salt iodization is a permanent and long-term solution to the problem. It eliminates iodine deficiency and continues to provide each individual with his/her daily iodine needs and prevents recurrence. Within one year of iodized salt containing the required iodine being widely available and consumed in a community, there will normally be a rapid decline in birth of cretins or children with subnormal mental and physical development attributable to iodine deficiency. Goitres in primary school children and adults will have started to shrink and even disappear altogether. Children will be more active and perform better at school.

21.2 Taking universal salt iodization to scale

The specific objective is to dovetail iodization into the prevailing salt production and distribution system in a country at minimum cost and disruption. The salt industry has obviously been a key player in enabling this major public health achievement. However, there is considerable variation in the production process and scale of this most ancient of industries. Salt manufacturing techniques and product quality vary over a wide range from cottage scale units producing a few hundred tons a year to very large fully automated plants producing several million tons.

The production of salt (sodium chloride) is one of the most ancient and widely distributed industries in the world. It can be produced by mining of solid rock deposits and by the evaporation of sea water, lake and underground brines by solar digging. Rock and solar-evaporated salt account for roughly 50% of production each. The requirements of Europe and North America are met mostly by mining while in Asia, Africa, Australia and South America solar evaporation is the main source. In some countries both forms are used. The extraction of salt from sea water consists of progressive evaporation of brine in large open ponds using solar heat and wind. As the brine evaporates its concentration rises and the constituent salts crystallize in a set order. During this process the sodium chloride fraction is separated from the brine over a fixed concentration range in a series of flat rectangular ponds and deposits as a uniform crust. This salt is 'harvested' by a variety of processes ranging from simple hand labour to the use of mechanized equipment to scrape the salt and transfer it through a series of conveyors for storage and draining [3].

Iodine is added as potassium iodate to salt after refining and drying and before packing. Iodization can often be linked with existing production and/or refining lines. This is typically done by spraying a solution of potassium iodate on the salt at a uniform rate followed by thorough mixing of the salt with the sprayed solution (Table 21.1).

Table 21.1 Methods of iodization and costs

	Suitability of application	*Key considerations*	*Operating cost ($/kg salt)*
Dry mix	High quality dry refined salt with potassium iodide or iodate	Suitable for large operations with continuous mixing	0.002–0.005
Drip feed	Low quality coarse crystal or powdered salt with potassium iodate	Typically installed on low-capacity salt grinders for continuous operation	0.005–0.01
Spray mix	Medium to high-quality powdered salt semi-dry with potassium iodate	Applicable to continuous refineries ahead of drying Applicable to portable units for field operation	0.01–0.03

For units with production >10,000 tons per year that are well organized with quality control systems, the integration of iodization has been relatively easy. Such large producers account for nearly 75% of all salt for edible consumption. However, a small but significant proportion of the salt is produced along coastlines or lake shores as a semi-agricultural operation by many small producers. The smaller units often operate with a minimum of organization and little or no quality control. They are scattered along the coast or lake shores and do not lend themselves to regulation by the government. Very often precise figures regarding even their location, extent of holdings and production statistics are not available. The producers may not be aware of IDD and of the potential of their product to be a carrier. Additionally they may be based in communities where consumer awareness is limited and, as business people, they are primarily interested in making a product that consumers will buy. The producers have limited financial means and lack of access to technical or financial assistance to institute quality iodization processes and to monitor quality. As a result the salt produced in these units is of poor quality. Additionally they have poor packaging practices or do not package the salt at all. Yet they are often the main salt supplies to the communities most at risk of IDD. This has complicated USI programmes.

Box 21.1 Overview of global progress

- More than 120 countries are implementing USI programmes.
- Globally, 70% of households are adequately consuming iodized salt.
- 34 countries have already achieved USI and another 28 are close to the goal.
- 84 million infants are protected annually from the risk of IDD.
- The number of countries where IDD remains a problem has dropped to 47.

Since the early 1990s, global efforts to introduce universal salt iodization world wide have resulted in impressive progress (Boxes 21.1 and 21.2). This progress has relied on effective multi-sectoral partnerships: Governments working with the salt industry, supported by international agencies and in functioning in coordination with the civic sector and expert groups. Each of these partners have gained experience from the past two decades, the lessons learned have been in turn, incorporated into the policy, programming and implementation frameworks that sustain USI (Box 21.2).

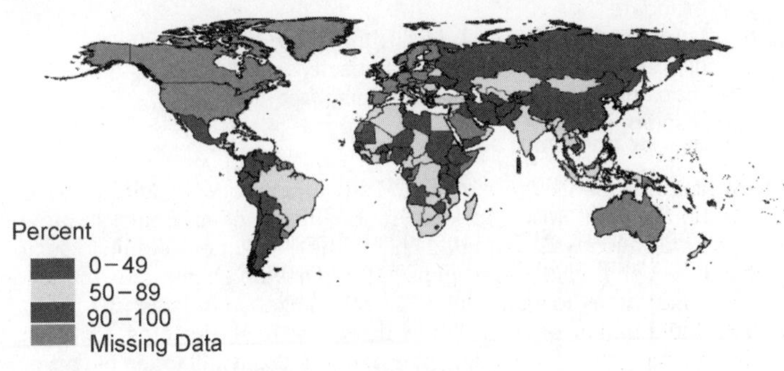

21.1 Households consuming iodized salt [4]

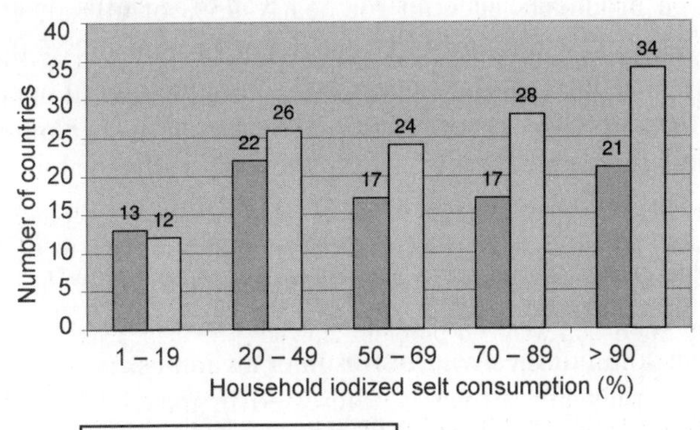

21.2 Progress in iodized salt coverage over the past decade [5, 6, 7]

Box 21.2 Universal salt iodization – country experiences[(a)]

A comparative review of the experience of 3 major countries in developing salt iodization programmes (India, Russia and China) indicates varying progress depending upon a number of factors but most importantly high-level government support.

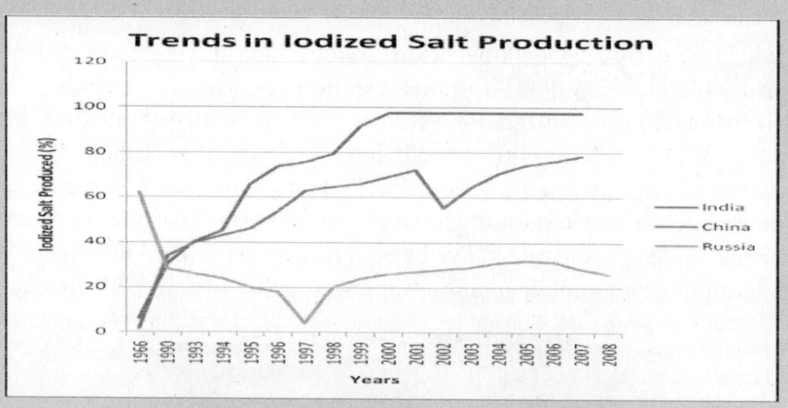

Trends lines extrapolated from available data.

As early as 1962, the Government of India (GoI) introduced iodization of edible salt. Under the National Goitre Control Programme, in effect from 1963 to 1982, however, salt iodization was *permitted* only in the domain of the public sector. In 1983, iodized salt production was opened to the private sector, thus marking the beginnings of a strategy towards universal salt iodization in India [8].

By 1996, India had issued state level bans in almost all states, including the major salt producing states forbidding sale of non-iodized salt for edible purposes. This was followed in 1998 with India instituting a national level legislation which banned the sale of non-iodized salt. This legislation was revoked in 2000 amidst political turmoil, and subsequently resulted in a drop of adequately iodized salt production from 70.3% in 1997 to 29.6% in the period 2000–2004. In 2006, Government of India reinstituted the ban on the sale of non-iodized salt for human consumption. Thus, India's production of iodized salt went from 4.1 million tons in 1999 to 1.69 million during the course of the interruption in legislation and then increased to 5.1 million tons in 2007 [9]. The accelerated increase was achieved due to special attention to increasing production of iodized salt and at consumption level monitoring iodine levels in salt within the legal frame work of state level legal bans).

In the former USSR, salt iodization was well established in an effort to eradicate endemic goitre which began in the 1950s. By the 1970s, goitre was declared virtually eradicated and with the problem "solved" prevalence not consistently tracked. With the dissolution of the USSR in 1991, the salt iodization programme also became fragmented as government infrastructures underwent major reorganization. In addition, during this period of decline, there was no investment into the salt production infrastructure further hampering the capacity to produce adequately iodized salt. Consequently, the USSR went from an era of iodized salt production of almost 1 million tons in the 1960s-1970s, of which Russia produced 318,000 tons and imported the remainder of their domestic demand from the Ukraine, through a period of decline. Such a trend had a negative impact and by 1997 Russia, as a country, produced less than 25,000 tons. Meanwhile, with the lack of iodized salt available, iodine deficiency re-emerged [10].

Numerous subsequent attempts to get legislation passed have failed. Nevertheless, the production of iodized salt has improved somewhat but production remains low (at approximately 130,000 tons in 2008, compared to an estimated domestic demand of 500,000 tons) and the household consumption of iodized salt is approximately 29% [11].

In both examples, national coalitions of organizations responsible for the IDD elimination oversight (government, salt industry, health and civic) have been either non-active/functioning or not established at all.

China, in contrast, is a study of dedicated government commitment at the highest level. Actual epidemiological evidence of the magnitude of IDD in China came to light in the 1960s which investigated the origins of endemic goitre and cretinism and showed that iodized salt was an effective intervention to address the problem. At that time an estimated 700 million people were at risk from iodine deficiency. In the 1970s, there were 35 million people with visible goitres and 25 million people with intellectual impairment due to iodine deficiency across the country [12]. Earlier efforts to deal with this public health problem were focused on highly endemic areas but were not entirely effective due to low government commitment, uneven salt iodization and, likewise, monitoring.

Spurred by the UN Summit for Children in 1990, where the Premier signed the declaration which had the elimination of IDD as one of its goals, China launched into an era of dedicated strategy to eliminate IDD by the year of 2000. The defining moment, however, was a high-level advocacy meeting in September 1993 held in the Great Hall of the People involving national and state stakeholders as well as international agencies. The meeting resulted in a State Council Leading Group on IDD Elimination which reaffirmed the commitment to eliminate IDD by 2000; the establishment of a National IDD Control Programme; a roll out of USI, regulation on iodized salt, including the creation of a salt monopoly to ensure iodized salt production, and the establishment of a multi-sectoral mechanism for social mobilization and advocacy. These key developments have sustained China's efforts. Universal salt iodization as the main strategy was adopted in the whole country in 1995 [13]. The result was an increase in iodized salt production from less than 3.3 million tons in 1993 to 8 million in 2005. Today nearly 96% of Chinese consume effectively iodized salt on a sustained basis.

(a) *Achieving Universal Salt Iodisation: Lessions Learned and Emerging Issues. Mannar M.G. Venkatesh, Bohac Lucie M. Published Proceeding in Volume 2 of the 9th International Symposium on Salt, Gold Wall Press, 2009.*

21.3 Components of effective USI programmes

While salt iodization is technically a simple process, its sustained large scale implementation calls for actions in the political, administrative, technical and socio-cultural spheres. Many countries have been moderately successful in this process, while others have struggled for several years to establish effective programmes. Available country experiences highlight certain key prerequisites:

21.3.1 Policy support

Several health and nutrition programmes compete for priority action by policy makers. Raising high-level awareness among high-level political leaders and bureaucrats regarding the problem and effectiveness of its control within a short period of time through salt iodization has been an important factor in generating political will to support sustained control and monitoring efforts. Evidence of political commitment to USI and elimination of IDD usually comes in the form of legislation that mandates that all salt for human and animal consumption be iodized, a national coalition or oversight body responsible for the programme that reports to the Minister of Health, and the appointment of a responsible executive officer for the IDD elimination programme [14].

21.3.2 Legislation and enforcement

For most developing countries an effective salt iodization programme needs to be supported by effective regulation, making iodization of all salt for human and animal consumption mandatory. The regulation must also require penalties for non-compliance.

21.3.3 Multisectoral approach

Salt iodization probably represents the first large-scale experience in national fortification of a commodity to eliminate a public health problem. While the responsibility for initiating, coordinating and monitoring an IDD control programme rests with the health sector, its planning and implementation calls for active involvement of other sectors like industry, trade, planning, transport, legislators, communication and education.

21.3.4 Involvement of the salt sector

Strengthening salt iodization and expanding it to cover all edible salt in the country is the key requirement to eliminate iodine deficiency in the country. The salt industry needs to be entrusted with the responsibility of dovetailing iodization into the prevailing salt production and distribution system, creating a standardized scheme for adequate iodization at minimum cost and disruption. Even where the extraction of the raw salt is done on a large scale its distribution and processing is often transferred to small processing plants at the consumer level.

As stated earlier, in countries such as India, while large producers account for nearly 75% of all salt for edible consumption in salt producing countries, a small but significant proportion of the salt is produced by many small producers with inadequate quality control. As an industry the salt sector must embrace USI and also seek to find ways to resolve bottle neck i.e. the sector needs to reconcile the challenges posed by the informal segment of the sector, which nevertheless hold a market share, as well as the inputs which are vulnerable to market conditions such as availability (procurement) and cost. New strategies will be needed to systematically identify ways in which small processors can comply with universal iodization requirements through a combination of advocacy, technical support, monitoring and enforcement. Small processors also need sustained and secure markets as well as a sustainable and secure procurement chain for raw materials and consumables like KIO3 (in convenient size packages and prices), salt packaging material, equipment and supplies. Support is also needed for preventive maintenance assistance, training and orientation and management. Such initial support "opens the door" to gain their support and compliance in the long term [15].The period of support is situation and country specific and determined by merits and demands within each country. However, it should be managed so as to not affect the commitment of other (larger) producers who already purchase their supplies and iodize at their own cost.

21.3.5 Public education and social mobilization

Goitre and cretinism provided the visual picture of iodine deficiency that gave it an easily identifiable reference. As IDD elimination progressed, these physical manifestations became far and fewer giving the impression that IDD problem had been solved. Yet iodine deficiency persists in its more common form – brain damage, to which the unborn foetus is especially vulnerable. In effect, IDD elimination programmes are threatened to be victims of their own success since a deficiency must be continuously addressed or it will re-emerge. Thus, on-going communication efforts are necessary. Ultimately, public education serves to solidify support for IDD elimination at all levels of the society and thereby creates a demand for iodized salt, a necessary component for the success of a USI strategy and for ensuring sustained demand and production of iodized salt.

21.3.6 Monitoring and evaluation

Systematic testing of iodine levels in salt at point of iodization and periodically at intermediate points in the distribution network, retail outlets and household level is essential for effective monitoring. Additionally, involvement of other sectors like NGOs, voluntary organizations and schools in monitoring iodine levels in salt, using low-cost field testing kits (Salt testing kits or rapid testing kits to provide a qualitative indication of presence of iodine in the salt using a dropper solution) is useful in generating pressure for adhering to the recommended level of iodine.

Box 21.3 Communicating the Message

- Relating IDD to brain damage, thereby creating an understanding of the functional outcomes beyond goitre and cretinism that result from iodine deficiency. These include mental impairment, the loss of IQ points, the impact on educational achievement and ultimately productivity
- Tailoring messages to the audience with a specific call of action they can take. The audience to be influenced ranges from top levels of government to the public health community to salt industry to community to the household
- Education at all levels must add to the supply push by creating a demand pull for iodized salt. Educated and motivated consumers who insist on iodized salt can become a force that salt retailers and processors cannot ignore and to whom they must respond by ensuring a steady uninterrupted flow of iodized salt. Conversely, unaware consumers will resist change and become a major obstacle to the programme by encouraging the circulation of unfounded rumours against iodized salt.
- Understanding the "common wisdoms" that exist in a community and correcting misinformation. Religious leaders and community leaders have been engaged to address culturally entrenched practices (i.e. washing of salt before use) which are obstacles to USI [16].
- Using multi-media to get IDD messages into popular culture [17].
- Integrating updated information about IDD into technical and educational materials of food inspection and control bodies, health-care training and academic curricula. [18].

While quality assurance of iodized salt occurs at the factory or production level, the testing of salt samples at the household level, done by UNICEF Multiple Indicator Cluster Surveys (MICS) in the Demographic Health Surveys (DHS), are useful to assess whether that iodized salt is reaching consumers or to detect potential leakage of non-iodized salt into the household, the latter issue being especially important to countries with mandated salt iodization.

The stability of iodine in salt and levels of iodization and packaging are also related to issues of quality assurance. Conditions of high humidity result in rapid loss of iodine from iodized salt, with iodine loss ranging anywhere from 30 to 98% of the original iodine content [19]. By refining and packaging salt in a good moisture barrier, such as low density polyethylene bags, iodine losses can be significantly reduced, during storage periods of over six months. Table 21.2 presents details on typical packaging methods of table salt.

Table 21.2 Typical packaging methods for table salt

	Salt variety	*Typical sizes*
Low density polyethylene sachets	Refined dry or semi-dry salt	0.5/1 kg
Paper/paper board	Refined dry salt	0.5/1 kg
Woven high-density polyethylene/ polypropylene	Unrefined crystal or coarse salt	10/20/50 kg
Polystyrene containers/paper board round cans	Refined dry or salt	0.5/1 kg

The salt industry has also been at the vanguard of innovation in testing equipment to allow for field testing of iodine levels in salt thereby enabling salt producers to monitor the quality of their product at source. These include the electronic checker (a modified filter photometer that converts the absorbance of the blue starch-iodate complex directly into a numerical read-out of iodine concentration in the salt samples) developed by the Salt Research Institute of the China National Salt Industry Corporation and the salt test kits or rapid test kits for checking iodine levels manufactured made by MBI Kits International. Work continues to refine such tools.

As a key component of any public health intervention, the monitoring of progress towards the goal and the evaluation of results, in this case the elimination of iodine deficiency is critical. Traditionally, testing for iodine deficiency relied on an assessment of goitre prevalence. However, a number of issues relating to the measurement of thyroid size (goitre) as well as the responsiveness to changes in iodine nutrition status have resulted in a move towards using urinary iodine excretion (UIE) as the standard mechanism of measurement [20].

In this regard, the key programmatic indicators [21] identified are as follows:

- Commitment to assessment and reassessment of progress towards elimination with access to laboratories able to provide accurate data on salt and urinary iodine,
- Regular laboratory data on UIE in school age children with appropriate sampling for higher risk areas,
- A database for recording of results of regular monitoring procedures particularly for salt iodine, UIE and if available neonatal TSH monitoring with mandatory public reporting.

21.3.7 Programme administration and coordination

While the responsibility for initiating, coordinating and monitoring the programme lies primarily with the Health sector, IDD control is a multi-sectoral activity that requires the motivation and active involvement of several sectors for specific functions:

Function	*Agency/Department*
• Planning	Ministries of Planning/Health/Industry/Information & Publicity
• Administration and Coordination	Ministry of Health
• Salt iodization, packing and distribution	Salt producers/processors/traders, Ministry of Industry
• Quality Control	Medical Research Institutes, Ministry of Health, Food Standards Institute, Food and Drug Administration Agency

• Information, Education and Communication	Ministry of Information and Publicity, Health Education Bureau, Ministry of Health, Medical and Nutrition Associations
• Legislation	Ministry of Health/Law
Monitoring and Evaluation	Ministry of Health
• Technical and Financial Support	Ministry of Finance, Multilateral and Bilateral development assistance agencies

21.4 USI – An example of successful fortification

Success with salt iodization will give the government, industry, consumer groups and other stakeholders a new confidence to address other more complex micronutrient problems using salt as well as other food carriers to deliver essential vitamins and minerals to the population. There is therefore much more at stake in the effort to achieve USI and eliminate iodine deficiency disorders in any country.

Salt enjoys unique advantages as a carrier of nutrients in most parts of the world in terms of universal coverage, uniformity of consumption and low cost of fortification. Encouraged by the progress made in several countries in implementing successful salt iodization programmes, efforts have been directed at examining the feasibility of fortifying salt with iron and other nutrients such as fluorine along with iodine [22]. With production, surveillance and monitoring infrastructure for iodization programmes already in place, such an integration and coordination, would enable resource savings and maximum efficiency. The commercial application of large-scale multiple fortification programmes would be a major breakthrough in establishing a cost effective delivery system for these nutrients to cover large populations.

21.5 Conclusions

In as much as tremendous progress has been made in making salt iodization indeed universal and global, the fact still remains that 2 billion people world-wide are still at risk of iodine deficiency. Although universal iodization has been generally accepted as a major public health intervention, 30% of households are unfortunately still are not using iodized salt.

It is clear that the foundation of a USI program requires mandatory iodization and this can be achieved only when there is strong government commitment. Recent reports by the Copenhagen consensus, which rate salt iodization as one of the top investments with a benefit cost ratio of 30:1, provide a strong argument to be directed at national policy makers in countries where national commitment has not been made [23]. In addition, in those countries which have existing USI programs, a reaffirmation in the form of commitment of both human and financial resources for salt iodization programs, would not only assure sustainability but also mark the national ownership of the program and the goal.

Strengthening salt iodization and expanding it to cover all edible salt in the country is the key requirement to eliminate iodine deficiency in a country. There is no other activity that draws together the productive sector of the society, the government sector, the political party sector, civic society and the general public such as iodine deficiency elimination does. It has taught valuable lessons in collaboration between government, industry, international organizations, the community at large and other sectors. It has also offered insights into building and sustaining an intervention politically, technically, managerially, financially and culturally.

References

1. DE BENOIST B, MCLEAN E, ANDERSSEN M , and ROGERS L (2008). 'Iodine Deficiency in 2007: Global Progress since 2003', *Food and Nutrition Bulletin*, **29**, no.3, pp. 195–202.
2. UNICEF, WHO (1994). 'World Summit for Children: Mid-decade goal- Iodine deficiency disorders', report from UNICEF and WHO Joint Commiteee on Health Policy Special Session, Geneva: UNICEF, WHO.
3. VENKATESH MANNAR MG and DUNN JT (1995). 'Salt Iodization for the Elimination of Iodine Deficiency', ICCIDD/MI/UNICEF/WHO.
4. UNICEF (May 2008). 'Sustainable Elimination of Iodine Deficiency,' New York: UNICEF.
5. UNICEF (2002), 'State of the World's Children 2002', New York, UNICEF.
6. UNICEF (2009), 'State of the World's Children 2009', New York, UNICEF.
7. Global Scorecard 2009 (2009) Retrieved from Network for Sustained Elimination of Iodine Deficiency, www.iodinenetwork.net
8. WHO, UNICEF, ICCIDD (2007, Third ed.), Assessment of iodine deficiency disorders and monitoring their elimination: A guide for programme manager, Geneva, WHO.
9. NDAO I, NDIAYE B, MILOFF A, TOURE N and A, N (2009). 'Tools to Improve Monitoring, Compliance and Profitability of Small Salt Producers in Senegal', Micronutrient Forum - Abstracts & Poster, Beijing: Micronutrient Forum.
10. LING J (2007). 'Achieving and Sustaining USI: Getting the Message Across to Change Policy, Attitudes and Behaviour', *SCN News*, **35** ISSN 1564-3743, pp. 37–42.
11. AKUNYILI DN (2007). 'Achieving and Sustaining Universal Iodization: Doing it Well Through Regulation and Enforcement. Lessons Learned from USI in Nigeria', *SCN News* **35**, pp. 43–47.
12. SHARMANOV T, TSOY I, TAZHIBAJEV S, KULMURZAYEVA L, OSPANOVA F, KARSYBEKOVA N, et al. (2008, February Vol. 27, no. 1). IDD Elimination Through Universal Salt Iodization in Kazakhstan. *IDD Newsletter,* **27**, no. 1.

13. DIOSADY L, ALBERTI J, MANNAR M, and FITZGERALD S (1998). 'Stability of iodine in iodized salt used for correction of iodine-deficiency disorders', *Food and Nutrition Bulletin*, **19** no. 3, pp. 240–250.
14. SULLIVAN K, SUCHDEV P, and GRUMMER-STRAWN L (2007). Achieving and Sustaining USI: Doing It Well Through Quality Assurance, Monitoring and Impact Evaluation. *SCN News*, **35**, pp. 48–53.
15. WHO, UNICEF, ICCIDD. (2007, Third ed.). *ibid*
16. HORTON S, ALDERMAN H, and RIVERA J (2008). '*Challenge Paper 2008: Hunger and Malnutrition.* Fredericksberg: Copenhagen Consensus'.
17. SUNDARESAN S (2008, June 23). Sustained Elimination of Iodine Deficiency: Progress, Sattus, Challenges and Way Ahead. *Presentation at the meeting of the Board of the Network For Sustained Elimination for Iodine Deficiency.* Ottawa, On, Canada: Network for Sustained Elimination of Iodine Deficiency.
18. VIR S (2009). 'Advocacy and Demand Creation for adequately iodized Salt - Lessons Learnt and Ways Forward', *Review of Salt Iodization in India,* New Delhi: Network for Sustained Elimination of Iodine Deficiency.
19. GERASIMOV G (2002). '*Iodine Decificency Disorders in the Russian Federation: A Review of Policies towards IDD Prevention and Control and Trends in IDD Epidemiology (1950–2002).* Moscow: web publication UNICEF.
20. GERASIMOV G (2009, May 11). 'Barriers to USI in Russia. *Presentation at the Satellite Session on IDD at the Micronutrient Forum*', Beijing, China.
21. QIAN M (2009, May 11). 'Universal Salt Iodization and Sustained Elimination of IDD in China', *Presentation at Satellite Session on IDD at the Micronutrient Forum*, Beijing, China.
22. YIP R, CHEN Z, and LING J (2004). People's Republic of China. In B.S. HETZEL, *Towards the Global Emilimination of Brain Damage Due to Iodine Deficiency* (pp. 364–395), New Delhi: Oxford University Press.
23. BEHRMAN JR, ALDEIMAN H, HODDINOTT J (2004). Hunger and malnutrition. Copenhagen Consensus Challenges and Opportunities. Copenhengan.

22

National iodine deficiency disorders control programme of India

Sheila C. Vir

Sheila C Vir, MSc, PhD, is a senior nutrition consultant and Director of Public Health Nutrition and Development Centre, New Delhi. Following MSc (Food and Nutrition) from University of Delhi, Dr Vir was awarded PhD by the Queen's University of Belfast, United Kingdom. Dr. Vir, a past secretary of the Nutrition Society of India, is a recipient of the fellowship of the Department of Health and Social Services, UK, and Commonwealth Van den Bergh Nutrition Award. Dr Vir worked briefly with the Aga Khan Foundation (India) and later with UNICEF. As a Nutrition Programme Officer with UNICEF for twenty years, Dr. Vir provided strategic and technical leadership for policy formulation and implementation of nutrition programmes in India.

22.1 History and current policy

The National Iodine Deficiency Disorders Control Programme (NIDDCP) of India, formerly known as National Goitre Control Programme (NGCP), is a central-assisted programme of the Government of India (GoI), which is being implemented in the country since 1962 [1]. The NGCP programme was launched following a prospective study undertaken in school children in the Kangra Valley of Himachal Pradesh which conclusively demonstrated (Figure 22.1) that iodized salt was effective in reducing goitre [3]. Iodization of edible salt was proposed to be the solution for prevention and control of goitre in the country. Potassium iodate was recommended to be the more suitable fortificant for iodization of salt than potassium iodide for Indian climatic conditions [2–6]. NGCP initially focused in addressing the problem of goitre primarily in the sub-Himalayan region, which was considered to be the only goitre endemic region. The three objectives of NGCP were (i) survey to identify goitre-endemic regions in the country; (ii) supply of iodized salt in place of ordinary salt in the identified endemic regions; and (iii) assessment of impact of goitre control measures in the form of resurveys over a period of time [2].

Evaluation of NGCP by the Nutrition Foundation of India in the year 1981 [2] presented a number of recommendations for strengthening the NGCP. In 1984, based on the evaluation findings and the surveys conducted by the Central Goitre Survey team of the Ministry of Health as well as the

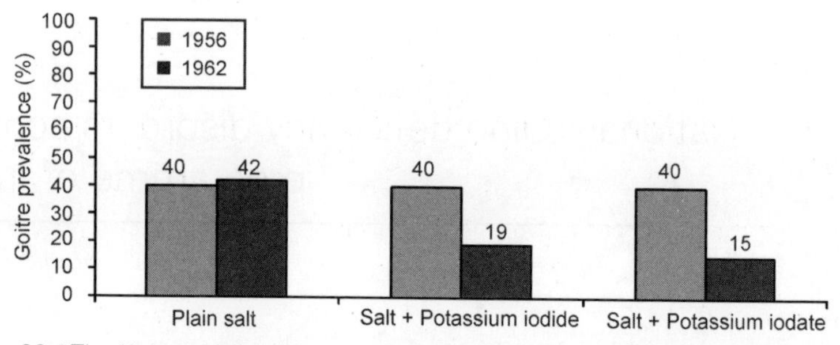

22.1 The Kangra Valley Study – iodized salt and goitre prevalence [3]

1984 recommendations of the Central Council of Health and Family Welfare, it was decided to implement the programme for compulsory iodization of salt for human consumption in the entire country. The participation of the private sector was recommended. The programme was launched in a phased manner in the entire country with effect from April 1, 1986 with a higher priority to the regions identified as goitre endemic.

The nomenclature of the NGCP programme was changed to the National Iodine Deficiency Control Programme (NIDDCP) in August 1992 with a view to address not only goitre but a wide spectrum of iodine-deficiency disorders (IDD) like mental and physical retardation lowering of IQ in children, deaf-mutism, cretinism, still-births, abortions, etc. The goal of NIDDCP is "to reduce the prevalence of iodine-deficiency disorders below 10 percent in the entire country by 2012" [1]. Universal salt iodization (USI) was the strategy adopted under NIDDCP. Box 22.1 presents the major events resulting in launch of NGCP, NIDDCP and USI.

The Central Government issued a notification banning the sale of non-iodized salt for direct human consumption in the entire country with effect from 17th May, 2006 under the Prevention of Food Adulteration Act 1954. Box 22.1 presents the major milestones of the NIDDCP and Universal Salt Iodization in India.

The NIDDCP strategy, as per the policy guidelines issued by the Ministry of Health and Family Welfare, Government of India, in 2006 [1], focuses on enhancing production, demand and supply of iodized salt for ensuring universal consumption by the population in the entire country. Following are the primary components stated to be part of the NIDDCP:

- Surveys to assess the magnitude of the iodine-deficiency disorders.
- Supply of iodized salt (the government in the policy document uses the term "iodated" and not iodized) in place of common salt.
- Health education and publicity.
- Laboratory monitoring of iodized salt and urinary iodine excretion.
- Resurvey after every 5 years to asses the extent of iodine deficiency disorders and the impact of iodized salt.

Box 22.1 Major milestones – NIDDCP and Universal Salt Iodization, India

- 1955 – Kangra valley experiments and iodization plants installed
- 1962 – Launch of the National Goitre Control Programme (NGCP)
- 1983 – Extended from public sector to private sector collaboration
- 1984 – Compulsory iodization entire country
- 1986 – Launch of national programme coverage – phased manner
- 1992 – NGCP renamed as National IDD Control Programme (NIDDCP) and a policy to cover entire country with iodized salt supply.
- 1994 – Acceleration of USI following endorsement of USI by UNICEF / WHO Joint Committee on Health Policy
- 1996 – GoI – Universal Salt Iodization: minimum iodine at production level – 30 ppm, consumption level – 15 ppm
- 1996 – State level ban notification (under the Prevention of Food Adulteration Act or PFA) on sale of non-iodized salt of edible purposes issued in majority of states, including the three primary salt producing states
- 1998 – National Legal Ban Notification under the PFA – banning sale of edible non-iodized salt
- 13th Sept 2000 – GoI lifted the national ban on sale of non-iodized salt for edible purposes
- 17th May 2006 – Notification re-issued the national ban on sale of non-iodized salt for direct human consumption

Government of India [1] reports that 263 out of 324 districts of 28 states and 7 Union Territories (UTs) surveyed to be IDD endemic with a total goitre rate of over 10 percent. These surveys confirm that no state in the country is free from iodine deficiency. NIDDCP continues to be a cent percent centrally assisted program and is an integral part of the National Rural Health Mission (NRHM). The Ministry of Health & Family Welfare is the nodal ministry for policy decisions on NIDDCP. The Central Nutrition and Iodine Deficiency Disorders Cell at the Directorate General of Health Services (DGHS) is responsible for the implementation of NIDDCP in the country. For effective implementation of the NIDDCP, the government by 2006 has established a network of 31 IDD Cells at state level in all states and Union territories except for three (Table 22.1). In 21 of these 31 IDD Cells, laboratories have been established and following functions are proposed to be undertaken by the IDD Cells [1].

1. Checking iodine levels of iodized salt with wholesalers and retailers within the state and coordinating with the Food and Civil Supplies Department.
2. The distribution of iodized salt within the State through open market and public distribution system.
3. Creating demand for iodized salt.
4. Monitoring consumption of iodized salt.
5. Conducting IDD surveys to identify the magnitude of IDD in various districts.
6. Conducting training.
7. Dissemination of information, education and communication.

Table 22.1 An overview of results of state goitre surveys and state-level infrastructure of NIDDCP [1, 7]

State/UT	*Total districts*	*Total districts surveyed*	*Total districts endemic*[(c)]
Andhra Pradesh[(a)]	23	12	11
Arunachal Pradesh[(a, b)]	11	11	11
Assam[(a)]	23	18	14
Bihar[(a)]	37	14	14
Chattisgarh	16	2	2
Goa[(a)]	2	2	2
Gujrat(a, [b)]	25	16	8
Haryana[(a, b)]	19	11	10
Himachal Pradesh[(a, b)]	12	10	10
Jammu & Kashmir[(a)]	15	14	14
Jharkhand	18	9	8
Karnataka[(a, b)]	27	20	6
Kerala[(a)#]	14	14	12
Madhya Pradesh[(a)]	45	14	14
Maharashtra[(a, b)]	35	29	21
Manipur[(a, b)]	9	8	8
Meghalaya[(a, b)]	7	4	4
Mizoram [(a, b)]	8	3	3
Nagaland[(a, b)]	8	7	7
Orissa[(a, b)]	30	8	7
Punjab[(a)]	17	3	3
Rajasthan[(a)]	31	4	4
Sikkim[(a, b)]	4	4	4
Tripura[(a, b)]	4	3	3
Tamil Nadu[(a, b)]	29	29	18
Uttar Pradesh[(a, b]	71	29	23
Uttaranchal[(a, b)]	13	9	9
West Bengal[(a)]	18	5	5
Andaman and Nicobar Islands[(a)]	2	2	2
Chandigarh[(a, b)]	1	1	1
Daman & Diu[(a, b)]	1	1	1
Dadra & Nagar Haveli[(a, b)]	1	1	1
NCT Delhi[(a, b)]	1	1	1
Lakshadweep[(b)]	1	1	0
Pondicherry	4	4	2
Total	582	324	263

[(a)] States with IDD cells established
[(b)] States with laboratory attached to IDD cells
[(c)] Endemic district – The district is declared as endemic district if the total goitre rate is above 5% in the children of the age group 6–12 years surveyed.

Supply of iodised salt is expected to be monitored by food inspectors under the Prevention of Food Adulteration (PFA) Act within the state. An evaluation undertaken by the National Institute of Health and Family Welfare recommends measures for satisfactory functioning of the state IDD cells [7].

The Salt Commissioner's Office (SCO), commonly referred as the Salt Department, under the Ministry of Industry and Commerce, is responsible for adequate production and distribution of iodized salt to the entire country. "Salt" is a Central (federal) subject in the Constitution of India and the SCO is responsible for controlling various aspects of salt industry. Earlier one of the primary roles of the SCO was issue of licenses to salt manufacturers. With the discontinuation of policy of issue of licenses to iodized salt manufacturers in 1996, a major task of the SCO to issue licenses has ended. SCO provides technical inputs for setting up salt-iodization plants, refineries as well as laboratories for monitoring quality of iodized salt at production level. Additionally, the office of the Salt Commissioner is the nodal government department responsible for ensuring appropriate distribution of iodized salt to the entire country. SCO is headed by the Salt Commissioner with its head quarters at Jaipur (Rajasthan) and a team of deputy/assistant salt commissioners located at five regional offices based at Chennai, Mumbai, Ahmedabad, Jaipur, and Kolkata.

22.2 Universal salt iodization (USI) – an integral part of NIDDCP

In 1994, at global level, UNICEF–WHO Joint Committee on Health Policy (1994) endorsed universal salt iodization (USI) as a safe, cost-effective and sustainable strategy to ensure sufficient intake of iodine by all individuals [8]. Following this, effort for supplying iodized salt was accelerated in the entire country. In 1994, the Salt Commissioner's Office, under the overall guidance of NIDDCP, directed efforts for accelerating universal salt iodization (USI) for elimination of IDD. The goal of USI programme in India, as per the international guidelines, initially was to ensure that over 90 percent population in the country consumes adequately iodized salt. In the 11th Five Year plan (2007–2012), the goal was revised to ensure 100 percent consumption of adequately iodized salt [9]. Following are the primary programme components of USI:

- Ensure accelerated production of iodized edible salt with minimum 30 ppm iodine at production level and minimum 15 ppm iodine at consumption level.
- Monitor iodine levels in salt (production to consumption) level, including implementation of the legal measures.
- Create demand for iodized salt.
- Assess impact on a continuous basis and organise required training for survey and laboratory activities.

22.3 Increasing production of iodized salt for edible purposes

22.3.1 Salt production in India

Salt is produced in India by solar evaporation from sea water in the east and west coastal regions of Gujarat, Tamil Nadu, Andhra Pradesh, Orissa, Maharashtra, Karnataka and West Bengal and from the sub-soil brine inland sources of Rajasthan. The major of common salt or raw salt produced in the country is in Gujarat (72%), Rajasthan (14%) and Tamil Nadu (11%), while the remaining quantity is from several other states along the Southeast and Southwest coast [10]. The total quantity of raw salt produced in India is approximately 17.5 MMT and almost one-third or 6.0 MMT of the total salt produced is for edible consumption (including livestock), 9.5 MMT is used for industrial applications, and the balance is allocated for export [11].

Salt production takes places in salt fields and the ownership patterns of these fields vary enormously. Small units operate below 10 acres either in private land or land leased from the government. The medium-sized units operate between 10 and 100 acres of land. The large units operate above 100 acres. The rationale adopted by the Salt Department to classify salt production units as small, medium and large is not based on the quantity of salt production but the "salt cess" which is linked to the size of salt fields. Of the total estimated 11,500 salt production units, only 822 iodized salt production units are reported to be registered with the SCO by 2009.

22.3.2 Production of iodized salt – public and private sector partnership

Production of iodized salt commenced in 1955 by the Government of India (GoI), and by 1981, a total of 15 iodization plants with a total production capacity of 225,000 tonnes per annum [12] were installed – nine plants in salt-producing states of Gujarat and Rajasthan and six plants in two non-salt producing states of Assam and West Bengal. The fortificant instructed to be used is potassium iodate [3]. This is based on the experience of Kangra Valley study. The concentration of iodine in salt was standardized initially at 25 parts per million (ppm) which was increased to a minimum level of 30 ppm in the year 1988.

Salt-iodization programme in early phases was confined to only the government-managed public-sector undertakings. In 1984, the programme was opened up for private sector collaboration since it was apparent that such a partnership with private salt industry was critical to meet the increased targets of iodized salt production – target was fixed at a low level of 0.7 MMT for 1986 since iodized salt was initially supplied to a very small identified goitre belt. Following ongoing-goitre surveys in the country, a larger number of districts were identified goitre endemic and these regions were included under the National Goitre Control Programme which resulted in higher requirement as well as a higher target for iodized salt – a target of 3.0 MMT. Between 1989 and 91, the NGCP shifted its focus from undertaking goitre surveys to accelerating and sustaining high level of production of iodized salt and simultaneously creating demand for iodized salt [12]. With the objective to supply iodized salt in the entire country, the target for production of iodized salt was increased to 5.2 MMT to meet the requirement of country's population, including the live stock. The total requirement was calculated at the rate of 6 kg/per person/year which takes into consideration requirements for livestock. A number of measures, as presented in Box 22.2, were taken since the launch of NGCP, to accelerate production and access to iodized salt [12, 13, 14].

Box 22.2 Important programme measures taken for accelerating salt iodization in India

- In 1984, permission extended to private sector to produce iodized salt. Launch of public–private partnership.
- Subsidy introduced for potassium iodate – 1st April 1986 to 1st April 1992.
- Higher priority was allocated for iodized salt transport by rail – ranked second to defence movement. Subsidy was given for using rail transport. Rail zonal scheme was introduced – relaxed in 2006.
- Since 1986, the Salt Commissioner's Office was identified as the nodal agency for monitoring quality of iodized salt at production level and prior to rail loading. The latter was linked to payment of subsidy to iodized salt manufacturers using rail transport for distribution of iodized salt to the identified districts/states.
- Inclusion of goitre control in 1986 in the "20 Point Programme" of the Prime Minister under "Health for All by 2000 AD".
- In 1986, customs duty on the import of iodine was reduced from 40% to 25%.
- In 1988, the Prevention of Food Adulteration Act (PFA) was amended to specify that iodized salt should contain not less than 30 ppm iodine at retail level.
- In 1989, the Ministry of Health approved the "Smiling Sun" logo for easy identification of iodized salt by the public. The logo is registered with the Salt Department. Use of logo, however, is not mandatory.
- Upto 1995, focus on state-level bans under on sale of iodized salt under the Prevention of Food Adulteration Act (PFA).
- In 1998, first time a national legal ban on sale of non-iodized salt for edible purpose issued.
- 2006, re-issue of the national legal ban which was lifted in 1999.

The second SAARC conference on children in South Asia held in Colombo, Sri Lanka, in September 1992 reiterated the earlier resolutions made at the 1990 World Summit for Children when "Universal access to Iodized Salt by 1995" was adopted as one of the goals. Between 1994 and 95, the Government of India's efforts to universalize iodization of salt assumed new dimensions with the international focus on USI for elimination of IDD. There was intensive effort to mobilize private salt producers for accelerating production of iodized salt to meet the goal of USI.

A significant increase in the establishment of iodized salt plants was the result of this effort—from only 15 plants producing 0.2 million tons of iodized salt established in 1983 to as high as 822 registered salt iodization plants by 2007-08. The number of unregistered iodization plants has also increased during this period. The total installed capacity of these plants for production of iodized salt is estimated to be about 13.83 million metric tons (MMT) [10, 11]. The capacity to produce iodized salt in India is estimated to be almost twice the 2009 revised country target of production of 6.0 MMT iodized salt which includes 5.2 MMT for only human consumption. On the other hand, the earlier target was stated to be 5.2 MMT to meet both human and livestock requirement. The production of iodized salt in 2008–09 is reported to have increased to 5.37 MMT (Table 22.2) as compared to 4.9 MMT in 2007–08 [12]. The total iodized salt produced is not used entirely for edible purposes within the country but is diverted to some extent to industry and is also exported. Moreover, the estimated total production of iodized salt refers to the production of salt fortified with iodine, irrespective of levels of iodine. This implies the total production of iodized salt of 5.37 MMT includes both adequately and inadequately iodized salt. Gujarat produces almost 60 percent of the iodized salt in the country (Table 22.2).

In the last decade, there has been a significant increase in the demand for powdered packaged salt, both refined and non-refined. The common perception that all the packaged powdered iodized salt is "refined" salt is not correct. The production of refined salt has been steadily increasing. By 2007, a total of 42 refineries, with the capacity to produce 3.76 MMT of refined iodized salt or 69.2% of the edible salt requirement of the country, were reported to be functioning. In 2009, the SCO reported an increase in the number of refineries to 65 with a much higher installed production capacity of 5.74 MMT of iodized salt [12]. These refineries are increasingly producing and selling good quality non-iodized common salt at a high price to the industries such as tannery, detergents etc .

Table 22.2 Iodized salt produced (MMT) 2008–2009 [12]

State	*Iodized salt production ('000 tonnes)*	*Non-refined iodized salt ('000 tonnes)*	*Refined iodized salt ('000 tonnes)*
Total	5368.04	3165.98	2202.06
Gujarat	3677.82	1779.70	1898.12
Rajasthan	846.36	747.16	99.20
Tamil Nadu	713.42	508.68	204.74

Figure 22.2 presents details on the target and production of iodized salt from 1970 to 2009. As indicated in Fig. 22.2, the target for iodized salt production in the initial phase of NGCP progressively increased since additional districts were continuously being identified to be goitre endemic and were gradually added to the programme. Following the 1984 policy to iodize all edible salt in the country, iodized salt supply targets were increased phase-wise up to 1990. Production of iodized salt accelerated in 1984 and there was a continuous increase in the production except for a drop in the production level in 2003–04 which has been attributed to the after effects of Tsunami (Figure 22.2).

One of the major constraints of the USI programme is the regular production and supply of Bargara salt (big crystal salt produced in the

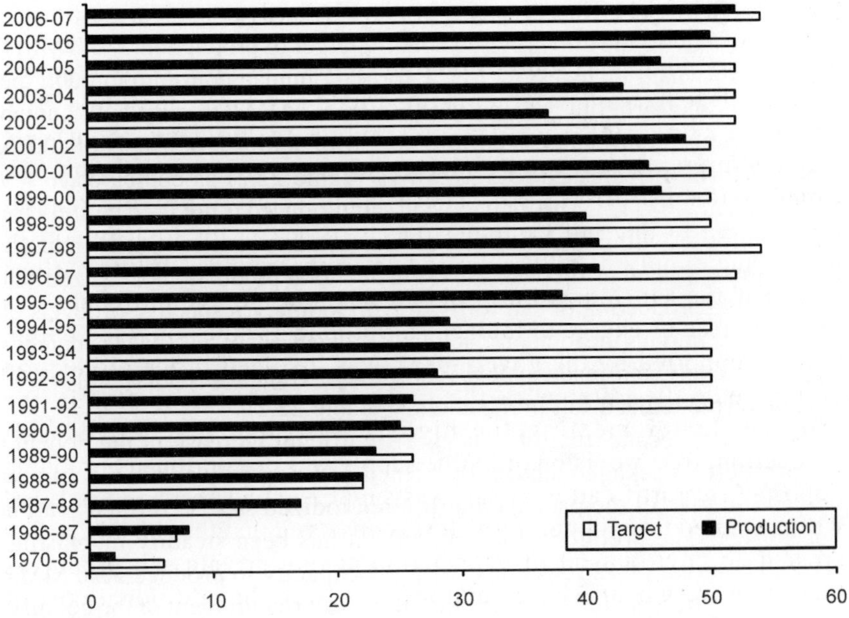

22.2 Target and production of iodized salt (Figures in million metric tonnes (MMT))

Rann of Kutch in Gujarat) which forms 22% of the total edible salt produced in the country. Due to unique chemical properties of Bargara salt, this variety of salt cannot be produced in small crystal size or crushed into powder and packaged. Bargara salt made into powder form becomes hard and lumpy within a few weeks of crushing. Bargara salt crystal is sold at a much lower cost and continues to capture the rural market of large states of Madhya Pradesh and Uttar Pradesh (UP). The study of salt trade in UP state in 2001 revealed that 49.3% of salt entering the state is bargara salt and very often this is the only type of salt available and sold in open market in remote rural areas or urban slums [15]. Such a supply situation is often misinterpreted to conclude that rural population prefers to purchase and consume bargara salt and not powdered salt. Moreover, conditions of storage, transport and marketing of bargara salt is invariably unhygienic and crystal salt, often covered with dust, is sold in non-packaged conditions at a low cost. The consumers traditionally wash and dry bargara salt prior to cooking. Such a process results in loss of iodine since the fortificant is primarily incorporated in the superficial layer of bargara salt and therefore gets washed off. Bargara salt with negligible or no iodine is at times the only salt available to consumers, especially for those below poverty lines.

22.3.3 Source of iodine and cost of iodization

There is no indigenous source of iodine in India. All the iodine required for the salt iodization program is imported from Japan and Chile [13]. Iodine is converted to potassium iodate in India by 18 private manufacturers of potassium iodate who are registered with the Salt Commissioner's office [16]. These manufacturers provide regular information to the Salt Commissioner's office on the total import of iodine and supply of potassium iodate in the country. In the earliest stages of the salt iodization program in India, potassium iodate was provided free of charge to iodized salt producers since only the public sector, supported by the government, was involved in the production of iodized salt. Later with the inclusion of private sector in the programme for meeting the high requirement for iodized salt production, free provision of iodine supply was discontinued but iodine imported for fortification of salt was supplied at a subsidized rate and was exempted from import duty. It was observed that the subsidy policy created an environment of expectation among private salt producers that the government would continue to absorb the additional cost of fortification with iodine since it was a public health intervention. The subsidy policy was observed to result in lack of ownership of the USI programme by iodized salt producers. Such an attitude was considered to be a risk factor for sustained production of iodized salt. The policy of subsidy was withdrawn by the Government of India in 1992.

The total potassium iodate requirement as fortificant for salt iodization in India is 250 MT (1 kg potassium iodate for 20 tons of salt) and is manufactured primarily by 14 of the 18 registered producers of the fortificant who are mostly located in the states of Gujarat and Mumbai. India, also, remains an exporter of potassium iodate. Fluctuating international price has adversely affected potassium iodate business. There has been an increase in the global prices for both elemental iodine and potassium iodate. Price of potassium iodate in India in 2009 is quoted as Rs 1050 per kg (about US$ 200/kg) compared to about Rs 600 per kg (US$ 14/kg) about 6 years back and $ 8.5 per kg in January 1995 [13, 16]. As presented in Fig. 22.3, the cost of iodization is estimated to be only about 2% of the total cost of production of iodized salt or about 25 paise (1–2 US cents) per person per year. The issue of escalating cost of potassium iodate in the international market remains a concern since it can have an adverse effect on the sustainability of the USI programme [16].

22.3.4 Transport and supply of iodized salt

Salt Commissioner's office, in coordination with railways, follows the 'zonal scheme' system developed for distribution of iodized salt by rail to

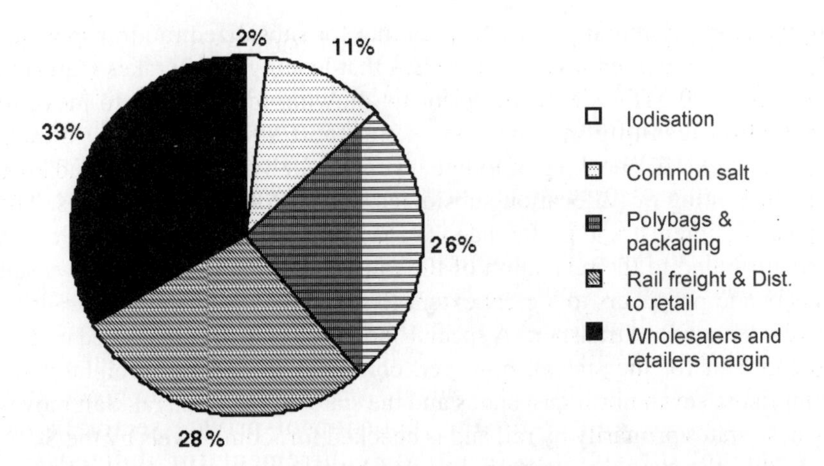

22.3 Cost of iodized salt – percentage distribution of various components

all parts of the country. This has been relaxed since 2006 resulting in removal of quota of iodized salt supply fixed for each state by the SCO and the Railway Department. The revised policy has resulted in flexibility in salt trade movement. Movement of iodized salt by railways is entitled to concession in tariff and is accorded priority for movement; non-refined iodized salt is given 'B' category which is only next to the priority given to the movement of defence items which moves under category A. No such preference is given to refined iodized salt moving by rail. SCO, in consultation with Ministry of Railways and State Governments, arranges for the priority rail movement of iodized salt from the production centre to the States and Union Territories. Salt Department, as per the policy, is expected to check iodine levels in salt prior to certifying and sanctioning rail rakes for subsidized transport of iodized salt. However, there is no such policy or authority with the Salt Department for checking iodine levels in salt that is being loaded at the production or distribution centre for road transport nor there is any system to check iodine levels in salt supply entering the state by road movement. This results in a gap in monitoring mechanisms for checking iodine levels in salt being transported by road and marketed for human consumption [13, 17].

In the past two decades, there is a consistent increase in the usage of road transport for moving iodized salt. In 2009, it is estimated that 55% salt moved by rail and 45% by road. Selection of transport by rail or road is based on factors such as distance and cost involved. It is not economical to use rail transport for distance below 500 km. Producers/traders are increasingly noted to be opting for road transport of iodized salt and not rail transport since the producers not only find it economically advantageous but also convenient since the road movement is not governed by any monitoring policy which adversely hinders their business interest. On the other hand, the salt traders are increasingly moving away from opting for subsidized rail transport for the following two reasons: (i) the policy that loading of full rakes (carrying capacity 2500 MT) is essential prior to allowing the rail rake to move to destination resulting in time loss in transport which adversely affects business; and (ii) checking of iodine levels in salt by the SCO is mandatory for sanctioning of "allocation subsidized quota" for use of rail rakes. The increasing interest and preference for road transport as compared to rail is also attributed to the relaxation of the rail zonal scheme which allows salt traders and producers to a great extent to select the destinations of trade as well as the mode of transport. A special "nominee system" (appointed traders procure salt for the states), however, continues to operate in eight states comprising seven north-east states and the state of West Bengal. Salt moves to these states primarily by rail and is checked for iodine levels by the SCO.

Within the state, salt trade is handled by the wholesalers and retailers. Figure 22.4 presents an overview of the salt trade chain. The wholesalers, private business persons, are a critical small group which control salt business within a state and are expected to follow the legal guidelines of procuring and selling salt as per the PFA. The number of wholesalers trading in salt business varies from state to state. A salt trade study undertaken in the largest state of Uttar Pradesh reveals that a total of about 344 salt wholesalers supply edible salt to over 180 million populations in the state [15, 18].

In an effort to ensure accessibility of iodized salt at a low cost to population below poverty line, as presented in Table 22.3, about 16 states have introduced the policy of subsidized iodized salt supply through the public distribution system or PDS [19]. The iodized salt supply policy through the PDS, subsidized on non-subsidized is continuously being reviewed and is often revised by the state governments. The advantages and limitations of subsidy system for ensuring the long-term interest in sustainability of the USI programme needs to be periodically examined by the state authorities since there is always a risk of leakage of subsidized iodized salt for marketing to neighbouring states as well as the problem of dependency on subsidy for procuring iodized salt.

22.3.5 Monitoring of iodine levels – production level

Defining standards for iodine fortification and the legal framework for fortification

In India, establishment of standards under the Prevention of Food Adulteration (PFA) Act of 1954 governs the quality of edible iodized salt in the country. The Act has been amended a number of times with reference to the provisions for labelling and packaging standards [1, 13]. Under the Prevention of Food Adulteration (PFA) Act, iodine levels for fortification is defined by taking into consideration the average iodine requirements of

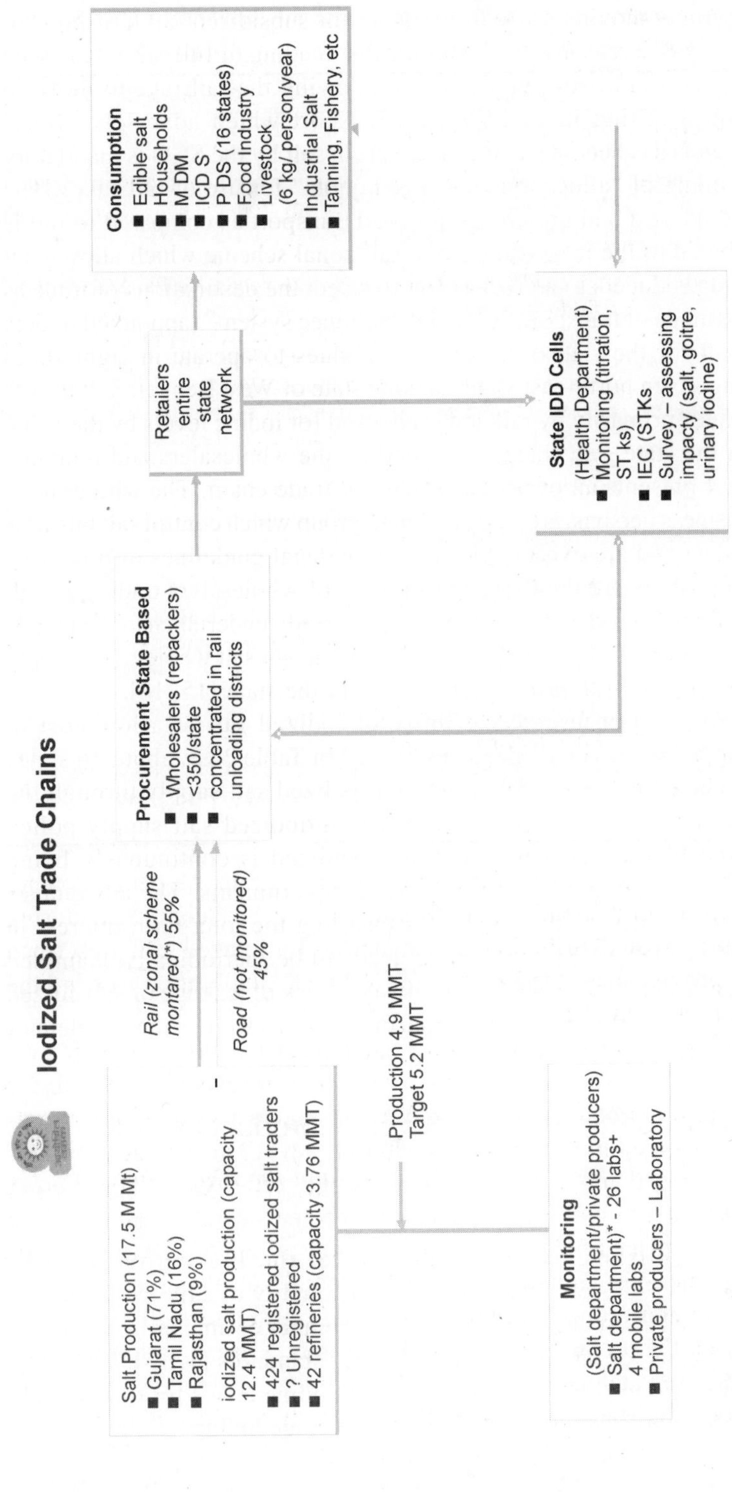

Iodized Salt Trade Chains

Salt Production (17.5 M Mt)
- Gujarat (71%)
- Tamil Nadu (16%)
- Rajasthan (9%)

iodized salt production (capacity 12.4 MMT)
- 424 registered iodized salt traders
- ? Unregistered
- 42 refineries (capacity 3.76 MMT)

Rail (zonal scheme montared) 55%*

Road (not monitored) 45%

Procurement State Based
- Wholesalers (repackers)
- <350/state
- concentrated in rail unloading districts

Retailers entire state network

Consumption
- Edible salt
- Households
- M DM
- ICD S
- P DS (16 states)
- Food Industry
- Livestock (6 kg/ person/year)
- Industrial Salt
- Tanning, Fishery, etc

Production 4.9 MMT
Target 5.2 MMT

Monitoring
(Salt department/private producers)
- Salt department)* - 26 labs+ 4 mobile labs
- Private producers – Laboratory

State IDD Cells
(Health Department)
- Monitoring (titration, ST ks)
- IEC (STKs
- Survey – assessing impacty (salt, goitre, urinary iodine)

22.4 Iodized salt trade chain

Table 22.3 Iodized salt sold at subsidized rate through the Public Distribution System (PDS) system – situation mid-2009 [12]

State	*Cost (Rs/kg)*	*Comment*
Andhra Pradesh	2.50 for non-refined alt 4.00–4.50 for refined salt	–
Arunachal Pradesh	0.75 / head	State government provides transport subsidy from rail head to retail shops
Assam	3.50 for unpacked salt 5.00 for poly pack	–
Chhattisgarh	0.25 to PDS card holders	Procurement price Rs. 2.32 per kg
Delhi	5.50 for refined salt	
Gujarat	0.50 for iodized salt	Distributed to BPL / tribal areas of 11 districts. Procurement price = Rs. 1.29 per kg)
Himachal Pradesh	5.50 for refined salt	Transport subsidy to hard and inaccessible areas is Rs. 1.99
Haryana	3.50	
Jharkhand	0.25 for iodized salt	Two kg salt per month to 23.64 lakh BPL families
Karnataka	3.00 for iodized salt	–
Orissa	1.80 for loose 3.80–5.40 for poly pack	–
Rajasthan	1.00 for iodized salt	Distributed to 5.62 lakh card holders in 6 tribal dominated districts. Procurement price = 1.68 per kg
Sikkim	2.90 for crushed iodized salt in loose	–
Tripura	3.50 in poly pack	–
Tamil Nadu	2.50 for iodized salt	Distributed to BPL population
Uttar Pradesh	–	Iodized salt in PDS shops by choice of shopkeeper

population, average estimated consumption of 10 gram salt per person per day as well as an estimated 50% loss due to weather conditions during transit, storage and distribution. The standards for iodized salt, prescribed under the provisions of the Preventions of Food Adulteration Act and the rules, are presented in Box 22.3.

Since 1984, for ensuring availability of iodized salt with adequate level of iodine, state/UT were encouraged to issue state-level notification, under the Prevention of Food Adulteration Act, to ban the entry and sale of non-iodized salt for edible purposes. Such state-level ban notification was considered critical and was accorded a very high priority in 1990s in order to monitor marketing of iodized salt within a state. Strategically, highest emphasis was placed for such ban notifications in the three primary salt-producing states, viz. Gujarat, Tamil Nadu and Rajasthan in order to prevent movement of non-iodized or inadequately iodized salt for edible purposes by road from the production sites to the various districts within the state or transport of inadequately iodized salt out of the salt-producing states to the neighbouring states. Intensive efforts were directed for issue of state-

Box 22.3 PFA standard prescribed for iodized/iodated salt [1]

"Iodated salt means a crystalline solid, white, pale pink of light grey in colour, free from visible contamination such as clay, grit and other extraneous adulterants and impurities."

Salt Quality

Sodium Chloride – not less than 96.0 % by weight on dry basis

Matter insoluble in water – not more than 1.0% by weight on dry basis

Matter soluble in water other than sodium chloride – not more than 3.0% by the weight on dry basis

Iodine Content

(a) At manufacturing level – not less than 30 parts per million (ppm) on dry weight basis.
(b) At distribution – not less than 15 ppm on dry weight basis.

Anti-caking agent – It may contain aluminium silicate to an extent of 2.0% by weight. Total matter insoluble in water in such cases shall not exceed 2.2% and sodium chloride content on dry basis shall not be less than 97.0% by weight.

Packing of iodated salt – The iodated salt (iodized salt) manufactures have been directed to pack iodated salt only in HDPE or polythene-lines jute bags of permitted capacity, i.e. 50 kg for bulk

level bans. In 1992, 22 of the 32 states and union territories had banned the entry of non-iodized salt for edible purposes while by 1996 all the three salt-producing states had also issued the ban notification. By 1997, all states and union territories, except part of Andhra Pradesh, Maharashtra, Kerala, Goa and Pondicherry, had issued the state-level ban on the sale of non-iodized salt for edible purposes [13, 20].

A national-level ban on the sale of non-iodized salt for human consumption was issued in 1998. On September 13, 2000, the Government of India lifted the central ban on the sale of non-iodized salt for edible purposes. This ban under the Prevention of Food Adulteration Act 1954 was subsequently re-instated with effect from 17th May, 2006 [21]. The legal ban specifies banning the sale of non-iodized salt for direct human consumption in the entire country. Box 22.4 presents the gazette notification. As per the GoI policy, food inspectors in each state are responsible to monitor the implementation of the PFA act including salt samples testing at the designated Central Food Laboratory based at Ghaziabad, Kolkata and Banglore. Salt samples are advised to be collected from producers and traders throughout the distribution channel. In case a salt sample is found not to be of the prescribed standard at the retail level, all responsible persons associated with iodized salt trade including the salt producer as well as retailers are considered offenders and are subject to non-bail warrants or imprisonment for not less than six months and fine up to 1,000 Indian Rupees.

Monitoring at production level

As presented in Figure 22.4, Salt Department or the Salt Commissioner's

Office is responsible for monitoring the quality of iodized salt produced by the registered salt iodization units. The Salt Department provides the monitoring support to the salt manufacturers and iodized salt producers through its five regional offices and over 100 field offices, including a network of 26 fixed laboratories and three mobile laboratories [22]. In addition, each iodized salt producer is responsible for checking iodine levels in salt during the production process.

It is mandatory for each iodized salt producers to have a laboratory or titration facility attached to the iodized salt production unit. However, monitoring guidelines developed by the Salt Department for iodized salt producers regarding checking iodine levels in salt by the titration method are often not known or ignored or only partially adhered to by iodized salt producers [16] resulting in ad hoc method used for sampling salt for testing iodine levels. Very often, the salt iodization units depend on salt-testing kits and not the approved titration method for periodical checking of iodine levels in salt during the production process. In addition, external monitoring is undertaken by the SCO only with reference to issue of permits to salt traders for the sanctioning of the allocation quota for subsidized rail transport system. A major gap in monitoring mechanism is the total absence of a system to monitor iodine levels in salt produced by non-registered iodization units or transported by road. Such a gap in the monitoring system, to a great extent, results in incorrect trade practices and increase the procurement and marketing of non-iodized salt or inadequately iodized salt by wholesalers of salt based in various states.

22.4 Advocacy and demand creation for increased production, universal access and consumption of adequately iodized salt

Intensive efforts are being made by the Government of India since 1989 to increase demand for iodized salt along with increasing production of iodized salt [13]. During this period, following a systematic study by the Ministry of Health, in collaboration with UNICEF, the logo of "smiling sun" for iodized salt was developed for easy identification. This logo was approved by the Ministry of Health in 2004. The logo is registered with Salt Commissioner's Office. Use of this logo (Figure 22.5) is not mandatory but the logo is being widely used by iodized salt producers on iodized packets for facilitating easy identification and promotion of use of iodized salt [23].

One of the major components of the NIDDCP is "health education and publicity" for iodized salt. Government of India uses print and mass media such as TV and radio to create public awareness. Since 1993, efforts are ongoing to sensitize politicians and policy makers to move away from the notion that iodine-deficiency results in merely a cosmetic problem of goitre

Box 22.4 The Gazette of India

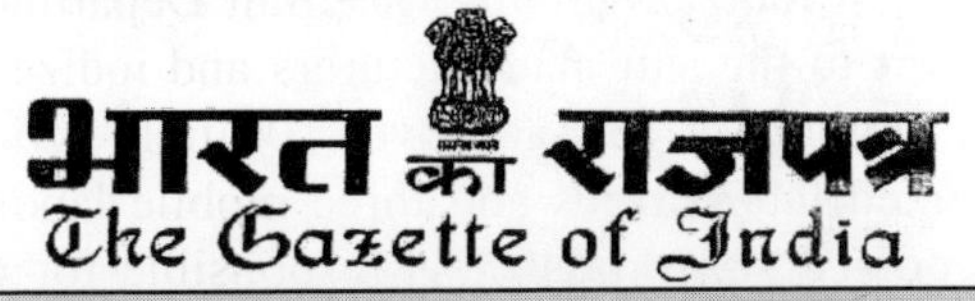

New Delhi, November 17, 2005

MINISTRY OF HEALTH AND FAMILY WELFARE
NOTIFICATION
New Delhi, the 17th November, 2005

G.S.R. 670(E)–Whereas draft of certain rules further to amend the Prevention of Food Adulteration Rules 1955, was published, as required by the Proviso to sub-section(I) of section 23 of the Prevention of Food Adulteration Act, 1954 (37 of 1954), at pages 1 to 3 in the Gazette of India, Extraordinary Part II, section 3, sub-section (i), dated the 27th May, 2005 under the notification of the Government of India in the Ministry of Health and Family Welfare (Department of Health) number of GSR 340(E), dated the 27th May, 2005, inviting objections and suggestions from the persons likely to be affected thereby before the expiry of a period of sixty days from the date on which copies of the Official Gazette containing the said notification, were made available to the public;

And whereas the copies of the said Gazette notification were made available to the public on the 27th May, 2005;

And whereas objections or suggestions received from the public within the specified period on the said draft rules have been considered by the Central Government;

Now, therefore, in exercise of the powers conferred by section 23 of the said Act, the Central Government after consultation with the Central Committee for Food Adulteration Rules, 1955, namely:

1. (1) These rules may be called the Prevention of Food Adulteration (8th Amendment) Rules, 2005.
   (2) They shall come into force after 6 months from the date of publication in the Official Gazette.
2. In the Prevention of Food Adulteration Rules, 1955,–
   (i) in rule 42,–
      (a) for sub-rule (v), the following shall be substituted, namely:–
         "(v) Every container or package of table iodised salt or iron fortified common salt containing permitted anticaking agent shall bear the following label, namely:–

IODISED SALT/IRON FORTIFIED COMMON SALT*
CONTAINS PERMITTED ANTICAKING AGENT
*Strike out whichever is not applicable.

      (b) in sub-rule(zzz), after clause (21), the following clause shall be inserted, namely,–
         "(22) Every container or package of common salt shall bear the following label, namely:–

COMMON SALT FOR IODISATION / IRON FORTIFICATION/
ANIMAL USE/PRESERVATION/MEDICINE/INDUSTRIAL USE*
*Strike out whichever is not applicable

   (ii) after rule 44H, the following rule shall be inserted namely:–
      "44L Restriction on sale of common salt No person shall sell or offer or expose for sale or have in his premises for the purpose of sale, the common salt, for direct human consumption unless the same is iodised:
      Provided that common salt may be sold or exposed for sale or stored for sale for iodisation, iron fortification, animal use, preservation, manufacturing medicines, and industrial use, under proper label declarations, as specified under clause(22) of sub-rule (zzz) of rule 42";
   (iii) in rule 49, in sub-rule(10), for the words "Edible common salt or iodised salt or iron fortified common salt", the words "Table iodised salt or table iron fortified common salt" shall be substituted.

[F.No.P. 15014/4/2005-PH(Food)]
Rita Teaotia, Jt. Secy.

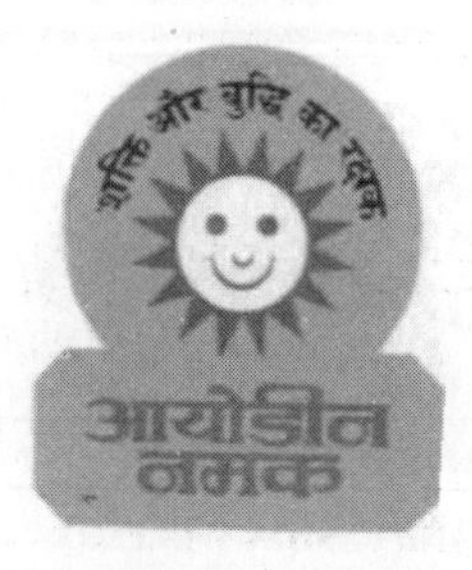

22.5 "Smiling Sun" logo for iodized salt, India

but to appreciate the serious adverse implications of iodine deficiency on brain development of unborn child, IQ levels of children (a decrease of average 10–13 IQ points is attributed to iodine deficiency), school performance as well as national productivity. Active support is sought from the politicians for the USI programme implementation and a number of events are organized every year on 21st October, the Global IDD Day.

Since 1993, communication efforts are being directed to reach iodized salt producers and sensitize them of their social responsibilities regarding protecting brain and young minds of children and mobilizing them to procure and sell salt only with the recommended minimum levels of iodine [13]. In 2003, such communication efforts were extended to include iodized salt wholesalers. Promotion of powdered or fine crystal packed iodized salt, both refined and non-refined, was emphasized. It is evident from experiences documented in mid-2000 (Box 22.5) that it is critical that communication strategy sensitizes the state-based wholesalers and mobilises them to appreciate their social responsibility and follow the correct trade practices of procuring only adequately iodized salt. Salt-testing kits have proven to be very effective communication and semi-quantitative testing tools.

22.5 Innovative efforts to accelerate USI

Intensive innovative efforts were made in 1993–96 in selected 13 states including all north-east states to establish an effective monitoring and management information system linked to the primary health care network [7, 23, 24]. As per the system, salt samples were tested using the salt-testing kits at health sub-centre levels by the auxiliary nurse mid-wife (ANM) and information obtained by ANMs was put together at block primary health care centre level and finally at the district health unit. The evaluation findings [7, 23] reported that such a monitoring mechanism created pressure on salt traders and was effective. The system is reported to have been discontinued in all the states except for the states of Gujarat and Sikkim.

Between 2003 and 2008, successful experiences from two states of India – Uttar Pradesh and Tamil Nadu – have been reported. In the state of Uttar Pradesh, the strategy focused on monitoring of iodine levels in salt at the wholesalers as well as at the household level through a network of the middle and high school children. Figure 22.6 presents an overview of the strategy. These two primary actions complemented each other and proved effective not only in monitoring iodine levels in salt procured and consumed but also in alerting the entire salt trade chain of their social responsibilities and the legal guidelines. The impact was positive in influencing sale, procurement and in turn production of adequately iodized salt [18].

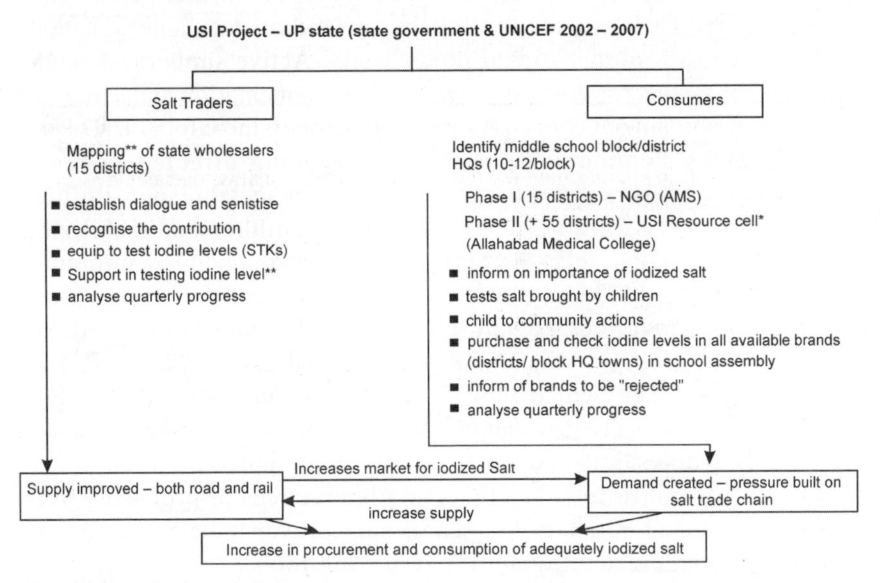

22.6 Overview of the strategy

Moreover, as presented in Box 22.5, monitoring of iodine at school level (over 20,000 salt samples per quarter) acted as a catalyst in the creation of demand for adequately iodized salt and also equipped the public to "discard" salt brands, locally packaged or otherwise, with inadequate level of iodine. The impact was evident in a few months. Figure 22.7 presents the impact at the wholesalers' level while Fig. 22.8 presents the impact at the consumption level [18].

In the state of Tamil Nadu, a state-based consumer organization was involved in the task of monitoring presence or absence of iodine in salt at retailer and household level. Over 0.1 m salt samples were tested in a period of three years resulting in a significant impact on increasing iodized salt supply and consumption [16].

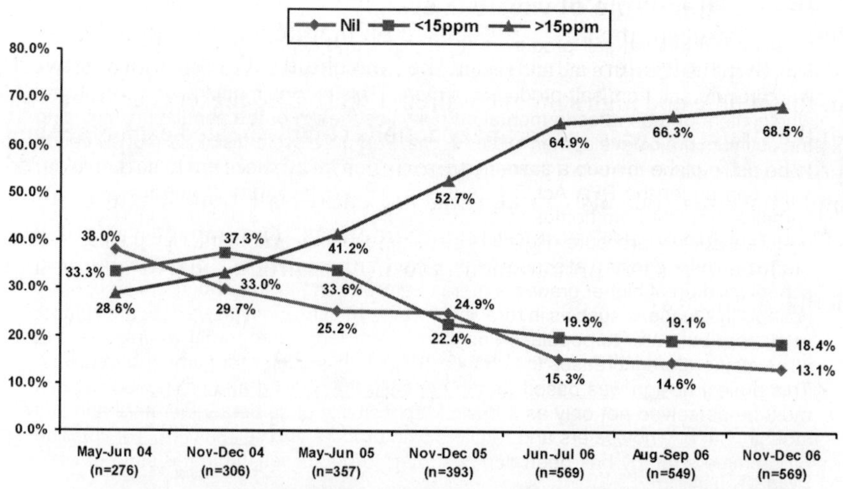

22.7 Trends in procurement (30 months) of iodized salt at wholesaler level in the state of Uttar Pradesh [18]

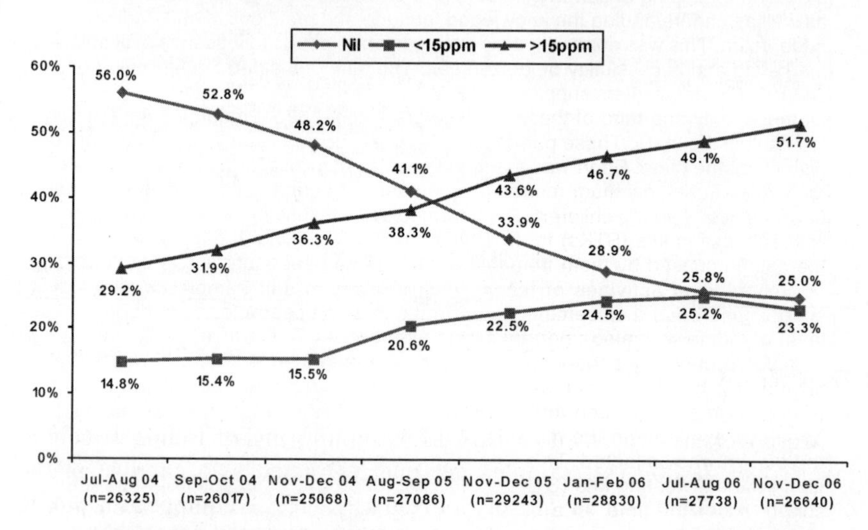

22.8 Trends in consumption (30 months) of iodized salt at wholesaler level in the state of Uttar Pradesh [18]

It is evident from these innovative activities that monitoring of iodine levels in salt, using salt testing kits, resulted in creating demand as well as in improving supply. Intensive ongoing monitoring of iodine levels in salt at community or at school level positively influences trade practices and results in an accelerated shift in reducing supply of salt with nil iodine, improving availability of iodized salt as well as increasing awareness and consumption of iodized salt.

Box 22.5 Uttar Pradesh innovative strategy – recognizing the strategic role of wholesalers

Pressure on iodized salt producers to produce and supply only powdered packed iodized salt can be achieved and sustained by working with the network of wholesalers who procure salt from salt-producing regions. This implies mapping and sensitizing wholesalers of their roles in mental and physical health of the population, including the optimum brain development of newborns. Further, a system simultaneously needs to be put in place to keep a sustained pressure on the wholesalers to adhere to the legal ban under the PFA Act. Three to six monthly testing of iodine levels in salt samples, brought from homes by school children of middle and high school grades, generate such a pressure. Retailers become cautious and market only those salt brands which are tested at school level to have an adequate level of iodine. Involving school children of higher grades is more useful as compared to working with primary schools in situations such as in rural India where middle and high schools are smaller in number but cater to population coming from a larger geographical area. Such a strategy therefore increases the chances of influencing a larger number of retailers. This project design was based on the principle that buying and selling iodized salt must be perceived not only as a basic responsibility of salt manufacturers and salt industry but of wholesalers and retailers who procure and sell salt [14, 18, 25]. The programme strategy has been demonstrated to be successful in the state of Uttar Pradesh (UP).

As a first step for the implementation of the above strategy in the state of UP, a study on mapping of salt wholesalers and understanding the salt trading system as well as understanding the knowledge, attitude and practices of salt traders was undertaken. This was done with a view to accelerate efforts to influence availability, marketing and accessibility of iodized salt. The study revealed that a total of only 344 primary wholesalers supplied salt to the entire state of 180 million populations. Of these, only one-third of these wholesalers – about 126 – marketed 80% of the total salt in the state. These primary traders were located in only 15 of the total 70 districts of the state. Effort was made to sensitize this core group of salt traders of their roles in the optimum mental development of young children and in school performance of young children. The informed salt wholesalers were also equipped with salt-testing kits (STKs) for facilitating routine checking and for ensuring that the salt purchased by them from salt producers had adequate iodine content.

School-level activities of testing iodine levels in salt samples brought by school children and disseminating information on salt samples with inadequate level of iodine was also undertaken simultaneously. The activity of testing salt samples brought by school children was complemented with another action of six monthly testing of open and all available packaged branded salt purchased from local markets. Each and every brand of packed salt and 2–3 samples of open salt available in the markets of the administrative block headquarters of the district was collected. This was followed by testing of these samples of salt using the salt-testing kits (STKs) in the presence of school children during the school assembly time. In a block with 100,000 populations, on an average a total of 12–15 brands of packaged salt were available in a particular block head quarter market. Children were informed of the specific iodized salt brands with nil or low levels of iodine and were informed of the importance of discontinuing its usage. These children were encouraged to disseminate the information of salt-testing results in their neighbourhood and community.

Over 217,000 salt samples, about 26,000 salt samples per quarter, were brought to school by school children and these were tested for iodine content using the salt-testing kits. Community was reached through the launch of "school child-to-community" approach. The households with salt samples not having adequate levels of iodine were visited by a group of students to sensitize them about the importance of iodine. Such a comprehensive programme strategy also resulted in protecting the business interest of wholesalers since demand was generated in the community for powdered packaged salt with adequate level of iodine.

The school activities resulted not only in influencing consumption of iodized salt, but also in galvanizing the entire chain linking consumers, retailers and wholesalers. Pressure resulting from school-based activities had an immediate impact on reduction in procurement of salt with nil iodine (Fig. 22.7). The school efforts were complemented by equipping the wholesalers to test iodized salt using STKs and technical support to get selected salt samples tested by titration method in a laboratory especially set up in a medical college for providing salt testing service to wholesalers. The impact was noted in the shift in pattern of sale of iodized salt. In less than 2 years, salt procured with nil iodine decreased from 38% to 15.3% and salt marketed with adequate iodine level increased from 28.6% to 64.9% (Figures 22.7 and 22.8).

It is evident from the innovative efforts of the two states, Tamil Nadu (TN) and Uttar Pradesh (UP), that even if public is made aware of the significance of iodized salt and convinced to consume only adequately iodized salt, the consumers are not in a position to distinguish adequately iodized salt from non-iodized or inadequately iodized salt due to the misleading practice of incorrect labelling regarding iodine content. A communication strategy, promoting consumption of powdered packed adequately iodized salt, needs to be complemented with actions for introduction of a mechanism to check iodine levels in salt. Such a combined effort is essential to guide consumers to purchase the right product at an affordable cost and not to be misled by false labelling which is a malpractice followed commonly by non-refined iodized salt manufacturers or re-packers [18, 25]. Measures are required to be introduced for equipping consumers with information for "rejecting" those salt brand packages which are found to have inadequate level of iodine. Use of low-cost salt-testing kit (costing about US $ 0.20 for testing 100 samples) produced by MBI Chemicals of Chennai, India [26] has proved to be not only a semi-quantitative monitoring tool but a very effective communication tool (Box 22.5).

Box 22.6—Testing Kit

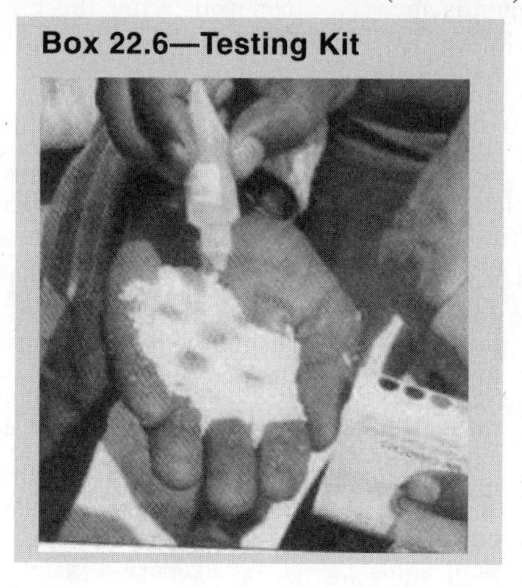

22.6 Elimination of IDD – impact and progress

(i) Monitoring system at consumption level

As per the NIDDCP policy, the task of monitoring iodine level in salt and impact on iodine nutrition status at consumption level is the responsibility of the state governments. The procedures adopted for sample collection and testing are clearly laid out in the existing protocols and guidelines of the government [1] but implementation of these guidelines is a low priority and has a number of weaknesses [7]. According to the NIDDCP Policy, each state under the Government of India centrally sponsored scheme, is encouraged to establish an IDD Cell (Table 22.1) along with laboratory facility for routinely monitoring iodine content of salt and assessing urinary iodine excretion. The network of state-based IDD cells are linked to the National Reference Laboratories established at the Bio-Chemistry and Biotechnology division of the National Centre for Disease Control or NCDC (earlier referred as the National Institute of Communicable Diseases) at Delhi, for training medical and paramedical personnel for undertaking monitoring iodine content of salt and urine. In addition to this, four regional IDD monitoring laboratories have been set up at Hyderabad (National Institute of Nutrition) for southern India, Kolkata (All India Institute of Public Health and Hygiene) for East, New Delhi (AIl India Institutes of Medical Sciences) for the western regions and NCDC for the northern states. These four regional centres have been assigned the responsibility for undertaking regional training and providing support in monitoring iodine contents of salt, measurement of urinary iodine levels as well as for conducting Thyroid Function Test (TFT).

Recent evaluation by the National Institute of Health and Family Welfare (NIHFW) recommends measures for improving the challenging task of strengthening the monitoring system through the network of IDD cell [7]. In addition to IDD cells, the food inspectors at states/provinces are assigned the responsibility to collect samples, under the PFA, and to organise testing of iodine levels at the designated laboratories for testing. Testing of salt is considered a low priority task by food inspectors. In 2009, under the NIDDCP, salt-testing kits are being supplied to voluntary health worker, referred as ASHA (Accredited Social health Activists) built-in for monitoring iodine levels in salt at household levels as well as at ICDS centres and schools.

(ii) Progress in access and consumption of iodized salt

An analysis of the progress of USI programme presented in Figure 22.9 indicates that iodized salt consumption with adequate level of iodine (over 15 ppm) has remained stagnant in the past decade. A sharp increase in iodized salt consumption to 70 per cent was reported in 1996 by the evaluation study conducted in 1996 in eight states (three salt-producing states Gujarat, Rajasthan, Tamil Nadu and non-salt-producing states Manipur, Karnataka, Bihar, Himachal Pradesh, Madhya Pradesh), by the Ministry of Industry [23,25]. Consumption of salt with nil iodine was reported from only 11% households. The substantial increase trend in iodized salt consumption, observed in 1996, is attributed to monitoring system which was introduced at consumption level using the primary health care network [23, 26].

In 1998–99, there was a decrease in percentage households consuming iodized salt. This decrease is attributed to lifting of the national ban notification during this period resulting in weakening of the monitoring system at the production level. Additionally, discontinuation of the primary health care system linked monitoring system of mid-1990s also is considered responsible for the decrease observed. As presented in Fig. 22.9, since 1999 there is no increase in the pattern of consumption of adequately iodized salt in the last decade [27, 28]. According to the National Family Health Survey NFHS-3 [27], conducted during 2005–06, (report published in 2007), 76% of people consume iodized salt while only 51.1% households consume iodized salt that is adequately iodized (containing a minimum of 15 parts per million of iodine) while 25 percent households consume salt with inadequate iodine. About 24% population consume salt with nil iodine. As per the two large national surveys (Table 22.6) consumption of adequately iodized salt has remained stagnant at 50% [27]. This implies 50% of the estimated 26 million children born each year, i.e. as many as 13 million are unprotected against iodine-deficiency disorders and are at risk of brain damage.

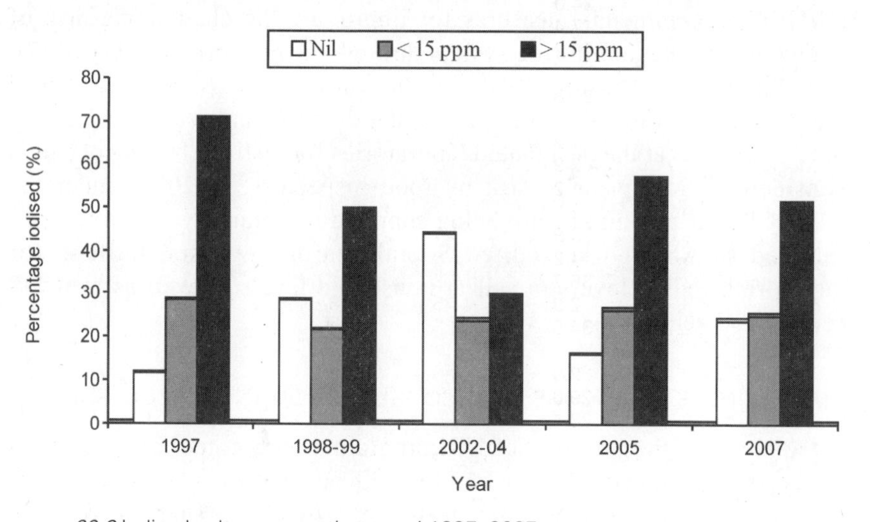

22.9 Iodized salt consumption trend 1997–2007

The situation regarding consumption of iodized salt varies widely among states (Table 22.4). In 14 out of 29 states, over 90% population are reported to consume salt with some iodine. States consuming salt with adequate level or at least 15 ppm of iodine varies between 31.0 per cent (Andhra Pradesh) and 93.8% (Manipur) and only the state of Manipur meets the criteria of USI goal with over 90% population being reported to be consuming salt with recommended minimum level of iodine. The situation

Table 22.4 Consumption of iodized salt-state-wise data from two national surveys [27, 28]

State	Iodine content of salt					
	None (0 ppm)		Inadequate (<15 ppm)		Adequate (≥15 ppm)	
	NFHS 2 (1998–99)	NFHS3 (2005–06)	NFHS 2 (1998–99)	NFHS 3 (2005–06)	NFHS 2 (1998–99)	NFHS 3 (2005–06)
Andhra NFHS 3	36.8	40.0	35.7	29.0	27.4	31.0
Arunachal Pradesh	0.8	1.2	15.0	15.2	84.1	83.6
Assam	1.8	2.8	18.2	25.4	76.9	71.8
Bihar	22.9	5.3	30.1	28.6	47.0	66.1
Chhattis-garh	–	21.0	–	24.1	–	54.9
Delhi	6.1	8.1	4.5	5.9	82.9	86.0
Goa	37.3	22.7	20.2	12.5	77.9	64.8
Gujarat	29.5	27.9	14.2	16.4	56.1	55.7
Haryana	19.5	28.2	9.2	16.5	71.0	55.3
Himachal Pradesh	3.2	5.9	6.2	11.6	90.5	82.5
Jammu and Kashmir	24.8	9.5	22.3	14.7	52.9	75.8
Jharkhand	–	7.3	–	39.1	–	53.6
Karnataka	24.1	34.0	32.4	22.7	43.4	43.3
Kerala	47.6	17.4	13.2	8.7	39.3	73.9
Madhya Pradesh	25.0	41.2	16.3	22.4	56.7	36.3
Mahara-shtra	32.0	25.8	6.9	13.3	60.1	61.0
Manipur	2.3	1.2	9.7	5.0	87.9	93.8
Meghalaya	6.7	2.9	30.0	15.2	63.0	81.9
Mizoram	0.7	1.2	8.0	12.9	91.2	85.9
Nagaland	10.9	2.2	21.2	14.5	67.2	83.3
Orissa	29.6	23.9	35.1	36.5	35.0	39.6
Punjab	16.7	14.2	7.8	11.2	75.3	74.6
Rajasthan	37.1	36.7	15.3	22.5	46.3	40.8
Sikkim	3.1	2.9	17.5	18.8	79.1	78.3
Tamil Nadu	62.7	34.5	15.8	24.2	21.2	41.3
Tripura	–	2.9	–	21.7	–	75.5
Uttaranchal	–	29.0	–	25.1	–	45.9
Uttar Pradesh	22.7	23.4	26.9	40.2	48.8	36.4
West Bengal	11.3	6.7	26.5	24.2	61.8	69.1
India	28.4	23.9	21.6	25.0	49.4	51.1

regarding consumption of salt with adequate levels of iodine of over 15 ppm is remarkably better than the national average in eight northern states as well as in the eastern states of West Bengal, Bihar and Jharkhand.

It is evident from Fig. 22.10 that the mode of transport of salt to a state seems to influence the availability of adequately iodized salt. Availability of salt adequately iodized is much higher in states where iodized salt is transported from salt-producing centres primarily by railways since a policy to monitor iodine levels in salt for the allocation of rail wagon quota exists. On the other hand, the adverse impact on the availability of adequately iodized salt in the absence of such a monitoring mechanism for salt moving by road transport is also evident. This is well-reflected in the poor consumption of iodized salt pattern in most of the salt-producing states

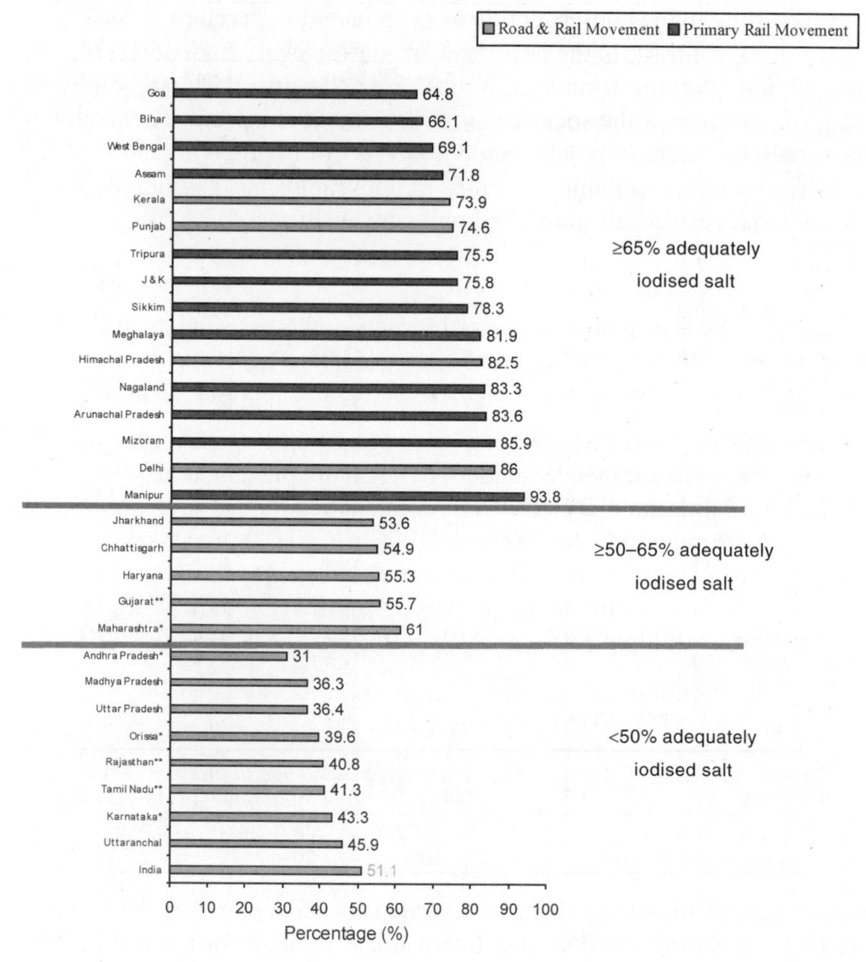

22.10 State-wise profile of availability of adequately iodized salt and mode of transport used for iodized salt supply

(Andhra Pradesh, Orissa, Tamil Nadu, Karnataka and Rajasthan) as well as in other states (Uttar Pradesh, Haryana, Madhya Pradesh, Maharashtra, Andhra Pradesh, and Karnataka) where road transport is the primary mode of transport for procuring iodized salt.

Analysis of nation-wide data with reference to socio-economic situation [27] indicates that a disproportionately large percentage of the rural poor continue to be deprived of adequately iodized salt. Iodized salt consumption shows a wide variation – higher in upper socio-economic group and much lower in the poorer socio-economic group. This is possibly due to the fact that in the absence of an appropriate system for monitoring of salt moving by road, iodized salt (often non-refined packaged or open salt or bargara salt) which contains inadequate iodine is procured and sold at a lower cost resulting in the poorer section of the population purchasing such low-cost salt. In contrast, in the north-eastern states, a very high percentage of households (varying from 71.8% to 93.8%) consume adequately iodized salt, irrespective of the socio-economic status. It is therefore evident that in situations where only adequately iodized salt is procured and sold for edible purposes, economic situations of households has negligible impact on iodine levels in salt purchased and consumed.

(iii) Status of iodine nutrition

Since 1999, besides goitre survey, iodine nutrition is assessed by measuring urinary iodine excretion. As per the Policy [1], IDD survey at district level is recommended to be conducted by using the method of population proportional to size (PPS) sampling in the age group of 6–12 years children. The indicators recommended under NIDDCP are presented in Table 22.5. The cut-off presented By NIDDCP corresponds to the epidemiological criteria recommended by WHO/UNICEF/ICCIDD for assessing the severity of IDD based on the prevalence of goitre in school-age children and for assessing iodine nutrition based on urinary iodine concentration of school-age children [30].

Table 22.5 IDD prevalence indicators and criteria for classifying IDD as a significant public health problem [1]

Indicator	*Severity of public health problem*		
	Mild	Moderate	Severe
Goitre grade >0	5.0–19.9%	20.0–29.9%	≥30%
Median UIE (Microgram/l)	50–99	20–49	<20

Iodine nutrition surveys have been carried out and reported by the National Institute of Nutrition (NIN), and International Council for Control of IDD (ICCIDD) and the Human Nutrition unit of the All India Institute of Medical Sciences (AIIMS). In 2003, NIN carried out a survey in forty selected districts of various states located in five different regions (Southern, Northern, Eastern, North Eastern and Central) of India to assess the impact of NIDDCP on the prevalence of IDD [29]. Districts with a higher percentage of goitre prevalence, prior to the launch salt iodization programme, were selected for the study. The findings revealed that the overall prevalence of total goitre declined significantly from 14–69% during 1984–94 to 2–40% in 2003, especially in the north-eastern regions. The prevalence of total goitre was ≥10% in half of the districts and ≥5% in 37 out of 40 districts surveyed. The median urinary iodine excretion levels among 6–11 year children was observed to be <100 μg/L only in 9 out of 40 districts (Table 22.6). IDD survey undertaken by ICCIDD during 1999–2006 in seven states (Kerala, Tamil Nadu, Goa, Rajasthan, Bihar, Orissa, Jharkhand), presented in Table 22.6, indicates that the situation is much better in Kerala and Jharkhand with median urinary iodine being over 100 μg/l and only about 8-10 percentage of subjects having urinary iodine <50 μg/l.

Table 22.6 Status of iodine deficiency – regional surveys [3]

Strata	Year	Coverage	Urinary iodine Median (μg/L)	(% <50 μg/L)
Kerala	1999–2001	State	123.3	8.2
Tamil Nadu	2001–2002	State	89.5	22
Goa	2001–2002	State	76	36.2
Rajasthan	2002–2003	State	138.7	16.9
Bihar	2003–2004	State	85.6	31.5
Orissa	2003–2004	State	85.4	32.2
Jharkhand	2006	State	173.2	10

22.7 Elimination of IDD – challenges ahead

India has been recognised as one of the sixteen "make or break" countries which require intensive efforts to accelerate the USI programme for achieving the global goal of USI. It is evident from Figure 22.11, that the consumption of adequately iodized salt in India is much lower than other Asian countries [31].

For addressing the goal of USI, and for sustained elimination of IDD, the following programme issues are critical.

- Ensuring higher political commitment and urgent enforcement of legal ban that was re-instated on 17th May, 2006. Advocacy to increase attention to the implications of iodine deficiency on increasing risk of brain damage to unborn children.
- Shifting the focus from merely iodized salt to "adequately iodized salt". Strengthening of the monitoring system at consumption level to ensure universal consumption of iodized salt with minimum 15 ppm iodine at household level.

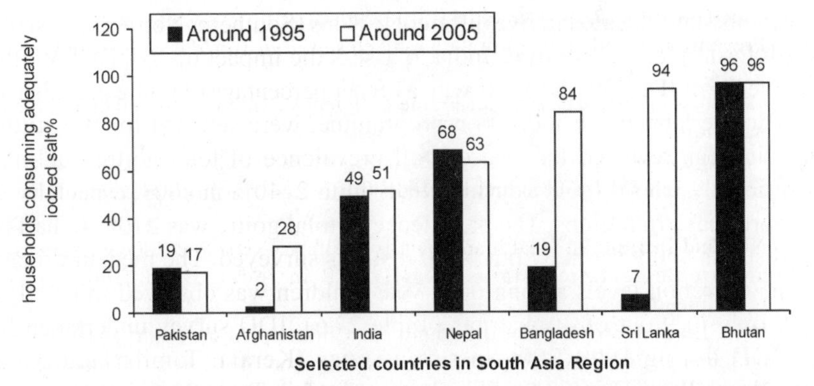

22.11 Progress in households consuming adequately iodized salt in South Asia [31]

- Integrating IDD programme activities in broader health-nutrition programmes. Active promotion of powdered packed or fine crystal (includes both refined and non-refined) iodized salt through traders network, school system, Integrated Child Development Services (ICDS), Maternal and Child Health (MCH) programme.
- Complementing quality iodized salt production efforts with actions to reach wholesalers of salt by urgently mapping, reaching and sensitizing wholesalers in each salt producing and non-salt producing states – it is estimated that not more than 300–350 salt wholesalers operate in each state and need to be recognized as critical partners in the NIDDCP.
- Institutionalizing mechanisms at state/district levels not only for creating demand for iodized salt but for exerting and maintaining pressure on salt trade chain – from consumption level to levels of retailers, wholesalers and producers by establishing a system of monitoring and regularly disseminating information at every level. Equipping consumers with information on iodine levels in salt that is available in local market so that they are in a position to "reject" and not purchase inadequately iodized salt.

References

1. Revised Policy Guidelines on National Iodine Deficiencies Disorders Control Programme (2006). IDD and Nutrition Cell, Directorate General of Health services, Ministry of health and Family Welfare, Government of India, New Delhi.
2. Nutrition Foundation of India (1998). The National Goitre Control Programme. A blue print for its intensification.
3. AIIMS / Salt Department, GoI / ICCIDD / MI/ UNICEF (2008). Salt for freedom and iodized salt for freedom from preventable brain damage.

4. SOOCH SS, DEO MG, KARMARKAR MG, KOCHUPILLAI N, RAMACHANDRAN V (1973). Prevention of endemic goitre with iodized salt. *Bull World health Organisation* **49**, pp. 307–312.
5. HETZEL BS (1989). The story of iodine deficiency. An international challenge in nutrition.
6. PANDAV CS, CHAKRABORTY A, SUNDRESHAN A, ANSARI MA, JAIN P, AGUAYO V, AYOYA M (2008). Salt for freedom and iodized salt for freedom from preventable brain damage.
7. National Institute of Health and Family Welfare (NIHFW) (2006). Evaluation and implementation status of NIDDCP in India. Brief findings and recommendation.
8. UNICEF and WHO, "World Summit for Children: Mid decade goal – iodine deficiency disorders". Report from UNICEF and WHO Joint Committee on Health Policy, Special Session, Geneva 27th January 1994.
9. Government of India, Ministry of Women and Child Development (2006). 11th Five Year Plan. Report of Working Group on Integrating Nutrition with Health (2007-2012).
10. Directory of iodized salt manufacturers, salt refineries, potassium iodate manufacturers and iodization plant fabricators, Government of India, Office of Salt Commissioner, ministry of Industry, Department of I.P.P. (2006).
11. Salt Department (2009). Personal Communication on "Particulars of iodization plants commissioned upto 30th September 2009.
12. Salt Department (2009). Personal Communication, October 2009.
13. USI: Universal Iodization India – Progress and Current Status (August 1996), salt Department, Ministry of Industry.
14. VIR SC (1995). Editorial: iodine deficiency Disorders in India. Ind J. Public Health 32, pp. 132-134.
15. Salt Trade in Uttar Pradesh – mapping of wholesalers and major traders and KAP study. Government of UP and UNICEF 2001.
16. VIR S (2007). Universal salt Iodization (USI) in India – Current Situation and Proposed Actions. Consultancy report presented to UNICEF, December 2007.
17. Salt Department and Ministry of Industry and UNICEF (1993). Universal Salt Iodization – We must act now.
18. VIR S, DWIVEDI S, SINGH R, MUKHERJEE A (2007). Reaching the goal of Universal Salt Iodization (USI): Experience of Uttar Pradesh. Food and nutrition Bulletin **28**(4), pp 384–390.
19. Salt Commissioner Office (May 2009). Personal Communication.
20. Salt department and UNICEF (February 1995). Banning Sale of Edible non – iodized salt – An urgent measure.
21. The Gazette of India, Ministry of Health and Family welfare Notification, New Delhi, 17th November 2005.
22. Monitoring system at production level, USI (India). Salt department, Ministry of Industry (August 1996)
23. Evaluation of Universal Salt Iodization in India—A mid term Evaluation , Indian Institute of Health Management Research for the Ministry of Industry, March 1998,
24. Iodine deficiency Disorders control programme, UNICEF-Department of Health Project Document, Ministry of Health and Family welfare, July 1993.
25. VIR SC (2008). How to increase consumption of iodized salt in India: a situation analysis. ICCIDD Newsletter, **30**(4): 7–10.

26. CHANDRASHEKHAR, MBI CHENNAI. International Workshop on Micronutrient and Child Health , Human Nutrition Unit, AIIMS, 20-23rd October 2009, New Delhi.
27. National Family Health Survey (NFHS 3), 2005-06, Volume I, International Institute for Population Sciences 2007.
28. National Family Health Survey (NFHS 2), 1998-99, Volume I, International Institute for Population Sciences.
29. VIJAYARAGHAVAN et al. Current status of IDD in select districts of different regions of India, National Institute of Nutrition 2003.
30. WHO, UNICEF, ICCIDD (2007). Assessment of iodine deficiency disorders and monitoring their elimination. A guide for programme managers Geneva, World Health Organization, 2007.
31. UNICEF (2009). Sustainable Elimination of Iodine Deficiency. Progress since the 1990. World Summit for Children.